THE SOURCE BOOK OF
Plastic Surgery

THE SOURCE BOOK OF
Plastic Surgery

COMPILED AND EDITED BY
FRANK McDOWELL, M.D., Sc.D.

Professor of Surgery, University of Hawaii;
Professor of Clinical Surgery, Stanford University;
Editor-in-Chief, Plastic and Reconstructive Surgery

THE WILLIAMS & WILKINS COMPANY
Baltimore

This book is sponsored by the

Educational Foundation of the American Society of
Plastic and Reconstructive Surgeons, Inc.

Copyright ©, 1977
The Williams & Wilkins Company
428 E. Preston Street
Baltimore, Md. 21202, U.S.A.

Made in the United States of America

Library of Congress Cataloging in Publication Data
Main entry under title:

The Source book of plastic surgery.

"Sponsored by the Educational Foundation of the American Society of Plastic and Reconstructive Surgeons."
   Bibliography: p.
   Includes index.
   1. Surgery, Plastic—Addresses, essays, lectures. 2. Surgery, Plastic—History—Sources. I. McDowell, Frank,
1911–   . II. American Society of Plastic and Reconstructive Surgeons. Educational Foundation. [DNLM: 1. Surgery, Plastic— History. W011.1 S724]
RD118.S67   617'.95'08   77-23946
ISBN 0-683-05766-9

Composed and printed at the
Waverly Press, Inc.
Mt. Royal and Guilford Aves.
Baltimore, Md. 21202, U.S.A.

PREFACE

"Who am I? Where did I come from?"

This primeval cry has been ever with us, unchanged, down through the ages. For the plastic surgeon, many of the answers will be found in this book.

The principal thing that differentiates the modern plastic surgeon from his predecessor, the ancient Egyptian pounding a hole in someone's head to let the sick spirits out, is, of course, the knowledge that has been developed in the interim. But that knowledge has not flowed in a continuous stream or trickle; rather, it has been created in single steps or blocks — some of them quite large. This book brings to you many of the most important building blocks which comprise plastic surgery, *in the authors' own words!*

Many have decried the lack of a definitive history of the now well-established specialty of plastic surgery — as well they might. Such a history could take any one of several forms but, as Emerson pointed out, in the end "there is no history, only biography." There is no better way to learn history than to study the men who made it and their contributions which comprise it. As far as plastic surgery is concerned, you have most of this history now in your hand. You will find the reading of it a thrilling experience, as you learn of the self-doubts of these men, their missteps, their uncertain exploratory attempts — and then see an important block of knowledge suddenly emerge, well created and definitively proven for all men in all times.

You will probably marvel, as I did, that some of these gigantic blocks of knowledge are so simple — so simple that they now seem self-evident. I hope that when the young men who represent the future in our field see this, they will take heart and vow to make similar efforts of their own. For though some of the advances of the future will be made by teams of persons pooling complex knowledge from many different fields with computers, working in sophisticated laboratories with incredible equipment under the aegis of infinite financing, that is not the sole path to progress — perhaps not even a viable one. In the future, if we are to believe the past, the most important new advances will arise as new concepts in the imagination of a single brain — and they will emerge only if that brain is prepared to recognize them. When each is brought forth, the rest of us will say, in effect, "How incredibly simple and obvious! Why didn't I think of that?"

Another reason, and a really essential one, for reading this book is Santayana's axiom, "those who cannot remember the past are condemned to repeat it." Who has gone to a medical meeting, or read an issue of a medical journal, and not found proof of this?

Have a good read.

Frank McDowell, M.D., Sc.D.

Honolulu, Hawaii
January 1977

You have to learn what others have done
because you won't live long enough to
make all the mistakes yourself.

ACKNOWLEDGMENTS

The meteoric papers of these distinguished investigators are the *raison d'être* for this book, of course. Only secondary to them are the fine commentaries and biographies herein. The editor is grateful to all who wrote them, and particularly to Robert Goldwyn and Blair Rogers for their multiple, fine contributions.

Many of these articles were originally reprinted in the pages of *Plastic and Reconstructive Surgery* during the past decade or two, and that would not have occurred except through the encouragement and support of members of the editorial board throughout that period. Eventually, all of this led to many requests, particularly from more recent readers of the *Journal,* that we assemble all of this material in one volume for continuity and quick reference. The Educational Foundation of the American Society of Plastic and Reconstructive Surgeons strongly supported this endeavor. In completing it, we decided to include a few milestone papers which had not been reprinted in *PRS*.

We are most grateful to the publishers and the editors of all the journals where these articles first appeared, for the opportunity to reproduce them here.

Finally, all of the above put together could not have resulted in a real book in your hands without the high skills and the unfailing efforts of key persons in the Honolulu editorial office — especially Mary McDowell, Kitty Dabney, and Barbara Kramer.

—F. McD.

CONTENTS

SECTION I
THE ORIGINS OF FREE SKIN GRAFTING

SECTION II
THE ORIGINS OF RHINOPLASTY

SECTION III
THE ORIGINS OF CLEFT LIP REPAIRS

SECTION IV
THE ORIGINS OF CLEFT PALATE REPAIRS

SECTION V
CROSS-LIP FLAPS

SECTION VI
OTOPLASTY

SECTION VII
FACIAL FRACTURES

The Origins of Free Skin Grafting

The Pinch Graft

THE FIRST FREE SKIN GRAFTS

Prologue

1869 was a year!—especially in Paris. Napoleon III, through his designer, the Baron Haussmann, had just transformed the medieval city into one of broad avenues, parks, sophistication, and great beauty. The new Place d'Opera and the Etoile were unique; there was no equal to the Place de l'Concorde, or the Rue de Rivoli. Gargoyles appeared atop the new Opera, and the 1867 Paris World's Fair had been a great success.

Gounod, Bizet, Offenbach, and Thomas poured forth a succession of melodies— Flaubert, Dumas, and others, books—Courbet, Corot, and Millet, new paintings with light in them. A young artist, one Manet, had recently created a furor with his *Picnic on the Grass.* Just now, he was beginning to paint with his friends Renoir and Monet, but the misty deliquescence of the Impressionists was yet to come. Manet's friend of the cafes, Emile Zola, had written two books and was developing a rebellious spirit. Jules Vernes' new book *Twenty Thousand Leagues Under the Sea* was the talk of the town.

True, the French had withdrawn from Mexico, leaving Maximilian to his fate, and had lost much of their political influence in Europe. But the Suez was about to open! Though the Second Empire had become weak politically, weak militarily, it was strong in construction and culture. Paris was the veritable center of art, fashion, and diplomacy—interested in the entire world and everything going on in it.

Abroad, Moussorsky had finished his moody *Boris Godunov,* Mendeleev his periodic law. From the new world came Mark Twain's *Innocents Abroad* and the first electric washing machine—from the old, Marx's *Das Kapital.* Grieg's piano concerto was thrilling, Brahm's first Hungarian dances vivacious, but the intoxication of the city came more from a stream of lilting waltzes—especially Strauss's new *Tales from the Vienna Woods.*

Newspapers undoubtedly featured the displacement of Disraeli by Gladstone, Chulalongkorn being crowned King of Siam, and the Meiji restoration in Japan. The end of an era was signalled, however, by deaths— Rossini, Kit Carson, Foucault, Purkinje, Hector Berlioz. Less evident, as always, was the beginning of a new era. Who could know the destinies of newborns named George Arliss, Gandhi, Neville Chamberlain, Harvey Cushing, Flo Ziegfeld, Maxim Gorky, Frank Lloyd Wright, or Booth Tarkington?

Paris was not only "the city of light" but also a medical and surgical mecca. General anesthesia had been used for years; J. L. Championniere had brought Lister's antiseptic surgical technique across the channel the year before. Operations on the extremities, head, and neck were common; abdominal operations of larger magnitude than ovariotomies and bladder stone removals were beginning. About the university and the hospitals walked Charcot, Littré, Brown-Sequard, Pasteur, Denonvilliers, Giraldes, Guerin, Sedillot, Nelaton, and many more. Claude Bernard, a member of the Academy of Sciences for some years, had just been appointed Senator by Napoleon III. Paul Broca, father of brain surgery, was chief at one of the medical centers, the Hôpital Necker.

And now, at the session of the Imperial Society of Surgery, a young Swiss surgeon from Geneva, currently working at the Hôpital Necker, arises to speak. He seems to be saying something about trying to heal wounds with "seeds of skin." Shall we listen? *Mais oui!*

——*F. McD.*

2

— 511 —

dant l'anesthésie, et d'éviter l'écoulement du sang dans le pharynx et dans la bouche. Les préceptes du savant président de la Société de chirurgie ont été suivis en 1868 par M. le docteur Thomas (de Tours) dans une opération habilement conduite, et qui a été l'objet d'un rapport de M. Verneuil à la Société de chirurgie.

J'avoue que la lecture de ce rapport de M. Verneuil ne m'a pas converti.

On ne peut que dans des cas exceptionnels, malgré les précautions indiquées, prévenir l'écoulement du sang dans le pharynx pendant les derniers temps de l'opération. D'un autre côté, l'hémorrhagie, lorsqu'elle a lieu, se produit plutôt vers l'extérieur que vers la gorge, ainsi que je l'ai observé chez mon dernier malade. Malgré cela, j'aurais été fort inquiet si ce malade eût été sous l'influence du chloroforme pendant cette hémorrhagie.

Le procédé recommandé par mon savant collègue ne me parait donc acceptable que dans un nombre de cas fort restreint. Il ne met pas toujours à l'abri des dangers de l'hémorrhagie, mais il a le mérite, lorsque tout se passe selon le vœu de l'opérateur, de soustraire le malade à de grandes souffrances.

Cet avantage est malheureusement compensé par des cicatrices très-apparentes, qui détruisent l'harmonie et la régularité du visage. Les *douleurs passent*, les *difformités restent*.

M. CHASSAIGNAC. L'ablation de deux plateaux du maxillaire supérieur donne une voie suffisante pour pénétrer jusqu'au polype; aussi faut-il rejeter l'ablation complète du maxillaire supérieur. Quant aux incisions qui, partant de l'angle de l'œil, suivent l'aile du nez et divisent la lèvre supérieure sur la ligne médiane, je les ai inaugurées depuis longtemps, et dans un cas où j'ai opéré de cette manière, en rejetant le nez tout entier du côté gauche, le polype envoyait des prolongements dans les sinus frontaux et maxillaires.

M. ALPHONSE GUÉRIN. J'ai eu l'occasion de voir, il y a peu de temps, le petit malade présenté par moi il y a trois ans à la Société; c'était la première fois qu'on ruginait la base du crâne sur une certaine étendue. La guérison est restée complète.

M. GUYON fait un rapport verbal sur le travail suivant de M. Reverdin.

Greffe épidermique. — Expérience faite dans le service de M. le docteur Guyon, à l'hôpital Necker. — Messieurs, la communication que j'ai l'honneur de faire à la Société de chirurgie a trait à une question de pathologie bien vulgaire, en appa-

Page 511 of Bulletin of Imperial Society of Surgery of Paris, 1869. Reverdin's presentation begins near the bottom of this page.

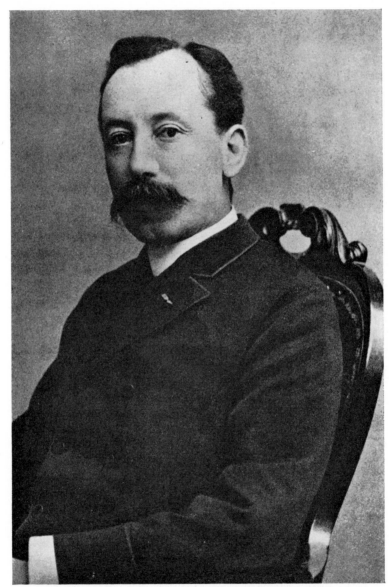

Jacques Reverdin, circa 1870. (Courtesy of Madame Dubois, Chief of Centre d'Optique et d'Electronique de l'Assistance Publique de Paris).

GREFFE EPIDERMIQUE—EXPERIENCE FAITE DANS LE SERVICE DE M. LE DOCTEUR GUYON, A L'HÔPITAL NECKER

J. L. REVERDIN, M.D., *Paris*

(*Bull. Imp. Soc. de chir. de Paris 10:511–515, 1869*)

Translated from the French by
ROBERT H. IVY, M.D.

Gentlemen: The communication which I have the honor to make to the Society of Surgery pertains to a very common question of pathology, apparently well understood, but which still presents some obscure and interesting points for elucidation. I refer to the cicatrization of wounds by second intention.

All surgeons know that while in the very great majority of cases, wounds that reach the stage of granulation heal by their borders, in a few exceptional cases one sees islets of epidermis forming on the wound surface more or less distant from the edges. The formation of these central islets has a remarkable and well-known influence on the length of time required for cicatrization. They shorten it considerably.

This fact being noted and admitted, the interpretation remains; here, opinion is not unanimous. Some, and Billroth is very affirmative on this point, believe that always in such cases a thin layer, even very thin, of the malpighian net-work has been left in place here and there. Their reasoning is based on the fact that it is in burn cases above all that the central islets are observed.

Other pathologists do not regard these conditions as indispensable.

For example, a short time ago, I had occasion to observe an instance of this nature. It concerned a mechanic who had his right thumb crushed. As a result it became necessary to amputate the thumb back to the metacarpo-phalangeal articulation. After cicatrization had commenced, we saw forming in the center of this wound several epidermic islets which remarkably hastened the process of repair.

Some time later, observing an extensive wound whose cicatrization was very slow, and remembering the patient just mentioned, the idea occurred to me to try the experiment which is the subject of this communication.

The patient involved is a man 35 years old who, on October 16 last when falling from a ladder, tried to save himself by catching his left elbow on an iron bar. The skin was cut near the bend of the elbow and torn away in its entire thickness as far as the middle of the forearm, thus forming a large flap which rapidly underwent complete necrosis. The resulting raw surface consisted of cellular subcutaneous tissue and, at the external part of the limb, of aponeurosis abraded in places. This wound soon began to granulate, but it was not until November 14th that one could begin to distinguish at its edges a little epidermic border. During the succeeding days this border spread slowly.

November 24th I tried the following experiment: I removed with the point of a lancet from the right arm of the patient, two small slivers of epidermis, being as careful as possible not to encroach on the dermis. The first sliver was very small, the second about a square millimeter in dimension; the resulting little wound of the forearm merely presented a rosy appearance. I placed my two epidermic slivers in the middle of the wound, their deep surface in contact with the granulations, a short distance apart, and I supported them with some of the diachylon bandelettes which served as a dressing for the patient. The next day, the segments were found to have remained in place despite a fairly abundant suppuration; they appeared to be a little swollen and whiter than on removal.

November 27, the epidermic slivers still remained in place. I detached by the same procedure as before, a slightly larger epidermic sliver 3 to 4 square millimeters in area and placed it on the wound at a distance from the first two.

November 28, the implants seemed to be adherent. I could rub the wound in their vicinity with a small piece of lint without detaching them.

November 30, the two first slivers seemed to be more pale, thinner, and appeared to be extending at their borders.

December 1, the two first slivers have united and formed a little pale white plaque; there has evidently grown a small epidermic zone around each of them. The third implant holds well, its edges present a narrow pale border.

In the days that followed, this pale border extended more and more, while presenting the same aspect; the islet formed by the junction of the first two implants likewise extends. Finally, December 7, the three implants have united to form a little pale and thin islet quite analagous to the epidermic border which has formed along the edges of the wound.

To-day, December 8, it is observed that the islet has notably enlarged since yesterday.

Such are the facts that I have the honor to submit to the Society of Surgery. I report them now as a matter of record, but I pledge myself to pursue these researches, as follows: It will be necessary to examine from the clinical point of view, in which of these wounds and at what period of evolution of these wounds, this experiment, which I voluntarily designate as epidermic graft, can succeed.

As a matter of fact, in a second experiment made on a wound not yet in a stage of cicatrization of its edges, the epidermic implant has remained with little or no adherence for several days, but its edges have curled away from the raw surface and finally it has come away with the dressing. I will also investigate the point at which this little operation can be applicable and of practical utility. Finally, I will have to study as closely as possible the histological process: Is it a simple result of contact, of environment? Is there proliferation of the transplanted elements? Here are many questions, which deserve some researches that I intend to undertake.

DISCUSSION

M. Trélat: M. Reverdin, in his work, and at the time of presentation of the patient of M. Guyon, believes that epidermic proliferation must be attributed to the graft. In order for this experiment to have a real value, it would be necessary for it to be repeated a great many times, and that it nearly always succeeded. It is necessary, in fact, to exercise on this point a very great amount of reserve. The spontaneous formation of epidermic islets on the surface of extensive wounds in process of cicatrization is a fact frequently enough observed, and one can see in the patient that I present to you a similar cicatricial islet, developed spontaneously on the surface of this large wound of the forearm.

M. Guyon: A single experiment can prove nothing and while M. Reverdin has, with my advice, presented this patient it was to attract attention to the subject and as a matter of record. The communication of M. Trélat proves that the purpose has been attained, and that the question of the epidermic graft is to-day a matter worthy of discussion.

M. Tillaux: If it has been demonstrated that one could, on the spot, provoke the

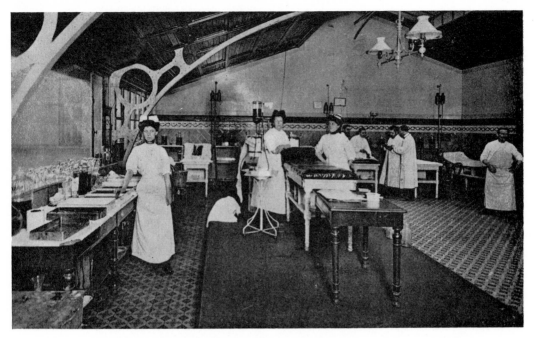

Operating room, Hôpital Necker, Paris, 1880. (Courtesy of Madame Dubois, Chief of Centre d'Optique et d'Electronique de l'Assistance Publique de Paris).

formation of cicatricial islets, M. Reverdin has rendered a great service to surgery. I have had in my practice a woman who, following burns, was left with a wound of the thigh four times the area of the hand.

M. Després: One must avoid here a confusion that could arise: It is not a question of grafting epidermis, but of joining by autoplasty a fragment containing a part of the superficial layer of the dermis; the scars borne by the patient at the place from which the so-called epidermic graft has been removed prove that a substantial portion of the dermis and the mucous or malpighian layer in their entire thickness have been included. The proliferation of the epidermis alone would be such an extraordinary phenomenon from a histologic point of view that it is necessary to avoid all confusion.

M. Guyon: If confusion apparently exists in the title of the work, it does not exist in the work itself. M. Reverdin indicates well that it involves the epidermis with its malpighian layer.

M. Blot: From the practical point of view

the question of the epidermic graft, or that of the malpighian or mucous layer, appears to me to be of no importance. To remove a piece of dermis from the arm or elsewhere to unite it to the surface of a suppurating wound which is slowly cicatrizing, just to save a little healing time, is to expose the patient, above all in our hospitals, to the danger of erysipelas.

M. Leon le Fort: I share completely the opinion of M. Blot and Després. The recent wounds borne by the patient from which the epidermis had been taken were re-covered by a reddened crust showing that at least a bloody discharge had followed. Therefore, the epidermis alone had not been removed; a fragment had been taken comprising capillaries and a door opened for erysipelas. As to the utility of the method, it is without importance, even granting that one can cast here and there a sort of seed which by germination on the spot will result in cicatricial islets. This cicatrix will have, like all others, a tendency to contraction, and this autoplasty cannot replace that to which, for example, one has recourse to prevent the scar retraction of an eyelid which could result in ectropion, or one of the face causing a deformity.

M. See: If M. Reverdin only takes the epidermic layers, including the mucous or malpighian layer, this experiment has, from the physiologic standpoint, more importance than accorded it by M. Després, since he would have demonstrated germination and proliferation of a tissue composed only of cells, and it is then a question not only of a graft, but of a veritable inoculation.

COMMENTARY BY DR. CLAUDE DUFOURMENTEL

Jacques Louis Reverdin was a Swiss surgeon born in Geneva in 1842, but he studied medicine in Paris where he became Interne des Hôpitaux in 1865. This title was, and still is, very difficult to obtain in France, especially for a non-French student.

He was the intern of Guyon in 1869, and it is in his surgical department of the Hôpital Necker that he tried and succeeded in grafting small and very thin pieces of skin on open wounds. Thus he could obtain healing of large defects which had resisted all other treatments known at that time.

His chief, Felix Guyon, was at that time a young (38 years old) chief-surgeon at the Hôpital Necker, one of the six large general hospitals in Paris (then and now). He was specially interested in urinary diseases and in 1876 he became the first professor at the Faculty of Paris of this new specialty. He created many instruments still in use. The Hôpital Necker became under his direction a world-famous center of urology. Guyon

supported Reverdin's work, but several surgeons doubted that he succeeded in really grafting skin. They thought that he had only stimulated healing. But, during the next months, several other surgeons tried his method and came to realize that it worked. The quality of the scar obtained by grafting such small and thin pieces was, of course, rather poor.

Shortly after the publication of the first cases of skin grafts by Reverdin, the war of 1870–1871 between France and Germany started. Although Swiss by nationality, Reverdin served in the French army at the head of the "Swiss ambulance" in Paris, treating many wounded soldiers. After the war, he went back to Geneva where he became chief surgeon of the Hôpital Cantonal de Geneve and Professeur de Pathologie externe et ʾde Medecine operatoire at the University.

For 34 years thereafter he continued his work in Geneva as a teacher and investigator. During this time he was noted for his investigations on the internal secretions of the thyroid gland and experimental production of myxedema, an honor which he shared with his countryman, Theodor Kocher of Berne. He also created the needle for sutures which bears his name and is still very commonly used in Europe.

In 1881 with Picot and Prevost he founded the *Revue Medicale de la Suisse Romande*, which he then edited for 38 years. He died at the age of 86 years, in 1928, after a most remarkable career.

Claude Dufourmentel, M.D.
178 Rue Courcelles
Paris 17, France

The Full-Thickness Graft

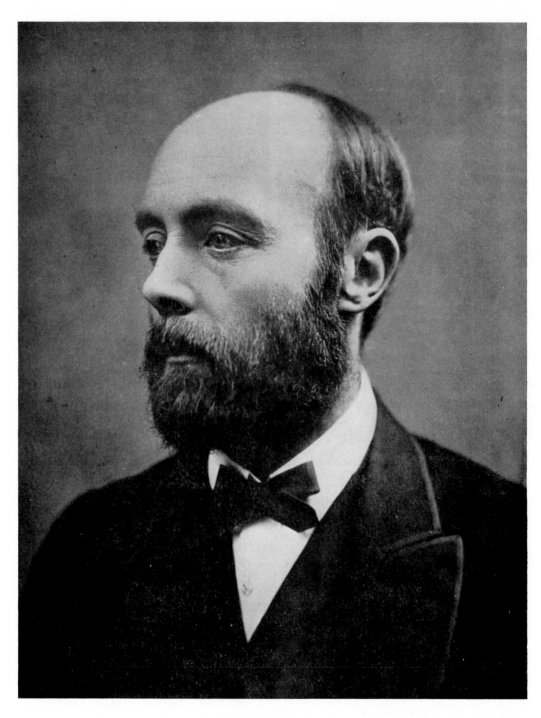

GEORGE LAWSON
1831–1903

THE SURGEON OCULIST AND HIS FOURPENNY GRAFTS

Two years after Reverdin demonstrated his "seeds of skin" in Paris, George Lawson presented patients before the Clinical Society of London in whom he had successfully performed free full-thickness grafts of skin the size of a fourpenny (32 mm, approximately the dimension of a current U. S. halfdollar) and a threepenny (16 mm, about the size of a current U. S. penny). This antedated the paper by Wolfe, and also Krause's, by some years. Lawson's paper was nearly forgotten until Sumner Koch called attention to it in 1941.

We are indebted to Mr. and Mrs. Eric Peet for photographing the original article for us, and for searching many places until they found this superb portrait of Lawson.

The paper is exemplary, a model for authors, a dream for editors. It is presented herewith in its entirety, as it appeared in the Transactions of the Clinical Society of London, *4:* 49, 1871.

FRANK McDOWELL

VII.—*On the Transplantation of Portions of Skin for the Closure of large Granulating Surfaces.* By GEORGE LAWSON. *Read November 11, 1870.*

I have brought before the Society this evening two out of three patients in whom I have successfully transplanted portions of skin taken from the inner side of the arm. In each case the new skin became rapidly united to the granulating surface.

During the process of union the pieces of skin underwent certain changes in their appearances, to which I shall shortly allude. They never, however, became apparently lost amidst the surrounding granulations, as has happened to many of the transplantations of minute portions of skin, but they maintained during the grafting period their own entities; and as soon as their new means of vitality were established, they threw out from their circumferences granulations which rapidly cicatrised, and contributed greatly to the closure of the wounds.

CASE I.

The first patient was a poor woman, æt. 42, in the Middlesex Hospital, who had been under my care on and off for over four years, suffering from a large, irritable, and extremely painful ulcer of the left leg. She had been twice an inmate of the hospital, but she had been each time discharged before the wound was healed; and on resuming her duties, the ulcer had very shortly regained its original size, and completely incapacitated her for work. She was admitted for a third time last August, when on account of the great dimensions of the ulcer, which was a large oval of about the size of the palm of the hand, and also from its excessive pain and its apparent inability to heal, she was willing to have her leg amputated.

Under treatment, however, the wound assumed a healthy appearance, and cicatrisation went on favourably up to the beginning of September, when the reparative process seemed to be almost arrested, and the size of the wound remained nearly stationary.

On September 22 I transplanted a portion of skin taken from the inner side of the arm, and in three weeks from that date the wound was completely united. As soon as the portion of new skin had established its vitality, granulations sprouted from its circumference, and these continued to spread in circles and to become skinned over until the whole gap was closed.

11

Case II.

The second case was in a man, æt. 24, a patient in the Middlesex Hospital, who had a large varicose ulcer, which no doubt would have healed by rest and ordinary treatment. He had suffered for two years and a half from an ulcer of the leg, which would heal for a time and then break out again. The size of the ulcer when admitted was three inches long, and one and. three-quarters wide. The man was kept in bed under treatment until the wound presented a healthy granulating surface, when I transplanted a piece of skin from the inner side of the arm, of the size of a fourpenny-piece, after it had been removed from the arm. The new skin very shortly united, and granulations rapidly sprang from its circumference which closed the wound in about eighteen days from the time of its transplantation.

In each of these cases the ulcers of the leg were completely healed before the wound in the arm, from which the skin had been removed, had cicatrised.

Case III.

Destruction of the Skin of the left upper Eyelid from Lupus. Complete Ectropion. A new Tegumentary Covering for the Lid formed by transplantation of Pieces of Skin from the Arms.

J. H., æt. 22, was admitted into the Royal London Ophthalmic Hospital on October 14, 1870, suffering from complete ectropion of the left upper eyelid, the tarsal edge being drawn up to the lower line of the eyebrow. The loss of skin which had occasioned this deformity had been produced by lupus. The eye suffered so much from the exposure consequent on the inability to close the lid over it, that the man was willing to submit to any operation to obtain relief.

On the following day I dissected down the lid from its attachments, and in order to keep it in position, I adopted a plan first suggested by Mr. Bowman, and pared at two points the corresponding tarsal margins of the lids, and united them by two fine sutures, and thus obtained a fixed level surface upon which to transplant some new skin as soon as the granulations were ready to receive it.

October 18.—As the whole of the upper eyelid presented a healthy granulating surface, and the tarsal margins were firmly united, I transplanted a piece of skin of the size of a silver threepenny-piece, which I removed with a pair of scissors from the inner side of the arm, and placed it on the nasal side of the lid, as at that spot the granulations looked most vascular and healthy. A piece of transparent isinglass plaster was laid across the lid to keep the piece of skin *in situ*, and over this a fold of lint with a compress of cotton wool was placed, and the whole was kept in position by a Liebreich's bandage, which was drawn firmly across both eyes. Before fastening the bandage, a compress of cotton wool on lint was also applied over the sound eye, as it was essential that both eyes should be excluded from light, in order to prevent any disturbance of the lid on which the new skin had been planted, from that constant rolling of the globes which goes on when one eye is allowed to remain open and be used by the patient.

First Day after Transplantation, October 19.—The piece of skin seen through the transparent plaster, which was not removed, looks very white, but shows no other evidence of diminished vitality.

Second Day, October 20.—The plaster was removed; the skin was not so white as yesterday, and its edges seemed to be clinging to the wound. I now transplanted another portion of skin of the size of a fourpenny-piece on to the outer portion of the lid. This I excised from the right arm of the patient—the wound left by its removal was exactly the size of a sixpence.

In speaking of the changes which daily took place in the appearance of the skin, I shall still refer only to the first portion which was transplanted, as the other went through exactly the same stages before it was firmly engrafted.

Third Day, October 21.—The first portion of skin which was transplanted presents to-day a peculiar rosy tinge, which is very marked when contrasted with the whiteness of the piece which was engrafted yesterday. Its edges are more vascular than the centre, and they seem to adhere closely to the granulations.

Fourth Day, October 22.—The whole of the skin has a rose tinge, deeper than yesterday, and its edges are distinctly vascular.

Fifth Day, October 23.—The cuticle is beginning to desquamate; in other respects the appearance is the same as yesterday. Granulations are springing up around it, and cicatrisation of the raw surface of the lid is proceeding rapidly.

Sixth Day, October 24.—The cuticle has completely desquamated, and the piece of skin looks vascular throughout. From this time the healing process was very rapid, and on October 29 the whole of the raw surfaces of the lid were completely skinned over.

Remarks.—The cases which I have related show that pieces of skin of the size of a sixpence can be easily engrafted on granulating surfaces; it remains for experience to decide how much larger portions can with safety be transplanted, and what are the conditions under which these transplantations can be most satisfactorily conducted. When once these facts are thoroughly ascertained, the present treatment of burns, and of deformities arising from a large destruction of skin, will be completely changed. We shall no longer allow extensive granulating surfaces to be closed over by an indrawing of the surrounding skin, but we shall freely transplant portions of skin from those parts of the body where there is a redundancy, and I have no doubt but that the time will come when we shall beg portions of skin from a parent or a friend who is willing to give of his abundance for the relief of a suffering child or a neighbour.

The conditions which seem to me essential for the grafting of large portions of skin are—

1st. That the new skin should be applied to a healthy granulating surface.

2nd. That skin *only* should be transplanted, and that special care should be taken that there is no fat adherent to it.

3rd. That the portion of skin should be accurately and firmly applied to the granulating surface.

4th. That the new skin should be kept in its new position without interruption, and that it should be lightly covered with a layer of lint, and over this a small compress of cotton wool, for the purpose of maintaining its warmth, and thus to assist in retaining its vitality until it has established its new life.

Lastly.—I would mention that the new skin thus engrafted, not only soon becomes vascular, but it acquires sensibility. In each of the cases I have related, there was no sensation for the first 8 or 10 days, but after that date, the new fragment of skin became sensitive, and could appreciate the slightest touch of any blunt instrument applied to it.

COMMENTARY BY MR. ERIC PEET

George Lawson, the author of this interesting paper, was born on August 23, 1831, the son of a partner in a firm of merchants in the city of London. He received his medical education at King's College, London, and took the Diplomas of the College of Surgeons and the Society of Apothecaries at the age of 21. Among his resident appointments at his hospital was that of House Surgeon to Sir William Ferguson who was then the most brilliant operator in London. In 1854 Lawson entered the army, the war between England and Russia being imminent. When war was declared he was sent first to Gallipoli and then to Varna where he contracted typhoid and became very ill. After a severe hemorrhage he was regarded as moribund and was asked if he had any last wishes to send to his family. To this he replied that he had no intention of dying and, contrary to expectation, he recovered.

He continued to serve with distinction in the army. As became a pupil of Dr. Snow, he was an ardent advocate of the use of anesthetics, against which some of the miliary authorities of the old school were prejudiced, and his was the only inhalar of the third division. In May 1855 he contracted typhus and was invalided home. After recovery he settled in London, turned his attention to the study of the eye, and became Clinical Assistant at the Royal London Ophthalmic Hospital, Moorfields. In 1863 he was elected Assistant Surgeon to that hospital and shortly afterward Assistant Surgeon to the Middlesex Hospital. He ultimately became Senior Surgeon to both institutions. Although best known as an ophthalmic surgeon, he also held a high place in general surgery. He was one of the pioneers of antiseptic surgery. In 1888

he was appointed Surgeon Oculist in Ordinary to Queen Victoria and continued to attend Her Majesty in that capacity during the rest of her life.

George Lawson died in 1903.

This is a brief story of this brave and chivalrous man and I am indebted to the libraries of the Middlesex Hospital and Moorfields for this information about him.

The article he wrote on skin transplantation is equally remarkable and contains ample evidence of his knowledge and foresight. It is not known whether he was aware of Reverdin's publication of 1870. It would seem that the grafts he employed were full-thickness grafts and that he left the donor area open. He was evidently well aware of the importance of removing all subcutaneous fat. Those of us who read his article, nowadays, although none of us would follow his technique, must have a feeling of admiration for a talented pioneer and a sense of humility in ourselves.

Eric Peet
Oxford, August 1967

EDITORIAL ADDENDUM

A fine biography appeared recently, entitled *George Lawson: Surgeon in the Crimea* (Constable & Co. Ltd., London, 1968). The book was written by Victor Bonham-Carter and Monica Lawson (grandaughter of George Lawson), and was based largely on his letters from the Crimea. It mentions that he was author of several authoritative works on eye medicine and surgery but, curiously, does not contain the words "skin graft" anywhere. When I corresponded with Monica Lawson about this, she was apparently unaware of her grandfather's famous contribution in this field.

F. McDowell

The Split-Skin Graft

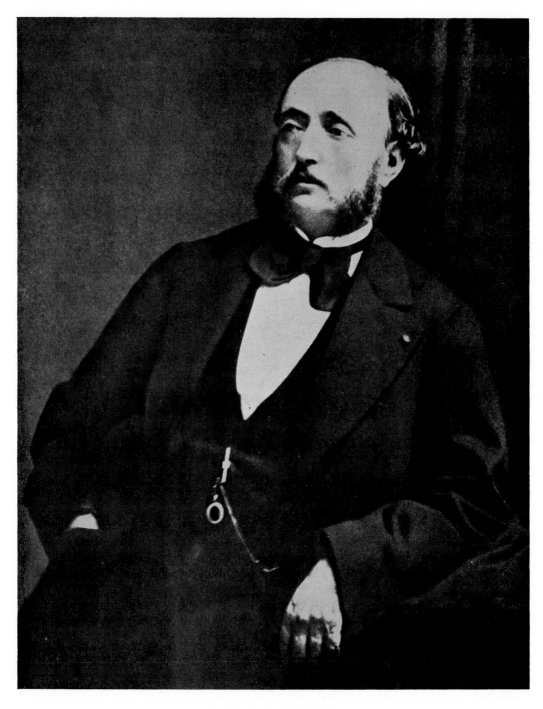

L. X. E. L. OLLIER

(Courtesy New York Academy of Medicine. From p. 274, *Médecins célèbres*. Mazgalon et cie, Geneva, 1947.)

GREFFES CUTANÉES OU AUTOPLASTIQUES

L. X. E. L. OLLIER, M.D.

Paris, France

Instead of grafting small pieces of epidermis of 2, 3 and 4 square millimeters, as reported by M. Reverdin, M. Ollier grafts large sheets of 4, 6, 8 square centimeters, comprising not only the superficial layers of the skin but the total thickness of the dermis. His objective is, not to create multiple centers of epidermization, but to substitute for the ordinary epidermic pellicle of scars a membrane incorporating the essential elements of normal skin, possessing the characteristics of the latter.

The scar resulting from sowing little islands of epidermis on the surface of a wound differs in no way from ordinary cicatrization. The epidermization of its granulations is more or less hastened, but the process is the same. It takes place by the gradual extension of epidermis over the most superficial layer of granulation tissue.

M. Ollier causes the connective tissue of the dermis to play the principal role in his skin grafts, and in order to demonstrate that the connective tissue has its own aptitude for grafting, he cites a periosteal graft that he has applied 20 days ago, to the surface of an ulcer—a 6-centimeter layer of periosteum detached from a leg which he had just amputated. This is the first time that he has transplanted periosteum in man under such conditions; he cannot yet predict the result from the standpoint of the osteogenic qualities of the transplanted periosteal graft.

M. Ollier has been able to study the late results of these dermo-epidermic grafts as compared with grafts comprising only a part of the dermis which he has practiced for the

From Bull. Acad. Med. de Paris, *1:* 243, 1872. Translated from the French by Robert H. Ivy, M.D.

past 2 years; but his experiences on the large grafts, comprising the entire thickness of the skin, are still too recent for a definite report.

He has applied the dermo-epidermic grafts to prevent reattachment of fingers after a syndactyly operation, following extensive burns of the hand. He has also applied them in the cure of old cicatrices, in interrupting by means of the transplanted tissue the continuity of the scar. In these cases, a year later one can recognize the graft by its greater suppleness and its normal color in contrast to the violaceous hue of remaining scar tissue. But the results appear to him more complete and more persistent when the entire dermis is transplanted, as he practices today. When one undertakes to oppose scar contracture by a cutaneous graft, one should not be satisfied to apply the graft on the excoriated or freshened scar surface; one must excise the scar tissue and apply the dermic graft to the healthy underlying tissue, once a layer of granulation has formed. One must not cover the scar tissue, one must replace it. Then only, the graft will be a veritable autoplastic procedure which will be indicated when sliding flap autoplasty is not applicable, on account of the extent of the scar or the disposition of the parts.

To procure cutaneous grafts, M. Ollier obtains them either from the patient himself, or from limbs amputated on account of accident in healthy individuals. When taken from the same patient, one can freeze the part by a refrigerant mixture. M. Ollier has been able in the past to employ periosteal grafts in animals 24 hours after death if maintained several degrees below zero (*C*). Without being able to establish at the present time the extreme limits of viability of cutaneous grafts, he believes that these conditions will be approximately analogous to those he has determined for the periosteal grafts.

To assure the success of the grafts, it is necessary to immobilize the operated region with a silicate bandage or by any other apparatus which will prevent all movements of the area and sliding of the graft on the wound. The silicate dressing has not only the advantage of immobilizing but of maintaining the graft under favorable environment (temperature and moisture) which favors its adhesion.

Colored illustrations shown the Academy, demonstrate the aspect of the grafts, their proportions, and the modifications that they bring to the status of the cicatrix. In one of these pictures, one sees the portions of skin detached after congealing by the refrigerant mixture, grafts of 25 days duration, contrasting by their natural coloration with the violaceous background of the rest of the scar which results from the ordinary process of healing.

L. X. E. L. Ollier, M, D.
Department of Surgery
Hôtel Dieu
Lyon, France

COMMENTARY BY SUMNER L. KOCH, M.D.[1]

Like Reverdin, Louis Xavier Edouard Leopold Ollier (1830–1900) came from a family with a background of scientific interest and achievement. Among his ancestors were a grand chancellor of the University of Toulouse, a number of magistrates, and 4 generations of physicians. His father was a physician in Vans in the department of Ardeche, where Ollier was born on December 2, 1830. A brother, a cousin, and two nephews were practitioners of medicine.

Ollier began the study of natural science at Montpellier, studied medicine at Lyon, and served as interne in the hospital of Lyon. He received his doctor's degree at

[1] Koch, S. L.: The transplantation of skin. Surg. Gynec. & Obst., *72:* 1, 1941.

Montpellier in 1856. The following year, attracted by the great name of Claude Bernard and interested in the problem of growth and reproduction of bone as a result of the influence of his teacher, Bonnet, he went to Paris to attempt to settle the question of the osteogenetic function of the periosteum. . . .

Ollier began his own experiments by raising a flap of periosteum from the surface of the tibia of a young rabbit, leaving the flap attached at its base and turning the free end of the flap over the deep flexor muscles of the leg. In 6 weeks the flap had become a loop of bone. He continued with other experiments, twisting the base of the flap to compress its blood vessels, dividing the pedicle 3 days after raising the flap, and finally transplanting free grafts of periosteum into the subcutaneous tissues of the thigh. In each case new bone was formed at the site of the transplant. He "entered Chauveau's laboratory a sceptic; when he had completed his first series of experiments he was convinced of the osteogenetic properties of periosteum."

In 1860, at the age of 30, he was called to the chair of clinical surgery at Lyon and appointed senior surgeon at the Hôtel-Dieu. After 8 years of patient experimental investigations—on the periosteum, on the medulla, on the bone itself, on the effect of experimental fractures, on the effect of injury to the epiphyseal lines of growth—he published the results of his observations in two volumes entitled *Traité expérimental et clinique de la régénération des os et de la production artificielle du tissu osseux*, a classic on the subject of growth and development of bone.

Throughout his long career as professor of surgery at Lyon he continued his experimental and clinical studies with unflagging interest and energy. In a memorial written by Eugene Vincent in the *Archives provinciales de chirurgie* the list of contributions to surgical literature made by Ollier or inspired by him in the years from 1868 to 1900 occupies 11 pages. Almost 100 of them were contributed by Ollier himself.

He died on November 25, 1900, in his 70th year, in the midst of a family reunion and only 24 hours after he had performed a number of operations at the Hôtel-Dieu and made the rounds of his surgical service. He had received almost every honor the surgical profession of his own and the other nations could bestow upon him.

Ollier's contribution to the subject of skin transplantation appeared in 1872 in the *Bulletin de l'Academie de Medecin* under the title *Greffes cutanées ou autoplastiques*. He went much farther in his conception of the problem than Reverdin, for he did not simply attempt to create new islands in granulation tissue from which epithelium might grow but carried out complete excision of scar tissue and its replacement with skin. He specifically stated that he used large grafts "4, 6, 8 centimeters square, and larger, including not only the superficial layers of the skin but the entire derma." For 2 years previous to his use of such "dermo-epidermiques"

grafts he had used strips containing only a part of the derma . . .; in this respect also he had gone farther than Reverdin, but he favored grafts of whole thickness skin. . . .

One cannot read Ollier's paper carefully without realizing that he deserves credit for the first description of the graft of intermediate thickness, and that he shares with Lawson the credit for the initial successful use of the graft of whole thickness skin. Finally, it is interesting to note that he laid a free graft of periosteum from an amputated leg over a granulating surface, for he considered the connective tissue as the active element in the growth of a graft. We do not know the result of this procedure but it indicates that his interest in the transplantation of skin was closely related to his long continued study of periosteal transplants and bone growth.

Sumner L. Koch, M.D.
Chicago, Ill.

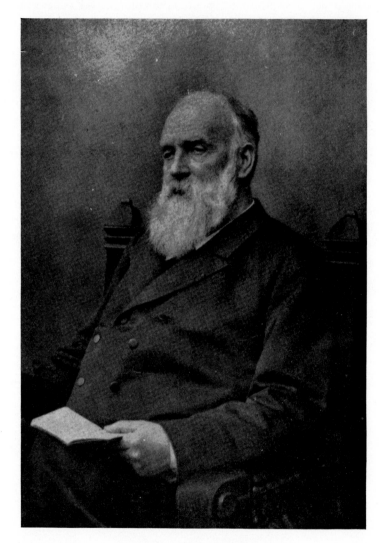

PROF. DR. CARL THIERSCH

UEBER DIE FEINEREN ANATOMISCHEN VERANDERUNGEN BEI AUFHEILUNG VON HAUT AUF GRANULATIONEN

(About the fine anatomical changes in the healing of skin over granulations)

PROF. DR. CARL THIERSCH, *Leipzig, Germany*

(*Verhandl. deutsch. gesellsch. chir.*, Berlin, *3:69, 1874.*)

Translated from the German by
DR. AND MRS. HANS MAY

Gentlemen! Anyone who has—at any time—studied the process of wound healing will always remain interested in this topic, and as soon as some new light is thrown on it he will return to his former love, although with subdued enthusiasm in his later years. Therefore, the beautiful invention of Reverdin's seemed to me an invitation to take up again my earlier researches in the healing process of wounds.

First of all, it seemed important to find the material on which to study this process of the healing of skin over granulation tissue in various stages. The opportunity arose soon: a patient had lost most of the skin of his leg after scalding. The surface defect consisted partly of granulation, and partly of ulceration of 4 years' duration; the patient came to the clinic at a time when Reverdin's method was already much in use amongst physicians.

After the healing process had reached its limit, the relatively large granulating area was closed by using numerous modifications of the method of skin transplants. This took a very long time. Finally, after a year and some days, the patient was discharged with his new skin coverage. But, as may have happened to others of my colleagues in such cases, he returned after a few months with the same extent of surface granulation as before. By various coincidental events the skin grafts had been lost.

Under these conditions the patient wished an amputation and I saw no other way out; but I selected this case for research and starting 3 weeks before the planned amputation, I transplanted small pieces of skin from time-to-time, the last ones 18 hours prior to the amputation. I applied only one of the modifications in this case, in order not to complicate the object of my research, i.e., I transplanted 1 cm square pieces of the entire skin, in which I had carefully removed the subcutaneous fatty tissue from the lower side. This seemed to me of advantage for anatomical investigation as the transplanted piece of skin is easily recognizable in its various parts.

The amputation was performed, the amputated member was injected with Gerlach's injection solution, and the skin was put in fixation. Unfortunately, I only fixed it with alcohol; it would have been better to use other methods of fixation, as alcohol causes different shrinkage of transplanted skin on underlying granulations—and so it happened that part of the transplanted pieces became detached. Yet, in the fine cuts of the specimen which were later stained in various ways, I was able to see many things which were new to me. Anyway, my results are very fragmentary, much remains obscure to me, and I restrict myself today to present to you the main points of my research.

1. The healing process takes place without a structureless substance of adherence (*fibrin—Ed.*).
2. If the graft takes, the healing process occurs under anastomoses of vessels, which can be seen 18 hours later (i.e., the connection be-

tween the blood vessels of the granulation and the skin graft occurs through intercellular ducts, which are immediately filled with blood derived from the vessels of the granulations and which circulates forth and back within the transplanted skin).

3. Nevertheless, the vessels of the transplanted skin undergo secondary changes, whereby they adapt themselves more or less to the structures of the granulations.

4. In some cases the transplant does not heal in its full thickness, but only the deep layer which is next to the fibrous tissue heals while the upper layer becomes necrotic and is rejected. I noticed that the sweat glands were enclosed in this deep layer.

Concerning the first point: the absence of structureless adhesive substance—I can be brief. There is no structureless fibrin layer, which supposedly plays a role in the healing process of wounds. Such a layer is non-existent here; the parts are directly joined together, except for the colorless blood cells which penetrate everywhere into the tiniest crevices. A molecular coagulation between the layers of attachment naturally can not be excluded; this may even be considered as a prerequisite to any adherence.

Coming to the second point (anastomoses) —it certainly is a striking fact that one can inject the capillaries of the skin graft 18 hours after the transplantation through vessels derived from the granulations, a proof that a close fusion has taken place. There is no mistake about it! The assumption that the injected solution could have escaped through tears in the vessels of the granulation tissue and could have found its way into the vessels of the skin graft, is not permissible. Everybody who has been working with injections knows that extravasated injection-solution never penetrates into vessels. The fact that the transplant can be injected completely from the granulation vessels after 18 hours is proof that a ductular connection has been established.

Closer observations lead to the following result:* between the clearly marked vessels

* The discusser demonstrates the anatomical part of his paper by means of a blackboard-drawing.

of the skin on one side, and those of the granulations on the other, there shows in low magnification ($\times$60) a pale, reddish, translucent zone of uneven thickness which, according to its position, belongs to the cellular coating of the granulations. At higher magnification ($\times$400), one can observe that this transparent reddishness is caused by a dispersion of the injected solution into intercellular ducts which are connected with the vessels of the granulation tissue. I did not observe myself the anastomosis of the host and graft vessels in this first stage, but it must be there. After a few days, some of the intercellular ducts become transformed into true vessels with the help of granulation cells, while the majority of the ducts disappear. Now, even with a small magnification, the connection between granulation and skin vessels can be seen. The process is, therefore, similar to that described by me for the other kinds of wound healing.

Before the second week one can see that (to use a not quite appropriate expression) the graft vessels are to some extent affected by the granulation vessels. They become wide, bulgy, start sprouting. In short, they assume embryonic characteristics. During the third and fourth weeks, the former structure returns and one sees vessels which have regressed partly, and others which did so entirely. (This circumstance caused Dr. Thierfelder, one of my young friends and colleagues, to come to the conclusion, as he was visualizing only this later stage, that the vessels of the transplanted skin must be either entirely, or almost entirely, reformed.) One finds the vessels in such a condition that it is difficult to decide whether they are newly formed, or preexisted. Then comes the question if the transplanted skin contains only newly formed vessels; that is, if the immediate anastomoses did not occur or had regressed. There is still a possibility that new capillaries grow into the intercellular mesh of the transplant from the granulations (as mentioned above) causing interstitial tissue-spaces to become filled with colorless blood corpuscles.

But this would rarely be enough to keep small transplants alive, which consist of the full thickness of the skin. The small piece will fall off, or only its lower layer will take, while the upper layer becomes demarcated as a scab.

I have seen this repeatedly. One finds the transplanted skin with the papillary and epithelial layer being cast off, but underneath is the deeper layer of the graft well joined with the granulations. This deeper layer forms (as one can see on the specimen) the transition to the subcutaneous tissue and includes fat lobules and sweat glands.

I belong to those who consider it likely that the coverage of granulating surfaces is carried out by already existing epithelium, which is demonstrated by the fact that the deep layers heal in, while the upper ones become rejected. It sometimes happens that a transplanted piece of skin takes for 6 to 8 days, and then falls off. The granulating surface is exposed again and the healing of the graft appears to have failed. But after another 8 to 14 days there appears epithelium. I suspect now that this epithelium may be the product of the healed-in sweat glands.

Allow me some more short remarks about the techniques of skin transplantation, and of the prospects of this operation for the future.

Good skin material, for transplantation to the granulating surface, can be found in the epithelial coverage at the rim of the wound. One takes flat, thin cuttings with a razor blade from this rim, and transplants them at random. The resulting defects of the rim restore themselves within 2 to 3 days.

Concerning the future of Reverdin's invention, I have to mention also its drawbacks, which I had called to notice before. The purpose of transplantation is to hasten the epithelialization of a granulating surface, which otherwise would become cicatrized.

In the first case, (*Ed. note: "epithelial"* grafts?) the result of the operation is usually lasting, especially in protected spots. The granulations shrink beneath the transplanted skin so that the transplanted pieces move closer together, even forming some sort of an elevation if they crowd together. Yet, the coverage of the wound surface is permanent.

In the second case, however, (*Ed. note: thicker grafts?*) as in the above mentioned amputation case, there is no (or hardly any) shrinkage of the scar of the granulating tissue beneath the skin grafts. Beneath the grafts remains loose, granulating tissue; the connection between them can be separated through any insignificant injury and, sooner or later, all is as it was before. Therefore in cases in which the method should have been a real advantage, the results are dubious.

Will it be possible to overcome this? Perhaps. On vertical sections of granulating tissue one can distinguish clearly two layers, a ground layer of rather firm fibrous tissue with a horizontally situated mesh of vessels, and from this horizontal vascular-fibrous tissue layer much softer and more vascular granulation tissue arises in a vertical direction (proud flesh).

If this part is deprived of the possibility to change into a scar (i.e., if the change of the soft vascular granulations into a firm, sparsely vascularized small cicatricial papilla does not occur) the recurrence of the granulations, which had been covered by skin grafting, is just a matter of time. There is nothing else to suggest but to remove the superficial part of the granulations and to transplant the skin directly upon the firm base. After slicing the granulations down, one waits until the bleeding has stopped and transplants the skin upon the freshly created wound. The vessels and the tissues of this wound surface are apt to promote immediate inflammatory adhesions. My researches in this direction are still incomplete, but, in all probability one should not only wait until the bleeding has stopped, but should add another few hours, during which the wound surface (perhaps protected by Lister's dressings) develops the first stages of inflammation.

In this way it may be possible to get a permanent take of the transplanted skin, since a fresh wound surface (*Ed. note: the undersurface of the graft*) is brought in contact with the inflamed surface of the exposed base of the granulations.

This reminds one of the ancient Indian rhinoplasty, in which a piece of skin was taken from the gluteal area and transplanted upon the freshened nasal stump. But before this piece of skin was transplanted, it was pounded *in situ* with a wooden shoe until it was considerably swollen. The old Schreger (certainly a marvelous surgeon but not free from the natural-philosophical "Anschauungen" of his epoch) believed that through pounding the vitality of the skin was enhanced. Nowadays, however, we might think, that soft pounding causes the beginning of inflammatory self-proliferation. Thus a fresh and an inflammatory-prepared wound surface come into contact, but with one difference. In the Indian rhinoplasty the surface of the stump was fresh and the piece of skin to be transplanted was prepared, while in our proposed skin transplantation, the opposite happens—the transplant is fresh, and the base is inflammatory-prepared.

Whether it would insure success to incite an inflammatory reaction in both surfaces before they are brought into contact with each other, is something that must be further investigated.

Prof. Dr. Thiersch
Department of Surgery
University of Leipzig
Leipzig, Germany

BIOGRAPHICAL SKETCH OF CARL THIERSCH, BY DR. HANS MAY

Carl Thiersch was born on April 20th, 1822 in Munich. He went to school there and graduated in 1836 to study medicine at the Universities of Munich, Berlin, Vienna and Paris. He received his Doctor of Medicine degree in 1843. In 1848 he was appointed prosector in pathological anatomy at the University of Munich. In the same year, he married the beautiful daughter of the great German chemist, Justus von Liebig.

In 1854, Thiersch was called to the chair of surgery at the University of Erlangen, and in 1867 he was appointed professor of surgery at the University of Leipzig. When the Franco-Prussian war broke out in 1870, he was made consultant surgeon to the armies of Saxony and served in this capacity until the end of the war in 1871.

After his return to Leipzig came his most fruitful years as surgeon, teacher, researcher and writer. He was the first German surgeon to recognize the importance of Lister's antiseptic method and introduced it to the Leipzig Clinic in 1867. This was the year of Lister's first publication on this subject and of Thiersch's first year at the Clinic.

His contributions to the medical literature were many and included his monograph on *Epithelial Cancer* (Engelmann, Leipzig, 1865), and his articles and papers before the German Surgical Congress on *Wound Healing* and on *Skin Transplantation.* He recognized that granulations were unstable tissues to graft skin upon and advised slicing the granulations down to the base before covering the latter with epithelial sheets, which were taken with a razor-knife. The skin of the donor area was held flat and under tension during this procedure.

Many national and international honors came to him. He was one of the pillars of the Deutschen Gesellschaft für Chirurgie and became its honorary member shortly before his death. He died on April 18th, 1895, a few days before his 73rd birthday.

REFERENCES

Thiersch, C.: Ueber die feineren anatomischen Veranderungen bei Aufheilung von Haut auf Granulationen. Arch. klin. Chir., *17:*318, 1874.
Thiersch, J.: *Carl Thiersch, sein Leben.* Johann Ambrosius Barth, Leipzig, 1922.

CARL THIERSCH, MICROSCOPY, AND SKIN GRAFTING

Perhaps fame begets a reputation for sagacity! Or, so it would seem in the early history of skin grafting.

The members of the Imperial Surgical Society of Paris were obviously unimpressed by the faltering presentation of the 27-year-old interne from the Necker Hospital. Perhaps Reverdin's youth was a factor, or his slight build, or his lack of involved explanations and animal experiments. True, he was awarded the gold medal that year in the competition amongst the internes of Paris—but this was for his work on anthrax and facial furuncles, not for skin grafting. Had Reverdin's work not been published automatically in the proceedings of the Society, it would probably have been lost (budding authors, please note).

As it was, the printed paper attracted some attention in London and in Lyon. The following year, on November 11, 1870, G. D. Pollock reported before the Clinical Society of London success in 8 of 16 cases in which he tried small Reverdin grafts to obtain healing of raw surfaces. The next paper on the program was George Lawson's classic, in which he described so lucidly his large and successful full thickness skin grafts. It is not known whether Lawson was aware of Reverdin's work before that hour. At the time, Lawson was a 39-year-old surgeon on the staff of Middlesex Hospital and of the Royal London Ophthalmic Hospital who had written two well-known books on ophthalmology. His future efforts were concentrated in that direction.

In Lyon, Professor Ollier, the 40-year-old chairman of the department of surgery, applied his keen investigative mind to the subject. No doubt, his interest was engaged by Reverdin's paper. But where Reverdin simply planted seeds of skin in a granulating bed, Ollier cut sheets of skin 4, 6, or 8 centimeters square, and larger, including not only the superficial layers but also considerable amounts or even the entire thickness of derma. He carried out complete excision of scar tissue and replacement of it by these larger skin grafts.

During all of this occurred the great Franco-Prussian war of 1870–71, furnishing wounds and amputations to be covered. The various German states loaned their armies to the North German Confederation, and these were formed into 3 great armies converging on Paris from 3 directions. The consultant surgeon of the armies of Saxony was the famed Prof. Dr. Carl Thiersch, chairman of the surgical department at the University of Leipzig. When the war ended, the German Empire was formed; the first Kaiser, Wilhelm I, was crowned in the Hall of Mirrors at the Palace of Versailles, just outside of Paris.

It would not have been incongruous for the King of Saxony to bring his august friend, Prof. Thiersch, to this ceremony. One wonders if he did, and if Thiersch met Reverdin or Ollier, or saw patients in Paris who had been treated by skin grafting.

However that may be, Thiersch did start experimental work on skin grafting soon after his return to Leipzig. Being a dexterous microscopist, he studied biopsies and was particularly interested in the minute anastomoses between the blood vessels of the graft and of the recipient bed. He came to the correct conclusion that in granulating wounds it is best to slice off the soft granulations down to a firm base before applying skin grafts. His other conclusion, however, was that thin grafts from the scar epithelium around the rim of the wound were the best to use, and the most likely to produce permanent healing. This erroneous conclusion gained widespread acceptance due, no doubt, to the great fame of Dr. Thiersch. He reinforced this view in later papers (1886, 1888) in which he advised cutting grafts with a razor blade in lamellae as thin as possible. This mistaken concept, surrounded by irrelevant evidence but supported by none, held back the development of split skin grafting for more than half a century.

Thiersch's other contributions were considerable. With Carl Ludwig and Wilhelm His he created the golden age of the medical school at the University of Leipzig. He used skin grafts to line flaps intended to replace the total thickness of the cheek, lip, or nose. Also, he grafted the donor beds from which flaps were rotated. He was the first in continental Europe to put Lister's principles in practice on a large scale. Lister was so impressed that he came to visit Thiersch in Leipzig, and was even more impressed when he attended one of Thiersch's lectures and found the King of Saxony sitting with the students, listening. Another surgeon who came to Leipzig to be inspired by Thiersch was a young unknown from New York, W. S. Halsted.

There are two facets to Thiersch's great error. One is the omniscience which we tend to attribute to the great and which they sometimes attribute to their own statements—especially the silliest ones. The other is the obvious failure of the editor; this article was crying for the pencil. It would have required courage for any editor to stand up to so great an authority, but how much better it would have been for everyone, Thiersch included, if the editor had just used that pencil!

—*Frank McDowell, M.D.*

The next two papers, on full-thickness skin grafts, appeared 4 and 22 years, respectively, after Lawson's paper on that subject. Yet, the English often call these "Wolfe grafts" while the Germans may refer to them as "Krause grafts."

A NEW METHOD OF PERFORMING PLASTIC OPERATIONS

J. R. WOLFE, M.D., F.R.C.S. ED.

Glasgow, Scotland

(Reprinted from Brit. M. J., *2:* 360, 1875)

It is now nearly three hundred years since Tagliacozzi published his great work on *Plastic Operations;* and, notwithstanding the admiration which the work of the Bologna professor had elicited, it is remarkable how comparatively little has since been done for the cultivation of plastic surgery. The reasons are obvious. The fact is that, in operations on the nose, eyelids, and face—the most interesting regions for improving deformities—Tagliacozzi's method of taking flaps from the arm has been generally abandoned, on account of the extreme discomfort which it involves; and the practice of taking flaps from the forehead or face having been the only one in vogue, the procedure came to be considered more serious. In addition, when we take into account the elements of failure, from shrinking of the flap, from erysipelas or gangrene, it is not to be wondered at that surgeons are generally chary of resorting to the expedient, except in great emergencies. It amounts to this: we are to cut skin off the face to repair the face; and, in doing so, we run great risk of failure. To render plastic operations on the face more acceptable, and to bring them within a wider scope of utility, the following conditions must be fulfilled. 1. We must take a flap from the arm, or from any other part but the face. 2. We must seek to eliminate the elements of failure. I propose, in this short communication, to indicate the means of fulfilling both these conditions.

First, Tagliacozzi laid down the rule, which has ever since been considered as the primary law, and *sine quâ non* to the success of the operation, that the flap must retain its connection to the adjacent living structure by a pedicle which is to be severed only after complete union and cicatrisation of the raw surfaces. This pedicle has, in my opinion, been a source of great embarrassment to surgeons, and tended rather to retard the progress of plastic surgery. From my observations on transplantation of structures from the lower animals and on skin-grafting, as well as on plastic operations, I have long held it demonstrated, that in most cases the pedicle is not essential, if indeed it do contribute anything, to the vitality of flap. This being once established, we are henceforward free to choose our bit of skin from any part of the body we may find suitable.

My next endeavour has been to eliminate the elements of failure. The principal cause of failure I find to be in the subcutaneous structures. If we wish a skin-flap to adhere to a new surface by first intention or agglutination, we must be sure that it is cleared of all areolar tissue, and properly fixed in its new place. The following case will illustrate the points referred to.

Formation of the Lower Eyelid with Skin from the Forearm—P. C., aged 25, a quarrier, was admitted into the Glasgow Ophthalmic Institution, with his face, eyes, and eyelids injured by an explosion of powder. I showed the man recently to the Edinburgh meeting of the Association, as an instance of conjunctival transplantation from the rabbit.* The right upper eyelid, which was strongly

* This patient had to undergo several operations before his eyes were rendered serviceable and his face presentable. Left eye: 1. Artificial pupil; 2. Conjunctival transplantation from rabbit. Right eye: 1. Paracentesis for onyx and hypopion; 2. Skingrafting on upper eyelid; 3. Plastic operation on lower eyelid. All these operations were done without chloroform.

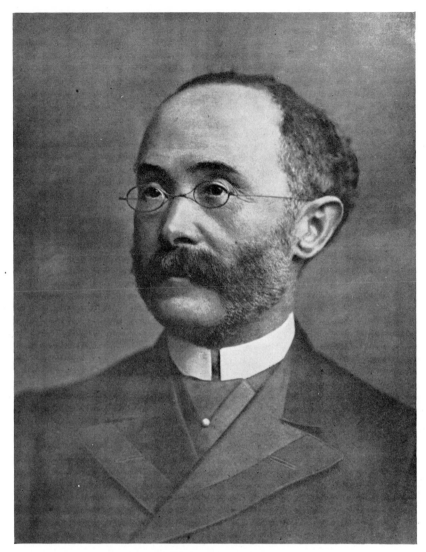

J. R. WOLFE, M.D., F.R.C.S., ED.

Surgeon to the Glasgow Ophthalmic Institution; Lecturer on Ophthalmic Surgery
in Anderson's University

everted, I partially succeeded in correcting by skin-grafting. The lower right eyelid being completely everted, its integument totally destroyed, and the skin of the face consisting of discoloured cicatrices not by any means suitable for plastic operations, I formed a new lower eyelid in the following manner. The edges of the upper and lower eyelids having been vivified, I introduced three ligatures into the border of the lower eyelid, which I en-trusted to my assistant. By means of these ligatures, he used traction, whilst I dissected the whole of the cicatricial tissue, and thus liberated the subjacent structure. The liga-tures were then introduced into the upper eye-lids, and the edges of the upper and lower eye-lids were thus united. I then elevated the edges of the wound, preparing them to re-ceive the new flap like a watch-glass. The skin required for the formation of this eyelid was two inches in length and one inch in breadth, which I took from the forearm. To test the principles above indicated, I divided my flap into three portions. The first I removed, along with the cellular tissue, as close to the dermis as compatible with the integrity of the flap. The other two portions, after removing them from the forearm, I turned up; and with a cataract-knife I sliced off the areolar tissue, leaving a white surface, which I applied to the eyelid. The difference between these flaps was very remarkable. The two flaps, which were previously prepared, healed by agglutination, without exhibiting even the slightest tendency to desquamation of the cuticle. Twenty-four hours after the operation, the surfaces looked pale; but the next day the temperature was normal, and appearance healthy; whilst that part which was applied without previous preparation looked rather livid the first day, improved the next two days; the fourth day, it began slightly to suppurate; and, after a hard struggle for life, a portion of it only remained, while the rest shrank. This however, will not compromise the result of the operation, which may be considered satisfactory.

The dressing consisted of gutta-percha tissue applied next to the skin, a graduated lint-compress, and a bandage to maintain immobility of both eyes. The union was so rapid and so perfect, that I separated the upper from the lower eyelid on the fourth day.

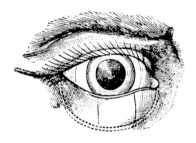

This figure was taken eight days after the operation, when union was complete. The thicker upper dotted line represents the elevated dissected edge, and the thinner lower dotted line shows the point of insertion of the

new skin. The vertical lines mark the division of the flap. The two outer and larger portions have been prepared before application; while the smaller, placed at the inner canthus, has been applied without previous preparation.

In conclusion, I would recommend this method to the profession, from its simplicity and safety, for trial, not only in similar cases, but also for the cure of congenital blotches on the skin of the face, which are not amenable to any other treatment.

John R. Wolfe, M.D.
Glasgow Ophthalmic Institution
Glasgow, Scotland

COMMENTARY BY MR. ERIC PEET

The author of this historical paper, John Reissberg Wolfe, was born in Breslau about 1824. He received his medical education at Glasgow University, where he graduated M.D. in 1856. He later studied in Paris. I learn from my enquiries that he took part in the Sicilian campaign of 1859 and took the title of "Senior Surgeon, Garibaldi's Staff and Inspector of Military Hospitals of the Italian Army." He received a personal letter from Garibaldi after the campaign was over, thanking him for all that he had done for liberty and the Italian people.

Returning to Scotland, he practiced in Montrose; in 1863 he was appointed Ophthalmic Surgeon to Aberdeen Royal Infirmary. On the death of Glasgow's first great eye surgeon, McKenzie, who founded the Glasgow Eye Infirmary, Wolfe returned to Glasgow. Disappointed at not being appointed to the staff of the Eye Infirmary, he founded (as it were) an institution of his own, The Glasgow Ophthalmic Institution, which is now the Eye Department of the Glasgow Royal Infirmary. He acquired a considerable reputation in the ophthalmic world. In 1893 he left Glasgow for Melbourne, where he practiced for some time, but 8 years later he returned to Scotland and went into retirement. He died in December 1904.

The article he wrote is full of interest. When first read through it is puzzling, because of the terminology he used. The term *free graft* was not in use in those days.

It is difficult to imagine the operations which he performed, on the patient he describes, without a general anesthetic and one wonders how such patients were sedated.

In the illustration reproduced, the outer two sections of the lower eyelid were applied as (what we today would call) Wolfe grafts; the inner portion was a graft of whole thickness skin with some areolar tissue on its deep surface. This inner portion evidently underwent a considerable degree of necrosis, as we would expect.

The experiment is surely a remarkable one on a conscious patient. The truth of Wolfe's conclusions regarding the importance of removal of all subcutaneous tissue from whole thickness free grafts has been passed down to us. This principle is one which entitles John Reissberg Wolfe to an honored name in the annals of plastic surgery.

Eric Peet, F.R.C.S.
Department of Plastic Surgery
The Churchill Hospital
Headington, Oxford
England

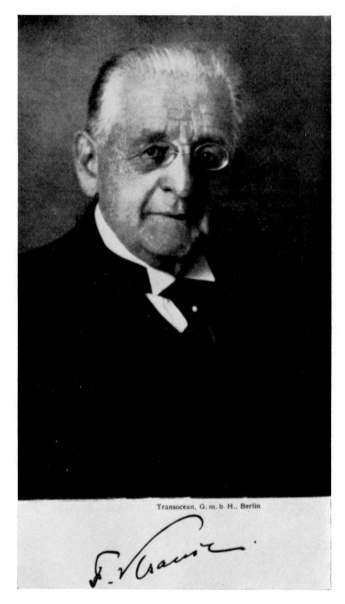

Transocean, G. m. b H., Berlin

Prof. Dr. Fedor Krause

THE TRANSPLANTATION OF LARGE UNPEDICLED SKIN FLAPS

PROF. Dr. FEDOR KRAUSE

Altona, Germany

(Translated from the German by Dr. and Mrs. Hans May)

In cases of large traumatic surface defects of the limbs the usual procedure to avoid amputation was, until now, a method devised by Maas and Wagner, whereby the defect was closed with large pedicle skin flaps which, for the arm, were taken from the trunk and for the leg and foot, from the opposite lower extremity. It is unfortunate that Thiersch's skin grafting was not sufficient for these extensive cases.

The transplantation of pedicled flaps, however, is quite cumbersome for the patient. The extremities must be immobilized in a plaster cast until the flap has healed sufficiently into the new area so that the pedicle can be severed without risking the viability of the flap. This has not been possible before the 10th to the 14th day, the forced position is extremely troublesome, and in cases of the leg there are additional difficulties as the flap can not be made too large; the new scar adds another handicap for workmen, who constitute the majority of patients for this procedure.

For these reasons, I have covered such defects for the past 2 years with non-pedicled skin flaps consisting of the entire thickness of the cutis (i.e. I have applied the method which one used to call "The Second Indian Method". The difference, however, is that with the "Second Indian Method," the subcutaneous fat-tissue was left attached to the flap, while, following Wolfe's technique, I use only the cutis together with the epidermis.)

The favorable results stimulated me to follow this technique also in old, very large leg-ulcers which, off and on, broke open; also in plastic operations of the face, particu-larly in cases after extirpation of large sections of the facial skin for lupus or cancer.

The healing in of the severed skin flaps is almost certain, provided meticulous technique is followed. My experience consists of 21 cases in which more than 100 skin flaps were used; of these, only 4 died completely. It does not depend upon the size of the excised skin pieces. Elliptiform flaps of 20 to 25 cm in length, and 6 to 7 cm in width, do not show any more difficulties of healing in than do smaller ones.

The main thing is for one to operate completely aseptic and dry and for bleeding on the recipient area to be stopped with compression.

The base to be covered must be a fresh wound, as after excisions of tuberculous or malignant lesions, or must be changed until wound conditions are healthy. In the latter case, traumatic wounds or ulcers must be cleaned before the operation is carried out. The latter is preceded by the application of a tourniquet to the limb and by rendering the operating area aseptic. In addition, granulations must be thoroughly scraped off with a sharp spoon. After the whole area has been scrubbed again with sublimate* solution, all sublimate is rinsed off with sterile saline solution. The area then is dried with sterile compresses.

From now on, the operation proceeds completely bloodless. The instruments and the hands must be completely dry. In granulating wounds the base is excised with a knife. Depending upon the time that has passed since the injury, the base may be infiltrated more or less from cicatricial changes; such infiltrated layers are removed,

From Verhandl. deutsch. Gesellsch. Chir., Berlin, *22:* 46, 1893.

* *Editor's note:* Mercuric chloride solution.

if this seems advisable, so that tissue as normal as possible will form the base for the skin graft. It does not matter whether depressions will result from this procedure; they become effaced soon, as we see also after Thiersch's transplantations. The same technique is carried out in treating large chronic leg ulcers. In these cases the tibia is also chiseled off, whenever it is found to be thickened. The wound is now covered with a pressure dressing, and the tourniquet is released.

In the meantime, the part of the body which serves as the donor area is disinfected. This should not be done too energetically. I try to avoid brushing hard and scrubbing the skin. The sublimate solution is rinsed off with sterile saline solution and the skin is dried. Only dry hands and dry instruments as well as sterile compresses, are to touch the donor area. The skin of the median-anterior side of the arm and forearm, or the anterior side of the thigh, or occasionally the trunk, is used as a donor area. To close the resulting defect immediately with sutures, the flaps are cut elliptiform; only after they have been removed are they cut according to pattern.

To remove these large cutis grafts from the subcutaneous fat-tissue, the entire flap is circumscribed with an incision. With an anatomical forceps, the lower point of the elliptiform flap is lifted up and dissecting is carried out with a knife, cutting more or less vertically against the cutis to be removed (i.e. just the opposite way from which pedicle skin flaps are dissected). After a sufficient piece of the flap has been dissected, the free end is doubled over so that raw surface comes to lie upon raw surface. This avoids unnecessary touching of the raw surface with the fingers, and one grasps the doubled over skin piece with the fingers for continuing the dissection. Such details assure success.

If necessary, flaps are taken from the entire length of the upper arm, forearm, or thigh and of such width in their broadest part that the immediate closure of the defect with sutures can be accomplished. Hence, in stout people, subcutaneous fat tissue must be excised for this purpose. Autogenous skin is always used. In this way very large flaps can be severed in a few minutes. The thin, delicate layer of fibrous tissue between cutis and subcutaneous tissue is taken with the flap. It does not matter if here and there fat-tissue remains attached to the flap.

The dissected skin flap, which shrinks immediately to $2/3$ or even less of its size, is placed immediately upon the raw surface. Bleeding of the recipient area has been stopped in the meantime by compression or by torsion of some of the vessels; ligatures are not used because the threads, being foreign bodies, interfere with the nourishment of the flaps (which, at first, is by diffusion from the recipient area). The flap is cut, if necessary, according to pattern and is pressed with gauze compresses upon the base. Soon it becomes glued to the recipient area; after the thin layer of blood has become coagulated, the gauze compresses are removed.

To suture the flaps to the surrounding skin is not necessary in limbs. In the face, I had to do this only once when I replaced nearly the entire upper lip with a graft taken from the upper arm (because the patient continually moved his mouth while coming out of anesthesia).

Whenever possible, the whole defect should be covered immediately with skin flaps. The dressing is applied, as follows: first, a 5 per cent sterilized iodoform gauze bandage is smoothly wrapped around, so that the flaps become fixed. Then follows an aseptic compression bandage; in extremities, splinting is necessary.

The first dressing is changed after 3 to 4 days. Blisters, which at times form on the skin flaps, are incised. In order to avoid tearing of the flaps, only the upper layer of the dressings is removed; then the entire limb is placed in warm boric water solution for one, or several, hours. On the face, grafts are covered with iodoform-boric Vaseline gauze; even then, one must be very careful when changing the dressings.

After 4 days the flaps look pale, or as a result of stasis, they may appear cyanotic. At times, they are swollen. After 7 to 8 days, there is a pink coloration which becomes more pronounced after 14 days, particularly so when one removes the dirty-gray epidermis, which always comes off. Here or there small superficial layers become necrotic or, in some places, even the whole thickness of the flap. But all in all, the flaps heal in well.

As mentioned, more than 100 large skin flaps have been grafted in 21 patients and only 4 became completely necrotic. Even if the superficial layers should become necrotic, the glandular appendages deep in the transplanted skin remain intact and regeneration proceeds from their epidermal linings. The skin flaps become regenerated, no matter **whether they are transplanted to muscle,** fascia, fibrous tissue, periosteum, dura mater or immediately upon the chiseled-off bone (be it corticalis, or spongiosa).

Depending upon the condition of the base which provides the nutrition of the flap, and depending upon the age of the patient, it will take 3 to 6 weeks, hardly any longer, for completion of the regeneration of the graft. Sensation, however, takes much longer to return.

Since with this method the entire thickness of the skin is transplanted, it is natural that, aside from the glandular appendages, the hair is also transplanted (as the follicles are practically all in the cutis). Therefore, it is possible to use parts of the scalp to replace missing eyebrows.

After regeneration, the skin is mobile. After excision of a little piece of transplanted skin for microscopic examination, it was astonishing to find that after 22 days a thin layer of beautiful yellow fat tissue had formed, although the cutis had been transplanted completely free of fat tissue upon the muscle fascia (i.e. the fat-tissue was newly formed).

I demonstrate to you a large number of photographs which will show clearly the results. The data are attached to the patients' charts. I shall endeavor to report about these details, as well as about the respective literature, in more detail.

Fedor Krause, M.D
Municipal Hospital
Altona, Germany

BIOGRAPHICAL SKETCH BY DR. AND MRS. HANS MAY

Fedor Krause was born in 1856 and died in his 81st year, on September 22, 1937. He began his medical studies in Berlin, subsequently spent several semesters in Halle and Frankfurt-am-Main, and graduated from Berlin University in 1879. The following 3 years were spent working at the Ophthalmological Clinic of the University Hospital under Julius Hirschberg, and at the Imperial Board of Health under Robert Koch. Later, he worked under Weigert at the Pathological Institute of the University of Frankfurt-am-Main.

He received his surgical training under the famous surgeon Richard von Volkmann at the University of Halle (1889–1892). The mighty personality of this illustrious man attracted the young Krause and left indelible imprints on his later life.

Krause's wide field of scientific interest included researches in ophthalmology and bacteriology; he published a monograph on tuberculosis of the bones and joints in 1891 and 1899. His inaugural thesis, in 1887, was on malignant neuroma; this entitled him to the rank of assistant professor, and he became an associate professor in 1889. In 1892 he was appointed chief of the surgical division of the Municipal Hospital of Altona (near Hamburg) and in 1900 he became surgical director of the Augusta Hospital in Berlin.

His chief interest now became surgery of the central nervous system, which at that time was in its infancy. He opened up many new paths, and must be counted among the pioneers in this field. In 1896, he published a monograph on neuralgia of the trigeminal nerve and the anatomy and history of that nerve. He was preceded by J. Eving Mears (of Philadelphia) and Horsley (of Richmond) in resecting the Gasserian ganglion but it was Krause who chose the extradural route, thus rendering the procedure less hazardous. (Coincidentally, Hartley, of New York, devised the same route independently within a few weeks after Krause's publication.) Although Krause considered extirpation of the Gasserian ganglion as the operation of choice in the treatment of tic douloureux, he also had performed preganglionic division of the nerve before Frazier and Spiller's publication on posterior root resection in 1904. In his epoch-making work entitled *Chirurgie des Gehirns und Rukanmarks*, which appeared in 1908 and 1911, he summarized his large experience in the entire field of neurosurgery.

One can consider his work on full-thickness skin grafting, which he presented before the Twenty-Second Congress of the Deutsche Gesellschaft fuer Chirurgie on April 13, 1893, as almost incidental. He was preceded by George Lawson, Surgeon-Oculist to Queen Victoria, and by John R. Wolfe, another ophthalmic surgeon who had immigrated to England from Germany and practiced in Glasgow. Fedor Krause undoubtedly deserves credit for having used full-thickness skin grafting on a large scale, and for having perfected and popularized the method.

Dr. and Mrs. Hans May

REFERENCE

1. Behrend, C. M.: Fedor Krause und die Neurochirurgie. Zentralbl. Neurochir., *2:* 122–127, 1938.

DIE TRANSPLANTATION BETREFFEND

PROF. OTTO LANZ, *Amsterdam, The Netherlands*

(*Zentralblatt fur Chirurgie, 35: 3, 1908*)

Translated from the German by
DR. LEO CLODIUS

During the time of my residency, I became unhappy with the fact that the donor area of a Thiersch skin graft was still an open wound, while the recipient area had already been healed for quite some time.

a thermocautery held close to the wound surface.

In the course of some castrations made necessary by prostatic hypertrophy, I have occasionally taken thin slices from the testicle with a razor and tried to ob-

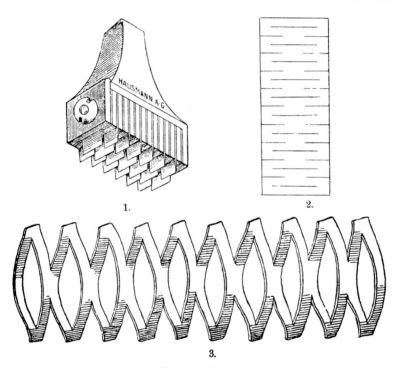

1.

2.

3.

Figures 1, 2, 3.

In an attempt to remedy this evil, I have tried various methods. In 1892 and 1893 I began to cover the Thiersch donor areas by freshly removed hernial sacs; later I tried to obtain rapid healing under crusts—by leaving the wound exposed to air, or by weak coagulation with

tain metaplasia of the glandular epithelium into surface epithelium by transplantation of the slices onto the defect to be covered.

None of the above experiments led to any usable results.

At this point I was reminded of a children's game our sisters used to play. By cutting serial incisions in a strip of paper (scarification) they could produce an inexpensive paper accordion. As a result, I ordered a stamp (Fig. 1) from my instrument maker (C. Fr. Hausmann, St. Gall), the effect of which is best seen in Figure 2 (incisions) and Figure 3 (pulled apart). A long Thiersch graft was then cut, halved, and each half stamped with the skin incisor. One half of the skin strip, expanded to form an accordion, was transplanted; the other half, also expanded, was replanted and was sufficient to cover the defect created at the donor site.

The construction of the stamp is such that it is easy to enlarge or to reduce the distance between the individual knives, by the interposition of dividers of varying thickness.

By the use of this stamp it is possible to cover both the area to be transplanted and the donor area with the skin strip removed all in one procedure. It may be used advantageously in cases where extensive wound areas are to be covered, or where only a small amount of skin is available for transplantation.

Otto Lanz, M.D.
Department of Surgery
University of Amsterdam
Amsterdam, The Netherlands

BIOGRAPHICAL SKETCH OF LANZ BY DR. LEO CLODIUS

Otto Lanz was born in Steffisburg, Switzerland, in 1865.

He graduated from medical school in 1889, after having attended the Universities of Geneva, Bern, Basle, and Leipzig. Thereupon, he became a surgical resident with Kocher in Berne. In 1894 he opened his surgical practice in Berne. In 1902 he was elected Professor of Surgery in the University of Amsterdam, Holland.

His special interests were (1) asepsis, (2)

surgery of the thyroid, and (3) appendicitis (Lanz's point in appendicitis).

In March, 1906, Lanz was probably the first to attempt a physiological operation for lymphedema of the leg. He fenestrated the deep fascia, which he considered to be the main barrier between the lymphedematous compartment of the extremity and the musculature. In addition, strips of fascia were threaded into the marrow of the femur. Lanz published this case in 1911, and reported a good result.

Professor Lanz was a friend of the famous Swiss painter Ferdinand Hodler. Once, Hodler asked his friend to put on the uni-

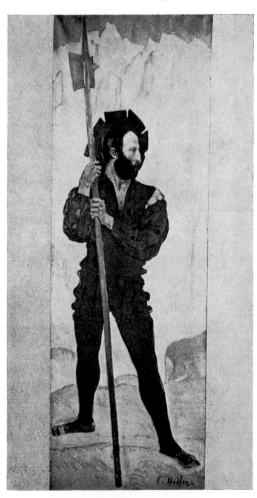

PROF. OTTO LANZ
1865–1935
(Painting by F. Hodler)

form of a Swiss lancer and to hold a halberd. Later on, Professor Lanz donated this painting to the founder of the instrument firm of Hausmann, as a token of his appreciation for the surgical instruments made by this company.

EDITORIAL NOTE

This paper, possibly the first description of the accordion (or "mesh") graft, was brought to our attention by Dr. Leo Clodius. The idea is apparently an obvious and a recurrent one. Later, it was published on several occasions (*e.g.* Lester Dragstedt, Surg. Gynec. & Obst., *65:* 104, 1937) and was common knowledge in the late 1930's and early 1940's (*e.g.* Brown, J. B., and McDowell, F.: *Skin Grafting of Burns,* p. 62. J. B. Lippincott Co., Philadelphia, 1943). Some of the drawbacks to this type of graft were discussed in a recent editorial in the *Journal* (*44:* 484, 1969).

Lanz was a man of catholic curiosity. Almost no two of his papers were on related subjects. It is curious, therefore, that he did not realize that donor areas of properly cut "Thiersch grafts" would heal rapidly without the necessity of suturing them, or grafting them. This was probably another example of a sometimes useful thing being invented for the wrong reasons.

—Frank McDowell

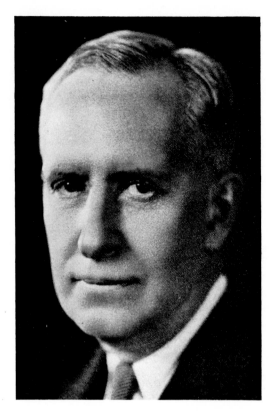

VILRAY PAPIN BLAIR
(in 1926)

JAMES BARRETT BROWN
(in 1930)

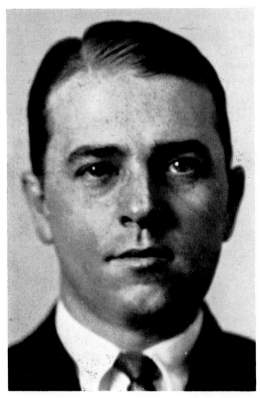

40

THE USE AND USES OF LARGE SPLIT SKIN GRAFTS OF INTERMEDIATE THICKNESS

VILRAY P. BLAIR, M.D., AND JAMES BARRETT BROWN, M.D.

St. Louis, Mo.

(Reprinted from Surgery, Gynecology, and Obstetrics, *49:* 82, 1929)

Early, quick, and permanent surfacing of burns and other cutaneous defects conserves health, comfort, function, time, and money; while unnecessary waiting spells economic waste.

The factors that might lead to a choice between the use of flaps or free grafts are not presented here, but having decided in favor of the latter, we should give serious consideration to the type of skin graft to be employed.

Next to the pedicle or sliding flap, a successful free skin graft of practically full thickness will most closely duplicate the natural surface, but a number of circumstances must be considered in each case: the type of the graft best fitted for the particular loss, the speed of the operation, the source of the graft, and the potential healing qualities of the patient—all have a bearing.

The full thickness graft is appropriate for a freshly made, clean raw surface where substantial protection, maximum mobility, minimum of subsequent contraction, and the most natural appearance are essential to a successful result. Circumstances permitting, the full thickness graft has usually been chosen to cover a contracted, healed surface, in which the full thickness of the scar must be cut through or removed to allow relaxation. Such an area may be situated on the front of the neck, on certain parts of the face, over the flexor surfaces of joints that can be extended, or the extensor surfaces of joints that can be flexed. The full thickness graft is also used in the correction of webbed fingers and for the release of arms fixed and grown to the trunk as the result of a burn.

On fresh granulating surfaces, on freshened scar surfaces in contradistinction to scar surfaces which have been completely excised, on surfaces that will resist subsequent contraction or in which allowance can be made for such contraction, if the appearance and demands of function do not contra-indicate their use, thinner grafts are chosen because of the comparative simplicity of their application and the greater certainty of the "take." On the back of the hand, except over the knuckles, and upon the subcutaneous muscles of the face, the orbicularis oris and orbicularis palpebrarum, a split graft of some thickness is, in most cases, the one of choice. Circumstances may make it necessary to vary any of these rules. The technique of application of the full thickness graft and its aftercare are both exacting and time-consuming. The graft itself is very susceptible to infection so that the patient must possess

From the Department of Surgery, Washington University School of Medicine.

Read before the Southern Surgical Association, White Sulphur Springs, W. Va., December 1928.

(*Ed. note:* The original paper was 16 pages in length with 27 Figures. It has been shortened for this reprinting, and the legends have been rewritten to correspond.)

good healing power. The wound produced by the removal of the full thickness graft must subsequently be closed.

The Ollier-Thiersch graft is theoretically supposed to include little more than the epithelial layer. If given half a chance such grafts will heal in close to 100 per cent in areas which are only relatively clean and in patients with somewhat lessened healing power. While it requires considerable time and skill to obtain a good full thickness skin graft of any size, very large thinner grafts can be quickly cut and, if one does not go too deeply and the dressing is properly applied, the resulting raw area is usually healed within 10 days when the first dressing is removed. In most instances it requires 3 weeks of exacting post-operative care to carry through a full thickness graft, but the successful thinner graft at most requires only protection for a few days after the primary dressing is removed. In many cases, moreover, if one wishes to form a lining for the antrum or for the conjunctival sac or to form a surface over de-epithelialized derma or the orbicularis oris or orbicularis palpebrarum, this lack of thickness of the graft is a very desirable quality.

Three factors associated with the use of the thinner graft, if ineptly applied, may seriously affect the final result: (1) the thinner graft may not give sufficient protection to a bearing surface; (2) the thinner graft, because of its thinness, will not correct the inequalities of the underlying surface; and (3) the thinner graft, if placed on a freshly made raw surface with a movable base and movable edges, such, for instance, as the subcutaneous tissue of the neck, may subsequently contract without any loss of epithelium, and the contraction may be as much as 60 per cent.

Contraction does not take place in the graft itself but in the layer of scar tissue which unites the graft to its new bed. In the full thickness graft the derma seems to a large extent to have the power to resist this potential contraction. If the thinner graft is laid on a freshly denuded scar base, on derma, on the periosteum, or on bare bone, or if the grafted area is surrounded by tense skin or scar, there may be little subsequent narrowing of the field. If the thinner graft is cut so as to include an appreciable amount of the derma, it seems to possess more of the good than the bad points of either the full thickness or the true Ollier-Thiersch graft, and it is this type of graft which we shall discuss here.

Having categorically presented the short-comings of the thick split graft it is only fair to reiterate its redeeming qualities. A graft of this type of large size can be easily obtained with relatively little damage to the area from which it is cut, the "take" is almost certain, and, if judiciously used, such a graft gives good protection and a fair final appearance. A graft aggregating one hundred square inches will heal as quickly and surely as one an inch square and not a great deal more time is required for the cutting (Fig. 1). Further, unless one cuts too deeply the defect resulting from the removal of one hundred square inches or more of graft will heal as quickly as that from a square inch graft. The more accurately and evenly the grafted area is

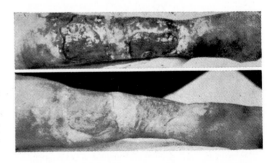

Fig. 1. (*above*) Ulcers in heavy scar base, 20 years duration. (*below*) Result of split skin grafting in one operation, with one small ulcer adjacent to one of the grafts regrafted 4 months later.

covered the more will the result approach the normal condition.

TECHNIQUE

Preparation of areas to be grafted. Acute purulent skin eruptions or acute pus infections of any kind are contra-indications to any plastic operation, and especially to free skin grafting. Therefore, a careful examination of the skin of the entire body is made before and on the morning of operation. A pimple or a boil, even on a remote part of the body, with sufficient induration to suggest the possibility of tissue necrosis or "core" formation, means that the host's resistance to that organism is low at that particular time; and we regard such a remotely located pimple, boil, or impetigo as a contra-indication to skin grafting. Acute tonsillitis is also a contra-indication. Almost all of the failures in our experience we have attributed to an unrecognized or an immediately developing infection of this kind. The chronic acne pustule, the simple inflammation about a comedo, and the acute pustule without induration are not regarded as sinister and receive little consideration unless they are located on the field of operation. . . .

. . . For preparation of healed cutaneous areas, ordinary cleansing care, the removal of all scurf or scales the day before operation, and the use of some antiseptic solution in the operating room are sufficient. . . .

. . . *The preliminary preparation of bare and granulating areas including indolent ulcers.* Unless it is the site of an aggressively active infection or of a locally impaired circulation, a granulating surface will, in time, epithelialize spontaneously; but, except for small defects, this is a waste of time and money. Ordinarily, in a patient of fair health, sluggish or dirty granulations can be quickly cleansed by absorbent dressings dampened with some sort of an aqueous solution changed every 8 hours, by rest, and by postural control of the return circulation. So long as it is non-irritating, the exact nature of the solution is probably not of great consequence. The important factors are: (1) that the dressing be damp and absorbent, not sloppy or allowed to dry in place; (2) that it be changed sufficiently often; (3) that it be firmly and comfortably applied. Regardless of the chemical content of the solution, the primary object is continuous drainage and pressure control of the circulation both within the granulations and in the associated area. . . .

. . . Success or failure in the use of grafts will depend more upon the healing qualities of the tissues than upon all other factors and influences combined, including good surgical technique. To secure the maximum benefit from a chemical antiseptic applied to the skin or raw tissues, it is imperative that special attention be given the primary factors already mentioned, and if the strength of the solution lessens tissue resistance then it is best to discard it entirely. A firm, bright red, easily bleeding, granulating surface that has but a slight mucus-like discharge and is free from surrounding induration or inflammation possesses a high potentiality for healing, and such granulations can usually be obtained by the simple plan of rest and frequently changed moist dressings as already described. Thin or moderately thick skin grafts have a distinct tendency to grow when put on such a granulating surface, but they will do much better if the granulations are sliced (not scraped) down to the underlying yellow scar base and the whole area is covered with large grafts put on with proper tension and pressure. If it is desired to use full thickness grafts it may be safer to cover the raw surface first with thinner grafts and to apply the full thickness grafts after the area is healed. In an indolent ulcer or an old granulating surface, all but the deepest layers of the mature scar base can be excised to advantage and either a graft applied immediately or a new, more healthy crop of granulations raised (Fig. 2).

The selection of the source, the cutting, the application, and the dressing of the graft and of the area furnishing the graft are all of importance and each should recive careful attention.

Source of the graft. The skin from which the graft is taken should be free from inflammation and it should be remembered that a graft of the thickness under consideration is apt to raise hair if it is taken from a hair bearing area. Such a development may be objectionable, especially for grafts put in the mouth. We have not a few patients who have to cut hair from these grafts. This surgery usually contemplates the improvement in appearance as well as in function; therefore, visible mutilations should be avoided if possible, especially in girls and girl babies. Today, the areas of skin ordinarily exposed are somewhat less restricted than formerly and this is especially true in athletes, so that now the areas left from

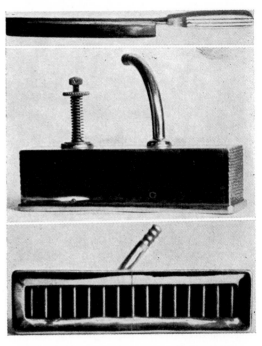

Fig. 3. Skin graft knife and suction retractor boxes, designed by authors for cutting large split skin grafts. Boxes are made in widths of 4.5, 7, and 9.5 cm; non-collapsible rubber tubing is used to connect the box to a strong suction machine. The knife is 18 cm long, 2 cm wide, made of a strip of razor steel set into a stiff back. It can be stropped on a piece of canvas with emery powder, as a sterile sharpening procedure.

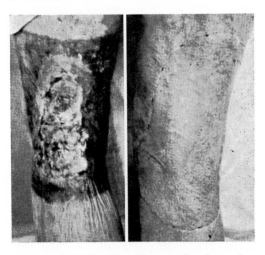

Fig. 2. Marjolin ulcer, 50 years after burn. Amputation was advised, but refused. (*right*) Result after excision, and grafting 4 weeks later.

which grafts may be taken are the inner and outer surfaces of the upper half or two-thirds of the thigh, the lateral surface of the buttock, and the front of the abdomen. In babies still in diapers the abdomen is the site of choice.

The cutting of the graft. When possible the graft is cut large enough to cover the area and to extend beyond its edges. Even if it requires more than one graft it is desirable to have as few as possible and to have them of even thickness. On a large thigh with a fair amount of subcutaneous fat, especially in women, good sized grafts of fairly even thickness can be cut with a long light razor-ground knife, the skin being held tense and flat by traction pressure of small straight-edged pans above and below the knife (Fig. 3).

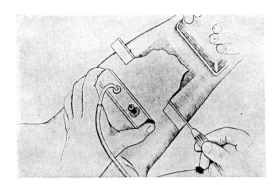

FIG. 4. Use of suction retractor. We always feel apologetic for using a special instrument but believe this has some justification. While this machine, in its present form, is not a substitute for manual dexterity in cutting grafts, one is enabled to cut grafts more quickly and to make them larger.

In thin muscular men, in thin patients with flabby muscles, and on the abdomen, especially of babies, pressure methods to tighten the skin are not satisfactory. In such patients a suction retractor is almost necessary to secure the type of graft that is desired. It is helpful in any case (Fig. 4).

Application of grafts. The grafts are applied as soon as the bed is prepared. Definable arterial or venous bleeders of any size may be caught and tied with split silk or No. 3* catgut, but this is usually not practical except in instances in which the scar has been entirely cut through or removed. In cases in which large areas are simply denuded hæmostatic pressure with gauze is maintained as the denudation progresses. When completed, the grafts are sutured in place and the surface pressure reapplied. The graft is put on to overlap the borders of the defect; if more than one graft is needed the borders of each piece overlaps its neighbor. This overlapping is possibly a prophylactic against future visible scar. The grafts are held in place, under about normal lateral tension, by continuous basting or whipping stitches of horse hair. A graft that is put on under normal

* *Ed. note:* 3-0 catgut.

stretch will be clearer and less muddy looking than one that has been allowed to contract. After the graft is sutured small holes are cut through it at appropriate intervals to insure drainage of blood and serum. A retained blood clot may be a source of failure.

DRESSINGS AND POSTOPERATIVE CARE

There has been more written on the dressings and postoperative care of skin grafts than on any other phase of the subject and in most of these contributions, many of which are a bit lengthy, the factors that we have found best to promote a quick, sure "take" either are not mentioned or are not recommended. These factors are (1) absence of virulent infection, (2) fixation, (3) pressure, and (4) provision for drainage.

Fixation and pressure can be obtained with any good, ordinary, well applied surgical dressing. Early slipping of the dressing may dislodge the graft. This is one reason why we suture the graft and why we are liberal in our use of adhesive plaster on the dressing. Any little secretion drying at the edge of the graft may block drainage or cause a dry dressing to stick and thus possibly detach the graft when the dressing is removed. Therefore, two layers of Vaselined gauze are applied next to the graft under the pad and, because Xeroform is supposed to be antagonistic to staphylococci which are present in all skin and all grafts, we make up the Vaseline with 3 per cent Xeroform. On a firm, even surface where pressure is easily applied, such as the forehead, we may use only dry gauze sponges next to the greased gauze. On uneven surfaces, on surfaces that lack a firm foundation, such as the front of the neck, or on the hand, large, flat, damp, marine sponges, which do not touch the bare skin, are applied evenly over the gauze pads. The whole dressing is fixed by a pressure bandage.

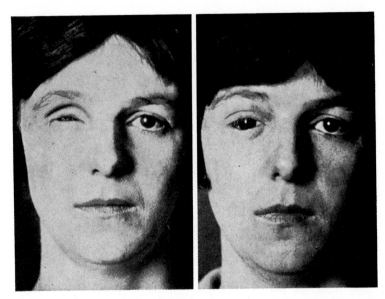

FIG. 5. (*left*) Contracted eye socket, 6 years after removal of globe. (*right*) Artificial eye in place, 6 weeks after orbit opened up and relined with split skin grafts put in over two wax forms.

In our original studies on the application of pressure dressings to skin grafts, the use of sponge rubber, inflated toy balloons, lambs wool, and damp marine sponges were included. In our experience we have found that the moist marine sponge has been the most practical distributor of pressure.[1, 2]

On a well prepared, healthy surface, the first dressing should be the last, but it is just as well to examine the wound at the end of 4 or 5 days, or earlier, if one has any doubt as to the healing quality of the grafted base. In some instances the dressing is allowed to remain 10 days before it is disturbed. Should a clot be found, the overlying graft is split with a sharp knife or scissors and the clots peeled out; then, if the graft is clean, there is fair probability that it will reunite to the base. Should there be an accumulation of serous secretion, yellow or clean, the detached part of the graft is cut away with sharp scissors and the area is considered not clean and is dressed accordingly. In such cases treatment consists in the application of an absorbent dressing very similar to the one used in the preparation of the granulation bed, at least daily inspection of the area, and the removal with sharp, fine, curved scissors of all raised edges of graft. . . .

. . . In certain sites such as within the mouth, on the eyelid, and on the lip, it is not practicable to obtain pressure by ordinary dressings. In these situations, if the graft is wrapped around a wax form, raw surface out, lateral tension of the graft is obtained by the traction of the graft on the wax or by the suturing under tension of the graft over the wax (Fig. 5). In turn the tissues to be grafted are sutured under tension around the graft covered form which furnishes the desired pressure.[2] Such grafts properly implanted in a newly made wound in the mouth will, if the patient is in fair condition and not subject to any acute infection, heal in close to 100 per cent of the cases in spite of the fact that the graft and the wound have been bathed in saliva.[3]

On two occasions the wax form of an eyelid graft was removed on the second day on account of discomfort in the eye—a complaint which should never be disregarded. The graft was lost in neither of these cases. . . .

. . . *Dressing of the donor area.* Discomfort in the area from which the graft has been taken may be caused by one of two factors: (1) infection which might rarely occur from organisms liberated from sweat and sebaceous glands at the time the graft is cut; (2) movement or pulling of the dressing. Ordinarily these areas are made comfortable by immediately applying six smooth, flat layers of Vaseline Xeroform gauze covered with a flat gauze pad, neither the gauze pad nor the greased gauze extending more than 1/4 inch beyond the raw area. The whole is then firmly strapped in place by means of adhesive plaster, which prevents any sliding or pulling on the raw surface of this deep dressing. Over this is bandaged a protective absorbent pad which may be changed as it becomes soiled. If two parallel grafts are taken from the thigh, a strip of uncut skin is left between the defects for the attachment of adhesive plaster. Ordinarily, at the end of 9 days, the blood soaked original dressing is lifted off or it is soaked loose by a wet pack. If the graft has not been cut too deep, the whole area is usually found to be healed. If in any place the cutting has gone down to the fat, healing at such spots will be delayed. If the patient walks about at this time it is well to reapply a firm pressure dressing under adhesive plaster to try to prevent the possible formation of small hæmatomata under the fresh thin epithelium. If it becomes uncomfortable before the ninth day, the dressing is soaked loose, and the area redressed with the greased gauze. If infection occurs, damp pressure dressings are used.

TREATMENT OF DEEP BURNS

Willis[4] and others have treated burns by immediate excision down to the sound tissue and then grafting the raw area, if necessary, when the wound has become sufficiently clean. In cases in which this can be successfully accomplished it is of real advantage. Regardless of the will to do so, in many cases whether from the extent of the burn, the condition of the patient, or the controlling circumstances, such treatment is at present impracticable. This should not, however, make one content with a practice all too prevalent of allowing these wounds to become deeply infected and to granulate and suppurate for months and possibly years before the wounds are covered with hard, distorting, limiting scars which, without later help, cripple the victim throughout life and later are too often the site of cancer (Figs. 2, 6, 7). Most joints so fixed by scar can be released by means of flaps or full thickness grafts.

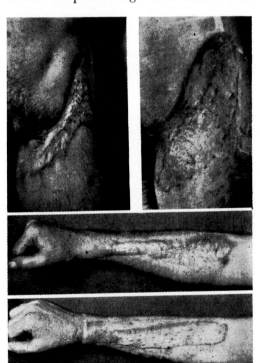

FIG. 6. Electrical burn scars of forearm and groin, excised and grafted in one operation. Total operative time, 1 hr. 55 min.

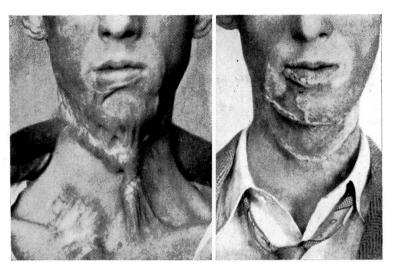

Fig. 7. Contractures of neck and lower lip, shown 2½ years after burn. Neck contracture corrected with full thickness graft, lip contracture with split skin graft.

This is not true, however, of the fingers which, during the slow healing process of a burn extending little deeper than the skin, often become so fixed by peri-articular thickening that a year or more of manipulation may be necessary to release them or they may never become released.

Immediately after the calamity of an extensive burn, relief of pain and preservation of life are the all-embracing considerations; but, as early as possible, means should be taken to protect the wounds from infection and to encourage drainage. The so-called open treatment of burns, which too often means a pus poultice under crusts, may be sufficient for superficial burns, but our observation of the late results of such treatment of deep burns makes us feel strongly that whenever possible some other plan of treatment should be instituted, especially when the full thickness of the derma is destroyed. When we have treated fresh burns we have usually been able to secure a healthy, firm, granulating surface within a month, and have the grafts healed in place within 2 weeks more. . . .

. . .In spite of many literary citations to the contrary, all our experiments with homo-grafts have ended in the graft being completely absorbed in from 3 to 6 weeks after it had healed in place, even when the bloods matched. Our observations, however, are incomplete as we have never tried the application of grafts from one young child to another of similar age nor have we grafted from one identical twin to another.*

ROENTGEN-RAY AND RADIUM BURNS

In the treatment of radium and roentgen-ray burns, the object should be the complete removal of the involved tissue, with an attempt to get beyond the limits of the endarteritis, the telangiectasis, and the active keratosis. Upon the type or degree of burn present, the size and depth of the necessary excision, and the location of the defect on the body, will rest the choice of method of repair. If free skin grafting seems indicated, full thickness grafts or thick split grafts may be used.

In those burns evidenced by change in color, by telangiectasis, and possibly

* Ed. note: This was done a few years later and reported a few years after that. cf. Brown, J. B.: Homografting of skin, with report of success in identical twins. Surgery, 1: 559, 1937.

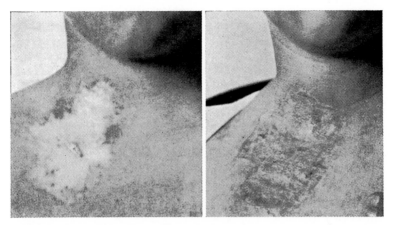

FIG. 8. (*left*) Radiation burn, from treatment of portwine stain. (*right*) Result 18 days after excision and application of split skin graft from thigh.

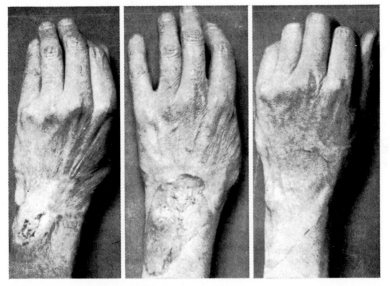

FIG. 9. *A*. Primary skin cancer, complicated by radium burn. *B*. Roughening in skin graft, a few months after deep excision and coverage with split graft. *C*. Result 16 months later, with complete function and smoothness.

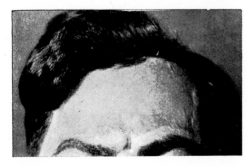

FIG. 10. Result of covering entire forehead with one split skin graft, after using forehead flap for facial reconstruction.

by some slight scaliness, the preparation of the bed for the graft may be done, as in healed burn scars, by slicing off the surface down to a very thin layer of derma and then immediately grafting with thick split grafts. If, in these areas, there are any smaller areas of excessive scaliness or keratosis, the excision should go deep and the defect in the graft bed should be closed with sutures to try to preserve smoothness if it is desired. Though trouble might possibly develop later in these areas, so far we have not had any. If it should occur, deeper excision and regrafting should be done (Figs. 8, 9).

LARGE FACE AND NECK BLEMISHES

We have treated large areas of damage to the skin of the face and neck, especially in women, such as oil or dirt filled superficial abrasions, large nevi or hairy moles, and scars resulting from trauma, acid or radiation, by dissecting off the lesion or scar down to the subcutaneous tissue and then, after allowing the area to granulate for 3 weeks, applying a thick split graft, as described under burns. If the scar is in the form of plaques, in or under the derma, as has occurred from long severe acne or smallpox, great improvement has resulted from dissecting off the damaged skin and the bases of the pits and applying the graft to a deeper plane of this blanket scar.

REFERENCES

1. Blair, V. P.: The full thickness skin graft. Ann. Surg., *80:* 298, 1924.
2. Blair, V. P.: The influence of mechanical pressure on wound healing. Illinois M. J., *46:* 249, 1924.
3. Blair, V. P.: The surgical restoration of lining of the mouth. Surg. Gynec. & Obst., *40:* 165, 1925.
4. Blair, V. P.: Value of debridement in treatment of burns. J. A. M. A., *84:* 655, 1925.
5. Blair, V. P.: A summary of the effects of repeated roentgen-ray exposures upon the human skin, etc. Am. J. Roentgenol., *13:* 139, 1925.

Epilogue

WARS AND SKIN GRAFTING: FROM BISMARCK
TO HITLER

The story of skin grafting is intertwined with the wars of this period. Reverdin's discovery came just before the Franco-Prussian War, at a time when Bismarck was making belligerent noises. Ollier's work was carried out during that war, doubtlessly stimulated by the open wounds that he saw. Thiersch also became interested in this work during that war, probably while trying to rehabilitate casualties.

The works of Lawson and Wolfe seem unconnected with any war but are, rather, expressions of that curious influence which ophthalmologists have had from time to time on skin grafting.

Before he vanished into neurosurgery, Krause's work seemed about to establish skin grafting as a routine part of the general surgical arsenal, at least in Germany. After this, however, a delayed reaction to Thiersch's influence set in and surgeons became obsessed with the erroneous idea that donor sites would not heal if the grafts were cut below the deepest pegs of the surface epithelium. They imagined more than they knew, cut grafts thinner and thinner, with the result that they became smaller and smaller and nearly useless for most clinical purposes. In the meantime, surgeons had come to realize also that full thickness grafts were nothing more than the trading of raw areas, at best. Skin grafting entered the doldrums.

In Blair's great opus of 1912, "Surgery and Diseases of the Mouth and Jaws," free skin grafting is mentioned in only a few scattered sentences. Wolff (*sic*) grafts are defined and not mentioned again. "Grafts made of thin shavings from the epidermis are used to cover raw surfaces from which the skin is missing. These are known as Thiersch grafts." Flaps were used for repairs, sometimes the beds were covered with Thiersch grafts dressed "with several thickness of silver leaf and then with two thicknesses of gauze, wet with a 10 per cent colloidal silver solution." (*Ed. note*—Silver has apparently long filled a psychological need of some surgeons in the treatment of open wounds. Recognizing that gold is too expensive for dressing large open wounds they may, nevertheless, feel that some advantage must be derived from using a noble substance rather than a base metal, or less.)

During the doldrums, Halsted and his group used small Reverdin or Thiersch grafts to cover defects from radical mastectomies. They may have been doing more skin grafting at that time than anyone else.

In World War I, flaps were the rule. Filatov (another ophthalmologist) published in 1917 the design of the tubed flap. J. F. S. Esser, however, introduced the use of the Thiersch graft wrapped raw side out around "stent" and buried to form an "epithelial inlay," particularly for the repair of contracted eyelids. Both of these procedures were quickly adopted and developed further by Gillies and his group. The Americans, under Blair, used flat flaps for the most part.

After this war, Blair developed methods for raising larger flaps with more certainty of survival, publishing "The Delayed Transfer of Long Pedicle Flaps" in 1921 (Surg. Gynec. & Obst., *33*: 261). Following this, he wrote "The Influence

51

of Mechanical Pressure on Wound Healing" (Illinois M. J., *46:* 249, 1924) and "The Full Thickness Skin Graft" (Ann. Surg., *80:* 298, 1924). These established the importance of uniform pressure over a graft to prevent hematomas and seromas under it, and to facilitate the ingrowth of capillaries from underneath. From great uncertainty, "takes" became more routine and free grafting for cosmetic purposes was possible.

Still, it was evident that full thickness grafts could never be used to cover large raw surfaces, to replace large areas of scar, or to release large burn contractures.

In the next few years, Blair and Brown established (by means of human biopsies) that "Thiersch Grafts" could not be cut thin enough to not include some derma. More important, they proved that donor areas from split grafts healed from deep islands of sebaceous gland and hair follicle epithelium, rather than from remnants of the surface epithelium. This opened up the possibility of transplanting considerable amounts of tough and "wearing" dermis with the graft; further, as it was not necessary to concentrate on thinness and trying to stay within the surface epithelium while cutting, it became possible to devise means of cutting much larger grafts. This they did. The 1929 paper on "Use and Uses of Split Skin Grafts" established, for the first time, skin grafting on a large scale useful in a large variety of clinical situations. Patients came from all over the world. The method which they devised for cutting split grafts is probably still the best for rapidly obtaining really large skin grafts.

Developments since then have consisted mainly of various mechanical devices for cutting grafts. The first, and still one of the most useful, was the dermatome developed by Padgett, just before World War II while Hitler was making belligerent noises.

With the papers by Reverdin, Lawson, Ollier, Thiersch, Krause, Blair and Brown, and Padgett (*cf.* Plast. & Reconstr. Surg., *39:* 195) we finish this series on skin grafting.

For biographical material on Blair and Brown, see Plastic & Reconstructive Surgery (*18:* 83, 1956—*38:* 284, 1966—*40:* 308, 1967).

—Frank McDowell, M.D.

SECTION II

The Origins of Rhinoplasty

TREATMENT OF FRACTURED NOSES IN ANCIENT EGYPT

(From Breasted, J. H.: *Edwin Smith Surgical Papyrus, in Facsimile and Hiero-glyphic Transliteration with Translation and Commentary*. University of Chicago Press, Chicago, 1930. Reproduced by permission.)

Editor's Note. The following are three case reports of *circa* 3,000 B.C., as copied from an ancient document by an unknown scribe in the 17th century B.C. This latter transcription is now known as the *Edwin Smith Surgical Papyrus*. The *glosses* contained herein were written by the scribe to explain the meaning of ancient terms to his 17th century B.C. readers. The *commentaries* contained herein were written by Professor Breasted, as he made his 1930 A.D. translation.

CASE ELEVEN

V 10–15

A BROKEN NOSE

TITLE

V 10

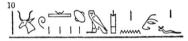

Translation

Instructions concerning a break in the column of his nose.

EXAMINATION

V 10–11

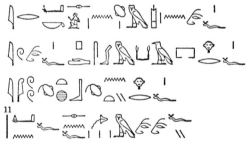

Translation

If thou examinest a man having a break in the column of his nose, his nose being disfigured, and a ⌈depression⌉ being in it, while the swelling that is on it protrudes, (and) he has discharged blood from both his nostrils, (concluded in diagnosis).

DIAGNOSIS

V 11

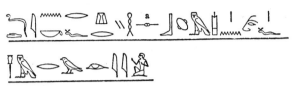

a The scribe at first omitted this *s* and afterward inserted it as a correction.

Translation

Thou shouldst say concerning nim : " One having a break in the column of his nose. An ailment which I will treat."

TREATMENT

V 11–14

Thou shouldst cleanse (it) for him [with] two plugs of linen. Thou shouldst place two (other) plugs of linen saturated with grease in the inside of his two nostrils. Thou shouldst put [him] at his mooring stakes until the swelling is reduced (lit. drawn out). Thou shouldst apply for him stiff rolls of linen by which his nose is held fast. Thou shouldst treat him afterward [with] grease, honey (and) lint, every day until he recovers.

Translation

GLOSS A

V 14–15

Explaining : Column of his nose

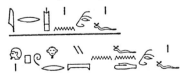

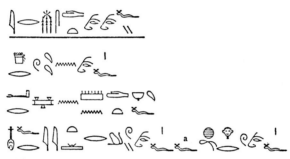

^a This *š* was omitted by the scribe in copying and was afterward inserted in the much too narrow space between *mš* and *d*.

Translation

As for : " The column of his nose," it means the outer edge of his nose as far as its side(s) on the top of his nose, being the inside of his nose in the middle of his two nostrils.

GLOSS B

V 15

Explaining : His two nostrils

^a This *f* is placed low in the line and there are above it and below it traces of erasures. As Smith himself noticed (Vol. II, p. ix, 2nd col.), the scribe originally wrote ⟨hieroglyphs⟩ and corrected it to *fḫ*. See commentary.

Translation

As for : " His two nostrils," [it means] the two sides of his nose extending to his [two] cheek[s], as far as the back of his nose ; the top of his nose is loosened.

CASE TWELVE
V 16–VI 3
A BREAK IN THE NASAL BONE

Commentary

This injury, while confined to the external bone, is certainly higher up than the preceding case, and in contrast with it quite certainly affects the bone. Thus these two cases of nose injuries are arranged like the wounds of the head in our treatise, which discussed first the injuries which were confined to overlying fleshy tissue without affecting the bones, and thereafter proceeded to fractures and similar injuries of the bones themselves. The case is interesting in that it is the first one we have met which involves setting the bone. The term for " set " is literally " cause to fall," followed by the words " so that it is placed in its position," or, more freely, " lying in its place." Not until after the nose is set does the surgeon cleanse the nostrils of the coagulated blood, called " every worm of blood." After the insertion into the nostrils of tampons of linen saturated with grease, this internal packing is externally reinforced by two stiff splint-like rolls, literally " posts " or " spars " of linen, probably laid one on each side, and " bound on." The three glosses are very instructive, especially the quietly rational explanation of " every worm of blood " as the coagulated blood " likened to a worm which subsists in the water."

TITLE

V 16

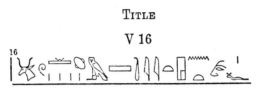

Translation

Instructions concerning a break in the chamber of his nose.

Commentary

As we shall see in the course of the treatment (V 17–20), our surgeon means the nasal bone by his curious designation " chamber."

EXAMINATION

V 16–17

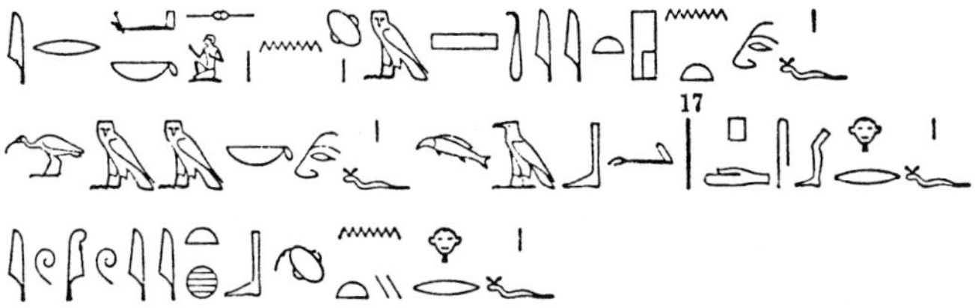

[hieroglyphic text]

Translation

If thou examinest a man having a break in the chamber of his nose, (and) thou findest his nose bent, while his face is disfigured, (and) the swelling which is over it is protruding, (conclusion in diagnosis).

DIAGNOSIS

V 17

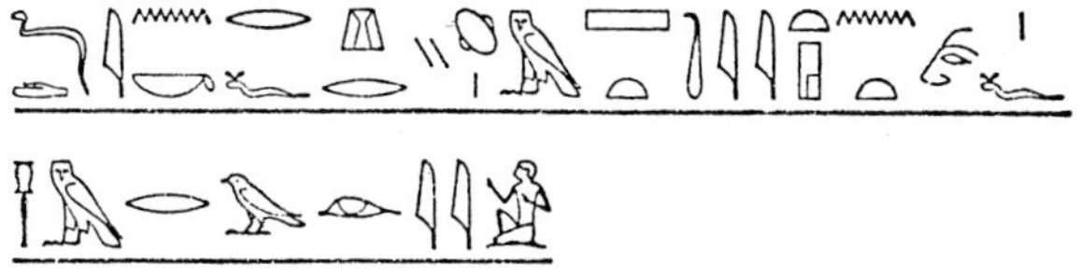

[hieroglyphic text]

Translation

Thou shouldst say concerning him : " One having a break in the chamber of his nose. An ailment which I will treat."

TREATMENT

V 17–20

¹⁸
^{sic}

¹⁹

²⁰

^a This word was omitted by the scribe, but the omission was discovered and the word subsequently inserted in the space over *k*, in red ink.

Translation

Thou shouldst force it to fall in, so that it is lying in its place, (and) clean out for him the interior of both his nostrils with two swabs of linen until every worm of blood which coagulates in the inside of his two nostrils comes forth. Now afterward thou shouldst place two plugs of linen saturated with grease and put into his two nostrils. Thou shouldst place for him two stiff rolls of linen, bound on. Thou shouldst treat him afterward with grease, honey, (and) lint every day until he recovers.

Gloss A

V 20–21

Explaining : Break in the chamber of his nose

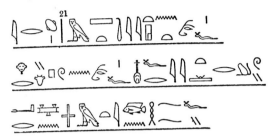

Translation

As for : " A break in the chamber of his nose," it means the middle of his nose as far as the back, extending to the region between his two eyebrows.

Gloss B

V 21–VI 1

Explaining : His nose bent, while his face is disfigured

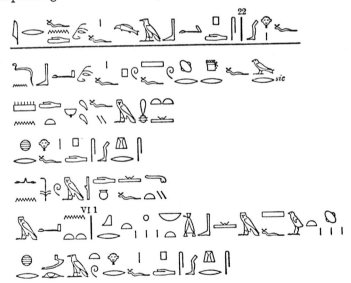

Translation

As for : "His nose bent, while his face is disfigured," it means his nose is crooked and greatly swollen throughout ; his two cheeks likewise, so that his face is disfigured by it, not being in its customary form, because all the depressions are clothed with swellings, so that his face looks disfigured **by it.**

Gloss C

VI 1–3

Explaining : Every worm of blood which coagulates in the inside of his
two nostrils

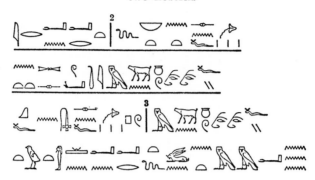

Translation

As for : " Every worm of blood which coagulates in the inside of his two nostrils,"
it means the clotting of blood in the inside of his two nostrils, likened to the *ᶜnᶜr·t-*
worm, which subsists in the water.

CASE THIRTEEN

VI 3–7

COMPOUND COMMINUTED FRACTURE IN THE SIDE OF THE NOSE

TITLE

VI 3

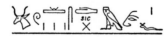

Translation

Instructions concerning a smash in his nostril.

EXAMINATION

VI 4–6

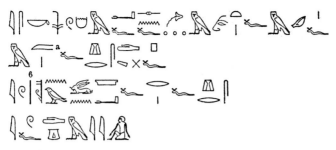

^a The text has ⌣, but the parallels elsewhere show clearly that the correct reading is ⌣ as given above. See commentary below.

Translation

If thou examinest a man having a smash in his nostril, thou shouldst place thy hand upon his nose at the point of this smash. Should it crepitate under thy fingers, while at the same time he discharges blood from his nostril (and) from his ear, on the side of him having that smash ; it is painful when he opens his mouth because of it ; (and) he is speechless, (conclusion in diagnosis).

DIAGNOSIS

VI 6–7

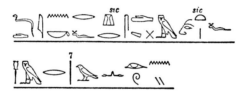

Translation

Thou shouldst say concerning him : " One having a smash in his nostril. An ailment not to be treated."

Commentary

As in the preceding three cases we have the diagnosis again reduced to a mere catchword, probably serving only as a memorandum, or possibly a student's note, to which the essential item, verdict 3, has been appended. See commentary on Case 5 (II 15) and discussion in the Introduction (pp. 46–48 and 73). The injury is so serious that it is regarded as fatal and no treatment is added.

COMMENTARY BY THE EDITOR

"Edwin Smith, after whom the papyrus is named, was born in Connecticut in 1822, the year that witnessed the first decipherment of Egyptian hieroglyphic by Champollion. Smith was one of the earliest students of Egyptian in any country. He studied hieroglyphic in London and Paris when the science was only a quarter of a

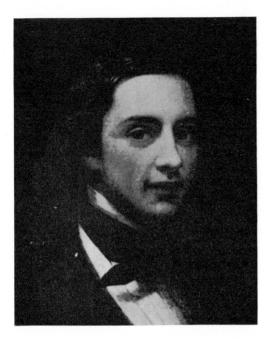

FIG. 1. Edwin Smith, after a painting by Francesco Anelli. (Courtesy of National Library of Medicine, Bethesda, Md.)

century old, and was probably the first American to learn scientifically the little then known about the Egyptian language. He then removed to Egypt and by 1858 was living in Luxor, where he remained for nearly twenty years.

"During his residence in Luxor, from 1858 to 1876, Mr. Smith met a number of the leading Egyptologists of the time and likewise many of the distinguished English travelers who so frequently visited the Nile in those days. . . . Birch refers to him as having descended with the British Vice-Consul into a tomb shaft ninety feet deep to bring up thirty mummies and their coffins for the entertainment of the Prince of Wales during his visit to Egypt in 1868." With these words, Professor Breasted introduces us to the extraordinary man who discovered this great papyrus, Mr. Edwin Smith (Fig. 1).

The papyrus was purchased in the necropolis of Thebes in 1862 from a pedlar, one Mustapha Aga, by Mr. Smith. In all probability, it was found in one of the tombs in the area. Smith recognized its surgical con-

tent and was aware of its importance, but at the time it would have been impossible for anyone to have prepared an adequate translation of such a highly technical text. Professor Breasted notes: "Among Mr. Smith's meager papers . . . I found a manuscript containing a remarkable attempt by Mr. Smith at a complete translation of the papyrus which now bears his name. When we recall how scanty was the knowledge of hieratic in the sixties . . . it is extraordinary how much of the document Mr. Smith has understood . . . of the eight fragments of the papyrus which, as we shall see, Mr. Smith rescued, he was able to place three with exactness and two more at least in their approximate connection."

After Smith's death, his daughter presented the papyrus to the New York Historical Society in 1906. In 1920, the Society persuaded the great Professor James Henry Breasted (Fig. 2) to undertake its translation. Dr. Breasted was the Director of the

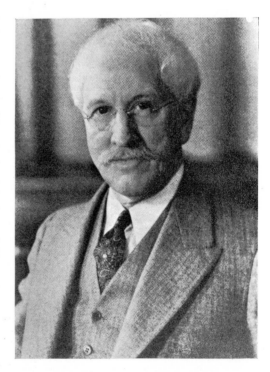

FIG. 2. Professor James Henry Breasted. (*From the National Cyclopedia of American Biography*, Vol. 29, p. 257. James T. White & Co., New York, 1941).

Oriental Institute of the University of Chicago and was, possibly, the foremost Egyptologist of the time. After one of the most detailed and scholarly studies that any papyrus has received, and with the medical assistance of Dr. Arno B. Luckhardt, the hieroglyphics and translation were published by the University of Chicago Press in 1930.

In this manner we have inherited the oldest surgical or medical record known to man. Dr. Breasted believed that this surgical treatise was written in the Old Kingdom (3,000–2,500 B.C.), presumably during the earlier part of that remote age. He even suggests that it may have been written by Imhotep,* (Fig. 3) and that it may be the "Secret Book of the Physician," quoted in the later Ebers Papyrus. The scribe who made this copy presumably did so to furnish a text for the use of the surgeons of his own day.

The Smith Papyrus is a fragment about 5 yards long and consists of 48 case reports —all of a surgical nature. They concern wounds, fractures, dislocations, ulcers, abscesses, and tumors. They are arranged in order, from head to foot; 27 cases are about the head (including these 3 of the nose, then come cases of the neck, upper extremities, chest, and spinal column—where the rescued portion of the papyrus ends abruptly.

Here, we find the word "brain" recorded for the first time in human language; the author describes the convolutions and the covering membranes. While most of the peoples of this period placed the seat of consciousness and intelligence in the heart or abdomen, this author describes paralysis resulting from an injury to the head and notes that it varies, depending upon which side of the brain is injured. He

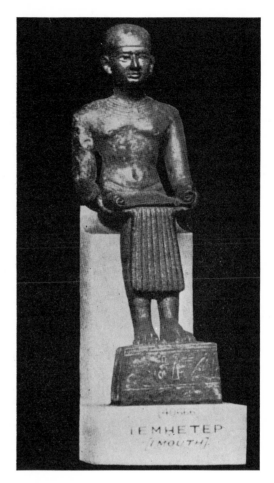

Fig. 3. Imhotep, as portrayed in an ancient statue. (Courtesy of National Library of Medicine, Bethesda, Md.)

recognized the heart as the center of a system of distributing vessels. "Its pulsation," he wrote, "is in every vessel of every member." Breasted remarked that the author of this papyrus "knew of the cardiac system and was surprisingly near recognition of the circulation of the blood."

He was logical and straightforward in his diagnoses. His decisions of whether to treat were obviously based on a vast experience, but his treatments were limited to the simple everyday items available. Lint was applied as an absorbent, as were swabs and plugs of linen. Bandages of linen were obtained from embalmers and adhesive plaster was used for bringing together the

* Imhotep was vizier to King Zoser (about 3,000 B.C.) and built the first of the Egyptian pyramids (at Sakkara). In addition to being a master architect, he was a physician of great renown. A century after his death, Imhotep was considered a demigod and much later, about 525 B.C., he was elevated to the status of the god of healing. Sir William Osler referred to him as "the first figure of a physician to stand out clearly from the mists of antiquity."

lips of a wound. Breasted translates one line: "Thou shouldst draw together for him his gash with stitching." Cauterization is recommended for ulcers and tumors. Splints or braces are mentioned several times. The splints were formed either of thin wood padded with linen, or of linen alone molded to the broken limb (probably with plaster or gum). Grease and honey were frequently applied to fresh wounds. Another favorite treatment was to "put him at his mooring stakes"—*e.g.* at rest, on a light diet, with moderation in all things.

The other great medical document of ancient Egypt is the Ebers Papyrus, probably from the same tomb as the Smith Papyrus and possibly written by the same scribe. The Ebers Papyrus, however, was a compilation of contemporary medicine, rather than a surgical text. The writer mentions cough, for example, and then proceeds to describe 21 prescriptions for it. The Ebers Papyrus is full of incantations to be chanted during the application of the treatment, or as the only treatment (a practice employed, it is believed, by some medical men in all ages). The cases described in the Smith Papyrus, however, were mainly the result of trauma; their cause was obviously not demoniac possession, but events well known to the patient and the author. He was mechanistic and logical in his diagnosis and treatment of them.

It is believed that Edwin Smith owned the Ebers Papyrus at one time and later sold it to Professor Georg Ebers, while retaining the surgical papyrus.

A most remarkable thing in the Edwin Smith Papyrus is that out of 58 examinations, the surgical teacher recommends treatment in only 42; he recognized that 16 were beyond his help. Professor Breasted wrote: "These discussions demonstrate the surgeon's scientific interest in the human body as a field of observation and disclose him to us as the earliest scientific mind which we can discern in the surviving records of the past."

—FRANK MCDOWELL

ANCIENT EAR-LOBE AND RHINOPLASTIC OPERATIONS IN INDIA

(From the Sushruta Samhitá, *c.* 600 B.C. Translated from the Sanskrit and published by K. K. L. Bhishagratna, Calcutta, 1907.)

EAR-LOBE OPERATIONS*

The exact middle point of the external ear should be pierced (with a knife) and the severed parts should be pulled down and elongated in the case where both the parts of a bifurcated ear-lobe would be found to have been entirely lost or eaten away. In the case where the posterior one of the two bifurcated parts would be found to be longer or more elongated, the adhesion should be effected on the anterior side; whereas the contrary should be the case where the anterior one would appear to be more elongated. Only the remaining one of the two bifurcated parts of an ear-lobe would be pierced, cut in two and adhesioned on the top, in the case where the other part would be found to be gone.

A surgeon well-versed in the knowledge of surgery (Shastras) should slice off a patch of living flesh from the cheek of a person devoid of ear-lobes in a manner so as to have one of its ends attached to its former seat (cheek).† Then the part, where the artificial ear-lobe is to be made, should be slightly scarified (with a knife), and the living flesh, full of blood and sliced off as previously directed, should be adhesioned to it (so as to resemble a natural ear-lobe in shape).

A surgeon, wishing to effect any sort of adhesion other than those described before, should first collect the articles enumerated in the chapter on Preliminary Measures to Surgical Operations, together with milk, water, Dhanyamla (fermented rice boilings), Suramanda (transparent surface-part of wine) and powders of earthen vessel. Then the hair of the patient, whether male or female, should be gathered and tied up in a knot, and the patient should be given a light food (so as to keep up his strength without hampering his digestion); after which his friends and relations should be asked to hold him firm.

Then having ascertained the particular nature of adhesion to be effected in the case, the surgeon should examine the local blood by incising, excising, scarifying or puncturing the affected lobes as found necessary, and determine whether the same is pure or vitiated. Then having washed the blood with Dhanyamla and tepid water, if found vitiated through the action of the deranged Váyu,‡ or with milk and cold water in the event of the same being contaminated by the deranged Pittam,§ or with Suramanda and warm water in the case of its being vitiated by the action of the disordered Kapham,¶ the surgeon

---

* *Editor's note:* These appear to have been for the repair of pierced ear-lobes which had split asunder under the weight of heavy ear-rings.

† *Editor's note:* Without doubt, this is the earliest known reference to a pedicle flap.

‡ Air.

§ Bile.

¶ Phlegm.

shall bring about the adhesion by again scarifying the affected parts of the ear, so as not to leave the adhesioned parts elevated (raised), unequal, and short. Of course the adhesion should be effected with the blood being still left in the parts that had been scraped.

Then having anointed them with honey and clarified butter, they should be covered with cotton and linen, and tied with strings of thread, neither too loose nor too tight, and dusted over with powders of baked clay. Then directions should be given as regards the diet and nursing of the patient, who may be as well treated with the regimen laid down in the chapter of Dvi-vraniyam.

Authoritative verses on the subject: The patient should be careful not to disturb the bandage and avoid physical exercise, over-eating, sexual intercourse, exposure to, or basking in, the glare of fire, fatiguing talk, and sleep by day. For three consecutive days the ulcer should be annointed with unboiled oil; and cotton soaked in the same substance should be placed over it, which is to be altered each third day, till healing. . . .

An ear-lobe should not be tried to be elongated just after the adhesion of its two severed parts, inasmuch as the centre of the adhesion, still being raw, might cause them to fall off again. Thus an ear-lobe under the circumstance should be gradually elongated, only when it would be found to be marked by the growth of hair on its surface, and the hole or the perforation has assumed a circular look, and the adhesion has become firmly effected, well-dried, painless, even and level in its entire length.

The modes of bringing about an adhesion of the two severed parts of an ear-lobe are innumerable; and a skilled and experienced surgeon should determine the shape and nature of each according to the exigencies of a particular case.

RHINOPLASTIC OPERATIONS

Now I shall deal with the process of affixing an artificial nose. First the leaf of a creeper, long and broad enough to fully cover the whole of the severed or clipped off part, should be gathered, and a patch of living flesh, equal in dimension to the preceding leaf should be sliced off (from down upward) from the region of the cheek and, after scarifying it with a knife, swiftly adhered to the severed nose. Then the cool headed physician should steadily tie it up with a bandage decent to look at and perfectly suited to the end for which it has been employed (Sadhu Vandha).

The physician should make sure that the adhesion of the severed parts has been fully effected and then insert two small pipes into the nostrils to facilitate respiration, and to prevent the adhesioned flesh from hanging down. After that, the adhesioned part should be dusted with the powders of Pattanga,* Yashtimadhukam,† and Rasânjana‡ pulverised together,§ and the nose should be enveloped in Kárpása cotton and several times sprinkled over with the refined oil of pure sesamum. Clarified butter should be given to the patient for drink, and he should be anointed with oil and treated with purgatives after the complete digestion of the meals he has taken, as advised (in the books of medicine).

Adhesion should be deemed complete after the incidental ulcer had been perfectly healed up, while the nose should be again scarified and bandaged in the case of a semi or partial adhesion. The

* Sappan wood.
† Licorice root.
‡ Barberry.
§ Some translations insert here: "As soon as the piece has grown fast, the attachment (to the cheek) is severed."—*Ed.*

adhesioned nose should be tried to be elongated where it would fall short of its natural and previous length, or it should be surgically restored to its natural size in the case of the abnormal growth of its newly formed flesh.

The mode of bringing about the adhesion of severed lips is identical with what has been described in connection with a severed nose with the exception of the insertion of pipes. The physician, who is well conversant with these matters, can alone be entrusted with the medical treatment of a King.

Thus ends the sixteenth chapter of the Sutra-Sthánam in the Sushruta Samhitá, which treats of the Piercing and Bandaging of ear-lobes.

ACKNOWLEDGMENT

The above material was made available through the courtesy of Mr. William Beatty, Librarian of the Archibald Church Medical Library of Northwestern University, Chicago.

COMMENTARY BY THE EDITOR

You have just read the original source material containing the first description of a pedicle flap and the first description of the surgical replacement of a missing portion of the nose. The latter was done with a cheek flap. "Indian rhinoplasty" with a forehead flap was first reported to the Western world from the same geographic area some 2,000 years later (although no one knows how many years or centuries it had been performed in the meantime).

If we believe the transplantation of tissue to be the essence of plastic surgery, then Sushruta must be "the father of plastic surgery." But he was more than the originator of this specialty. The image of this great man comes down through the millenia to us as probably the greatest surgeon and surgical teacher of pre-renaissance times. Sushruta considered these two facets of his life inseparable; he noted that a bungling surgeon is a public danger, saying "theory without practice is like a one-winged bird that is incapable of flight." *

So great is the image of Sushruta that some scholars believe that he was not one man, but that the writings ascribed to him were a composite description of the developments by numerous surgeons over many centuries. The consensus is against

this view, but it has not been possible to establish the exact dates of his work, or to even prove that he was one man. K. K. L. Bhishagratna, the translator of the Sushruta Samhitá (collection of teachings), remarks: "In a country like India, where life itself was simply regarded as an illusion, the lives of kings or commoners were deemed matters of little moment to the vital economy of the race; and all histories were looked upon as the embodiment of the flimsy vanities of life." The entire history of ancient India is thus clouded and is the subject of vexatious disputations amongst scholars on every detail. It is just possible, however, that the peoples of ancient India contributed more than any other group to the origins of medicine and surgery. For this reason, the reader may be interested in the following sketches, based on statements by various scholars, even though there is no unanimity of opinion.

THE VEDAS

The Sushruta Samhitá is believed to be part of one of the four Vedas (ancient Indian sacred books of "knowledge" or "lore"). The history of these is as follows.

In pre-Aryan times (before about 1,500 B.C.), the Indian subcontinent was inhabited by a darker-skinned and smaller race divided into two linguistic families,

* *Editor's note.* Score another first for Sushruta —the first critical evaluation of "the armchair surgeon."

Kolarian and Dravidian. The Kolarian languages are related to those presently used in southeast Asia (particularly the Khmer of Cambodia); there are striking resemblances between the Dravidian languages and latter day Finnish and Hungarian. Recent excavations have confirmed that the peoples of this Indus civilization built many populous and closely-packed cities, clustered around citadels which served as centers of government, religion, and as defense bastions. The findings indicate a high degree of excellence in art and in architecture, and have revealed scraps of a written language that has not yet been translated.

About 1,500 B.C., India was invaded from the northwest by a lighter-skinned and taller Aryan race who came, presumably, from the regions of the Caucasus and Iran. In some ways the conquering race was inferior to the conquered, but they brought with them several items of near-European origin, including their own language.

The language of the Vedas indicates that the first of them, at least, came into being within the first century or so after the Aryan invasion; the linguistic connection between it and ancient Iranian is very close. This language is now known as Vedic Sanskrit.

The term Veda embraces a body of writings, the origin of which is ascribed to divine revelation. The Veda forms the foundation of the Brahmanical system of religious belief. This sacred canon is divided into four collections: (1) the Rig-veda (or lore of praise and hymns); (2) the Sama-veda (or lore of tunes and chants); (3) the Yajur-veda (or lore of prayer and sacrificial formulas); (4) the Atharva-veda (or lore of the Atharvans, a high order of priests).

The term Ayurveda (meaning "knowledge of life") was given to the ancient Indian system of medicine, and it is believed to be a part of the Atharva-veda—which is much the youngest of the Vedas and the latest to be recognized as a sacred canon. Ayurvedic medicine is still practiced in some areas of India today and is based, primarily, on the Charaka Samhitá (medicine) and the Sushruta Samhitá (surgery). The Charaka Samhitá was probably the earlier of the two; some think it was composed as early as 1,000 B.C. It is predominantly a medical treatise and ascribes diseases as being due to disturbances of the three humors—air, bile, and phlegm. It shows many influences from the pre-Aryan Indus civilization and contains an enormous number of medicines of plant, animal, and mineral origin (including ephedrine, rauwolfia, and others). The Sushruta Samhitá was probably put together about 600 B.C. (about one century before Gautama Buddha). Both of these Samhitás are predominantly in metre, but partly in prose, and were probably transmitted down by word of mouth for quite some time. However, being religious texts which it was essential to preserve unchanged, they were subjected to various controls which made this transmission exceedingly exact. It is not known at what date they were committed to writing. According to Hindu lore, there were two great universities in India during the time of Buddha, one at Taxila and one at Benares; Sushruta is said to have taught surgery at Benares.

THE SUSHRUTA SAMHITÁ

The following quotations are from a translation by Anna Moreshvar Kunte in Bombay in 1877, with some omissions and parenthetical explanations inserted by your editor. The Samhitá begins:

"Now, hereafter, we shall narrate the chapter named the descent of knowledge of medicine, just as it was taught to Sushruta by the venerable Dhanvantari (the physician to the gods). Aupadhenava, Vaitarana, Aurabhra, Paushkalavata, Karavirya, Gopura, Rakshita, Sushruta, and his other friends in earnest addressed the venerable Dhanvantari.... 'Sire! we are moved with compassion, seeing human beings ... being afflicted with numerous bodily, mental, natural, and accidental maladies. We wish to be instructed in the Science of Medicine for the sake of public good.... Hence, Sire, we have come to you to become your pupils.'

"To them said the venerable man: 'Ye are welcome. All of you, my lads, shall be taught and made to meditate. Ayurveda is an Upanga of the Atharva-veda. The Self-born, after creating the universe, composed it in a thousand chapters, containing 100,000 verses. But, knowing the brevity of human life and the limitedness of human understanding, he reduced it to 8 divisions. These are: 1. Shalyam (surgery); 2. Shalakyam (disorders above the clavicles); 3. Kayachikitsa (diseases affecting the whole body); 4. Bhutavida (diseases of the mind); 5. Koumarabhrityam (diseases of children); 6. Agadatantram (antidotes); 7. Rasayanatantra (elixirs); 8. Vajikaranatantram (rules for increasing the generative powers). Which of these do you wish to be taught?'

" 'Sire,' said they, 'teach us all, but begin with surgery first.' *

" 'Be it so,' said he.

"They again requested him, saying, 'Sushruta, after consulting us all, shall ask you for explanations (in matters of doubt), and whilst he is made to understand we shall also try to do the same.'

" 'Well, then, my pupil Sushruta,' said he, 'the Science of Medicine has for its object the emancipation from disease of those who are afflicted by it.... Of all of the 8 parts of which the Ayurveda is composed, this (surgery) is the best, from the speediness of its operations, from its including the use of appliances, surgical instruments' (Figs. 1, 2), 'caustics, cauteries, and from its being common to the other parts (of the science)....'

" 'In this science, the use of edged instruments is considered to be predominant... (they) are used for 8 purposes—viz. 1. amputating; 2. opening; 3. scarifying; 4. puncturing; 5. exploring; 6. drawing; 7. evacuating; 8. sewing. A surgeon contemplating to operate in any of the above ways should first have ready the following: blunt instruments (forceps, etc.), sharp instruments, potential cauteries, virtual cauteries, catheters, horns, leeches, a dry gourd, a cauterizing needle, stuffing materials, strings, board, bandage, honey, ghee, fat, milk, oil,

soothing decoctions, injections, lotions, fan, cold and warm water, a frying-pan—able, steady, and attached servants.' ..... †

" 'Let the patient be seated, who has taken very little food.... The surgeon should stand with his face toward him and plunge his instrument... until matter comes out, and withdraw it, avoiding vital parts.... Boldness, rapidity of action, sharp instruments, operation without trembling, fear, or doubt, are always praiseworthy of the surgeon operating.... The operations for moles, ascites, piles, calculus, fistula, and mouth diseases are to be performed on an empty stomach.... The instruments should be so made that they... (are) of a good finish, strong, clean in appearance, with good handles, whether they be sharp or blunt.'

" 'Among these, the Svastika instruments ought to be about 9 inches long; their mouths should be respectively like those of a lion, tiger, wolf, hyena, bear, elephant, cat, hare, antelope, crow, heron, dog, jay, vulture, falcon, owl, kite, cock, bee, rat, mouse, or bullock—each half being united to the other by a nail of the form of a lentil-seed, being bent inward at the handles like the elephant-driver's hook. These forceps are recommended for the extraction of splinters lodged in bones.'

" 'The tubular instruments are... used for removing obstructions from the great canals of the body, or for examination of diseases, or as suction-tubes, or for the easy application of remedies... different tubular instruments are used in fistula, hemorrhoids, polypi, sores, urethral injections, enemas, retention of urine, ascites, inhalation for dyspnea, and obstruction of bowels.' ...

" 'The probe-like instruments are of various kinds and serve a variety of purposes.... Among them, the earthworm-like probe, the arrow probe, the serpent-hood probe, and the hook probe are... recommended for sounding, separating, loosening, and extracting foreign bodies. Probes having lentil-seed-like ends... are used for the extraction of foreign bodies from the large canals. There are 6 probes which are capped with cotton wool and are used for cleaning and wiping purposes.... There is a nasal-polypus probe which resembles the kolasthi.... There is the urinary catheter, which resembles the stalk of the Jasmine flower.'

" 'The lion-mouth forceps is for foreign bodies that can be seen, while for covered ones there is the heron forceps.... These should be

* *Editor's note.* The perspicacity of Sushruta and his class is here self-evident and undeniable.

† cf. "The one-man band." Plast. & Reconstr. Surg., *42:* 158, 1968.

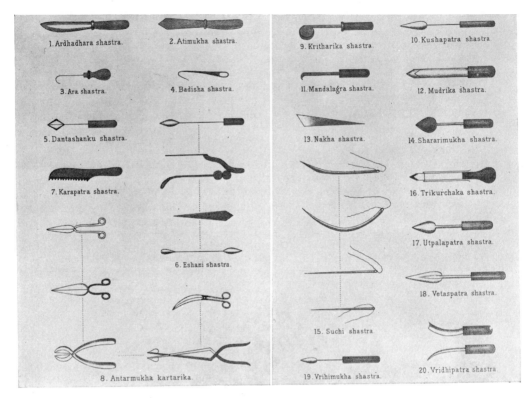

FIG. 1. Sharp surgical instruments described by Sushruta. *3*, Bent awl. *5*, Dental instruments. *7*, Bone saw. *8*, Various-mouthed scissors. *14*, Mouth cautery. *15*, Various needles, with thread. *19*, "Grain-of-rice" knife (for cataract removal?). *20*, Elevators. (From *A Short History of Aryan Medical Science* by Sir Bhagvat Sinh Jee, MacMillan Co., London, 1896. Reproduced by courtesy of National Library of Medicine.)

used gently.... The heron forceps is the best of all forceps, since its use never leads to accidents. It enters easily and is very easily drawn back. It lays a firm hold on splinters and removes them easily.' "

After the first part containing his initial instructions from Dhanvantari, Sushruta describes a great variety of operations. Aspiration is advised for ascites and hydrocele. For removing metallic splinters Sushruta mentions the magnet. Sutures should be of cotton, hemp, leather, horsehair, or animal sinews. Needles were straight or with various curves. The operation for extraction of cataract is minutely described, as are a number of other operations on the eye. The obstetrical section describes difficult labor, various forms of presentations, the use of obstetrical forceps, and gives directions for performing a Caesarian section.

The operation for stone in the bladder is described in great detail. The surgeon should "introduce into the rectum the second and third fingers of his left hand, duly anointed and with the nails well-pared." The fingers should be carried upward towards the middle line, bringing the stone "between the rectum and the penis when it should be so firmly and strongly pressed as to look like a tumor. An incision should then be made on the left side of the raphe of the perineum ... and the entire stone should be extracted with the help of forceps."

Sushruta had dissected human bodies and described the bones, muscles, and internal organs in considerable detail.

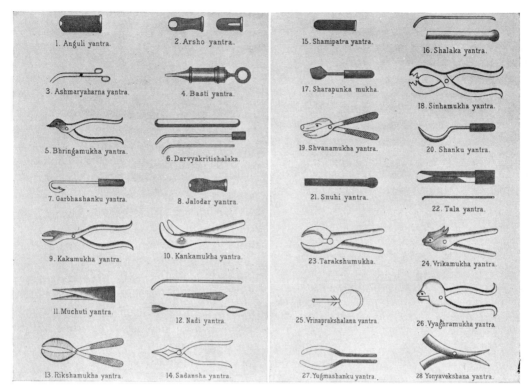

FIG. 2. Blunt surgical instruments described by Sushruta. *1,* Finger splint. *5,* Forceps with mouth of large black bee. *9,* Crow-mouth forceps. *10,* Heron-mouth forceps. *18,* Lion-jaw forceps. *23,* Hyena-jaw forceps. *24,* Scorpion-mouth forceps. *26,* Tiger-mouth forceps. (From *A Short History of Aryan Medical Science* by Sir Bhagvat Sinh Jee, MacMillan Co., London, 1896. Reproduced by courtesy of National Library of Medicine.)

AFTER SUSHRUTA

There is evidence that the early Buddhist missionaries coming to Greece brought their Ayurvedic medical knowledge with them and that Pythagoras (?580–498 B.C.), "the father of Greek medicine," obtained much of his knowledge from these *gurus.* In any event, after the conquests of Alexander the Great (4th century, B.C.) commerce with India was established and Indian medical science became part of the Greek heritage (Alexander, himself, had Indian physicians). Hippocrates and Galen borrowed heavily from Indian sources. Centuries later, Rhazes, Avicenna, and other Arabic physicians referred frequently to Sushruta.

In that greatest medical classic of recent times (*The Life and Times of Gaspare Tagliacozzi,* by Martha T. Gnudi and Jerome P. Webster), it appears not unlikely that knowledge of the work of Indian surgeons was an inspiration to the Brancas and to Tagliacozzi.

How, then, did this work (some of which was not repeated in Europe until nearly 2,000 years later) become lost to the Western World? The answer probably lies in the transmission by the spoken, versus the written, word. Although a number of physicians, both Western and Indian, brought fragments of Ayurvedic medical knowledge to the Western World from time to time, it was not written down in a complete, systematic form. The latter existed only in Sanskrit manuscripts in India; Western scholars were largely unaware of Sanskrit literature until the British entered India in the 18th Century. After that, a considerable time elapsed before they found this literature and were able to translate it.

In 1963, Dr. N. H. Keswani (Professor of Anatomy, All-India Institute of Medical Sciences, New Delhi) noted: "Most of the extant ancient texts, written exclusively in Sanskrit, have remained in manuscript form, waiting to be edited and translated. Many of the great works, already published, are accessible only to Sanskrit pundits. Most of the ancient medical texts have for years remained a closely guarded secret with the families of the Vaidyas (the surgical class), who looked with disdain upon the very idea of making their knowledge available to the World, and scorned at those who dared translate them into foreign languages."

The first translation of the Sushruta Samhitá was into Latin by Hessler in 1844, and later into German by Vellurs.

The first complete English translation was apparently the one by Bhishagratna in 1907, excerpted here. Keswani noted in 1963 that there are over 1500 medical manuscripts in Sanskrit, listed in Theodor Aufrecht's catalog, which have never been translated into a major, contemporary language. To anyone who has spent long hours pawing through Sanskrit dictionaries, as I have in preparing this commentary, this is a formidable, but worthwhile, task.

Through all of Sushruta's flowery language, incantations, and irrelevancies, there shines the unmistakable picture of a great surgeon. Undaunted by his failures, unimpressed by his successes, he sought the truth unceasingly and passed it on to those who followed. He attacked disease and deformity definitively, with reasoned and logical methods. When the path did not exist, he made one.

—Frank McDowell

THE DEVELOPMENT OF PLASTIC SURGERY FROM ANCIENT TIMES TO THE END OF THE EIGHTEENTH CENTURY

The story of rhinoplasty, and of all plastic surgery, during these 2,500 years is one of isolated peaks of accomplishment by a few individuals, connected by slender threads. There were, of course, biblical references as well as those of the ancient Greeks and Romans. The latter are, perhaps, best exemplified by Hippocrates, Celsus, and Galen—terminating with the writings of Paul of Aegina in the early part of the 7th century. During the ensuing Dark Ages in Europe, most of the developments occurred in the Arab school, with Albucasis (*c*. 950–1013 A.D.) giving us the best description of advances in surgery. (*cf.* Spink, M.S., and Lewis, G.L.: *Albucasis On Surgery and Instruments*. University of California Press, Berkeley, 1973)

With the Renaissance in Europe, probably the greatest developments in rhinoplasty were those of Gaspar Tagliacozzi. (*cf.* Gnudi, M.T., and Webster, J.P.: *The Life and Times of Gaspar Tagliacozzi*, Herbert Reichner Co., New York, 1950)

Tagliacozzi's book *De curtorum chirurgie per insitionem* is so long, varied, and detailed that no short excerpt could serve as an adequate example. It is, however, an important prelude to that which follows.

—F. McD.

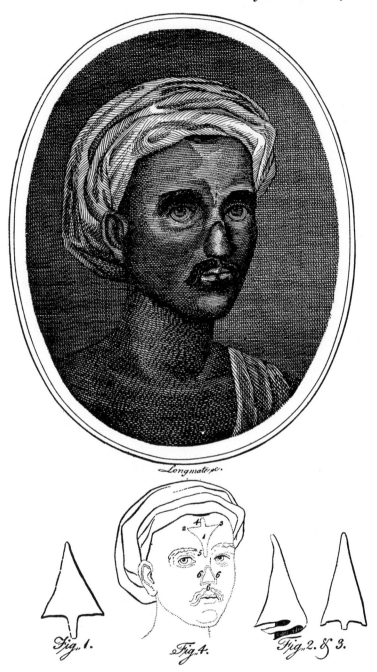

Longmate sc.

Fig. 1.   Fig. 4.   Fig. 2. & 3.

PLATE I

THE "B.L." BOMB-SHELL

Editor's note. After several thousand years of sporadic interest in plastic surgery, punctuated by the peaks attained by the Brancas and Tagliacozzi, the following letter by "B.L." appeared. Dramatically, suddenly, the imagination of the profession and laity alike was captured and stimulated. From this episode, one can date the beginning of a widespread interest in rhinoplasty, and in plastic surgery in general, throughout the Western world. Seldom, if ever, has any "Letter to the Editor" had such an explosive effect.

*(From Gentleman's Magazine, London, October 1794, p. 891)**

MR. URBAN,

Oct. 9

A friend has transmitted to me, from the East Indies, the following very curious, and, in Europe, I believe, unknown chirurgical operation, which has long been practised in India with success; namely, affixing a new nose on a man's face. The person represented in *Plate I.* is now in Bombay.

Cowasjee, a Mahratta of the cast of husbandman, was a bullock-driver with the English army in the war of 1792, and was made a prisoner by Tippoo, who cut off his nose and one of his hands. In this state he joined the Bombay army near Seringapatam, and is now a pensioner of the Honourable East India Company. For about 12 months he remained without a nose, when he had a new one put on by a man of the Brickmaker cast, near Poonah. This operation is not uncommon in India, and has been practised from time immemorial. Two of the medical gentlemen, Mr. Thomas Cruso and Mr. James Trindlay of the Bombay presidency, have seen it performed, as follows: A thin plate of wax is fitted to the stump of the nose, so as to make a nose of good appearance. It is then flattened, and laid on the forehead.

A line is drawn round the wax, and the operator then dissects off as much skin as it covered, leaving undivided a small slip between the eyes. This slip preserves the circulation till an union has taken place between the new and old parts. The cicatrix of the stump of the nose is next pared off, and immediately behind this raw part an incision is made through the skin, which passes around both *alae,* and goes along the upper lip. The skin is now brought down from the forehead, and, being twisted half round, its edge is inserted into this incision, so that a nose is formed with a double hold above, and with its *alae* and *septum* below fixed in the incision. A little *Terra Japonica* is softened with water, and being spread on slips of cloth, five or six of these are placed over each other, to secure the joining. No other dressing but this cement is used for four days. It is then removed, and cloths dipped in ghee (a kind of butter) are applied. The connecting slips of skin are divided about the 25th day, when a little more dissection is necessary to improve the appearance of the new nose. For five or six days after the operation, the patient is made to lie

* Reproduced by courtesy of the John Crerar Library, Chicago.

on his back; and, on the tenth day, bits of soft cloth are put into the nostrils, to keep them sufficiently open. The artificial nose is secure, and looks nearly as well as the natural one; nor is the scar on the forehead very observable after a length of time. The picture from which this engraving is made was printed in January, 1794, ten months after the operation.

Fig. 1. the plate of wax when flattened.

Fig. 2. and 3. the plate of wax in the form of the nose.

Fig. 4. 1. figure of the skin taken from the forehead; 2. and 3. form of the alae of the new nose; 4. *septum* of the new nose; 5. the slip left undivided; 6.6.6. the incision into which the edge of the skin is ingrafted.

Yours, &c.

B.L.

THE JAMES WALES BROADSIDES

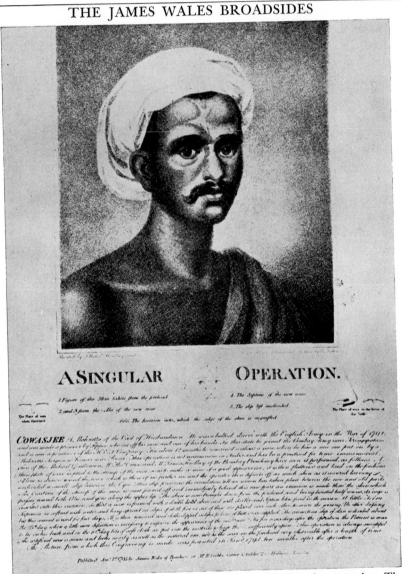

FIG. 1. The third of the James Wales broadsides about the Cowasjee operation. The first of these was published in Bombay some 6 months before the "B.L." letter, and contained almost the identical words to which "B.L." later signed his name.

Editor's note. The well-known artist, James Wales, who was a close friend of the British Resident in Poona (Sir Charles Malet), apparently did the drawings of Cowasjee.* He published at least 3 broadsides about Cowasjee's operation, all headed by his drawings, but containing minor variations. The first was published some 7 months before the "B.L." letter, on March 20, 1794 in Bombay; the engraving was done by R. Mabon and the name of the British surgeon in Poona was given (correctly) as Dr. James Findlay, instead of Dr. James Trindlay (as it appeared in the "B.L." letter). Otherwise, the wording of the broadside was identical with the later "B.L." letter. The second broadside was published by Wales in London on January 1, 1795, with an engraving done by Nutter of the same Wales drawing and a variation in the text—"when he had a new one put on by a Mahratta Surgeon, a Kumar near Poona." The third broadside published by Wales was under the same dateline (January 1, 1795) and place (London), but (for the first time) had legends alongside the small drawings of the operation. It is reproduced, in reduced size (Fig. 1).

* We are indebted to Prof. R. D. Choksey, University of Poona, who probably has more knowledge of this era than anyone and who has recently undertaken more research on this and corresponded with the Journal. Prof. Choksey notes that Cowasjee is not a Maratha name, but a Parsi name. He has sent us many interesting bits of information about the characters in the Cowasjee drama, which we hope to publish at a later date—together with the results of his further investigations.

A TRAVEL EXPERT CONFIRMS THE "B.L." LETTER

Editor's note. Thomas Pennant traveled extensively and wrote exhaustively on remote parts of the world. His works on Iceland, Tibet, and Japan were the most authoritative ones extant, as was this 3 volume description of India.

(From Views of Hindoostan, by Thomas Pennant. Hughs, London, 1798. Vol. 2, pp. 237–238.)†

I MUST by no means omit one branch of *European* surgery, that has of late been practiced with great success by a *Poonah* artist who has lately revived the *Taliacotian* art, differing only in the material, for he does not apply to the *brawny parts of porters*, &c. &c. to restore the mutilated patient. I am not master of the process, but am told it is by cutting the skin and muscles of the forehead on three sides and drawing it over the deficient part. If the bridge of the nose is injured, I presume that must be supplied by some ingenious invention. The *Hircarrah*, or *Madras* Gazette, of *August* 5, 1794, informs us that *Cowasjee,* two years before, fell under the displeasure of *Tippoo Sultan* who instantly ordered the nasal amputation. The sufferer applied to the great restorer of *Hindoostan* noses, and a new one equal to all the uses of its predecessor immediately rose in its place. It can sneeze smartly, distinguish good from bad smells, bear the most provoking lug, or be well blown without danger of falling into the hankerchief. It will last the life of the wearer; nor like the *Taliacotian* need he fear,

That when the date of *Nock* is out,
The drop of sympathetic snout.

† Reproduced by courtesy of the Sinclair library of the University of Hawaii.

ACCOUNT OF THE METHOD OF SUPPLYING ARTIFICIAL NOSES; AS PRACTICED BY THE NATIVES OF THE MALABAR COAST

Editor's note: This article indicates that "B.L." was a Mr. Lucas and that his letter was seen in Bombay at least 6 months before it was published in London.

*(Reprinted from Philadelphia Medical Museum, 2: 343, 1806)**

Most of our readers have, no doubt, heard of the formation and adaptation of artificial noses. In Europe this operation has been generally considered as visionary, and has afforded a fine theme for the ridicule of some of our wits of the first order. For example, Addison, Steele, and Pope have not overlooked the art of famed Taliacotius. This art, it appears, is actually practiced, and with great success, in the western parts of India by a cast of Hindoos, called Kamoos. An account of their method of performing this operation appears in a paper published in the Bombay Courier of the 4th April, 1795, which we have extracted for the information of the curious:

"It is much to be lamented that the Europeans, whose talents have been devoted to the literature of India, have applied themselves rather to the speculative than to the practical parts of knowledge; and that their discoveries, however meritorious, have been more curious than useful.

"Although we cannot agree with those who look to India as the source from whence Europe has derived every thing that is valuable in science, yet we must allow that it has been the fountain of much of our knowledge; and that the common practice of the necessary arts of life among an ancient people would yet afford us not a little instruction.

"The progress that has been made in surgery for several centuries past in Europe makes it little probable that any improvement could be expected from the natives of this country; but we think that in two operations we may still receive instruction. The first of these is the depression of the Chrystalline lens, when it becomes opake; and the second, the formation of noses. We may also remark that with instruments far more imperfect than ours they perform the operation of lithotomy in the very place which, by the consent of modern surgeons, is esteemed the best.

"The Hindoos certainly deserve the praise of making artificial noses in a superior way to any people in the world; an art, unfortunately for them, the more necessary, as in no part of the world is the practice of cutting off noses so common. The process of repairing them was recommended in Europe about three hundred years ago, and was said to have originated with the Calabrians, from who it was received by the surgeons of Bologna.

"The celebrated Taliacotius, so unjustly exposed by some of our wits to ridicule, wrote a volume of those unions of living matter, under the title of *'chirurgia curtorum per Insitionem Membrorum.'* We have never had access to this work; but we have reason to think ... that the operation in Europe was much inferior to the one in use in this country....

"We have seen a letter from Mr. Lucas, an ingenious surgeon of Madras, describing very particularly the operation of putting on noses, which in one case he himself performed with success. This differs but little from the Indian method practiced by the Koomas, a cast of Hindoos; with which, as it has been ably described by a gentleman who witnessed the process, we shall conclude these observations.

"Some religious ceremonies are first performed: beetel and arrack put into the patient's hands, he is then laid upon his back, his arms stretched along his sides on the ground. He is ordered, on no pretence whatever, to raise his arms during the operation; and they impress him with the idea that it cannot be successful unless he complies strictly with these injunctions. A plate of wax being previously formed into the shape of the defective nose, it is flattened and laid obliquely upon the forehead,

* Reproduced by courtesy of the John Crerar Library, Chicago.

so as to avoid the hairy scalp. The alae and septum of the artificial nose being placed upwards, the other extremity of it terminating at the indentation of the ossa nasi with the os frontis, the operator marks out a portion of integuments equal to the size of the flattened wax, and then dissects it from the pericranium, leaving a small slip undivided between the eyebrows, to preserve the circulation in the detached piece until an adhesion takes place between it and the stump of the nose; and immediately behind the incision he makes an incision, into which the edge of the integuments are to be grafted or inserted.

"As there remains a slip of teguments between the eyebrows undivided, the detached portion, when turned down, is twisted half round; so that its recent surface may be applied to the face of the scarified stump, and the edge grafted into the above-described incision, which extends along both alae to the superior part of the upper lip, into which the septum is inserted. Thus carefully grafting or inserting the scalp, it is kept exactly in this situation by a cement, called in this country Kitta, which is softened with a little water and spread on long narrow bits of cotton cloth; five or six of which are applied over each other upon the junction which forms an irregular triangle. The dressing for the wound on the forehead is pieces of cloth dipped in ghee; the patient is desired to lie on his back five or six days. Four days after the operation the cement is removed, and the junction only covered with cloth moistened in ghee or oil, which is renewed every day: neither stitches, sticking plaster, compress, nor bandages are required. About ten days after the operation, round dossils, made of soft old cloth, are introduced into the nostrils to prevent them from contracting too much, which would happen if this precaution were neglected.

"The connecting slip of integuments is generally divided about the twenty-fifth day; and on this occasion some more dissection is necessary to effect an exact union and to leave as little seam as possible on the superior part of the arch of the nose."

COMMENTARY AND ADJUVANTS

As in agriculture, the seeds of surgical knowledge must be sown at the right time in the right place. Never were the latter more opportune for the development of plastic surgery than in the London of 1794. The fascination with cutting things out or off was beginning to fade; those in the vanguard were restlessly beginning to think of how things might be put back on.

Fortunate was it that "B.L." published his letter in a popular magazine, where it fired the imagination of laity and profession alike. Fortunate, also, was it that the work emanated from the subcontinent which was the new center of attention for all Britons—That ancient and exotic colossus, India (which was to become the backbone of empire and replace the savage wilderness, with its spurious "Indians," which had just been lost).

After smoldering for 5,000 years, with an occasional spark, plastic surgery burst into flame with the "B.L." letter. As we shall see in forthcoming Classic Reprints, the developments which followed were rapid and numerous.

Let us see what the propitious circumstances of the Cowasjee incident were. If history should ever be ready to repeat itself, someone ought to recognize the pattern.

CORNWALLIS AND COWASJEE

Though the East India Company established its first outpost in India in 1613, Britain did not become a dominant force in India until the victory of Clive in 1757. From that time onward, strong efforts were made to expand trade and to consolidate control over the entire subcontinent. In 1772, Warren Hastings was appointed governor-general of Bengal, with headquarters in Calcutta.

During this time Charles Cornwallis (son of the first Earl of Cornwallis) was born in England in 1738. He attended Eton and Cambridge, served with the British army in

Germany in 1761, succeeded to the earldom in 1762, became governor of the Tower of London in 1770. Shortly thereafter, he was sent as a major-general to command the British forces in the American War of Independence. With his defeat at Yorktown, at age 43, the English cause in the United States fell. He returned to England for a few years, and then was sent out (in 1786) as governor-general of India.

His chief adversary, and obstacle to consolidation, was Tipú Sultán (Fig. 2), wily ruler of Mysore. Cornwallis, through the British Resident (Sir Charles Malet) in Poona (near Bombay), persuaded the Peshwa (prime minister) of the Mahrattas (peoples of central India) to assist the British in subduing Tipú in the south. Cornwallis' army, with his Mahratta allies, then moved south into Mysore where they engaged Tipú Sultán's armies before Seringapattan, near Bangalore. For food, Cornwallis depended upon Mahratta bullock drivers (who went along with him) to purchase or scrounge grain from farmers in the area and haul it to his armies. Cowasjee was one of these. Tipú Sultán, realizing that he had not the forces to defeat Cornwallis in combat, became desperate and tried to cut off supplies by striking such terror in the bullock drivers that they would desert and flee.

HOW COWASJEE LOST HIS NOSE(?)

Editor's note. The following is extracted from pp. 200–201 of *History of the Reign of Tipú Sultán* by Mir Hussein Ali Khan Kirmani.* This work existed only as a Persian manuscript until 1864, when it was translated by Colonel W. Miles. A limited printing was made in London, under the auspices of the Oriental Translation Fund, in 1864.

"During this time the Commander-in-Chief of the English, in the space of fifteen or twenty days, having put his army in order

* Reproduction of this rare item was made possible by the East-West Center Library of the University of Hawaii.

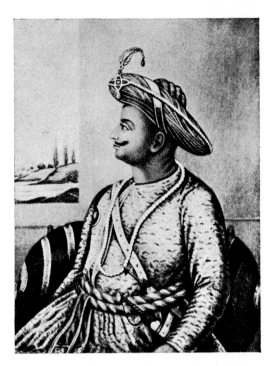

FIG. 2. Tipú Sultán (1750–1799), ruler of Mysore, son of Hyder Ali, opponent of British or Mahratta control in southern India. (From *Fort William-India House Correspondence, 1792–1795,* by Y. J. Taraporewala. Vol. 17, p. 510. National Archives of India, 1955. Courtesy East-West Center Library, University of Hawaii.)

(restored their materiel), marched towards Seringaputtun by the route of Burdi and Chen Puttun. But the infantry of the Commander-in-Chief of the Sultan's army who were posted in ambush in the forest of Makri, during the dark nights gained many signal advantages over the army of the enemy, and every night captured five or six hundred Bunjaras (men who carry grain about for sale,) with their bullocks laden with corn, and returned after cutting off the noses and ears of the men, and whoever brought in a nose received a hoon or a pagoda (as a reward), anyone who brought in an ear received a purtah (or half a pagoda), for every bullock with his load, five rupees; and for every horse two hoons were given. Every day, therefore, the Kuzzaks attacked the enemy in front and in rear, and exceedingly harassed and distressed their soldiers, often threw their followers into confusion, and almost all their bullocks laden with grain and stores were driven off and taken by them."

Editor's note. These terrorist tactics failed and Cornwallis forced Tipú (Fig. 2) to surrender shortly afterwards at Seringapattan—thus ending most of the effective resistance in southern India. Such were the by-products of building empire.

SOME OTHER PERSONS IN THE COWASJEE DRAMA

Editor's note. Mr. James Findlay and Mr. Thomas Crusoe were surgeons at the British Residency in Poona in 1793 and witnessed the operation on Cowasjee. Drawings of Cowasjee were made by Mr. James Wales, artist-in-residence at the Poona court, who later published and circulated broadsides publicizing the surgery.

Sir Charles Malet was the first British Resident (Advisor) at the Court of the Peshwas. The Peshwas were hereditary prime ministers of the Mahratta empire which, at the time, included most of central India and had its capitol at Poona (119 miles east of Bombay). On arrival in 1785, Malet noted that "the Peshwa Sawai Madhavrao is a boy of about 11 years old, of a slender habit, and small for his age."

The following excerpts from *A History of British Diplomacy at the Court of the Peshwas, 1782–1818** (by Professor R. D. Choksey, Ph.D., Israelite Press, Poona, 1951) are relevant.

"Malet became a very popular person in Poona Society. He introduced European arts, sciences and medicine. . . . It was Malet who introduced the famous artist James Wales to the Peshwa's Court. It was his enthusiasm which induced the Peshwa to establish a school of drawing in his palace. Drs. Crusoe and Findlay, the Residency Surgeons, contributed to the spread of English medical treatment. . . . Dr. Findlay gave lessons to the Peshwa in astronomy and ge-

* Courtesy of East-West Center Library, University of Hawaii.

ography and received handsome rewards from him.

"On the 2nd November, 1795, Uhthoff described to Sir John the various versions of the Peshwa's fall from the balcony of his palace to the fountain below, sustaining serious injuries. . . . Hard put to know the actual condition of the Peshwa, Uhthoff offered the services of Dr. Findlay, the European surgeon of the Residency. . . ."

Editor's note. Uhthoff was acting Resident, during Malet's absence.

"Sir Charles Malet had, as the reader will recall, the pleasantest abode in India. The abode was made livelier still by the members of the Wales family who were in Poona between 1790 to 1795. James Wales was the artist who came to India about 1790 to seek his fortune. He was destined to aid in leaving behind on canvas some of the great personalities of the Poona Court."

Editor's note. Wales was a Scot from Aberdeen who received his art education in Europe. He was greatly interested in archeology and devoted much time to making some of the first and best drawings of the now-famous ancient cave temples and carvings at Ellora and Elephanta. Near the end of his stay in India, Malet married Wales' daughter. Wales' stature as an artist was such that one must regard his portrayal of Cowasjee as an accurate one.

EPILOGUE

Nothing further has been found about the Cowasjee incident, or the persons associated with it. Much of the fragmentary material contained in this article has been obtained from unusual sources and is published here for the first time in medical literature. Professor Choksey, currently Chairman of the Department of History of the University of Poona, has kindly consented to undertake further researches into the matter.

—Frank McDowell

LETTER TO THE EDITOR (July 1971)

"MR. LUCAS" AND THE "B. L." LETTER

Sir:

Reconstruction of the nose by a forehead flap has been practiced successfully in India, of course, for many hundreds of years. But the knowledge only reached Europe at the end of the 18th century in the letter describing the operation on Cowasjee, signed "B.L." and dated October 9, which was published in October 1794.[1] From this "bomb-shell," "one can date the beginning of a widespread interest in rhinoplasty, and in plastic surgery in general, through the Western world" (McDowell,[2] 1969).

Zeis[3] (1863) had some caustic remarks to make about the failure to pass on this knowledge earlier. In a paragraph headed "On the lack of information about the art of making noses in India" he said: "When one thinks that the English have already lived for a couple of hundred years in India, one must be astonished that, if rhinoplasty has really been practiced there from time immemorial, the news did not reach Europe earlier than 1794. It is also remarkable that, in all this time, no English doctor living on the spot has investigated the history of our art in India, since there was a mighty long span between Susruta and the artist of Poona. Finally, it is not recorded whether, after the operation on Cowasjee, a similar operation has ever been carried out by an Indian surgeon. These are all questions which need an answer."

Part of the answer could have been given by Brett,[4] in a textbook of surgery published in Calcutta in 1840. "A tribe of Koomhars or Potters who reside at Kot-Kangra in the hills north of the Suttledge, have long been famed for their dexterity in this operation, and numbers of mutilated individuals resort to them; but from the cases I have witnessed I had no reason to admire their performances." He then gives a detailed account of his own technique. This information, however, would still not have been enough to satisfy Zeis, as Brett was working and writing at a time when the technique of rhinoplasty was well established in Europe. European modifications and improvements had been passed back to India, so that Brett was able to quote Dieffenbach, von Graefe, Liston, Dupuytren, and other surgical giants.

Zeis' rebuke would seem to have been justified when applied to the earlier surgeons in India. No record has yet been found of the involvement of Europeans in Hindoo surgery in the 18th century, apart from the Cowasjee operation and fleeting references to a "Mr. Lucas"—the elusive Mr. Lucas, who may have been the first European surgeon to perform a rhinoplasty in the revival of the Indian method, but "whose first name seems to be nowhere recorded" (Gnudi and Webster,[5] 1951).

There were 4 occasions when Lucas was mentioned:

1. A leading article in the *Bombay Courier* of Saturday, April 4, 1795 in which the editor laments that most Europeans have applied themselves rather to the speculative than to the practical parts of the knowledge of India—in particular to the Hindoo art of making noses. "We have seen a Letter from Mr. Lucas, an ingenious Surgeon of Madras, describing very particularly the operation of putting on Noses, which in one case he himself performed with success. This differs but little from the Indian method practised by the Koomas, a cast of Hindoos...."

2. An article in the *Philadelphia Medical Museum*[6] (1806) entitled "Account of the Method of supplying Artificial Noses; as practised by the Natives of the Malabar Coast." After an introductory paragraph, this article, apart from a few minor misprints and alterations in punctuation, quotes an exact copy of the *Bombay Courier* as above, including the sentence about Mr. Lucas.

3. In Carpue[7] (1816): "I am obligingly in-

82

formed by Major Heitland, of the Indian service, that in India, several years ago, in the time of Hyder Ali, Mr. Lucas, an English surgeon, was, in several instances, successful in the operation, which he copied from the Hindoo practitioners."

4. In Nélaton et Ombrédanne[8] (1904): "En 1803, Lucas tente en Angleterre la première restauration par la méthode indienne, et aboutit à un échec."

To take the last of these references first: Nélaton and Ombrédanne's account of the history of Indian rhinoplasty contains so many errors that it seems doubtful whether any part of it should be believed. Gnudi and Webster were unable to verify the reference to Lucas; they believed that the authors were confused by Carpue's account of an unnamed surgeon, who was said to have performed the nasal operation in London in 1803 without success.

If this reference is to be disregarded as unreliable, we are left with the first two references which tell us that Mr. Lucas was a Madras surgeon who wrote a letter, giving a very precise account of the operation, at some time before April 1795—and Carpue's account, which is more detailed.

Carpue's "Major Heitland" is identifiable, I think, as William P. Heatland (Dodwell and Miles,[9] 1835) who served in the Infantry in the Madras Presidency from 1782 until he retired as a Major on August 26, 1807. If Heatland's information was correct, Lucas must have been operating before Hyder Ali died. Hyder (Haidar), father of Tippoo (who ordered Cowasjee's nose to be cut off), died of a boil or carbuncle on December 7, 1782. During his last illness it was reported that "pregnant women were cut open and the babes extracted from the womb, their livers being applied as a poultice" (Le Fanu,[10] 1883).

It seems, therefore, that Lucas might have been working in Madras several years before the Cowasjee report of 1794. Search of the official list of the Officers of the Medical Establishments of India from 1764–1838 (Dodwell and Miles,[11] 1839) for the 3 Presidencies (Bombay, Madras, and Bengal)

FIG. 1. Page 35 from the "List of Inscriptions on Tombs or Monuments in Madras[12]...."

shows, however, only one Lucas—James Lucas, of the Bombay Presidency. He was appointed Assistant Surgeon on September 19, 1809 and died at sea on January 7, 1812. But among a list of the inscriptions on tombs in Madras (Cotton,[12] 1905) is recorded the death on March 23, 1797 of COLLY LYON LUCAS, Esq. "Chief Surgeon and a member of the Medical Board, aged 66 years." He is buried in St. Mary's Cemetery (Fig. 1), in Madras City, formerly known as the English Burial Ground on the Island.

Turning again to the official list, under the Madras Presidency, it can now be seen that there is an entry for COLLEY, L. Lucas (died 1797 in India); he had been appointed Assistant Surgeon in 1765 and Surgeon on April 14, 1786. This type of misprint (Fig. 2) is not uncommon in the early records, and is due to faulty transcription of reports from India by the clerks in the East India House (Crawford,[13] 1930).

Colley (Colly) Lyon (Lyons) LUCAS can now be identified from well-authenticated sources (Crawford,[14] 1914, Johnston,[15] 1917, and Crawford,[13] 1930). Many details are known of his professional career (Fig. 3) but very little is recorded of his personal

NAMES.	Assistant-Surgeon.	Surgeon.	Superintending or Head Surgeon.	Member of the Medical Board.	REMARKS.
Benza, Pasquil Maria (M.D.)	June 27, 1832				
Beauchamp, William	Novemb. 24, 1832				
Buchanan, R. H.	January 27, 1833				
Dedwell, E. Gustavus	July 7, 1833				
Balfour, Edward Green	June ... 2, 1836				
C					
Colley, L. Lucas	....1765......	April....14, 1786			Died in 1797 in India.
Corbitt, Michael	Nov. ... 3, 1785	January 15, 1793			Died May 7, 1798, at Prince of Wales's Island.

MADRAS SURGEONS.   76–77

FIG. 2. Pages 76–77 from "Alphabetical List of the Medical Officers of the Indian Army from the Year 1764 to the Year 1838."[11]

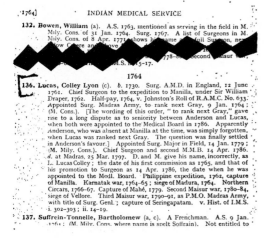

[1764]   INDIAN MEDICAL SERVICE

132. Bowen, William (a). A.S. 1763, mentioned as serving in the field in M. Mily. Cons. of 31 Jan. 1764. Surg. 1767. A list of Surgeons in M. Mily. Cons. of 8 Apr. 1771 shows his name as full Surgeon, ... M.S. ... 15–17.

1764

136. Lucas, Colley Lyon (c). b. 1730. Surg. A.M.D. in England, 12 June 1761. Chief Surgeon to the expedition to Manilla, under Sir William Draper, 1762. Half-pay, 1764, v. Johnston's Roll of R.A.M.C. No. 633. Appointed Surg. Madras Army, to rank next Gray, 9 Jan. 1764 ; (M. Cons.). [The wording of this order, " to rank next Gray," gave rise to a long dispute as to seniority between Anderson and Lucas, when both were appointed to the Medical Board in 1786. Apparently Anderson, who was absent at Manilla at the time, was simply forgotten, when Lucas was ranked next Gray. The question was finally settled in Anderson's favour.] Appointed Surg. Major in Field, 14 Jan. 1779 ; (M. Mily. Cons.). Chief Surgeon and second M.M.B. 14 Apr. 1786. d. at Madras, 25 Mar. 1797. D. and M. give his name, incorrectly, as L. Lucas Colley ; the date of his first commission as 1765, and that of his promotion to Surgeon as 14 Apr. 1786, the date when he was appointed to the Medl. Board. Philippine expedition, 1762, capture of Manilla. Karnatak war, 1764–65 ; siege of Madura, 1764. Northern Circars, 1766–67. Capture of Mahé, 1779. Second Maisur war, 1780–84, with title of Surg. Genl. ; capture of Seringapatam. v. Hist. of I.M.S. i. 302–303 ; ii. 14–19.

137. Suffrein-Tonnelle, Bartholomew (a, c). A Frenchman. A.S. 9 Jan. 1764 ; (M. Milv. Cons. where name is spelt Soffrain). Not entitled to

FIG. 3. Excerpt from the "Roll of the Indian Medical Service, 1615–1930."[13] (Editor's note. To me, the next to the last line in this sketch—"capture of Seringapatam"—is the astounding clincher in this research by Mr. Patterson. It places, indubitably, Mr. Colley Lyon Lucas as a military surgeon present at the exact moment and place where Cowasjee had his nose cut off.)

affairs. Born in 1730, he was appointed to the Army Medical Department on June 12, 1761 as Staff Surgeon to the 96th Foot. He was Chief Surgeon to the expedition to Manila, under Sir William Draper in 1762. He arrived in Madras in the "Grosvenor" in August 1762, to establish an Army Hospital (Dodwell,[16] 1930). He was then employed continuously in India, mostly in Madras, until his death in 1797. He was engaged in military campaigns until 1767; there seems then to have been a respite from war service for 12 years. He married Miss Martha Lee on May 12, 1776.

In 1779 he was again in the field, promoted to Surgeon Major, taking part in the Second Maisur War (1780–1784), and was present at the siege of Vellore. He was a well-known Freemason, the first Master of the Lodge of Perfect Unanimity which was constituted in Madras in 1786. On September 22, 1786 he was appointed Second Member of the Medical Board in Madras (Fig. 4); this post he held until his death, being absent only during the Third Maisur War (1790–1791) on deputation as Surgeon-General to the Madras Army. On January 9, 1794 he joined the Honorable East India Company Service (Madras) as "full" Surgeon, with the equivalent rank of Colonel— for which his wife was granted a pension after his death on March 25, 1797 (Crawford,[14] 1914).

Here, then, is a distinguished surgeon of Madras, Colley Lyon Lucas, whose career would fit with the little that we know of "Mr. Lucas." He would have been active "in the time of Hyder Ali," and there would

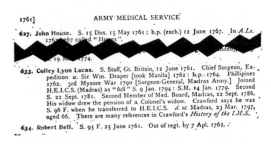

[1761]   ARMY MEDICAL SERVICE

627. John House. S. 15 Dns. 15 May 1761 ; h.p. (exch.) 12 June 1767. In A.Lr. 1761–67 called "Howes". ... ... 19 M ... 1774.

633. Colley Lyon Lucas. S. Staff, Gt. Britain, 12 June 1761. Chief Surgeon, Expedition v. Sir Wm. Draper [took Manila] 1762 : h.p.–1764. Phillipines 1762. 3rd Mysore War 1790 [Surgeon-General, Madras Army.] Joined H.E.I.C.S. (Madras) as "full" S. 9 Jan. 1794 ; S.M. 14 Jan. 1779. Second S. 22 Sept. 1781. Second Member of Med. Board, Madras, 22 Sept. 1786. His widow drew the pension of a Colonel's widow. Crawford says he was S. 96 F. when he transferred to H.E.I.C.S. d. at Madras, 23 Mar. 1797, aged 66. There are many references in Crawford's History of the I.M.S.

634. Robert Bell. S. 95 F. 25 June 1761. Out of regt. by 7 Apl. 1762.

FIG. 4. Excerpt from "Commissioned Officers in the Medical Services of the British Army, 1727–1898."

have been ample opportunity for Carpue's "Major Heitland" to make his acquaintance; they both served in the Madras Presidency.

Did Lucas carry out rhinoplasty by the Indian method? There was certainly no lack of opportunity. Surgeons in India writing after this time comment on the frequency of nasal mutilation and on the consequent experience of reconstruction—which was far greater than that of contemporary surgeons in Europe (Brett,[4] 1840; Hendley,[17] 1895, who worked in Jeypore from 1874; Keegan,[18] 1900, Residency surgeon at Indore for fifteen years from 1879). Smith,[19] writing in October 1897, recorded that he had operated on 6 cases during the past spring. However, no document has yet been found to confirm the report in the *Bombay Courier* (1795) that Lucas successfully carried out the operation himself.

The relationship between Lucas and the Cowasjee episode is another tantalizing problem. Here Pennant's[20] account in 1798 may be relevant. He notes that the news of Cowasjee's operation was published in Madras in *Hircarrah* or the *Madras Gazette* for August 5, 1794. The original drawing of this was published in Bombay on March 20, 1794. Could it be that Lucas, in Madras, saw the account in the local papers in August, and wrote a letter to Bombay to establish his prior claim? These, sir, and many other questions still await an answer.

Thomas J. S. Patterson, F.R.C.S.
Department of Plastic Surgery
Churchill Hospital
Oxford, England

ACKNOWLEDGMENT

I am grateful to the staff of the following institutions for their continuing help in solving this riddle. The Bodleian Library at the University of Oxford (particularly the Indian Institute Library and the Radcliffe Science Library), The India Office Library in London, the Library of the Wellcome Institute of the History of Medicine (London), and the Library of the United Grand Lodge of England.

REFERENCES

1. Gentleman's Magazine, p. 891. London, October, 1794.
2. McDowell, F.: The "B.L." bomb-shell. Plast. & Reconstr. Surg., *44:* 66, 1969.
3. Zeis, E.: *Die Literatur und Geschichte der plastischen Chirurgie*, p. 213. Engelmann, Leipzig, 1863. (freely translated)
4. Brett, F. H.: *Surgical Diseases*, p. 453. Calcutta, 1840.
5. Gnudi, M. T., and Webster, J. P.: *The Life and Times of Gaspare Tagliacozzi*, p. 314. Reichner, New York, 1951.
6. Philadelphia Medical Museum, *2:* 343–47, 1806.
7. Carpue, J. C.: *Two Successful Operations for Restoring a Lost Nose*, p. 40. Longman, London, 1816.
8. Nélaton, C., et Ombrédanne, L.: *La Rhinoplastie*, p. 21. Steinheil, Paris, 1904.
9. Dodwell and Miles: *Indian Army List, 1760–1834*. London, 1835.
10. Le Fanu: *A Manual of the Salem District of the Presidency of Madras*, Vol. 1, p. 72 (Footnote), 1883.
11. Dodwell and Miles: *Alphabetical List of the Medical Officers of the Indian Army from the Year 1764 to the Year 1838*. London, 1839.
12. Cotton, J. J.: *List of Inscriptions on Tombs or Monuments in Madras Possessing Historical or Archaelogical Interest*, p. 35. Madras, 1905.
13. Crawford, D. G.: *Roll of the Indian Medical Service, 1615–1930*, p. 258. London, 1930.
14. Crawford, D. G.: *A History of the Indian Medical Service, 1600–1913*. London, 1914.
15. Johnston, W.: *Commissioned Officers in the Medical Services of the British Army, 1727–1898*, p. 35. London, 1917.
16. Dodwell, H.: *Calendar of the Madras Despatches, 1754–1765*, p. 309. Madras, 1930.
17. Hendley, T. H.: *A Medico-Topographical Account of Jeypore*, p. 56. Calcutta, 1895.
18. Keegan, D. F.: *Rhinoplastic Operations*, p. 18. Balliere, Tindall, and Cox, London, 1900.
19. Smith, H.: Reports on medical and surgical practice in the Jullundur Civil Hospital, Punjab. Notes of surgical cases. Brit. M. J. *2:* 1180, 1897.
20. Pennant, T.: *The View of Hindoostan*, Vol. 2, p. 238. Hughs, London, 1798.

LETTER TO THE EDITOR (January 1972)

MORE ABOUT "B.L.," "MR. LUCAS," AND MR. CARPUE

Sir:

It was with great interest that I read Mr. Patterson's letter in the July 1971 issue. Although I have reached the same conclusion as Mr. Patterson (that Colly Lyon Lucas may have been the first Englishman to perform the Indian rhinoplasty), I disagree with him on a number of points because of some additional information that I have to disclose.

It disturbed me that the *Philadelphia Medical Museum (2:* 343–347, 1806) reprinted in 1806 an article from the *Bombay Courier* that had been published originally in 1795. The postal service between Bombay and Philadelphia might have been slow, but 11 years seemed too long a delay. When I glanced at the report in the *Museum,* I found it was in the section of the journal entitled *Medical and Philosophical Register.* (Today we might call the *Register* "International Abstracts and Reports," for it reproduced, in abbreviated or original form, reports of interest from other journals.) If one reads carefully the last two words of line 3 on page 347 of the *Museum,* he will see: *Europ. Mag. (i.e.* the reference for the article).

After considerable searching, I found the same article as it appeared in the *European Magazine* for August, 1797 *(32:* 87–88, 1797). Apparently, the editor of *European Magazine* had reproduced the article in turn from the *Bombay Courier* of 1795, shortly after it arrived by ship from India. It would seem that the editor of the *Museum* was so hard up for material (he was working on his second volume) that he decided to rehash an article that had been copied from the *Bombay Courier* of nearly a decade before. This would appear to explain the 11-year delay between the publication of the article in the *Bombay Courier* and the *Philadelphia Medical Museum.*

Secondly, Mr. Patterson was unable to locate Carpue's Major Heitland, but he did find a Major William P. Heatland in Dodwell and Miles' *List of the Officers of the Indian Army.* I have found a Major Heitland mentioned in the *Gentleman's Magazine* on two occasions *(84,i:* 200, 1814 and *87,ii:* 473, 1817). The latter occasion recorded the Major's death on September 25, 1817. The Public Record Office in London has the registered copy of this Major Heitland's will (Probate 11/1598/Folio 598) which begins, "This is the Last Will and Testament of Mr. William Peter Heitland of Fitzroy Street, Fitzroy Square, in the County of Middlesex, a Major in the Honourable East India Company Service." Thus, Carpue correctly recorded the name of the major who was incorrectly identified by Dodwell and Miles as Heatland, and who lived less than a mile from Carpue in London after his retirement from the Indian Army.

Thirdly, I disagree with Mr. Patterson that Lucas, after reading an article in *The Hircarrah* (or *Madras Gazette*) of August 5, 1794, fired off a letter to the editor of the *Bombay Courier* to establish his priority in performing rhinoplasties. The article in *The Hircarrah* is simply an announcement by A. B. Bone, *The Hircarrah*'s publisher, that subscriptions were available through his office to a print of Wales' painting of Cowasjee. I doubt that Lucas would have become incensed over this advertisement for engravings.*

Finally, whether Lucas performed one rhinoplasty (as the *Bombay Courier* stated) or several rhinoplasties (as Major Heitland said) is insignificant. Lucas deserves no more than a footnote in the history of plastic surgery, in my opinion. As fas as we know, Lucas never published his experience with rhinoplasty and he was not responsible for the rebirth of plastic surgery at the beginning of the nineteenth century. It was Carpue, I think, who reawakened the world to Tagliacozzi's work and who published the details of his own first two successful operations. It was Carpue's name that was constantly mentioned in the European medical literature of the time, and I believe it was Carpue's book that spread knowledge of rhinoplasty throughout the world. As Sir Francis Darwin said (*Eugenics Review 6:* 9, 1914):

" ... In science the credit goes to the man who convinces the world, not to the man to whom the idea first occurs. Not to the man who finds a piece of grain of new and precious quality but to him who sows it, reaps it, grinds it, and feeds the world on it."

M. Felix Freshwater, B.S.
Yale University School of Medicine
One South Street
New Haven, Conn. 06510

P.S. I would like to thank Jane Bebbington of the European Manuscripts Department, India Office Library, and Mr. Robin Price of the Wellcome Institute of the History of Medicine for their valuable advice and assistance.

---

* In the Sir Charles Warre Malet Collection at the India Office Library, I have inspected a subscription book for the 1794 Cowasjee print that probably belonged to Mr. James Wales, Malet's father-in-law (MSS. Eur. F. 149/97). The book is dated March 12, 1794 and says that the engraving would be published by the end of the month (*i.e.* March 31, 1794). The list of subscribers include Mr. James Findlay and Mr. Thomas Cruso of the Indian Medical Service, who are mentioned in the print. Four copies of the print were ordered for Sir Joseph Banks, Bt., one of Carpue's close friends who might have shown Carpue one of his copies and first awakened his interest in rhinoplasty. From B.L.'s letter of October 9, 1794 in the *Gentleman's Magazine (64,ii:* 891, 1794) it appears that he received a copy of Wales' print from a friend in India; therefore, B.L. could not be Mr. Lucas of Madras.

THE CASE OF THE ELUSIVE MR. LUCAS, THE MYSTERIOUS MAJOR HEITLAND, *ET AL*

Tracking the quarry through the bowels of the India Office Library in London, and through other early and rare records, it would appear that Mr. Patterson (PRS, *49:* 88, 1971) and Mr. Freshwater (*Letter to the Editor,* this issue) have established the identities of these gentlemen beyond all reasonable doubt. It must have been Colly Lyon Lucas who built the new nose from a forehead flap for Cowasjee at Poona. It seems likely that this was one of a series of similar operations done by him, as Major Heitland informed Carpue. In spite of Mr. Freshwater's objections to the idea, five gets you one that he wrote the "B.L." letter.

While welcoming Freshwater to the corps of investigators, I cannot agree with him that Lucas's role was insignificant and that Carpue's furtherance of the work of Tagliacozzi constituted the renaissance in plastic surgery which occurred about 1800. Tagliacozzi was known for the arm flap, not the forehead flap. In Carpue's preamble to his first forehead flap case (PRS *44:* 175, 1969) he is aflame from the recent reports of the Indian cases, scarcely able to await his first opportunity to try this. He says, "I can add no more to the history of the Indian methods; but what has appeared is sufficient to arrest the reader's attention . . . as it offers so great an improvement on the Taliacotian practice . . . ."

All of England at this time was excited about the ventures of the East India Company, and about the many new and fascinating items and practices arriving almost daily from this ancient and exotic land. Interest in medieval Italian surgery was, at this moment, undoubtedly low. Without Lucas, would Carpue have written his book about Indian rhinoplasty from forehead flaps? Would there have been a rebirth at this time and in this place of the art and science of plastic surgery? I think not.

But, about Mr. Freshwater's discoveries concerning the *European Magazine* and the identity of Major Heitland. Ah! Now those . . . .

—*Frank McDowell, M.D.*

European Rhinoplasty

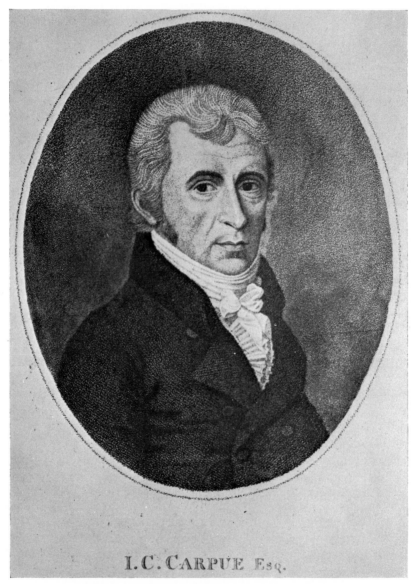

I.C. CARPUE Esq.

JOSEPH CONSTANTINE CARPUE, F.R.C.S.
1764–1846

AN ACCOUNT OF TWO SUCCESSFUL OPERATIONS FOR RESTORING A LOST NOSE*

J. C. CARPUE, F.R.C.S.,

York Hospital, Chelsea

(*Printed for Longman, Hurst, Rees, Orme, and Brown, London, 1816*)

On undertaking the first of the two cases to be hereafter narrated, I was induced to make such personal inquiries as were within my reach in this country, concerning the Indian method. I did myself the honour to write to Sir Charles Mallet, who had resided many years in India, and who obligingly confirmed to me the report that this had been a common operation in India from time immemorial; adding that it had always been performed by the caste of potters or brickmakers, and that though not invariably, it was usually successful.

Mr. James Stuart Hall, a gentleman who was many years in India, assured me that he had seen the operation performed, and that it was of tedious length. From Dr. Barry, of the India service, I learned that he also had seen the operation: that it occupied an hour and a half, and was performed with an old razor, the edge of which, being continually blunted in dissection, was every moment re-set. Tow was introduced to support the nose, but no attempt to form nostrils, by adding a septum, was made.

I am obligingly informed by Major Heitland, of the India service, that in India, several years ago, in the time of Hyder Ali (*Ed. note:* father of Tipú Sultán), Mr. Lucas, an English surgeon, was, in several instances, successful in the operation, which he copied from the Hindoo practitioners. . . .

I have heard that about the year 1803 the nasal operation, by the Indian method, was performed in London, without success. The patient, I am told, is still alive in India.†

I can add no more to the history of the Indian methods;‡ but what has appeared is sufficient to arrest the reader's attention, both as it offers so great an improvement on the Taliacotian practice, and as it illustrates the history of the operation in general. It cannot be otherwise, than that this discovery of its existence in the distant regions of India, should awaken our curiosity more earnestly than before, as to the place and date of its original use.

CASE 1

In the month of September, 1814, I was applied to by an Officer in his Majesty's army, whose nose was in a mutilated state, and who introduced himself to me by saying, "Sir, you see my unfortunate situation. I was informed, at Gibraltar, that you had performed the

† If the Gentleman who performed the operation is still living, and will favour the Author with an account of the cause of its failure, he will much oblige him.

‡ The Author will be very thankful for any communication on this subject, from persons resident in India, or who have resided in that country.

* *Editor's note.* The two case reports which we are publishing represent only a part of the book. This material was furnished to the Journal by Mr. William K. Beatty, Librarian of the Archibald Church Medical Library of Northwestern University in Chicago—who has been most helpful with several of these classic reprints.

operation for restoring a lost nose. I am in the army; and, having been bred to that profession, I wish to undergo the operation, in order to put myself again in condition for active service."

I readily consented; but, at the same time, apprized my patient that what he had previously heard was founded in mistake. I had long wished for an opportunity of performing the operation; and, for the space of fifteen years, had constantly recommended it to my pupils. I added that I considered it as by no means dangerous, and that it might be practised in either of two methods: the one, the Italian or, as it is commonly called, the Taliacotian, in which the part is supplied from the integuments of the arm; the other, the Indian, in which it is taken from the forehead.

The patient went to Egypt in the year 1801; but, becoming affected with a liver complaint, was obliged to return to Europe. At Malta, as well as previously in Egypt, mercury, the usual remedy in such a case, was employed. Being subsequently ordered home, he went to Ireland, where the same plan was pursued. Returning from Ireland to London, after being attacked by a sore throat, he consulted Mr. Heaviside, who was decidedly of the opinion that the sore throat was *Mercurial* and not *venereal;* and advised him to discontinue the use of mercury. Unfortunately, the gentlemen to whose care he committed himself were of a contrary opinion; hence, the mercury was persevered in. Very shortly after his consultation of Mr. Heaviside, his nose became affected: and, upon this, the mercury was increased; the practitioners being but the more convinced that the complaint was venereal. The consequence of this excessive use of mercury was that the septum of the nose began to slough, etc. The patient's constitution being, at the same time, greatly injured, the mercury was at length laid aside. Thus relieved

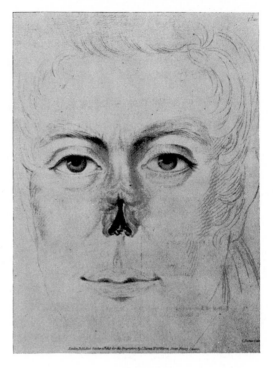

PLATE I

from the occasion of his sufferings, he gradually recovered his health; but with the loss of the septum, all the anterior part of the cartilage, and, in truth, the whole front of the nose, a small portion of the alae, or sides of the nostrils excepted. The nasal bones remained entire* (Plate I).

Considering that if my attempt succeeded, I should introduce into the London practice an operation, the propriety of which I had for fifteen years recommended to my pupils, I was the more anxious to have a case in which success would in all probability follow. Knowing that in India the operation was

* The mischievous effects of the abuse of mercury are beyond description. In my daily practice, I witness consequences even more melancholy than those experienced by this patient. The value of mercury in medicine is incalculable; and, in *Lues Venerea,* there is no cure without it. In the meantime, the mistaken or excessive use of it is one of the greatest and most prevalent scourges to which society is at present subject.

usually fortunate; but from the observations of Dr. Ruddiman, given in these pages, on the facility with which, in that country, divided parts unite, I was led to think that without adverting to the difference of climate, there were circumstances which rendered my prospects not equally favourable. In the case presented to me, the parts had sloughed from disease; in India they were divided by art, leaving a healthy base. In this case, too, the constitution had been impaired by the liver complaint and its improper treatment. The question to be decided was, is this a fair case for trial? I wished to determine that point; therefore, under pretext of preparing for the operation, I made incisions near the remains of the alae. The wounds healed; and, being satisfied, now, that I had healthy parts to act on, I had little doubt of complete success. I relied on adhesion taking place before the cold weather set in.

I next, after the practice of the Indian surgeons, to whom the whole merit of the method belongs, formed a nose of wax and commenced a series of experiments on the dead subject. I operated in that manner eleven times. At this period of the undertaking I consulted my friend, Mr. Sawrey, whose opinion coincided with my own. From him I received much assistance in planning and executing this new operation and in its subsequent stages; as likewise from my friends, Messrs. M'Lochlin, Morris, and Domville, surgeons of Greenwich Hospital. I also performed the operation in my theatre on the dead subject, before my pupils and a number of medical friends who obligingly attended, and who unanimously agreed to the propriety of the operation. At length, on the 23rd of October accompanied by my friends Messrs, Sawrey and Warren, and in the presence of Mr. Lamert, surgeon to his Majesty's thirtieth regiment of foot, who attended at the request of the patient, I proceeded to perform the operation.

The patient's forehead was unusually low. On that account, some days previously to performing the operation, I removed the hair, by the roots, from the scalp; the integuments of that part being required to form the septum or base of the nose. This portion of the integuments to be dissected, was my only subject of uneasiness; my fear being that the hair would grow and prevent adhesion.

Having well ascertained the size of the graft required, by means of a wax model which I then flattened and laid on the forehead. I drew the outline round it with red paint. I drew lines, also, on the sides where I was to make the incision and a line beneath for the septum. This done, the patient leaped upon a table and, laying himself on his back with his head supported by a pillow, refused to be held, saying "I hope I shall behave like a man!" Nor did he make the smallest complaint during the operation.

I now made an incision on the right, and then on the left; and dissected out a sufficient quantity of the face, with some muscular fibres of the *Compressor Nares,* and the *Levator* and *Depressor Labii Superiores Alaeque Nasi,* to receive what was to be dissected from the forehead. I made a simple incision for receiving of the septum, considering that the inner part of the integuments would certainly unite with the upper part; and that if, when adhesion took place on the upper part of the lip, hairs should grow on the lower part of the integuments intended to form the septum, and the old and new parts, in consequence, should not unite, I could then, with greater safety, dissect the roots of the hair from the part and bring it into contact with the lower part of the incision. My apprehensions, however, appeared ultimately to have been groundless; for both surfaces readily united and an excellent septum was formed.

The parts of the face being prepared for the reception of the new nose, I began that part of the operation which belongs to the forehead by making an incision along the lines I had drawn. I then dissected the integuments, merely leaving the pericranium. The angular artery on the left side bled freely; but the loss of blood was very inconsiderable and there was no occasion for tying the artery. The part which was dissected, and which hung down, became of a purple colour; and the patient, at this period, informed me that his forehead felt extremely cold. I applied warm sponges, which afforded great relief, and which were continued during the remainder of the operation.

My next steps were to make the *turn* of the dissected parts, and introduce the septum into the incision of the upper lip, where I confined it by ligature. After this, I brought the integuments exactly into contact with the integuments on the left side and fixed them also by two ligatures; and then I did the same on the right. I introduced lint to distend the nostrils and applied straps of adhesive plaster to keep the integuments in contact. Everything being thus done for the nose, my concluding care was to bring the edges of the integuments on the forehead and between the eyebrows as near together as possible and keep them so by means of adhesive plaster.

A brother officer of the patient having been in the room during the operation and kept an account of the time by his watch, I am enabled to state that it occupied exactly a quarter of an hour; the dissection having employed nine minutes and the ligatures six. After this, the application of the necessary bandages, changing the linen of the patient, sponging away the blood, and placing the patient in bed consumed twenty-two minutes more, making in the whole thirty-seven minutes. Short, however, as was the time, had it not been for my habit of frequently performing operations on English soldiers, I must have been astonished at the fortitude with which my pa-

tient went through this. When it was past, he observed that, "It was no child's play—extremely painful—but there was no use in complaining;" that he felt little or nothing after the dressings were applied. His resolution is the more worthy of observation because there was, in his case, no prior example of success, either in my own practice or in England, to support his confidence in me, or mine in the certainty of the result.

The patient, being put to bed, enjoyed some sleep. The room was kept very warm and a flannel laid on the patient's head. In the night there was hemorrhage, but not in any quantity. Perfectly quiet the next day. Pulse as before operation. Much inclination for food, but allowed only barley-water and warm jellies.

On the third day I took off the dressings. It will be supposed that I felt exceedingly anxious on this occasion; for, though I had every reason to expect adhesion, it was possible that it had not taken place. The parts, however, adhered; and I had the high satisfaction to hear the officer, before alluded to, exclaim from the foot of the bed, "My G--d, there *is* a nose!"

Adhesion, agreeably with my most sanguine hopes, had taken place in every part; and the nose was of the same colour with the face. Meantime, it was perfectly flat and rose and fell with every inspiration and expiration. This state of the nose, together with the wound of the forehead as it was left immediately after dissection, is represented in Plate III, in which Fig. 1 is the dissection or cicatrix on the forehead; Fig. 2 is the portion of integument dissected off to form the septum of the nose; and Fig. 3, the flat nose. The flatness of the nose alarmed me with a fear of its preserving a very unsightly appearance; and to remedy this I thought of procuring the air bladder of a fish, which I proposed to introduce into the nose and then inflate with the design of raising the point of the nose. My ap-

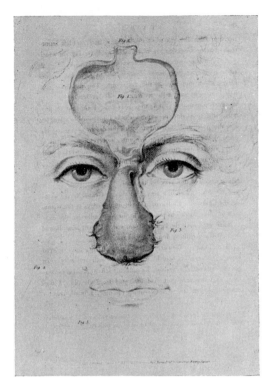

PLATE III

prehensions, however, on this, as in other parts of the cure, were groundless. Nature worked with me and raised the nose by her own means.

Fourth day. Cut away two ligatures and dressed the forehead which appeared in a very healthy state.

Fifth day. Nose in a very good state. Granulations formed on the forehead. Endeavoured to bring the edges of the wound as much into contact as possible by means of adhesive plaster.

Sixth day. All the ligatures removed. Patient now allowed meat, but particularly desired not to masticate.

Seventh day. Patient, having a good appetite, ordered broiled kidneys, of which he ate one with impunity. In proceeding with the second he suddenly felt a peculiar sensation, as if the new parts had separated from the old. I was immediately sent for. On examining the

nose I found that on the left side a small portion of the newly-united parts were divided. The greater part of the fissure was again made to unite; but a small part remained open, as it still does though, with time, its filling up is not to be doubted. The open part is represented at *a*, Plate IV, figures 2 and 3.

Eighth day. Room exceedingly warm. The heat oppressed us all, and the patient was near fainting. At this time the face lost its colour and the nose with it; but, on ventilating the room, the face regained its usual complexion and the nose also.

Ninth day. Nose became edematous. See Plate IV, figure 1.

Twelfth day. Nose very large, being much distended with edema; and compression appeared to do more harm than good. At this period Professor Assalini

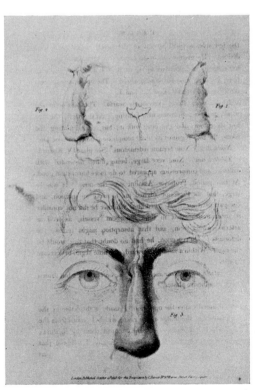

PLATE IV

saw the nose. It was so large that the Professor advised me to make an incision and cut part of it away. I asked him whether he did not consider it edematous; that in time absorbent vessels as well as arteries would form, and that absorption might remove the deformity? On reflection, he had no doubt that this would be the case. Within a month afterward, the nose began to decrease in size.

Twentieth day. Nose inclined to rise on one side; but drawn down by adhesive plaster.

Four months after the operation I made a dissection of the integuments on the bridge of the nose, which I united from the turn, which had disappeared, and confined them by ligature; being of the opinion that if, in this cold climate, I followed that part of the Indian method which consists in removing the turn, by which is carried on the circulation from the parent parts, the nose would slough; as seems to have been the case in the story related by Van Helmont, and in others referred to by the early writers. In no other particular of importance have I departed from the Indian method.

The edema at length subsided, but left the nose very flat. Subsequently, however, granulations formed and the nose experienced a healthy enlargement. To ascertain, from time to time, whether the nose, after being relieved from edema, increased in its projection from the face, I caused the patient to place himself in such a situation as allowed his profile to be drawn upon a wall; and, by making the comparison every two or three days, I had the pleasure to see its gradual increase demonstrated.

In the present state of the nose (Plate IV, figure 3), though there is neither bony or cartilaginous septum, yet the anterior or projecting part is solid and has every appearance of a natural nose. The nostrils are gradually growing big-

ger and the secretion takes place as usual. The forehead was healed in three months; and the size of the cicatrix is that which is represented in the plate (Plate IV, figure 3). I am happy to add that the nose is improving every day and that the trifling deformity which is still to be observed is capable, I trust, of being removed by a very simple operation.

CASE 2

At the battle of Albuera, in Spain, which was fought on the 16th of May, 1810, the right brigade of General Stuart's division was sent to the support of the Spaniards who were driven back from the heights they occupied on the right of the line; and while charging the enemy with the bayonet, a body of Polish horse lancers coming up unperceived (on account of the heavy storm of rain which, with the smoke from the firing, prevented anything from being distinctly seen) their flank was turned and they were charged in the rear. Some of the regiments, in consequence, were almost wholly destroyed, the enemy giving no quarter and slaughtering the wounded and fallen.

At this time, Captain (then Lieutenant) Latham, of the third foot, seeing one of the colours of his regiment in danger of being taken from the ensign who carried it, by four or five of the lancers, sprung to the spot; and in attempting to seize the colour he lost an arm by a sabre-cut. Still persevering, with the other hand he tore the colour from the staff; but not before he received five wounds, one of which took off part of his cheek and nose. One of the lancers now charged him through the others and, with his lance, hit him with such force in the groin as to throw him to the distance of some yards, al-

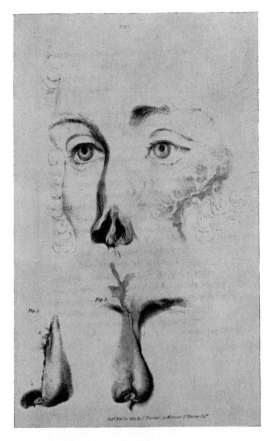

PLATE V

most in a state of insensibility, but still with the colour in his possession. . . .

In the state in which the nose was left by the sabre of the enemy, all the interior was exposed, as in Plate V, fig. 1. Exclusively of the disagreeable appearance produced, Captain Latham suffered from repeated colds and inflammations.

The right side of the alae remaining, the patient preferred a cicatrix in the middle of the nose to an amputation of the sound part. I consulted my friends, Mr. Astley Cooper, Mr. Sawrey, and Mr. Anderson, surgeon to the captain's regiment, who were of opinion with myself that the integuments taken from the forehead would unite with those which covered the side of the nose.

I made an incision on the forehead,

as in the former case; as also similar dissections. On making the dissection on the forehead, there was a very considerable hemorrhage; so much so, that I was compelled to tie an artery. When the flap hung down, instead of the part appearing purple, as in *Case 1*, an artery bled as freely as the temporal artery when opened. This, however, subsided and there was no occasion for a ligature.

The parts were brought into contact, as in *Case 1*, by means of five ligatures. The only difference was that the right side of the integuments, instead of being received into an excavation, was brought into exact contact and that the lip was not divided, but the lower part of the septum dissected away and the new part brought into contact and detained there by ligature. Adhesive plaster was applied to the forehead as before, and the usual dressings.

The patient had some fever the first night, but with a little sleep. More hemorrhage than in *Case 1*.

Second day. Free from pain. Little fever.

Third day. The part felt very uncomfortable. Removed the dressings. Much inflammation. Inner part of the integuments united but the skin did not adhere. Cut away the ligatures and brought the skin together by adhesive plaster.

Fourth day. Considerable suppuration from the internal parts. Forehead in a very good state. Adhesion complete between the eyebrows.

Sixth day. Parts became edematous, as in *Case 1*. On the side in which the new nose was inserted, the nostril drawn upward toward the cicatrix on the face as in plate V, fig. 1. The patient having lost a great part of his cheek on that side* I had great difficulty in applying

* The integuments, muscles, and part of the os malae, or cheek bone, were cut away by the sabre. These were a considerable time before they were

adhesive plaster to the contracted part; it occasioned inflammation, that part being exceedingly irritable.

Tenth day. The skin, which had been disunited by the swelling of the parts, restored to perfect union. Edema not so considerable; and, in this case, pressure seems of advantage.

In six weeks, forehead completely healed and a cicatrix as in Plate V, fig. 3.

At the end of two months, edema less considerable; and afterward continued to decrease. There remains, however, an edematous disposition.

On the 7th of October, in the presence of Messrs. Warren and M'Lochlin, I performed the second part of the operation, which consisted in making a longitudinal incision upon the top of the nose, from *a* to *b*, (See Plate V, fig. 2) and then, continuing the dissection across the bridge, under the new nose. After this, I dissected away a considerable portion of the under surface of the new nose, also from *a* to *b*; and then made a longitudinal incision in the new nose, from *a* to *b*; so that the new nose was made to fit as nearly as possible the excavation I had made in the old nose. I now brought the longitudinal incisions of the old and new noses exactly in contact, passed two silver pins through the integuments, and united them by the twisted suture. Then I applied adhesive plaster to the remaining parts. Forty-eight hours after the op-

completely cicatrized, as a considerable sloughing took place. The cicatrix at length formed, will be seen on reference to Plate V, fig. 1. The newly reformed parts are exceedingly irritable, and have frequently broken out.

eration, I removed the dressings; and, finding that a perfect adhesion had taken place, I withdrew the pins, and applied adhesive plaster. A little suppuration followed from the lower pin, but of no consequence. The parts were perfectly recovered in two days. In ten days, the time usually allowed, complete adhesion had taken place. A dissection of the new nostril remains to be made.

Captain Latham has enjoined me not to conclude this account of his case without recording some particulars of the generosity and benevolence of His Royal Highness the Prince Regent, which are intimately connected with it, which it is his pride to acknowledge, and for which he feels that he can never be sufficiently grateful. It will appear, from the following copy of a letter which I had the honour to receive from Major-General Bloomfield, by the hands of Captain Latham, that His Royal Highness not only condescended to place that gentleman under my professional care; but, further, to direct me to provide, at His Royal Highness's private charge, for the personal accommodation of my patient, during the cure. In addition to this liberality, since the operation has been performed, and it has been proper that Captain Latham should have the benefit of the air, His Royal Highness has been pleased to cause one of his carriages to attend him daily for that purpose.

J. C. Carpue, F.R.C.S.
York Hospital
Chelsea, England

BIOGRAPHICAL SKETCH OF CARPUE*

Joseph Constantine Carpue was born in London on the 4th of May, 1764. He was descended from a Spanish family.... His father, a gentleman of small fortune,

* Reprinted from Lancet, *1:* 166, 1846.

resided at Brook Green, in the county of Middlesex. He was intended for the church and received the elements of his education in the Jesuits' College at Douay. At the age of eighteen he was impressed with a strong desire to travel, and being limited in his resources, resolved to make the tour of the Continent of Europe on foot....

We have heard him tell of his having seen Louis the Eighteenth and Marie Antoinette at the dinnertable, waited on by the Duke of Orleans. And at a subsequent visit to Europe, of his having listened to the declamations of Danton, Marat, and Robespierre. On his return to Britain, he made the tour of Wales on foot, and subsequently that of the Highlands of Scotland.... To the end of life his delight in traveling continued unabated....

Whenever, during his travels, he entered a town of any magnitude, his practice was to make enquiry concerning the hospitals and other medical establishments, and the names of the professors of medicine and surgery; and to go at once and introduce himself to the latter. On these occasions he was invariably received with respect and courtesy, and put in possession of whatever information he desired, whether provided with letters of introduction or otherwise; and in many cases he made valuable friendships, as in the instance of Professor Graef of Berlin.

Having completed his classical education, Mr. Carpue ... resolved on becoming a surgeon; he commenced his medical studies under the direction of the late Mr. Keate and Dr. George Pearson, at St. George's Hospital, to which institution he was, for some time, house surgeon. He was then appointed staff surgeon to the York Hospital, at Chelsea, where he remained for twelve years....

His career as a lecturer on anatomy commenced in the year 1800, in the following manner. While at the York Hospital he omitted no opportunity of perfecting his acquaintance with anatomy and a gentleman, who was then studying medicine, one day said to him, "I wish I knew anatomy as well as you, Carpue;" to which Mr. Carpue replied, "If you desire it, I

will teach you." They then set to work diligently, and the result was so satisfactory to the pupil, Mr. Norman, that he insisted on the acceptance of twenty guineas by his teacher. This circumstance suggested to Mr. Carpue the first idea of becoming an anatomical lecturer, and the sum presented to him by Mr. Norman fixed the amount of his fee, which he never after altered....

His class was for many years full to overflowing. He delivered three courses of daily lectures during the year, and, with the exception of a few days in the summer season, without intermission. Twice in the week, in the evening, he also gave lectures on surgery. The original mind of our lecturer soon perceived the inutility of formal lectures, and the necessity of making each student, in his turn, take a share in the demonstration. He stood before his table, surrounded by his pupils, and illustrated the points of study by means of an extemporaneous diagram, and, as often happened, when subjects were scarce, he trusted to his practical descriptions and piece of chalk alone. From the latter circumstance, the gayer spirits of his day called him the "chalk lecturer," a title which, in after life, became one of affection....

An occurrence which took place at about the time of the commencement of Mr. Carpue's career as an anatomical lecturer, is worthy of notice, and we record it from an unpublished MS, in his own handwriting.

"Some time in the year 1800, three of the greatest men of their time, namely Mr. West, President of the Royal Academy, Mr. Banks, and Mr. Cosway (though last mentioned, not the least active in forwarding inquiry in regard to subjects of painting, sculpture, &c.) having agreed amongst themselves that the representation of the crucifixion did not appear natural, though it had been painted by the greatest artist of his age, wished to put this to a test.

They, therefore, requested me to nail a subject on a cross, saying that the tale told of Michael Angelo and others was not true of their having stabbed a man tied to a cross, and then making a drawing of the effect. Shortly after this application, a circumstance occurred at the college at Chelsea, which enabled me to comply with their request. A man of the name of Legg, one of the captains of the hospital, having had a dispute with a man named Lamb, a fellow pensioner, entered his bed-room with two loaded pistols, presented one to Lamb, and requested him to give him that satisfaction that one soldier had a right to demand from a fellow soldier. Lamb indignantly threw the pistol on the ground, when Legg fired the other pistol, and shot Lamb through the thorax. He immediately expired. I was at this time surgeon of the York Hospital, Chelsea. Mr. Keate, surgeon of Chelsea Hospital, not being in the way, I was sent for to examine the dead man. I found that the ball had divided the upper cava, which occasioned his immediate death. A jury sat on the body; the verdict was wilful murder. Legg declared that if the man were living, he would do what he had done, namely, shoot him. As Legg was in his perfect senses, there could be no doubt that he would be found guilty of murder and executed. Mr. Keate, surgeon general and surgeon at the hospital, was master of the College of Surgeons; to him I applied for the body when executed. Mr. Keate, who, as well as being one of the first surgeons of the age, was a most liberal man, and a great admirer of the arts, said I had come in a lucky moment, as he had received an order from government not to allow murderers to be exposed to public view. He promised to give the sheriff an order that the subject might be given for the purposes required. A building was erected near the place of execution; a cross provided; the subject was nailed on the cross; the cross suspended; when the body, being warm, fell into the position that a dead body must fall into, let the cause of death be what it may. When cool, a cast was made, under the direction of Mr. Banks, and when the mob had dispersed, it was removed to my theatre."

The cast is still in existence, and is preserved in the studio of Mr. Behnes....

The active practical pursuits in which he was engaged, left Mr. Carpue but little time for literary occupation; hence, his writings are few in number. In 1801, he published a "Description of the Muscles of the Human Body;" in 1803, an "Introduction to Electricity and Galvanism, with cases showing their Effects in the Cure of Disease;" in 1816, "An Account of Two Successful Operations for Restoring a Lost Nose;" in 1819, "The History of the High Operation for the Stone."

Mr. Carpue had the good fortune to be introduced to the Prince Regent, on the occasion of the illness of the Princess Amelia, at Worthing. The Prince took much interest in conversing with him on the subject of medical and physiological science; and, on several occasions after the Prince's accession to the throne, Mr. Carpue received a private audience from his Majesty on these topics.

In private life, Mr. Carpue was ... beloved by all who knew him.... He was ... an admirer of simplicity of manners and appearance. His disposition, in the latter respect, is evinced in the instructions which he has left for his funeral; that that ceremony shall be as private as possible, and as plain and simple as decency permits; and that everything in the shape of pomp or display shall be studiously avoided.

We cannot conclude this sketch of a most worthy and excellent man, and one distinguished in medical science, without having occasion to point out the accursed stain, the plague-spot of an honourable profession. Mr. Carpue was passed over by the Council of the College of Surgeons, when his turn to sit in that body arrived; he was cast aside by the self-elected, to make way, neither for an abler nor a better man. But this is not all; to the disgrace of all who possess the wretched privilege of appending the letters F.R.C.S. to their names, Mr. Carpue was not elected by the *Fellows* when *they* had an opportunity of placing him on the Council. He was never a Councillor of a miserably governed College. He was, however, a Fellow of the Royal Society, at the invitation of his friend, Sir Joseph Banks. He was not of the Council of the College of Surgeons, but *he was* the companion of his prince and of his king.

Editorial note. Mr. Carpue died in his 82nd year, apparently of pneumonia, on January 30, 1846.

RHINOPLASTIC OPERATION, PERFORMED WITH SUCCESS AT THE HOSPITAL ST. ELOI DE MONTPELLIER

PROFESSOR JACQUES-MATHIEU DELPECH

(Reprinted from Lancet, 4: 123, July 24, 1824.)

Charles Sychal, native of Toulon, a sailor attached to that port, aged 30 years, was admitted at the hospital St. Eloi in June, 1818. The alae of his nose were affected with ulcerations, which had a syphilitic appearance, as to the origin of which there was at first some doubt. Whether the patient feared that he should not be kept in the hospital, or from whatever other cause, he constantly denied that he had had any intercourse with women before the appearance of these ulcerations. He stated that his father had a gonorrheal running for seven years, for which he employed no remedy; and it was evidently his wish to persuade us that his disease was congenital. He had had in his youth eruptions about the thighs, and glandular enlargements, which had disappeared spontaneously. According to his own account, at the age of sixteen years, he had experienced pains in the inside of the nose, which were followed, a long time after, by the appearance of the first ulceration. The disease was of very old date, but it had made little progress when he was admitted, in the month of March, in the same year, at the hospital of Toulon, where its character was ascertained, and he was treated by a mercurial course in the form of pills; he took 120 during the two months he remained at this hospital; but he went out without deriving any benefit from this treatment.

We kept the patient at St. Eloi long enough to procure a certain effect from the internal exhibition of the sublimate, and to remove all our doubts as to the character of the disease....

The whole of the soft portion of the nose was destroyed, with the exception of

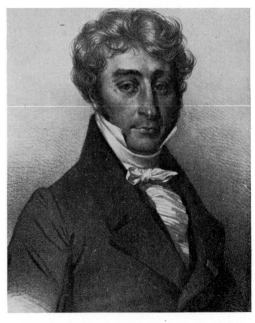

FIG. 1. Prof. Jacques-Mathieu Delpech (1777–1832) of Montpellier. Delpech was noted for animal grafting, autoplasty, this work on rhinoplasty, and original research on congenital deformities and wound healing. He went to Montpellier after losing out to Dupuytren in the contest for the Sabatier chair of clinical surgery. Later, he returned to Paris where he founded an orthopedic clinic. He died of a gunshot in the streets of Paris on October 19, 1832, "fired by a certain Demptos, an idiot." (Courtesy National Library of Medicine.)

Editor's note. The four short articles published here give a good picture of the state of rhinoplastic surgery "after Carpue." There were many speculations, of course, about the possibilities in this new field.

a narrow ridge round the nostrils, which was formed by a remnant of cartilage; a cicatrix confined this ridge, and pressed it towards the centre of the two openings. . . .

The patient was accordingly operated upon on the 4th of June 1823, in the following manner:—

Having placed him upon a strong chair, exposed to the light, we traced with ink the incisions which were to be made to receive the edges of the flap which was to repair the breach of the nose. We then cut out a paper model in the form of the portion of skin to be engrafted, and laying this model down on the forehead, and transposing it from one side to the other, we marked it out with ink; the forehead not being very open, we were obliged to encroach a little upon the part of the skin covered with hair, which was to form the lower part of the nose.

Everything being thus arranged we made the incisions as they were marked out round the breach; but our line having been placed on all sides in the convexity formed by the interior inclination of the remnant of cartilage, in order to prevent any deformity, we avoided cutting perpendicularly the whole of this excess and removing it entirely; we contented ourselves with paring the cicatrices, so as to augment the surface to which the flap was to be adapted.

The flap was then dissected, care being taken to make it as thick as possible, without however laying bare the coronal. This portion of skin had the form of an ace of spades reversed; the small portion destined to represent the cartilage answered to the tail of the spade, and its point was represented by the pedicle of the flap which was prolonged between the eye-brows and the internal angle of the eyes. This prolongation was extended to the point where the turning down and

twisting of the flap could be made without difficulty.

Three curved needles, with a single thread in each, were passed across the extremity of the little prolongation destined to make the lower edge of the cartilage, and around the loss of substance which had been made opposite the central point of the edge of the upper lip; and these three points of suture having been secured, this central portion of the bottom of the flap was adapted, and fixed the rest. Four similar points of suture were made on each side of the flap, and successively secured; they united the whole circumference, with the exception of the upper point formed by the pedicle. Everywhere the proportion of the thickness of the parts was exact, and their adaptation perfect without employing any other means.

During this part of the operation, the wound of the forehead was kept covered to prevent the blood flowing on the parts on which we were operating; it was afterwards dressed with simple dressing, some compresses, and a bandage.

The operation was concluded. We had taken great care not to make any useless waste of the forehead in a transverse direction, while we took, however, what was necessary to extend from one ala of the nose to the other. The distance was great, and when the flap was adapted, the transverse retraction which it experienced, and to which nothing was opposed, reduced its extent in that direction, to the interval which separated these two points in a straight line without any elevation; it seemed that this portion of skin was much too narrow, and only fit to form a sort of valve before the opening of the nose. The assistants thought that the operation would be unavailing, from this cause, and pressed us strongly to put some lint under the flap, in order to push it forward, and even to stretch it. We did not participate in their fears, and we yielded only from complaisance; we put behind the central point of the flap a few bits of lint, which we removed the next day without replacing them, lest by doing violence to the flap we should produce mortification. We had learnt to place confidence in the efforts of nature, and our confidence was not disappointed.

The operation was long and painful, owing to the minute attention which it demanded. Immediately after it, we gave the patient two grains of opium, which were repeated at night. He suffered pain for the first four hours after the operation. . . .

On the 1st of August, the traces of the engrafted nose were entirely lineal; and the resemblance or imitation of the original nose was the astonishment of every one who beheld it. The wound of the forehead was nearly cicatrised and the deformity arising from it very slight.

The portion of skin taken from the forehead, which was soft, undulating, like a valve without action or consistence, has acquired the density of a nose furnished with cartilage; and it is the adhesion of the cellular surface which suppurated, to which this astonishing change is alone attributable.

We will explain at a future opportunity our ideas on this singular property, which always manifests itself in parts which have been subjected to suppuration, and which is as curious as it is important, in directing our proceedings in a variety of interesting circumstances.

Upon quitting us, this young man went to Toulon, where he still resides, and where he has been an object of general curiosity and astonishment, so happily has nature been imitated in his artificial nose.

M. GARENGEOT'S STORY

(Reprinted from Lancet 1: 233, Nov. 16, 1823.)

Among the stories of adhesions of the separated nose, the following, which is related by* M. Garengeot, a French surgeon, whose high reputation procured for him a seat in the Royal Society of London in the year 1728, is one of the

* Dr. Balfour, of Edinburgh, has published a case of adhesion, almost as extraordinary as that related by M. Garengeot. On the 10th of June, 1814, a man came to him with half the index of the left hand wanting. Dr. B. inquired what had become of the amputated part. The man told him that it had been struck off by the stroke of a hatchet, and that he had never looked for it, but he believed it would be found where the accident happened. Dr. Balfour despatched a man, who accompanied the patient to search for it. In about five minutes, the man returned with the piece of finger, which was white and cold, and looked like a piece of candle. Without the loss of a moment, Dr. B. poured a stream of cold water on both wounded surfaces, to wash away the blood from the one, and any dirt that might adhere to the other, and then applied with as much accuracy as possible, the

most marvellous. "In the month of September," says M. Garengeot, "a soldier of the regiment of Conti coming out of L'Epée Royale, from an inn in the corner of the street Deux Ecus, was attacked by one of his comrades, and in the struggle had his nose bitten off, so as to remove almost all the cartilaginous part. His adversary perceiving that he had a bit of flesh in his mouth, spat it out into the gutter, and endeavoured to crush it, by trampling upon it. The soldier, who, on his part, was not less eager, took up the end of his nose, and threw it into the

wounded surfaces to each other. On the 2d of July the re-union of the parts was complete, and Dr. B. remarks that 'the finger was, in fact, the handsomest the man had;' an observation, which reminds us of the predilection of the wag, who, being condoled with on the loss of his leg, replied, that he was sorry for it too, for it was his *favourite* leg.

shop of M. Galin, a brother practitioner of mine, while he ran after his adversary. During this time M. Galin examined the nose which had been thrown into his shop, and as it was covered with dirt, he washed it at the well. The soldier returned to be dressed, M. Galin washed his wound and face, which were covered with blood, with a little warm water, and then put the extremity of the nose into this liquor, to heat it a little. Having in this manner cleansed the wound, M. Galin now put the nose into its natural situation, and retained it there by means of an agglutinating plaster and bandage. Next day the union appeared to have taken place; and on the fourth day I myself dressed him with M. Galin, and saw that the extremity of the nose was perfectly united and cicatrized."

(*Editor's note.* The above was first printed in M. Garengeot's book, *Traite des operations de chirurgie,* published in Paris in 1731.)

EXAMPLES OF REUNION OF PARTS TOTALLY SEPARATED FROM THE REST OF THE BODY

(Reprinted from Gazette de Santé, No. 9, Mar. 21, 1817.)

Sir:

The issue of March 1st of your interesting paper offers two examples of reunion of parts totally separated from the rest of the body. This physiological phenomenon is thus, today, well established, and one can, without exposing himself to the ridicule which was so unjustly directed toward Garengeot, report similar feats. Those with which I am going to entertain you are doubtless almost unbelievable, but they were attested to me by an eye witness, a man too high above the common man to let himself be deluded by old wives tales, General P . . . . , my brother-in-law, who was commander-in-chief of the troops ruled by Daoulet-rao-Scindah, long-time sovereign of the Mahrattas of Bérar.

Amputation of the nose being a punishment widely used in India, doctors have been searching all over the world for a remedy for this hideous deformity. Two methods are used to operate on a cut-off nose. The first consists of turning down on the nose a portion of the skin of the forehead, following the procedure you have described in your issue of September 1, 1816, and which has been employed with such success by M. Carpue, member of the Royal College of Surgeons of London. The second method consists of grafting, in place of the cut-off nose, a piece of skin and cellular tissue taken from the buttock.

A non-commissioned officer of cannoneers of the army of General P . . . . . had been particularly hated by one of his officers. Taking advantage of the absence of the general, and of a slight error the non-commissioned officer had made, this one cut off his nose. The unlucky mutilated one had recourse to the Indians known for operating to restore the nose. This is the process which they usually aimed for.

The amputation of the nose was already old and the wound had commenced to cicatrize. The borders were freshened. They chose a place on the buttock which they beat with hard blows with an old shoe, until this repeated percussion had produced a suitable inflation. They then cut from this inflated part a piece of skin and cellular tissue in a triangular form which they transferred to the wound of the nose, and which they affixed with adhesive plaster. This living graft reunited marvelously, and General P . . . . . had this man in his service a long time following this operation.

Another actual and extraordinary deed

came to me from the same source. General P . . . . . , traversing a friendly country, had strictly forbidden any kind of looting. Someone brought in a man caught stealing. The general ordered the thief's ear cut off instantly. This man was a Brahmin, as were nearly all the scribes attached to the Indian army, and this infamous punishment caused a great furore, which was appeased with money. Meanwhile it was a question of replacing the ear which had been thrown out and lost. An ear was bought from an outcaste. This was cut off and grafted to the place of the ear of the Brahmin; this graft united. One might remark, in passing, that in this circumstance necessity made the Brahmin forget the horror usually inspired by an outcaste.

Many attempts have been made to do grafts on animals. I, myself, did several experiments of this kind on rabbits. None of these united. This lack of success is probably due to the cause you have indicated. (See the March 1st issue).

H. Dutrochet, D.M.
Chareau, near Château-Regnault
March 5, 1817

RHINOPLASTIK

oder

Die Kunst den Verlust der Nase Organisch zu Ersetzen

DR. CARL FERDINAND GRAEFE

Berlin

(*Editor's note.* This, the first book on rhinoplasty, was published in Berlin in 1818. It was 208 pages in length and listed 55 previous articles and books on the subject, the most recent one being Carpue's work. The following two plates from Graefe's book may be of interest to the reader, as they illustrate the standards which were in vogue then, and for the next several decades, in rhinoplastic surgery.)

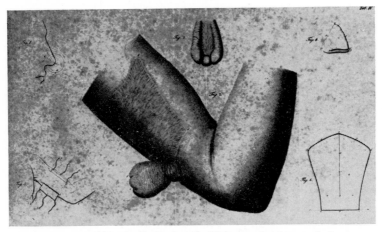

Fig. 2. Plate IV from *Rhinoplastik,* by Graefe. This was the first, and the most complete, illustration of the arm-flap rhinoplasty after the great work by Tagliacozzi. (Courtesy National Library of Medicine.)

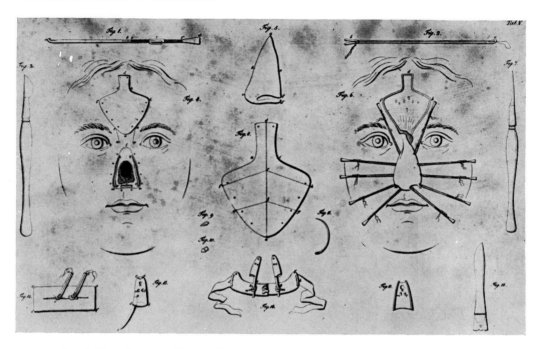

FIG. 3. Plate V from *Rhinoplastik*, by Graefe, illustrating his refinements and the status in 1818 of the "Indian" forehead-flap rhinoplasty. (Courtesy National Library of Medicine.)

SUCCESSFUL ATTEMPT OF RECONSTRUCTION OF A NOSE FROM A COMPLETELY SEPARATED PIECE OF SKIN FROM THE LEG

PROF. DR. BÜNGER, *Marburg, Germany*

(*Journal der Chirurgie und Augenheilkunde, 4: 569, 1822.*)
Translated from the German by

DR. HANS MAY

The main reason for my decision to select such an unreliable method of nasal reconstruction in a 30-year-old, unmarried, female patient, Wilhelmine M . . . , was a lupus which had been uncontrolled for 15 years and had destroyed the mobile part of the nose, the skin of the remainder of the nose, adjacent parts of the cheeks, inner canthi, and the forehead skin above the root of the nose. No other method was applicable because of the extent of the lesion.

In previous years I had succeeded in reconstructing a nose with parts from the cheek, but doubted if this were possible in this patient.

Six years ago I mentioned to the patient the possibility of reconstruction of her nose, news which she liked to hear. At that time the lesion was limited to the mobile part of the nose. I was thinking of a flap transfer from the upper arm, as all attempts by other physicians and myself to achieve epidermization were fruitless. Hence, the patient lived in seclusion in the country.

However, as soon as certain news of successful nasal reconstruction *via* Berlin* and England† (including my own successful case) reached the patient, she became encouraged. In spite of the extent of the lesion, reconstruction might be possible in her. She came to tell me that she was not afraid of pain and wished the reconstruction carried out. As desirable as this seemed to the brave, formerly beautiful, but now so desperate, girl, it seemed to me impossible to help her. Nevertheless, I decided to remove the diseased parts of the cheeks to test her healing capacity.

The cure was started by removal of a large (4-groschen sized) piece of skin from the right cheek, and two weeks later of a smaller piece of the left cheek. When, after a certain time, both attempts proved successful in obtaining barely visible scars and the lupus did not recur, I became encouraged (together with the patient) to dare more than this—to remove the remainder of the diseased skin of the upper lip and the lesion over the nasal bones and, perhaps, to replace the missing skin immediately with skin taken from other parts of the body.

I considered first the forehead flap for coverage, but gave up the idea—because it would not yield a sufficient amount of skin and, secondly, I was afraid of a purulent infection (the resulting scar of which might add to the patient's deformity). Flaps from the cheeks and the arm were also out of consideration because they would not yield enough skin either. I was also considering another

Editor's notes: *Von Graefe, C. F.: *Rhinoplastik*. In der Realschulbuchhandlung, Berlin, 1818.

† Carpue, J. C.: *An Account of Two Successful Operations for Restoring a Lost Nose*. Longman, Hurst, Rees, Orme & Brown, London, 1816.

subject as donor, but this seemed dubious because of the various difficulties of immobilization of two subjects, even if it were only for a short time.

Nothing remained open to me now except the Indian method, by which a full-separated piece of skin is taken out of the buttocks and transplanted to the nasal stump. I had great doubts about this method, as I believed that if the transplant were lost the patient would be left with a not insignificant amount of pain in the donor area. Finally, however, I decided to use a piece of skin from the gluteal area.

The operation was carried out on the 26th of June. I was assisted by my colleague, Ullmann. Changing my mind, I did not use the gluteal area as the donor site because difficulties in the healing process might be encountered from sitting and lying on the back. Instead, I chose the upper lateral area of the thigh which (according to the well-known advice to increase the vitality of the skin*) was lashed with a leather strap until it became red and swollen. Then, the diseased skin was excised over the nose, inner canthi, and above the root of the nose. This caused considerable pain and much bleeding. It took an hour to stop the latter.

The skin at the thigh was removed in an oval shape, 4 inches long and 3 inches wide. The removed skin consisted of skin and subcutaneous fat tissue. The graft was quite thick; therefore I reduced it by removal of one-half of the thickness of fat tissue. It then was cut according to the paper pattern. The flap became blanched, it looked almost white and lost its warmth. Bleeding of the recipient area had recurred in the meantime; it

*Editor's note: See Dutrochet's description of this being done in India (Plast. & Reconstr. Surg., 44:288, 1969). This pounding of the donor site was a European import from India and was pursued by Thiersch in 1874 (Ibid. 41:365, 1968) and Krause in 1893 (Ibid. 41:573, 1968) in doing free skin grafting.

took another one and one-half hours to stop it.

I then placed the piece of skin upon the raw surface in the form of a nose and fastened it with stitches, but it looked shockingly white. The area was now covered with a pressure dressing of fluffed-up white charpie.† The donor area was pulled together with adhesive strips. A veil was laid over the patient's face and I instructed her to cup her hands over it from time to time and exhale upward.

On the second postoperative day I found the eyelids and the entire facial skin swollen and the scars at the cheek a bright reddish color. I lifted up the charpie capsule over the transplanted skin and found the new nose white as chalk, but free of discolored places. In spite of the fact that the patient complained of a great deal of pain at the donor site, I did not dare to change that dressing because I did not want to dim the patient's hope concerning the final outcome of the whole procedure.

On the third postoperative day, my colleague, Ullmann, and I went to the patient's bed—firmly convinced that the flap had died completely and would have to be removed. But, how I would have loved it if the patient's relations and several of my colleagues had been present! I could not believe my eyes when I found the flap scarlet red and swollen, after we lifted up the charpie capsule. We physicians stared at each other in disbelief to see the change of color in the flap from chalk white to scarlet red. Only the lower part of the graft, which was to form the tip and alae, was partially bluish discolored.

I was now in doubt whether I should remove the stitches. It seemed that the fusion between graft and recipient area, judging from the redness of the entire graft, came from the base and not from

†Editor's note. Lint.

the wound borders. However, we did not have much confidence in the consolidation of the wound edges, due to the necrotic areas. Therefore, we removed only 4 stitches. I was now so excited about the whole thing that I decided to do everything to preserve as much as possible of the transplanted piece. I decided against dry dressings. We finally agreed to irrigate the charpie dressing with a decoction of china tea and sabina* to which camphor was added. This was done hourly and a piece of dry linen was placed over it.

On the fourth day the situation did not look so good any more. The redness was paler and the suspicous area of bluish discoloration had increased, rather than decreased. All stitches were removed, whereby the flap proved to be firmly adherent to its base, but the borders had become dehiscent.

On the evening of the fourth day, the bluish discolored area became covered with vesicles, as happens to necrotic skin in other parts of the body. On the fifth day I was glad to notice no further extent of the necrosis and demarcation of the dead areas. With continued use of the decoction, a beautiful trench of living pus became visible and the lower part of the graft, which was supposed to form the nostrils and the septum and the alae, began to separate in the form of a half moon. The process of demarcation was complete on the ninth day. The necrotic area could now be removed, with the exception of a small corner where the excision caused an escape of a few drops of beautiful red blood.

After removal of the dead part, the border of the piece that had taken showed nice granulations. It was most amazing that the center part of this piece

---

Editor's note. Probably savin oil, which is produced from the bitter, acrid tops of the sabina (Eurasian evergreen juniper tree), and which causes inflammation of the skin and mucous membrane.

overhung the lower part of the nasal bones—*i.e.* it overhung the nasal cavity so that the *spina nasalis* of the upper jaw was almost covered by this piece. The decoction was continued until the fourteenth day, until all necrotic tissue was eliminated. The wet dressings were later replaced by periodic use of Balsam of Peru, with the use of a china and camille tea decoction during the day, and zinc ointment during the night.

At the end of the fifth week, a well-formed, flat scar concluded the healing process. The lower overhanging rim healed first, but the scar of this raw surface caused a curling of the protruding part into the nasal cavity. I found no way of preventing this.

I may mention also the appearance of small pustules over the part that had taken which, however, disappeared immediately after application of the decoction. Found beneath was a layer of newly formed epidermis so that the whole area looked quite living and beautiful. Finally, fine, fuzzy hair appeared—as one finds it on the leg.

Although the end result of this method was not quite satisfactory, yet, from the physiological point of view, it was most remarkable. Even if the reconstruction of the nose was only partially possible, the case proved again that completely severed pieces of skin can become regenerated—even if the separation had lasted for hours.

The transplanted piece did not show any evidence of change during the next year, except that it became white. I tried to counteract this by advising the patient to expose this part to the sun, while blocking off the surroundings.

Amongst several traveling physicians who saw this patient in this condition was Henke of Erlangen, who advised Schreger to include this case in his textbook on surgical operations, *Grundriss der Chirurgischen Operationen* (1819).

I was in a dilemma how to help the patient further in reconstructing the nose, for this seemed to be impossible. One year later I did remove the diseased part of the upper lip and tried to reconstruct it, together with the nasal tip and alae. I used an arm flap for coverage. The flap was severed after 7 days. There followed some breakdown. I was pleased to demonstrate before many witnesses that there was a strong tip and septum, but unfortunately, no alae. The latter were reconstructed later on with pieces of adacent parts of the cheek and were connected with the thigh and arm pieces. This connection left an inconspicuous scar.

I shall publish a follow-up of this case later on and present the necessary illustrations to the public.

Prof. Dr. Bünger
University of Marburg
Marburg-am-Lahn
Germany

COMMENTARY BY THE EDITOR

Compared to today, communications were rather poor in the early years of the 19th century, but that may have had advantages. Those physicians who were thinking ahead, who were doing clinical research, were not inundated by oceans of trivial and repetitious literature.

In the quiet little university town of Marburg/am/Lahn, Dr. Bünger was Director of the Anatomy Institute and (of course) practiced surgery. He was quite aware of Carpue's rhinoplasties in London, of von Graefe's in Berlin—and, curiously, of the short tale of an Indian rhinoplasty published by Dutrochet in the Parisian *Gazette de Santé* (certainly an obscure item). The latter is the only known prior record describing the use in India of a free flap of skin and fat from the buttock to the nose, and the flailing of the donor site to produce hyperemia before removing the tissue. This may have been the first composite graft.

The intrepid little anatomy professor had a patient in need of a nose, and decided to try the "Indian operation." The paper that you have just read is one which is almost unknown today, but it forms a tangible link in the historical chain of plastic surgery.

Heinrich Christian Bünger was born October 11, 1782 in Braunschweig and died in Marburg on December 13, 1842. His academic career began at Halle under Loder, then in Helmstädt under Beireis. Under the latter's influence, he became a staunch admirer of truth and investigation—and an enemy of dogma. He was described at the time as "venturesome." In 1810, he became a prosector in anatomy at Helmstädt, and moved to Marburg in the same position in 1811. Later that year, he became a privatdozent in surgery at Marburg. In 1813 he became Director of the Anatomy Institute;

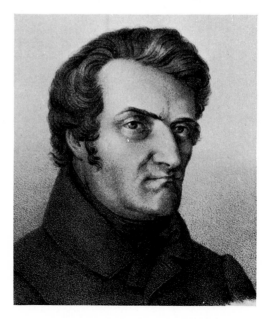

PROF. DR. C. H. BÜNGER

in 1815 he was made a full Professor of Anatomy. It was in this position that he wrote the above paper.

Later, he served for a time in various positions in addition to his posts in anatomy and surgery. These included Interim Director of the Obstetrical Service, Associate Professor of Medicine, Director of the Animal Welfare Service, Chief of Ophthalmology, Chief of Dentistry, and General Medical Advisor to the University.

The Anatomy Institute at Marburg was built according to Bünger's proposals and plans; during his life, it became especially rich in preparations demonstrating the nerves and the venous system.

Bünger has been described as a skilled and bold operator, possibly the first to ligate both common carotid arteries. In 1828 he published a work entitled "First successful removal of a common carotid aneurysm, with application of a ligature."

—FRANK MCDOWELL

Editor's note: The above material, and the drawing of Dr. Bünger, were made available by the kind assistance of Prof. Dr. W. Straub (present Dean of the Medical School) and Prof. Petry (present Director of the Anatomy Institute) of the Phillips-Universität, Marburg an der Lahn.

A Landmark Paper from America—The Beginning of Cosmetic Rhinoplasty

THE DEFORMITY TERMED "PUG NOSE" AND ITS CORRECTION, BY A SIMPLE OPERATION

JOHN O. ROE, M.D., *Rochester, N.Y.*

(Reprinted from The Medical Record, June 4, 1887)

The nose is the central and most prominent feature of the face; and on its shape, size, and appearance, to a great degree, depends the relative facial beauty of the person.

Physiognomists emphasize the importance of the nose in the category of anatomical conformations that are indicative of special traits of character; and regard it as a measure of force in nations and individuals.

Says Wells: "A skillful dissembler may disguise, in a degree, the expression of the mouth; the hat may be slouched over the eyes; the chin may be hidden in an impenetrable thicket of beard; but the nose will stand out 'and make its sign' in spite of all precautions. It utterly refuses to be ignored, and we are, as it were, compelled to give it our attention."

Even in ancient times much attention was given to its shape and appearance. Among the ancient Persians no man who had a crooked or deformed nose was allowed to sit upon the throne. Cyrus, it is said, had an asymmetrical nose, which was made a thing of beauty through the kind assistance of his emasculated attendants. In order to secure symmetrical and handsomely formed noses, in the children of the royal blood, the eunuchs who had charge of the royal offspring were accustomed to mould their noses into perfect shape (Mackenzie).

Considered from the profile point of view alone, noses are classified according to their shape by students of physiognomy into five main classes:

1. The Roman noses;
2. The Greek noses;
3. The Jewish noses;
4. The Snub or Pug noses; and
5. The Celestial noses.

These classes of noses, considered in the light of the characteristics of the race or class to which they are peculiar, are observed to indicate prominent traits of character, as follows:

The Roman indicates executiveness or strength; the Greek, refinement; the Jewish, commercialism or desire for gain; the Snub or Pug, weakness and lack of development; the Celestial, weakness, lack of development, and inquisitiveness.

"Le nez retroussé" of the French is applied to the Celestial nose, which is simply the pug lengthened and turned upward so as to form a gentle curve from the root to the tip.

The fact that the deductions of physiognomists almost completely harmonize with the anatomical and physiological facts in the case of the last two classes becomes striking, when we consider that those deductions have been made from observation alone.

Mr. Warwick says: "A snub-nose is to us a subject of most melancholy interest. We behold in it a proof of a degeneracy of the human race."

Tristram Shandy's father, regretting his son's misfortunes, remarked: "No family, however high, could stand against a succession of short noses;" and his grandfather "when tendering his hand and heart to the lady who afterward con-

Read before the Medical Society of the State of New York, February 1, 1887.

sented to 'make him the happiest of men,' was forced to capitulate to her terms owing to the brevity of his nose."

There are three conditions that may occur during the development of the nose that give it the appearance called snub or pug. They are: (1) excessive development of the alae and cartilaginous portions on the end of the nose; (2) a lack of sufficient development, or a sunken or flattened condition of the base and bridge of the nose, while the end of the nose may be but normally developed; (3) the combination, to a greater or less degree, of the conditions just mentioned. This last condition is the one most frequently found.

During development the nose and parts comprising the central portion of the face, as the ethmoid and sphenoid bones, and parts adjacent, are late in developing, and are also the last portions of the face to undergo ossification. At birth the nose, at its base and central portions, is flat and nearly level with the face, but later this depressed line is replaced by a more prominent one as the nose becomes developed. From this it will be seen that anything interfering with the proper development of these parts so as to cause them to remain in their infantile condition, while the end of the nose undergoes due development, will give the nose a snubbed and unsightly shape.

The best developed and most beautiful noses are one-third the length of the face. But noses often vary from this proportion, and in some instances an ill-formed nose is inherited, it being a special family mark. Ribot says, "that of all the features, the nose is the one which heredity preserves the best" (*Hereditary Traits*, Richard A. Proctor). But in other instances it is the result of diseased conditions affecting its growth and proper development during infancy and early childhood.

There are many conditions that operate to produce this result. The principal one is obstruction of the nasal passages which cuts off nasal respiration. During the inspiratory act of respiration and deglutition, when the nasal passages are obstructed, a partial vacuum is produced in the naso-pharynx. This suction force, being exerted on the inner side of the yielding cartilaginous nasal tissues, tends thereby to draw them inward, and thus in a corresponding degree retards or prevents their normal expansion and development. This obstruction of the nasal passages may also cause an enlargement or undue development of the portion of the nose below and beyond the obstruction, especially if this obstruction is composed of firm tissues, through interfering with the return circulation. The end of the nose thus becomes engorged, the vessels distended, and a marked thickening of the tissues takes place. The importance of attention to obstructed nostrils in infants, commonly called snuffles, is thus clearly demonstrated.

All chronic affections of the nose, even when unattended by obstruction of the passages, tend to produce by sympathetic irritation more or less congestion of the vessels of the end of the nose, and, by reason of these vessels having less power of resistance, an undue distention of them takes place; the surrounding tissues become thickened, and an enlargement of the end of the nose occurs. This is very commonly observed during the treatment of nasal diseases.

This diminished resistance of the peripheral vessels explains the effect of alcohol in the coloration and enlargement of the end of the nose in "old topers," which is so often observed. Alcohol produces congestion of, or sends the blood into, the capillaries and terminal blood-vessels. Since the capillaries in the nose have less resistance than the other superficial vessels of the face or

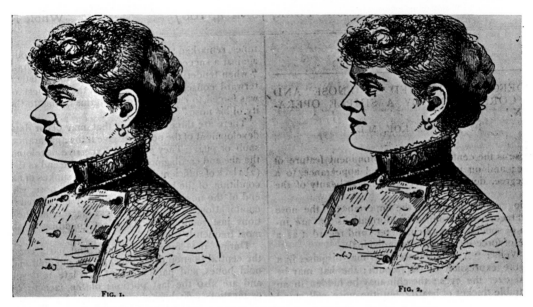

FIGS. 1 AND 2. (*Courtesy of National Library of Medicine, Bethesda, Md.*)

other parts, the effect of imbibition is first shown in the end of the nose.

A crooked or wrinkled septum will have the effect to lower the contour of the nose, as well as to cause an undue arching of the palatine vault.

A snubbed appearance may be given to the nose by injuries to its bridge or base, and also by ulceration and necrosis of the bones of the nasal chambers, especially the vomer, resulting in the removal of the support to the centre of the nose, which then falls inward.

The operation for the correction of the deformity under consideration is easily performed, although I can find no record of it, and have no knowledge of its having been proposed or performed.

It may be classed about the same as the operation for strabismus, and, like many other operations, is mainly to improve the personal appearance of the individual.

The operation consists in the removal from the end of the nose that tissue which is in excess, or which is disproportionate in amount to the other portions of the nose. In other words, we are to make the nose symmetrical from one end to the other.

In cases where the bridge is low and undeveloped, if the end is lowered, made smaller, and brought down so that the top of the nose forms a straight line from its base, or junction of the frontal and nasal bones, to the end, the nose ceases to be unduly noticeable or unsightly; and, although the nose will be smaller, it will appear much larger than before by reason of its being symmetrical and proportionate throughout.

The nose does not appear ugly by reason of the fact that its size is disproportionate to that of the face (for noses vary greatly in this respect), but by reason of the disproportionate relations to one another of the different parts of the nose itself.

In those cases in which the deformity consists in an undue enlargement of the end or cartilaginous portion of the nose, while the bony framework is normally developed, it will be seen that the main portion of the nose is straight until we come to the enlarged end, which suddenly tilts upward. Even in this class

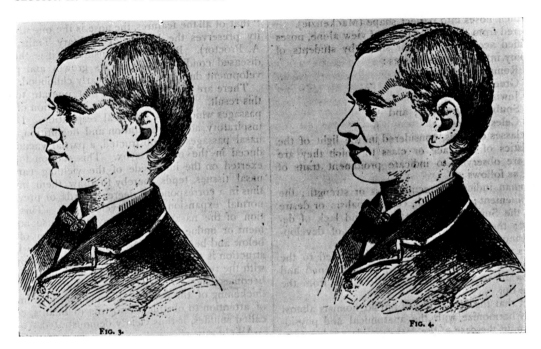

FIGS. 3 AND 4. (*Courtesy of National Library of Medicine, Bethesda, Md.*)

of cases it is not the end of the nose that really appears too large, but it is the base or bridge that appears too small or depressed.

This fact is shown by the foregoing illustrations, made from photographs taken in each case shortly before and shortly after the operation.

In Fig. 1 the bridge of the nose appears much lower than it does in Fig. 2, although it is of the same height. This is also true of Figs. 3 and 4.

The expression of the face in Fig. 2 is decidedly different from that of the face in Fig. 1. The same is also true of Figs. 4 and 3. This change is due entirely to the alteration made by removing the excessive tissue in the end of the nose. It will also be observed that in the case of the boy, excepting the nose, the features are the same in both pictures; and so in the case of the girl. This can be very easily demonstrated in the foregoing illustrations by comparing the shapes of the noses before and after the operation.

The operation is performed as follows:

We first deaden the sensibility of the interior of the end of the nose by cocaine (general anaesthesia being unnecessary) and then brightly illuminate this part.

If the tissue is to be removed from that portion where the mucous membrane is not too firmly adherent, the membrane should be dissected back, to be replaced after the operation.

The end of the nose is turned upward and backward, and held with a retractor by an assistant; then sufficient of the superfluous tissue is removed or dissected out to allow the nose to conform to the shape that we desire. Great care must, however, be exercised not to remove too much tissue, and also not to cut through into the skin, lest we may have afterward a scar or a dent in the external surface of the nose.

In some cases no after-treatment is required, but in others it is advisable to mould a saddle or splint, as it were, to the top of the nose, so as to make it, while healing, assume the shape we wish to obtain.

In some instances the large and unsightly end of the nose is not due to an excessive tissue but to a malformation of the cartilages of the alae, bulging outward with a corresponding concavity on the inside.

These noses can be very readily moulded into a handsome shape by cutting, with a small tenotomy knife, through these cartilages, in different places, sufficiently to destroy their elasticity. Then by inserting a silver or hard-rubber tube, of the proper size and shape, into the nostril, and conforming the saddle to the outside of the nose, we have it encased in an outside and inside splint that compels it to conform to the exact shape we desire.

While performing this operation and moulding the nose into shape, we must not neglect to preserve the nasal passages free and unobstructed.

Thus far I have performed this operation on five persons. I have, however, illustrations of but the last two, although all have been successful. With the first two patients it did not occur to me to have photographs of the nose taken before the operation, and the third patient would not permit it.

John O. Roe, M.D.
28 Clinton Avenue North
Rochester, N.Y.

COMMENTARY BY DR. JOHN MARQUIS CONVERSE

John O. Roe, M.D., LL.D. (1848–1915) was born at Patchgogue, Long Island in a family descended on both sides from English ancestors who were among the earliest settlers of Providence, Rhode Island. He graduated from the University of Michigan and received the degree of M.D. in 1870 from this University. Coming to New York, he matriculated at the College of Physicians and Surgeons, Columbia University, receiving his diploma in the class of 1871. After a year of graduate courses in New York, Roe entered upon the special practice of diseases of ear, nose, and throat in Rochester, New York. He soon recognized the necessity of additional training and to secure this went to Europe where, for a period of two years, he worked in clinics in Vienna, London, and Berlin, notably with Sir Morell Mackenzie. Returning to Rochester, he became laryngologist to the Rochester Hospital.

In 1887,[1] Roe gave this paper on an intranasal approach "without wounding the skin" for the correction of saddle nose deformity. In 1891,[2] the operation for the correction of what he termed "angular deformities" of the nose (hump nose)—also by a subcutaneous operation—was described by him.*

Roe appears to have been the first to describe the intranasal approach for corrective rhinoplasty. Aufricht,[3] in the first issue of *Plastic and Reconstructive Surgery* recounts the following incident: "An interesting and somewhat embarrassing incident happened when Jacques Joseph of Berlin, recognized as the foremost author of the principles and more or less classic methods of endonasal rhinoplastic operations, first presented his endonasal approach in Berlin in 1898. A physician from San Francisco, present at the meeting, afterwards told Joseph that two American Surgeons, Roe in 1887 and Weir in 1892, had used the endonasal approach previous to him. Unquestionably Joseph, who was a genius himself in this field, devised the method independently, making the report without knowing of the previous work of others."

In a paper entitled "The Correction of Nasal Deformities" published in 1908, Roe summarizes his experience and shows a

* *Editorial note.* This paper, which was really the first one on reduction rhinoplasty, is to be seen on pp. 131–135.

number of excellent results from various types of congenital and traumatic nasal deformities.[4] "There is no class of operations that demands in every case a more careful preliminary study of all the conditions presented—not only in respect to the abnormal state of the tissues to be operated upon, but also in respect to the possibility of obtaining the desired surgical result—than the operations required for the correction of nasal deformities." After reviewing the various causes of nasal deformity, Roe continues: "After this careful study of the cause and nature of the deformity, it is necessary to consider the possibility of obtaining the result desired in its correction and to advise intelligently as to the desirability of the operation and the probability of its being a success. It may be said on general principles that the correction of a deformed nose, in which so much is involved to both the patient and the surgeon, may be likened to matrimony, which 'should not be entered into unadvisedly or lightly, but reverently, discreetly, and advisedly.' "

"If the deformity of the nose is found to be associated with a local disturbance inside the nose, obstructing the passages, we should invariably remove or correct this local condition, whether it be deviation or thickening of the septum, enlargement of the turbinates, a polypoid or other growths, or even adenoids and large tonsils. To preserve perfect nasal respiration is of the utmost necessity, not only to the health and comfort of the patient, but to the satisfactory correction of the nasal deformity.

"While symmetrical relations of the different portions of the nose to one another are of the greatest importance, the symmetrical relation as to the size and shape of the nose to the general contour of the face must also be carefully considered, in order to approach the ideal from an artistic point of view.

"We are able to relieve patients of a condition which would remain a lifelong mark of disfigurement, constantly observed, forming a never-ceasing source of embarrassment and mental distress to themselves, amounting, in many cases, to a positive torture, as well as often causing them to be objects of greater or less aversion to others."

These quotations from Roe's writings could have been written in a present-day paper. Because of his technical skill and his esthetic sense, Roe achieved international fame. That he was amply recompensed for his surgery is suggested in the following letter written to my father, George Marquis Converse, M.D.

DR. JOHN O. ROE   28 CLINTON AVENUE NORTH
HOURS: 10 TO 2   ROCHESTER, N.Y.
                                         September 16, 1901

Dr. George M. Converse,
330 West 67th Street
New York, N.Y.
Dear Doctor:
    I am back from my vacation and have just received a letter from the father of the boy you wrote me about and whose pictures you sent me. He inquires about the assured success of the work and also wants to know the lowest cost. The expense attending such work depends upon the amount of work, also the nature of the work, which it is impossible to tell beforehand. Unless one takes one by the lump job it is impossible, especially without seeing the case, to give any where a correct estimate. There is as a rule much more work connected with these cases in order to bring about perfect result, than we count on beforehand, but I should say that as near as I can judge from the pictures and your description of the case, that $1000.00 would be a fair fee for a case of this kind, that is, taking it for granted that they are in comfortable circumstances. If they were wealthy they should pay considerable more. As you are well

acquainted with the people I write you for information in regard to them before replying to his letter.

By the way I wish you would kindly give me his name. Every word in his letter is perfectly legible but his name and that I am unable to make out with any degree of certainty.

Very truly yours,
John O. Roe

P.S. I have just discovered a printed card with his name on enclosed in his letter.

After 3 years of postgraduate study in Europe, my father decided to establish himself in the practice of medicine in New York City. He returned to his home in San Francisco two years later. It was during the New York period, in 1901, that he corresponded with Roe about one of his patients.

John O. Roe received many honors, in this country and abroad, but none touched him as much as the degree of LL.D. bestowed upon him two years before his death by his alma mater, the University of Michigan.

—JOHN MARQUIS CONVERSE, M.D.

REFERENCES

1. Roe, J. O.: The deformity termed "pug nose" and its correction by a simple operation. Medical Record, *31:* 621, 1887.
2. Roe, J. O.: The correction of angular deformities of the nose by a subcutaneous operation. Medical Record, *40:* 57, 1891.
3. Aufricht, G.: Development of plastic surgery in the United States. Plast. & Reconstr. Surg., *1:* 3, 1946.
4. Roe, J. O.: The correction of nasal deformities. Laryngoscope, October 1908.

RHINOPLASTY

A Short Description of One Hundred Cases

TRIBHOVANDAS MOTICHAND SHAH, L.M. *Junagadh, India*

(From the book by the same name, published by the Junagadh Sarkari
Press in 1889.)

Having had exceptional opportunities in the performance of rhinoplastic operations, I am enabled to put before the profession a brief account of some unfortunate cases of mutilated nose, their treatment and results. The Makrani outlaws, who carried on depredations against the Junagadh State for a period of nearly three years, had not unfrequently indulged in mutilating the noses of undefended and unarmed ryots* of villages. They have been only recently apprehended, and their unlawful career having been put a stop to, a cause of immense anxiety to the State and its subjects has ultimately been removed.

Mutilation of the nose is a practice for avenging wrong—real or imaginary—peculiar, I believe, to this country. No similar deeds are reported from Europe or America. In these countries loss of the nose is only a consequence of disease—chiefly syphilis. In other countries the chief modes of mortal revenge are homicide, either by poisoning, shooting, or wounding. But here, in this country, cutting off the nose is a special way of manifesting vengeance. Of all the organs of the body the nose is considered the organ of respect and reputation. The usual saying—when a person is told that he has no nose—means he has forfeited delicate feelings of honour. A person deprived of his nose is spoken of as a shameless fellow, and is looked down upon by society. A noseless person is not only thus execrated,

but is held as an unfortunate being, whose face ought not to be seen first on rising in the morning, or ought not to be confronted in the performance of propitious deeds and rites. Thus, people in India, who are deprived of their noses, feel the greatest humiliation; they try to shun society, and are even ready to sacrifice their life—no matter in what way the organ is lost, either by a natural disease or some criminal weapon.

In cutting off the nose, a razor, a knife, a sickle, or a sword has been used, and according to the sharpness of the instrument, the cut is a clean one or a ragged one. Besides these instruments, I have had a few cases in which teeth were the means employed. In one case the nose was merely lacerated, and in the others, a large portion of the nose was bitten right off.

Thus, according to circumstances, mutilation varies in its extent from the mere detachment of the tip of the nose, to the most thorough sweep of the whole of the soft parts of the nose. In the case of incomplete cuts, more or less of the cartilage of the nose is sliced away, both alae may be equally or unequally removed, and more or less of the septum and columna is also taken away. In the case of more complete cuts, the wound begins from the osseous bridge, the skin of which is sliced, besides a complete removal of the ala, septum, and columna. In some cases the deadly weapon encroaches more or less deeply upon the upper lip, and occasionally the cheek on one or the other side is also in-

* *Editorial note*. Peasants of India.

volved. Sometimes the injury extends to the lower lip and in one case (No. 76) besides the nose and upper lip the front upper teeth were excised. I have had cases of cut-nose of almost every variety and extent.

The resulting cicatrix causes varying degrees of disfigurement according to the extent of the cut. The free corner of the remaining ala has a tendency to be drawn up and inverted, and thus shortens the natural length of the nose. When the lip is wounded, it contracts during the process of healing and becomes everted, so as to expose the upper teeth and add materially to the ugliness of the lineaments of the face.

The apertures of the nasal passages have a tendency to diminution by the contraction, thickening, and inversion of their margins. In the case of a female Dhedh (No. 27) no trace of cartilage was left on the right, the cheek on which side was cut, and the right nasal aperture was

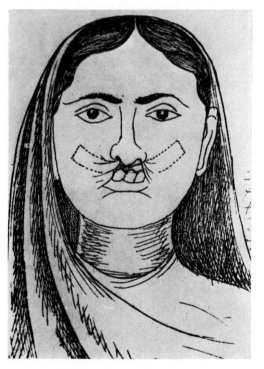

FIGURE 1

merely a small opening, outlined by a tense cutaneous border. The aspect of the face in such cases is hideous and shocking to a degree.

I have performed to date upwards of 50 Rhinoplastic operations, that is, formed more than 50 new artificial noses, besides some minor operations on the nose for trivial or separate injuries. For instance, a child was brought to the hospital with a very deformed nose by an accidental crush; the nasal bones were injured and discharged; the nose was consequently completely snubbed, the nostrils completely closed, and breathing was carried on through an opening in the middle of the flattened nose. The margins of this opening were pared and stitched, so as to close the aperture, and at the same time the passages of the nostrils were incised and kept patent by the introduction of plugs. In time, the pseudo-opening was closed, and the nasal passages restored, but the nose remained flattened. Several other noses were repaired for trivial wounds and bites. But noses which had to be repaired by a fresh skin flap were 24, from March 1886 up to the end of February 1887, and they are included in this paper. Among these, eighteen cases were due to the heartless Makranis, five cases were due to the callous hand of husband or paramour, and one owed its authorship to private feud and animosity. There were 19 males and 5 females.

METHOD OF OPERATION BY THE FOREHEAD FLAP

This includes the following steps: *1.* shaping; *2.* mapping; *3.* dissection; *4.* freshening the nasal margins; *5.* twisting and suturing; *6.* dressing; *7.* management of root.

1. First of all the proper shape of the lost nose is taken by means of paper. A piece of paper is placed on the nose, and part of the paper is cut answering to the shape and size of the lost nose. It is not so

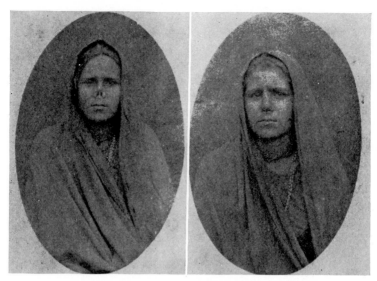

FIGURE 2

easy to cut paper of the required dimensions, as it may at first sight appear. Defects, which are not apparent when the paper is cut, become very evident when the nose is formed, and it requires some time and experience in acquiring tact for taking the proper measurements with paper. The key of success in Rhinoplasty lies in taking the proper form with paper. It varies not only with the actual loss of tissue in each individual case, but also according to the different shapes of noses. A natural nose may be small with rounded tip, or it may be large, with a thick and broad tip, or it may be thin and elevated, with sharp and elongated tip. Nostrils may also accordingly be rounded or narrow and triangular. The columna is measured with the flap. The columna ought to be of sufficient length so as to support the flap and preserve the natural height of the nose. The tip of nose is in-

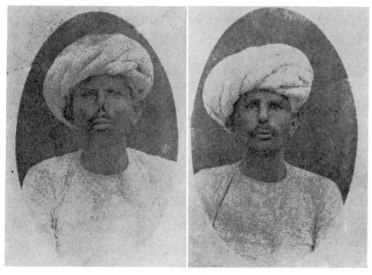

FIGURE 3

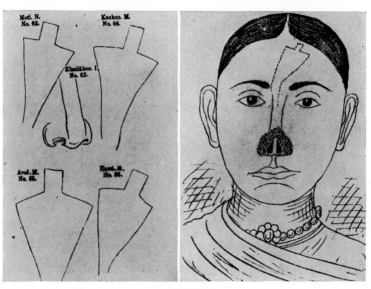

FIGURE 4

cluded in the columna. When the columna is short, the nose becomes acquiline. The angle between the columna and the flap should be, as a rule, obtuse and not a right angle. This affords a natural outline to the nasal aperture. It will be seen in most of the figures of forehead flap that the sides of flap on each side of the columna are standing. This allows the tip to be the most dependent portion of the nose.

2. After the paper measure has been framed, it is placed on the forehead and mapped out with ink lines along its edges. It depends upon the size of the forehead as to how the map is to be marked out. If the forehead is sufficiently broad, a vertical flap should be taken, which is likely to leave the smallest cicatrix. If it is narrow, an oblique flap inclined to one side or the other should be marked out. In many instances the flap (chiefly the columnar portion) extends into the hairy scalp, and I have included the hairy skin whenever unavoidable. Dr. Erichsen directs us to form the columna, even in the cases of forehead flap, from the upper lip by a subsequent operation. This appears to be unnecessary. The formation of a columna from the upper lip is, I have already pointed out, not without its drawbacks. In regard to it, the same authority says: "Indeed, this is the part of operation that I have always found most troublesome and requiring most attention."

3. When the patient is being anaesthetized, the scalpel is made to run lightly upon the lines, so that there may be no mistake in tracing them at subsequent stages of the operation. The flap is, when the patient is fully anaesthetized, dissected up. The former incision is deepened, and then with a few touches of the knife one corner is raised, and then the columna and the other corner are easily detached from the pericranium. Bleeding is effectually checked by haemostatic forceps and pressure with sponges. In most cases I have operated upon two patients at a time, and alternate dissection is carried on in one case while bleeding is controlled by pressure in the other. Time is thus greatly utilized. Dissection of the flap is thus carried on as it were in stages. It is desirable, I think, that time should be taken in dissecting the flap, so that circulation in the raised flap may have

sufficient time to be reestablished. When the flap is dissected I have watched it, in some cases, with great anxiety, as it felt cold and seemed dark livid. By degrees it attained again its natural colour and heat. The root of the flap is best left towards the inner corner of one or the other eyebrow, instead of keeping it in the central line. The incision to the side towards which the flap is turned should be a little lower. After the flap is dissected up to its root, it may be twisted over the freshened margins of nose, so as to see whether it covers the gap completely without undue tension. If it be found short or tense, a little further dissection will render it suitable to its new position.

4. After the forehead flap has been dissected, or during the intervals of its dissection, the margins of the mutilated nose have to be pared. Pinching the skin with artery forceps, a slice of the margin of the nasal aperture, is taken away from both sides. The skin or cicatrix over the prominent osseous nose is also detached. It is not carried as far up as the root of the nose. There is generally troublesome oozing of blood from the parts. The margins should be so pared as to be bevelled outwards. When the margins are bevelled outwards, the line of union is exquisite. When it is flat or inclined inwards, a groove is left at the line of union. The site, where the columna is to be planted, is also pared, and the margin of the septum should also be pared. Plugs should be kept in the nasal orifices, so as to prevent blood from passing inside the nasal passages.

5. When all bleeding has ceased, both from the flap and the vivified margins of nose, the former should be turned and applied to the latter, and united by sutures. Three or four silver sutures are required on each side, and two sutures for the columna. The first suture on each side should be passed, so as to bring the angle of the flap and nose together. In order to facilitate the introduction of sutures and also to avoid disturbance of the parts, while passing each separate suture, all the loops should have their respective ends entangled and kept loose; and when all sutures have been passed, they should be tightened one by one beginning with the lowest on each side— the columnar sutures preceding all. The columna should be so applied that its attached end may be raised upwards, so that its connection with the flap will form a nice tip of the nose. I used to apply one suture to the columna, but laterally I have applied with advantage two sutures, one at each corner of the columna. Care should be taken in stitching the angles of flap to the nasal corners, so that there may be perfect adjustment of level.

When more or less of the septum remains, it supports the nose flap, and gives it the natural lateral curve and central prominence of bridge, but in some cases no trace of cartilaginous septum is left, and even the osseous septum may have been mutilated. When there is no support in the centre, the new nose will be flattened out. A small pad of folded lint is therefore placed in the middle line over the margin of the osseous septum to afford central support to the flap. The flap will retain its shape, after it has been rendered stiff by inflammation and effusion.

The gap, in the forehead, left by the removal of the flap, is then to be shortened by applying sutures to the sides. The sides lowest towards the root and the highest corresponding to columna will be brought in approximation by sutures, and a more or less gap, according to the size of flap, will be left in the middle to be healed up by granulation. Harelip pins assist in narrowing the gap. The forehead wound takes the longest time to heal. The central ulcer often becomes flabby and elevated, and cicatrizes in the majority of cases very slowly.

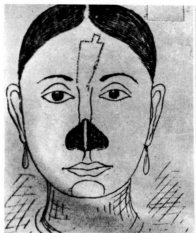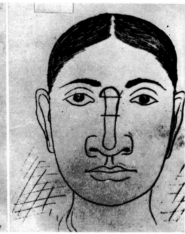

FIGURE 5

6. Rounded lint plugs are introduced into the nostrils. They will support the flap and aid in preserving the natural length of the columna. The thickness of plug varies with the size of the nostril. It ought to be about half an inch in length, and ought to be dipped in iodoform before introduction. Iodoform is then sprinkled over all the lines of the wound, and dry lint is put on. Adhesive straps are applied over all. It is satisfactory to record that secondary haemorrhage is rare, notwithstanding the immense vascularity of the parts.

On the next day after operation there is, in many cases, swelling of the lids and corners of the eyes, but it disappears in the course of four or five days. The first dressing is changed from two to ten days after the operation. If there be pain, tension, or suppuration, dressing is changed early; if there is no such necessity, it may be left undisturbed for days. Carbolic oil may be applied if there be particular stiffness of dressings. Sutures are removed after one or two weeks.

The secondary operation consists in first dividing the neck from the point of its attachment (vide Fig. 5, upper transverse line). A grooved director is passed underneath the free neck of the flap and the groove is directed obliquely upwards. It is then cut across by a bistoury passed along the groove with its edge turned upwards. On cutting across the neck, there is spouting of a blood vessel from the forehead side, which is not easy to be secured. A suture is applied, bringing the margins of the small wound together, so that bleeding is completely stopped.

The tail-end of the flap does not bleed immediately, but it looks blanched at first, and shortly when the tide of circulation is reversed, it begins to bleed. Next, its under-surface is excised as far down as it has become adherent to the nose. The amount of tissue to be sliced away depends upon the thickness of the tail and the prominence it forms upon the bridge of nose. Thirdly, the skin over the osseous bridge of nose, opposite the loose tail of flap, is excised, and a groove formed, to the edges of which the sides of the tail are stitched. In removing the skin of nose, two parallel longitudinal incisions are made and the lower end of the skin, thus marked out, is raised first, by transfixing it, and while excising this skin at its upper part, a small tongue of integument should be left. The end of the flap root is united with this tongue, so that the resulting union is very satisfactory. If no tongue is left and if the tip of the nasal groove is slanting or bevelled, the union of the end of flap is not entirely satisfactory. Before the points of suture are applied, the edges of the flap end should be pared and rendered regular. Sutures should be applied after all the bleeding has ceased. If haemorrhage continues, cotton or lint compresses may be applied, and the application of sutures may be postponed for the next day. After stitching, the usual iodoform and lint-dressing

and adhesive straps are to be applied. Instead of attaching the whole flap as directed by Dr. Bryant at the first operation, if the attachment of the tail of the flap is left for a secondary operation, at a subsequent period, the results are more satisfactory. Most of the noses after I adopted this method were excellent.

Tribhovandas M. Shah, L.M.
Junagadh Hospital
Junagadh, India

Mr. Shah was Assistant Surgeon and Chief Medical Officer at the Junagadh Hospital.

COMMENTARY BY DR. CHARLES PINTO*

Tribhovandas Motichand Shah was born in 1850 in a small town in the princely state of Junagadh. The odds were against him; he came from a poor home where life was a struggle for existence. Yet, out of the dim shadows of poverty and obscurity, overcoming obstacles, he literally earned his high school education.

Nineteenth century India was hardly the ideal place for a young man wishing to make a career in medicine. Everything was against him. There were only two medical schools in India at the time, one in Bombay, the other in Calcutta. The Licentiate of Medicine was the only qualification open to Indians.

Young Shah decided to make the trip to Bombay, a distance of about 400 miles; even the journey was an odyssey, involving such primitive forms of travel as camel-back. He enrolled in the Grant Medical College, Bombay, and obtained his Licentiate, only to come up against further frustrations— the absence of post-graduate training facilities, of opportunities for clinical experience, and (far more practical) problems of employment.

Dr. Shah, temporarily forced into a dead-end job of dispensing bottles of medicine in

a Government dispensary in the suburbs of Bombay, was undaunted. He migrated to Ahmedabad and obtained what clinical experience he could in a private hospital. Slowly, over a few years, he attracted sufficient attention for the Nawab of Junagadh to take a personal interest in him. The

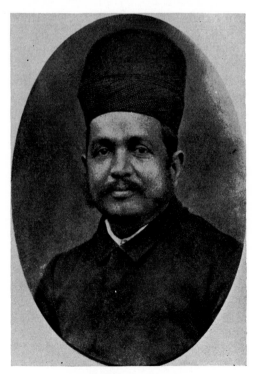

T. MOTICHAND SHAH

* Dr. Pinto is Honorary Professor of Plastic Surgery at The King Edward Memorial Hospital and the G. S. Medical College, Bombay, India.

Nawab induced him to return to Junagadh and appointed him Principal Medical Officer of the State Hospital there. Dr. Shah did not see himself in the role of a conquering-hero-returns-home. Instead, he saw his appointment as a splendid opportunity to work in a area of surgery that fascinated him—reconstructive surgery.

The opportunity proved to be a golden one; he had a wealth of clinical material at hand. The local gangster, Kadu Makrani, a notorious outlaw and public enemy No. 1 of the Nawab, had his equivalent to the latter-day gunning down of victims. He simply chopped off their noses!

The dacoit* must have been quite a terror, as the volume of work Dr. Shah could do was enormous. Indeed, in his introduction to his book, *Rhinoplasty,* he was to say that "within a comparatively small period of four years, I had the opportunity of performing more than a hundred rhinoplasties, a number that rarely falls to the lot of a surgeon during his lifetime." In fact, Dr. Shah performed more than 300 rhinoplasties.

The first record of his work was published in the Indian Medical Gazette (1888), soon to be followed by this monograph entitled *Rhinoplasty* (1889), which was illustrated with photographs and drawings of his labors. In using the median forehead flap and the cheek flaps, he actually initiated a renaissance of the techniques described by Sushruta (*circa* 500 B.C.) and Vagbhat (*circa* 400 A.D.) and also handed down to con-

Editorial note. One of a class of criminals in India and Burma, who robbed and murdered in roving bands.

temporary plastic surgeons the "Craft" of the legendary clay potters of Satara (around Poona).

We, today, can assess this contribution to modern plastic surgery for its intrinsic scientific value, but his reconstructive surgery was more than appreciated by the unhappy victims of the unpleasant brigand chief. There still exists a Gujarati proverb *"Kadu kape nak Tribhowandas Sande"* (Kadu, the local bandit cuts off the noses and Tribhowandas heals them). One can, therefore, understand Dr. Shah's popularity with the local population (folk songs were actually composed about his work).

One must also appreciate his versatility. He was a famous eye surgeon and did more cataract operations than he could keep count of. He wrote a treatise, *Advice to Expectant Mothers,* to educate his people on the value of maternal and child care. Finally, Dr. Shah wrote in Gujarati (the local language) *Sharir ane Vaidik Shastra,* a book on anatomy, physiology, pharmacology, and surgery. The outstanding feature of this was a comprehensive account of the pharmacological actions of Indian medicinal plants.

Dr. Shah died at the age of 54 years, of coronary thrombosis. He left two monuments. (1) He had carved 10,000 steps into a mountain face for pilgrims to reach a Jain temple, his personal expression of a deep commitment to his religion. (2) His work in rhinoplasty, which was his personal legacy to plastic surgery.

Dr. Charles J. Pinto
Pinto-ville, Dadar
Bombay 28, India

The First Reduction Rhinoplasty

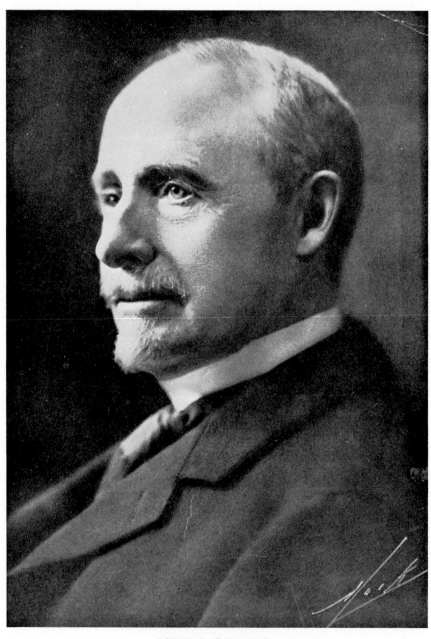

JOHN O. ROE, M.D.
(Courtesy of Rochester, N.Y., Academy of Medicine)

THE CORRECTION OF ANGULAR DEFORMITIES OF THE NOSE BY A SUBCUTANEOUS OPERATION

JOHN O. ROE, M.D., *Rochester, N. Y.*

(Reprinted from The Medical Record, July 18, 1891)

At a meeting of this Society four years ago I presented, as you may remember, a paper on "The Deformity Termed Pug-nose, and its Correction by a Simple Operation." *

It is my purpose to describe to you, in this short paper, an operation for the correction of angular deformities of the nose by a subcutaneous operation. This is an operation for the correction of a condition directly opposite to that deformity which formed the subject of my previous paper, and is applicable not only to the correction of angular deformities of congenital origin, but to the deformities resulting from injuries as well.

In all surgical operations about the face, it is as necessary to avoid mutilation of the skin as to correct deformity, since in many instances an operation might otherwise simply result in exchanging a deformity for an unsightly blemish. It is for this reason that many deformities of the face, and particularly of the nose, are allowed to go uncorrected, which are a *marque de reconnaître* for every one who sees them, and a constant source of annoyance to the persons themselves.

In describing the technique of this operation, I cannot make it more clear than by briefly reporting some cases in which I have performed the operation. Miss C_____, aged twenty-five, consulted me for a "winter cough," which was giving her much concern. While she was under treatment she often referred to her nose, and complained about an angular, bony projection on its top that not only gave her nose an unsightly shape, but so pierced the skin as to make it painful for her to wash or wipe her face. She was quite desirous of getting rid of this annoying projection, but was afraid an operation might leave an unsightly scar. In order to avoid this possibility, I suggested that the projection be removed by an incision from the inside of the nostril without wounding the skin, and this suggestion at once induced her to have the operation performed.

After anaesthetizing the part with cocaine, both by applying it to the interior of the nostril and by injecting some under the skin with a hypodermic syringe, I made a lineal incision completely through the upper wall of the left nostril, just in front of the nasal bone, between it and the upper lateral cartilage of the nostril, to the under side of the skin. This incision I widened laterally from the insertion of the upper border of the triangular cartilage half-way down the side of the nose, until I had a sufficiently large opening to permit the introduction of instruments freely. I then raised the skin from the bridge of the nose over the region where the operation was to be performed. After the skin was sufficiently freed from the top of the nose I inserted a pair of angular bone-scissors and cut off the projecting piece of bone until the top of the nose was perfectly straight and smooth. The operation was done with the

* Medical Record, June 4, 1887.

Read before the Medical Society of the State of New York, February 6, 1891.

strictest antiseptic precautions, and after completion I blew in some iodoform powder, through the opening, over every portion of the wounded surface. The skin was then allowed to drop back upon the bridge of the nose, and, by strapping it down with gentle pressure, the wound healed without the slightest formation of pus, and there was very little soreness. There was no mutilation of the interior of the nose, for even directly after the operation it was difficult to detect, by simply inspecting the interior of the nose, the incision that had been made. In a few days the nose was entirely healed, and the soreness had disappeared when the patient left for her home. About six weeks afterward she wrote me that she was highly delighted with the result. She no longer had to be constantly on her guard lest she should allow something to come against her nose, and she said that it felt as if she could beat it against a stone wall without hurting it.

Figs. 1 and 2 represent the appearance of the nose from photographs taken before and after the performance of the operation.

The second case was that of a young lady on whose nose I operated for a similar deformity, and in the same manner, and with a like excellent result. See Figs. 3 and 4, which are also from photographs taken before and after the operation.

The third case, an exceedingly interesting one, was for the correction of a deformity, resulting from an injury, the details of which are as follows: Mr. M_____, a gentleman residing in a neighboring city, was out one day on horseback. His horse, being very spirited, suddenly shied at a piece of paper flying in the street and threw him violently to the ground, directly under the horse's feet. The horse at the same time struck him with a shoe cork of one of its forefeet, directly in the centre of the top of his nose, producing a very severe fracture. His family physician, who was an excellent surgeon, was at once called. He found the nose so badly broken up that portions of the nasal bones were lying loose in the gaping wound. These he picked out, and after thoroughly cleansing the wound, brought the different portions of the lacerated skin together as well as possible, and carefully applied an antiseptic dressing. The following day the doctor telegraphed me to come and see the patient. I found the nose in as good shape as circumstances would permit. The vomer was, however, broken

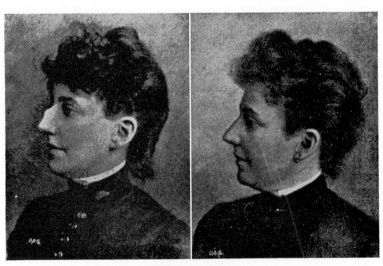

FIGURES 1 AND 2.

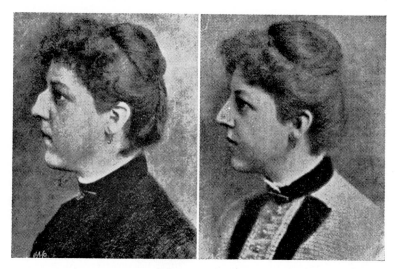

FIGURES 3 AND 4.

and crowded out of place. The swelling of the nose and face was by this time so great that it was not advisable to attempt any active interference lest it should prevent or disturb the healing of the lacerated skin.

In about five days the swelling had so much subsided that the real condition of the nose was apparent, and he then came to Rochester for further treatment. The septum was put in place, and held there by means of metallic splints wound with cotton; but it soon became apparent that the support to the bridge of the nose was so completely undermined, the lower portion of the nasal bones being destroyed, that the nose was quite sure to fall in, unless proper support could be applied at the right spot from the inside. The plan of transfixing the nose with pins to hold it up in place could be of no avail in this case, so the following plan was resorted to: A piece of brass spring wire was bent to form a spiral spring as shown in the illustration (Fig. 7). One arm was bent to lie along the floor of the

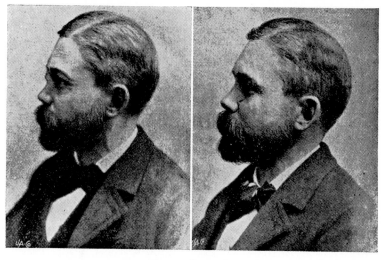

FIGURES 5 AND 6.

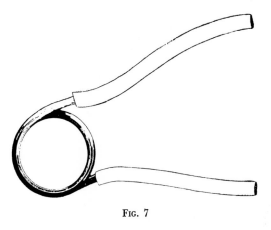

FIG. 7

nose; the other was bent to fit under the bridge of the nose. These arms were covered with snugly fitting rubber tubing, so as to make them soft and to prevent erosion. The arms were bent together before insertion, but when allowed to open they exerted an upward pressure, with the floor of the nose for the fulcrum or support. One of these springs was inserted into each nostril. This plan worked admirably. It kept the bridge of the nose elevated as high as the amount of tissue left would permit until the broken septum had become firm and the other parts healed so that the nose was self-supporting. This patient, before the accident, had a fine Grecian nose, but the loss of a large portion of the nasal bones converted it into *le nez retroussé*. The nose was, however, rendered very unsightly and conspicuous by the angular projection of the stumps of the nasal bones, where they were broken by the horse's shoe.

The operation for the removal of this projection was deferred for several months, in order that the nose might become thoroughly healed and firmly fixed in position.

On June last, the operation for the removal of this projection was made. As an impediment to the operation, however, there was the scar in the skin that

had become firmly adherent to the bone at the seat of the injury. This was thought to be an insurmountable obstacle to the success of my proposed operation.

I made an incision, similar to that described in the previous case, through the upper wall of the nose from the inside, to the under side of the skin; then with a very delicate knife, having a round, slender shank, I very carefully dissected this adherent skin from the bone, without cutting through the skin at any point. After the skin was raised from every portion to which it had become adherent, and also from that portion which was to be removed, I cut and drilled away the bone down as far as desired. The operation was done antiseptically, so that no inflammatory trouble followed, and the result was satisfactory in the highest degree. The skin has remained free and movable over the bone, and the scar of the skin is scarcely visible. The use of cocaine locally to the nostril and injected under the skin rendered the operation quite painless.

The patient, as you will observe by the cut (Fig. 6), which is from a photograph recently taken, has a very presentable nose, quite as good as could be hoped after so severe an injury. Fig. 5 represents the appearance of the nose before the operation.

Since the above-described operation was performed I have operated on two patients for angular deformity of the nose, with most excellent results in both cases. In one case the deformity was congenital; in the other it was the result of an injury incurred when the patient was quite young.

For the performance of this operation the application of cocaine to the interior of the nose, and injected under the skin, is, in nearly all cases, sufficient to render the operation quite painless, although general anaesthesia can be employed should it for any reason be necessary.

This operation is readily seen to be of great value in the correction of all kinds of angular deformities of the nose, from whatever cause, since it avoids all necessity of wounding the skin, and no after-treatment is required, other than the use, for a short time, of a light compress or bandage over the seat of the operation.

John O. Roe, M.D.
28 Clinton Avenue North
Rochester, N.Y.

Editorial note. The illustrations for this article were reproduced through the kind assistance of Dr. John Blake, National Library of Medicine.

EDITORIAL ADDENDUM

There is no doubt that this was the first description of a reduction rhinoplasty to enhance the appearance of a patient. It was, as can be seen, a crude and primitive procedure—but it was a beginning.

Dr. Roe's interests were varied. His last paper was on "Phlegmons of the Upper Respiratory Tract" but one of his obituaries states that he had "an especial reputation in plastic surgery of the nose." Another one notes that he had "an international reputation as a surgeon in affections of the eye, ear, nose, and throat, and more recently had been particularly successful in plastic work." He was a Fellow of the American Medical Association and of the American College of Surgeons, a founder of the Rochester Academy of Medicine, a member of the New York Academy of Medicine, and at one time was president of the American Laryngological Society. From the brief obituaries that one finds on him, however, it would appear that he was not particularly well known as a surgeon and that his work on rhinoplasty was relatively obscure.

For a time, it was thought that no good likeness of Dr. Roe existed; later it was found that the Rochester Academy of Medicine had a large sepia portrait of him on display. That likeness is reproduced here for the first time (by the courtesy of Mrs. Helen C. Frauel, Executive Director of the Academy).

—Frank McDowell

ON RESTORING SUNKEN NOSES WITHOUT SCARRING THE FACE

ROBERT F. WEIR, M.D., *New York, N.Y.*

(Reprinted from New York Med. J., *56:* 443, 1892)

The recent surgical endeavors to restore a sunken nose, whether this has occurred from traumatism or from the ravages of syphilitic disease, have, where the loss of support has involved the cartilaginous septum, proved so far unsatisfactory. Among the many attempts that have recently been put forth to overcome such deformities, the plan proposed by König and modified by Israel* has so far proved the best. It is, however, open to the objection that this procedure, as well as almost all the others that have been suggested, gives rise to a very serious and very disfiguring scarring of the face.

Israel's operation consists in that, at first, the cartilages and the extremities of the nose are separated by a transverse incision from the sunken bridge to allow the tip of the nose to resume its normal level, and then a frontal flap is detached from the forehead. This latter is composed of the skin, periosteum, and a layer of bone, which is separated by a chisel, turned down without twisting and with the skin surface beneath into the nasal gap, and sutured around the lowered extremity of the nose. The sides of the resulting gap in the forehead are also stitched together as far as possible. The exposed surface of bone in the transplanted portion, now looking forward, becomes in time covered with granulations, and finally by a cicatrix which, as it contracts, draws the skin on its edges

* Archiv f. klin. Chirurgie, *36:* 373.

inward so that the resulting scar is diminished to two thirds of its original width.

When the parts are soundly healed, the surgeon proceeds by a second operation to close the cleft on the lateral aspects of the nose. These are made beneath the skin of the sunken part of the nose and above the turned lower part of the frontal flap. The transplanted portion is drawn to one side with a sharp hook, and the skin over the old bridge of the nose is divided in the median line and a quadrangular flap detached by means of two transverse incisions made at the upper and lower extremities of the longitudinal one. The cutaneous cicatrix of the transplanted portion is now turned outward and the pre-formed flap from the sunken portion is applied to its raw surface and sutured in place. The opposite side is subsequently treated in a similar fashion. This completes the operation.*

* Israel, in the *Deutsche med. Wochenschrift,* January 14, 1892, admits that his method, even where successful, is attended by three drawbacks—viz., that the hollow between the forehead and nose is obliterated; that the nose itself is broadened; and that a more or less wide cicatrix longitudinally scars the nose.

He has, therefore, modified somewhat his procedure. The pedicle of the nasal flap is cut through at the end of three weeks and so deeply inserted in the subjacent skin that the physiological sinking between the glabella and the root of the nose is restored. He finally draws the lateral flaps of skin at his final operation so far toward the median line over his transplanted bone as to cover the same in this way with skin. To do this satisfactorily, however, one should, in cutting the forehead flap, make the skin and periosteum cut broader than the bony piece, so that this latter could, so to speak, be entirely enveloped by skin when in its new place.

From the College of Physicians and Surgeons and the New York Hospital.
Presented at the meeting of the New York Surgical Society on January 13, 1892.

Besides the scar that is the unavoidable result of this operation, there is a disappointment not infrequently met with in that the small portion of bone detached from the os frontis and carried downward in the flap to fill up the gap of the sunken portion of the nose becomes absorbed and disappears, resulting in a reproduction of the deformity. This I have seen occur in two instances, and I now show to you a patient in whom this mishap occurred.

It is not difficult to overcome the deformity which results from the flattened bony ridge of the nose by division by a chisel of the ossa nasi, first in the median line and subsequently at the line of their attachments to the superior maxilla, or by the use of forceps, to fracture their attachments to the same bone. The sunken bridge can then be raised and held *in situ* readily by a pin crossing the nose and secured by clamping on it a shot at each end, pressure on the shot clamp being guarded against either by the interposition of a small pad of iodoform gauze or, what I like better, of a small square of a

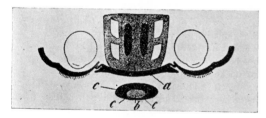

FIG. 1. *a*, the skin of the sunken nose; *b*, the frontal osteo-cutaneous flap, skin surface beneath; *c*, the cicatrized raw surface of *b*.

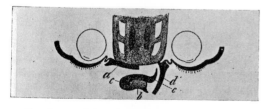

FIG. 2. *a* and *b* as in Fig. 1; *c*, the turned-down skin flap from the transplanted osteo-cutaneous portion, confronting a refreshed surface; *d*, corresponding to that of the raised skin of the originally sunken part of the nose.

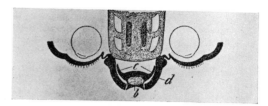

FIG. 3. The operation completed on both sides.

thin shaving of sterilized cork. This little retention apparatus can easily be worn from five to ten days without giving rise to any perceptible scar.

The chiseling of the sunken nasal bones can either be accomplished by a small incision, beveled in its character, through which a narrow engraver's chisel can be introduced, and the section then be made from without, or the section of the bones in the median line and laterally can be accomplished, but with a little more difficulty, without any external incision, by the chisel being carried up through the nasal passages. If an external incision is made, the little mark—thanks to the suggestion of Packard, of Philadelphia, of making it of a beveled nature— is quite imperceptible. But when we come to the question of the restoration of the sunken central cartilage, I have considered until recently that such an improvement was one of the most difficult things in nasal surgery, and I was not sufficiently pleased with the plan I presented in 1880* of taking flaps from the cheek to continue it further. Another procedure was therefore tried in the following case:

Four years ago a young man, about twenty-six years of age, with a history of syphilis, presented himself to me with a nose sunken to a level of his frontal prominences from depression of the nasal cartilages and bones from the aforementioned affection. His right ala nasi was doubled in on itself and was almost obliterated, while his left one projected markedly forward (Fig. 4).

* See Medical Record, March 13, 1880. Weir: On the Relief of the Deformity of a Broken Nose by some New Methods.

Upon cogitation, I submitted to him the difficulties of the case and said that I was willing to resort to experimental surgery upon him to be conducted in the following manner: I entertained then the idea, following upon the gratifying results that had occurred in the insertion of bones belonging to another individual, as had been successfully practiced by Macewen and Poncet, that in the present conditions a bony support might be inserted under the nasal skin and left there, with the hope that the same might become organized and form a permanent portion of the man's economy. After some deliberation I concluded that the breast bone of a fowl, from its angular shape, would best imitate the form of the nose and give the most satisfactory support. I determined, therefore, to use the same in this patient's case, but I considered it essential that both sides of the bone used should have vascular supply, and, moreover, that the new bone that I introduced should not be exposed at any point in the nasal cavity.

A triangular incision was therefore made in October, 1889, with the apex meeting just above the ends of the nasal bones and its legs running down on each side to the base of the ala nasi. The incision was made into the skin tissue, but not into the cavities of the nostril. The knife was then so employed as to split the skin belonging to the tip of the nose and the alae in a downward direction, and also similarly in an upward direction nearly to the level of the frontal bones. This was accomplished without entering the nasal cavity, save in one small spot which was closed afterward by catgut sutures. I had prepared in this way a bed for my bone, and had, at the same time, skin of sufficient thickness and looseness to cover over the new piece of bone after it had been inserted. At this period of the operation a young duck which had been chosen was killed, and its breast bone, deprived of periosteum, was cut into a shape of nearly an inch and a half long. The angular character of the bone was preserved by taking the projecting vertical sternum of the duck for one side of this new nasal support and one of the attached lateral portions for the other side, cutting away the second lateral portion as not being required. This gave me a triangular portion composed of two very thin layers of compact structure of bone.

I will ask attention later to the character of the support, which was trimmed in such a way on its sides that the broader portion was fitted downward and its narrower portion was at the upper end and rested upon the nasal bone. The skin accommodated itself without any tension over it and was secured by sutures. The restoration of the nose was remarkably satisfactory (Fig. 4).

Three weeks passed. The patient's delight was great, and mine was greater. Unluckily, soon after, he complained of an increased discharge from his nose, and I felt, by means of a probe introduced through the nostril, that the lower layer of tissue which I had carefully preserved had yielded at a small point. At the end of the seventh week a swelling appeared at the root of the nose, culminating in a little abscess which discharged and left a persistent ulcer. In brief, at the end of eight weeks I felt that my procedure was not a success, and thought it was necessary to remove this foreign body. I reopened the old incision, exposed the bone on its right side first, and appreciated that on its left side there had been a good many firm adhesions of the bone to the tissue, and resolved that I should only take away the right portion of the bone, which was undoubtedly loose and useless. Unfortunately, in my endeavors to divide the bone along its central portion so as to leave in the left half of it, I could not avoid such an amount of motion as to loosen considerably this portion of the support. Two weeks later, as a result, I think, of this surgical traumatism, I was compelled to remove the left half also.

The examination of the first portion removed, as well as the second one, showed that in numerous points along the edges vascularization had advanced to a distance of as much as half an inch into the substance of the bone. Along the portion which corresponded to the free border of the nose, whence the bone had been cut at the time of the operation, there was also vascularization running similarly into the substance of the bone.

It seemed that if my selection of a bony support, instead of being two thin layers of the compact structure, without any cancellar bony tissue, had been one where the conditions were more equalized or reversed, or if, perhaps, instead of such a large piece in an intact condition, there had been put in one that had numerous perforations in it, so that the vessels could have reached the more distant portions of bone, success might have been achieved. The outcome of the case was simply that by the V-shaped incision the tip of the nose had been dropped down nearer to a level, and also by the

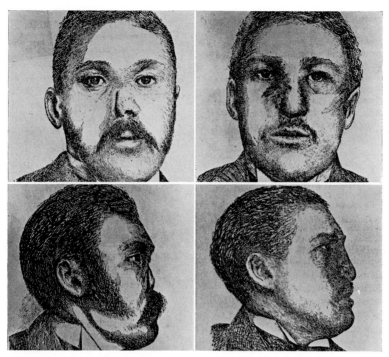

Fig. 4. (*above*) A young man, about 26 years of age, with a history af syphilis and a sunken nose. (*below*) After operation. Implantation of a duck's sternum.

inflammatory action set up by the procedure an increased thickening of the nasal tissue had resulted, which persisted for a year afterward and which caused, in the patient's estimation, a decided improvement over his original condition.

I was prepared in January, 1891, to repeat this operation, with the above modifications, in the person of a young woman, twenty-four years of age, who had a somewhat similar condition, though to a less degree, caused by syphilis, with total destruction of the septum. Her appearance is well represented in the accompanying figure (Fig. 6). I, however, learned from a work which then came to my notice, entitled *De la prothèse immédiate,* that its author, C. Martin of Lyons, had remedied this deformity in several cases by the use of an internal support of platinum, and that the procedure had received the distinguished indorsement of the celebrated Ollier of Lyons.

Martin, in this work, gave the details of three cases where, after the nose had been separated from within the mouth from the bony parts immediately surrounding the nasal aperture, a support of narrow platinum had been inserted, one leg of which rested upon the nasal bones and the other two legs had, by sharpened points (Fig. 5), been inserted into the superior maxillae on each side just within the line of the alae nasi. On this support the restored nose lightly rested. No external incisions were resorted to whatever. No inconvenience resulted from the retention of this narrow piece of platinum, and in the reported cases the patients had worn the support for two, three, and four years, respectively. Platinum is, as is known, an inoxidizable material, unirritating, strong, and capable of being soldered, in which latter point aluminum, which might be thought of, is defective. Therefore, in the case which was then under my considera-

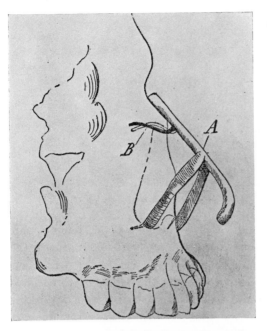

FIG. 5. Martin's platinum support for a sunken nose.

jaw cut through and the nose separated from the periphery of the osseous opening of the nasal cavity up to the middle of the nasal bones.

A platinum support,* made for me by the skillful hands of a dental friend, Dr. S. L. Benson, and depicted in Figure 5, was introduced, the broad portion resting on the nasal bones and the two upper wires soldered to it, passing laterally up under the nasal bones. This was resorted to so that the support should not be tilted away from its bony support at this point. Two little openings were made on each side of the alae in the superior maxillae by means of a fine awl, and the pointed ends of the lateral legs of the platinum support were inserted therein. (These lateral portions should be above the level of the alae so as not to interfere with their muscular motions.) The lifted-up nose was then allowed to sink on these supports, which was accomplished without any traction or pressure.

One or two stitches were made in the line of the incision of the mucous border of the mouth, and within a week the swelling which resulted from the operation had passed away and the success of the operation, so far as concerned the sufficiency of support, was demonstrated. The

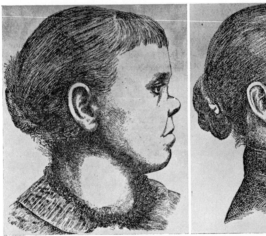
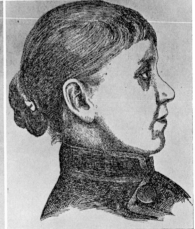

FIG. 6. (left) A young woman, about 24 years of age, with total destruction of the saeptum caused by syphilis. (right) After the insertion of Martin's nasal supporter.

tion I determined to test the efficacy of this method.*

On February 9, 1891, this procedure of Martin's was carried into effect. The upper lip was raised and its mucous attachment to the

---

* Of which Ollier (Revue de chirurgie, 1890, p. 828) said that he preferred the sample autoplasty over the metallic apparatus of Martin to the use of osseous or periosteal flaps.

patient has now worn this for nearly a year without the slightest discomfort, and, without being exactly a thing of beauty even in the improved condition, is a source of joy to herself from that time to this. The platinum support

---

* These should be, according to Martin, half a millimetre in thickness and seven millimetres in width. These are curved on themselves and soldered together by gold solder, or sometimes cut in one piece.

can be seen by inspection through the nostrils. It is firm, gives rise to no trouble or discharge whatever, no tenderness, and the patient would not know it was there unless she had been told of it or had discovered it by digital examination. I have resorted to the method twice since with equally favorable results. In the second case the patient has worn the support eight months without irritation. The last case, one week old, is shown you this evening.*

Some few more words may be permitted in connection with this department of surgery. In 1885, some time prior to the publication of Roe's able article on the subject of The Deformity termed Pug Nose and its Correction by a Simple Operation (Medical Record, June 4, 1887), wherein a similar procedure is advocated—

I was called upon to relieve the distress that was occasioned in the mind of a gentleman well known in social circles by the presence of a nose which he considered with some justice (Fig. 8) to be unduly large. This goodly sized organ was intensified by a somewhat receding chin and diminutive mouth. He had become so much perturbed in mind concerning the unsightliness of his nose that it became more than an operation for the relief of a cosmetic annoyance. It seemed to his physicians and relatives essential to the preservation of the balance of his mind that some attempt should be made to relieve him of what he persistently dwelt upon as a distressing deformity. With the consent of his attending physicians, Dr. Satterlee and Dr. Polk, I took out a triangular portion of the saeptum narium (Fig. 8), fully a quarter of an inch in width at the columna, its apex running up and encroaching upon the ethmoid saeptum. The nose, moreover, at this point was forced downward toward the face and the cartilage and the divided columna sutured together by fine sutures. To accommodate this sinking of the nose, by means of my nose forceps† (one blade inside the nose and the other outside), the nasal bones at their lower borders were also crowded backward and inward and then to a slight degree flattened.

This operation was done with most gratifying success (Fig. 8). The nasal prominence at the

* In this case a variation in the support was made, as seen in Fig. 7. The plate of platinum is shorter, less than an inch in length, and the legs were made of sharpened, hard platinum wire.

† Medical Record, loc. cit.

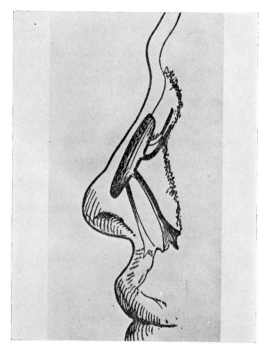

FIG. 7. A modification of Martin's nasal supporter, to be used when the nasal end is firm and only the central part requires elevation.

tip, particularly the unsightly portion in the otherwise fairly straight nose, was diminished, and the patient's mental relief was correspondingly great for a time. However, at the end of a couple of months, with the aid of incessantly looking at himself in the glass, he arrived at the conclusion that something more should be done to his nose—this time that the slightly increased breadth of the nostrils should be remedied. This was very readily accomplished by an incision along the curve made by the attachment of the nose to the cheek, and there slicing off a small beveled portion of the nose and re-uniting the divided edges by sutures. This was followed by no apparent cicatrix whatever.

A year later this monomania, for such it was, developed itself in a further desire to have something more done to the nose. This I was unwilling to do, because I considered it a first-class nose as it was, but only upon the intercession of his family, which they, moreover, clinched by giving me voluntarily a statement in writing that the operation was done at the patient's and their own request, did I consent to accomplish what he wished, which was that the nose should now be shortened. The nose had by the previous operation been rendered less prominent, and its lateral dimensions had been reduced satisfactorily, but, from being brought

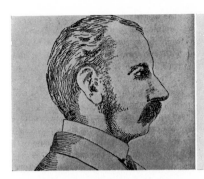
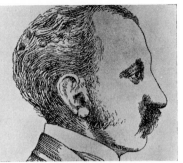

Fig. 8. (*left*) Gentleman with an unduly large nose, which I operated upon in 1885 (some two years prior to Roe's first report). (*right*) Condition after first operation, which consisted of resection of a triangular portion of the saeptum narium (its base ¼" in width at the columna, its apex above at the ethmoid saeptum) and moving the nasal bones inward and backward.

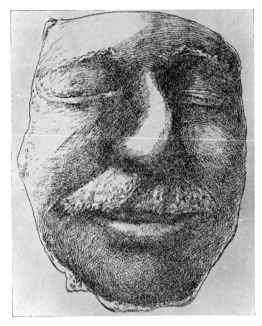

Fig. 9. A twisted nose.

a little closer to the line of the face, it struck him as being a little longer. His aim in life was then to have this nose made shorter—a problem for which I could find no help in my reading. It was, however, accomplished in the following way:

The columna was divided in the line of the old cicatrix. The ala on each side was separated from the cheek through the previous almost invisible cicatrices. After dissecting off the anterior portion of the columna from the cartilage, this dissection was carried along exterior to the lateral cartilages, so that the thick skin constituting the knob of the nose, for a distance of, say, half an inch above its tip, was freed from the subjacent cartilages and tilted upward. The cartilages were then trimmed off and shortened as required and the skin replaced. The result was a very satisfactory one.

This completed the surgery of his nose, with one slight exception, which took place several months later. The original opening inward of the nose had intensified the naturally slight hump that many of us have at the junction of the bony and cartilaginous structures. This he insisted upon being removed, and it was done by a slight beveled incision on one side, which permitted, after raising up the skin, careful chipping off of the offending cartilage by means of a fine engraver's chisel. The wound healed without a perceptible scar. I would remark here that I have since twice removed such humps by incisions conducted, as had lately been published by Dr. Roe,* by getting beneath the skin from the nasal passages, and, with properly shaped knives, or chisels, which I like better, have cut off sundry portions of the projecting mass.

This interior incision is much more difficult and unsatisfactory than the one I resorted to in the case just given; but in women it probably is the better one.

For the relief of twisted noses, meaning those bent in the cartilaginous portion (Fig. 9), or where even the osseous portion has been deviated also on the same side, requires much more interference than is supposed. The bent portion of the bony part I yet like best to accomplish by

* Medical Record, July 18, 1891.

means of a fine chisel introduced through the skin, chiseling off the nasal bones on both sides from their maxillary attachments, and cutting through the saeptum. This is all accomplished through one opening. It rarely requires a second opening on the other side.

Sometimes the replacement of the bony deviation carries with it and remedies the deviation of the cartilaginous saeptum; but, as a rule, I have found the cartilaginous saeptum requires to be very freely divided. This division, in my hands, has been most certainly done by the introduction of a knife somewhat similar to an angularly bent iridectomy knife, which should cut through the cartilage up to the very skin; of course, not through it, but as near as possible to the bony junction, and going backward some distance in the cartilaginous saeptum. This is to be supplemented by one or two similar incisions through the cartilaginous saeptum, running likewise to the skin at points lower down. In one case I found it necessary to join these incisions running from the front of the nose backward in the cartilaginous saeptum, by an incision parallel to the free border of the nose, by which the two incisions were joined deeper in the nose, and in that way a movable portion of the cartilaginous saeptum was left for me to act upon.

But it must be distinctly understood that in conducting an operation for this end a perfect restoration must be accomplished at the time of the operation, and it must be capable of being maintained without any force, or retention pads, or apparatus. A deviation that requires force to hold it in position, while the patient is yet under an anaesthetic, is sure of defeating the aim of the operator. It is best, therefore, to overdo the operative procedure, either by force or freedom of incision, so that the nose will retain its proper shape at the conclusion of the surgical work. In addition, it must be emphasized that further improvement must not be hoped for by the use of pluggings of iodoform gauze or plugs of other material introduced into the nostril or nostrils. They are only serviceable, in my opinion, to prevent the nose from slipping out of position by incautious movements or other accident. Plugging with iodoform gauze I like best for the interior retention work, because it accomplishes at the same time an antiseptic purpose. I have been much pleased also with the plugs that have been made of cork and covered with collodion, as suggested by Dr. French, of Brooklyn, which I used in one case successfully in conjunction with him, where a deviated nose, with an imperfectly operated upon hare-lip, was brought into proper shape

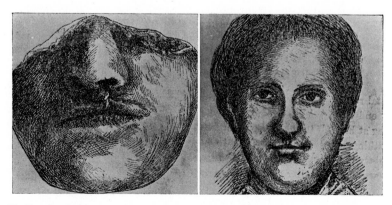

Fig. 10. Result of the operation described, on the patient shown in Fig. 9. (The hare-lip operation was done over again at the same time.)

by this free division of the saeptum. At the same time the hare-lip operation was done over again in a more satisfactory manner. (Fig. 10).

I may say here, in this class of nasal deformities, that the flattening of the nose, which is sometimes associated with a successfully treated harelip, can be relieved by the same incision under the lip, freeing the nostril on the side, and holding the restored nostril in position by a suture, which, securing itself in the cartilage of the ala of the flattened side, is passed across the saeptum to the cartilage on the other side, which is to be left fixed to the jaw bone. This suture was, in two of my cases, retained *in situ* in this way for a week or ten days with a satisfactory result.

Robert F. Weir, M.D.
37 West Thirty-Third Street
New York, N.Y.

COMMENTARY BY THE EDITOR

This paper of Weir's is nearly incredible! Although Roe's first halting efforts at reduction rhinoplasty were published a few months earlier, this is the paper that describes the beginnings of the logical step-by-step rhinoplasty in use today—the one that bears the imprint of the master surgeon.

Let us skip lightly over the divertissements—his description of the platinum prosthesis (the silicone of that day)—his story of bringing the live duck to the operating room (certainly antedating the bringing of pigs to the O.R. for liver perfusions in our time). What are the basic and lasting advances described herein? Why, they are the fundamentals of corrective rhinoplasty!

First, he tells of elevating a depressed dorsum by narrowing the nose.

For the third patient in this paper, he improvises an entire reduction rhinoplasty, step-by-step. At the first operation, he removed the hump and lowered the dorsal line, then narrowed the nose. In such a situation, we all know now that the tip is apt to overbalance the resulting nose—but this was virgin territory then and Weir had to improvise a second operation. This he did by alar base excisions, the procedure that has come down to us as "the Weir operation." The tip was still not reduced enough, however, so he improvised a third operation to expose the alar cartilages and reduce them in size in all directions.

Several months later, Weir had the first experience (in this same patient) with the development of the secondary deformity now known as "parrot nose." For this, he did the first secondary rhinoplasty, "carefully chipping off of the offending cartilage by means of a fine engraver's chisel."

This patient's preoccupation with small details of nasal contour was so great, and Weir's sensitivity to these feelings so acute, that he was able to diagnose a syndrome that had never occurred before. This condi-

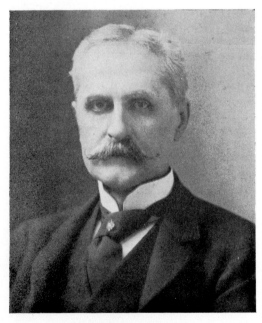

ROBERT F. WEIR, M.D.
1838–1927
(Courtesy of the New York Academy of Medicine)

tion, common enough today, is one in which at first the patient seems to be seeking merely a perfect nose—but it later becomes evident that he is, in reality, seeking to have his nose operated upon forever. This psychological-crutch condition Weir called "monomania;" perhaps a better name would be "rhinomania."

Not content to conclude his paper with just the principles of reduction rhinoplasty, and the building-up of sunken noses by rhinoplasty, Weir tossed in a section on straightening twisted noses—another first. He concludes this with two maxims, which could well be framed and displayed now in every operating room in which rhinoplasties are done.

"A perfect restoration must be accomplished at the time of the operation, and it must be capable of being maintained without any force, or retention pads, or apparatus."

"Further improvement must not be hoped for by the use of pluggings of iodoform gauze or plugs of other material introduced into the nostril or nostrils."

Born in New York in 1838, Weir attended the Free Academy—but let him tell the story of why he entered medicine to become a surgeon.

"I had graduated, the youngest in my class, from the just established New York Academy (later the College of the City of New York) and had started as a clerk for my father, who was an apothecary in Grand Street.... Perhaps this training inclined me to the practice of medicine, but I have always been convinced that two incidents determined my career. The first was the experience I obtained from the painful ingrown toe nail of my big toe. It plagued me so badly for several months until my father took me one Saturday to the office of Dr. James R. Wood, whom I had frequently seen in the store and who was generally known by all the neighborhood as "little Dr. Jim Wood." His office was at the corner of East Broadway and Market Street (and these were fashionable streets then). There he held once a week a sort of clinic for his serious students. Thither I went in due time, and was ushered into his sanctum. He examined my stripped toe and while explaining to the embryo medicos the nature of my trouble,

slyly took up a pair of pincers, and quickly placing one jaw of this under the nail, clamped the upper jaw to and pulled the nail out. I gave a jump and a wild yell, but it didn't hurt so much as I thought it would, since the nail had been considerably loosened by the prolonged inflammation and suppuration. I went home relieved and in telling my father of it, I said: I'd like to be able to do like that." (This impression was augmented when a few months later, his father sustained a Pott's fracture and was treated by the same Dr. Wood.) "The next day I announced my firm determination to become a surgeon."

The story of Weir's career is well told in Stark's recent article "Friendship of Three Giants" (*Plastic & Reconstr. Surg., 40: 599, 1967*) and there is no need to repeat it. Suffice it to note that Weir became Professor of Surgery at the College of Physicians and Surgeons—and then president of, successively, the New York Surgical Society, the Practitioner's Society, the New York Academy of Medicine, the Greater New York Medical Society, and the American Surgical Association. In 1905, the Royal College of Surgeons of England decided to institute honorary fellowships. The first 3 were bestowed, in a ceremony that year, upon Dr. Weir, Dr. W. W. Keen of Philadelphia, and the Prince of Wales.

At the first convocation of the American College of Surgeons, held in the Gold Room of the Congress Hotel on the evening of November 13, 1913, that new college bestowed its first honorary fellowships upon 5 outstanding surgeons. President Finney conferred them upon Sir Rickman Godlee of London (then President of the Royal College of Surgeons), William S. Halsted of Baltimore, W. W. Keen of Philadelphia, John Collins Warren of Boston, and Robert F. Weir of New York.

When Weir died in 1927, he had probably been accorded more honors than any surgeon up to that time. His writings throughout the years would indicate that, though his interests ranged widely throughout the body, his inventive mind was at its best when devising plastic and reconstructive surgical procedures. It is more a mark of the preoccupations of medical historians, than of Weir's, that he is listed by them as "the father of appendicostomy."

Perhaps it is time that the leaders of the American Surgical Association, the New York Academy of Medicine, the American College of Surgeons, and the Royal College of Surgeons be made aware of the nature of the most significant and lasting contribution made by this master surgeon whom they honored so wisely—more wisely than they knew.

—FRANK MCDOWELL

CORRECTION OF THE SADDLE NOSE DEFORMITY BY RECONSTRUCTION OF THE NASAL DORSUM OUT OF THE CHONDRO-OSSEOUS SIDEWALLS OF THE NOSE

DR. VINCENZ V. CZERNY, *Heidelberg, Germany*

Excerpt from "Three Plastic Operations"
(Deutsche Gesell. f. chir., 24: 211, 1895)

Translated from the German by
DR. URSULA SCHMIDT-TINTEMANN

It is well known that the correction of the saddle nose deformity has been tried in various ways and has been the subject of repeated discussions. For a slight depression of the nasal dorsum I tried to achieve this goal by using a one-stage operation which resulted in minimal disfigurement by a hardly-visible scar on the dorsum of the nose.

In two cases, I first cut the skin of the dorsum of the nose in the midline—from the glabella to the tip—and then dissected the skin off both sidewalls. Then a half-elliptical, full-thickness flap (*i.e.* out of the triangular cartilage and the nasal bone) was constructed out of each sidewall of the nose, with the base in the midline of the nasal dorsum. According to a little paper pattern (that had been cut to the height of the nasal defect) the chondrous part of the sidewall of the nose was sectioned with a strong little knife and the osseous part with a fine chisel, first on one and then on the other side.

Then both flaps (which were lined by mucosa on the inside and covered by periosteum on the outside) were turned upwards towards the sagittal plane on the nasal dorsum, so that their periosteal surfaces met. The vascular supply of the flaps was secured from the septum. The free margins of the flaps were approximated by a few interrupted catgut sutures. (Turning the flaps upwards is a little difficult and could be facilitated somewhat by a wide Pean artery forceps.) The skin edges over this elevated nasal dorsum were closed by a running silk suture.

To reconstruct the nose as close to normal as possible, and support the elevation of nasal dorsum, a mattress suture was placed through the nose and the chondrous septum immediately above the alae nasi.

This method of correction is useful only in saddle nose deformities of lesser degrees, without major distortion of the nasal tip—those in which the osseous and chondrous structure of the sidewalls are intact and the septum is not perforated, for the latter has to support and nourish the new dorsum of the nose.

CASE REPORTS

Case 1

1. F.R., a 20-year old male from a healthy family (without a history of rickets or lues) had suffered a depression of the osseous nasal skeleton through a fall on his nose, when he was 3 years old.

Editorial note. This is, I think, the first description of building up the nose by turning up flaps from the lateral walls on septal hinges and suturing them back-to-back.

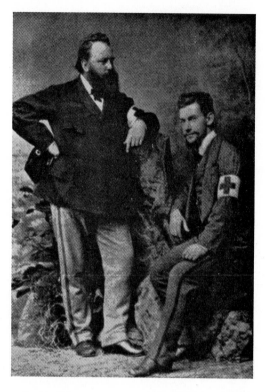

FIG. 1. Vincenz Czerny (*right*) with his teacher Billroth (*left*) during the Franco-Prussian War of 1870–71. (From p. 171 of *Heidelberger Chirurgie 1818–1968*, Springer-Verlag, Berlin, 1968. By permission.)

Findings

The nose showed a marked depression and flattening, with a simultaneous widening in the region of the bony nasal dorsum; the nasal tip appeared to be pulled upwards, the nostrils wide open. Both nasal fossae were somewhat narrow superiorly, the conchae were moderately hypertrophic, the septum was not perforated, and the mucosa was edematous with a mild pharyngitis. Hearing was normal, the other organs unremarkable.

Operation on May 4, 1894

A cut approximately 5 cm in length was made in the midline, extending from the glabella to the tip. Then a small flap (composed of periosteum, bone, and cartilage) was developed from each side of the nasal roof in the region of the nasal bones and upper lateral cartilages. The two flaps were joined in the sagittal plane, like an open book, so that they touched each other with

their periosteal layers; the free margins were united with 3 catgut sutures. The skin incision over this new nasal dorsum was closed by silk sutures. Zinc paste splint.

Progress note

Removal of the skin sutures on the third day; discharge of the patient on the 6th day after primarily healing. According to the report and photography of February 1895, the patient is satisfied with the result, the nasal depression is almost (although not completely) corrected, the former widening is markedly reduced, and the cutaneous scar is hardly visible.

Case 2

2. G.M., 12 years old, from a healthy family, had had periostitis of the maxillary region at the age of 4 years (which had originated in the incisors and caused a purulent infection extending to the nose). After cessation of the infection, the dorsum of the nose gradually sank in to its present form.

Findings

Slender, anemic boy, deeply depressed saddle nose deformity, the skin was freely mobile over it. The alae formed normally, both nares

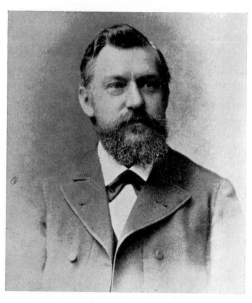

FIG. 2. Prof. Vincenz v. Czerny, at about the time this article was written. (Courtesy of Dr. Weisert, Director of the University of Heidelberg Archives.)

patent, the septum was not perforated. The tonsils were markedly hypertrophic.

Operation on February 25, 1895

(Under chloroform anesthesia, as described previously.) The osteo-chondral flaps were of poor resistance and therefore did not form a very stiff structure for the nasal dorsum. Finally, the tonsils were removed with the "button-knife." Healing took place without complications, so that the boy was discharged on March 5.

Progress

On March 11, he presented with a small abscess of the left side of the nose; this was incised. The nose looked good and had gained so much, that the saddle deformity had been corrected to almost a straight nasal dorsum. The patient presented again on June 19. The saddle nose was improved, but was not as good as immediately after the operation.

Dr. Vincenz v. Czerny
Das Akademische Krankenhaus
Heidelberg, Germany

COMMENTARY BY DR. URSULA SCHMIDT-TINTEMANN

Vincenz v. Czerny was born on November 19, 1842 in Bohemia, the son of a pharmacist. He received a broad education in the natural sciences at the Universities of Prague and Vienna. At the latter, he first met the great surgeon Billroth, in 1868.

Billroth stimulated Czerny's enthusiasm for surgery (Fig. 1) and made him do independent research, in which animal experiments played a fundamental role. When only 29 years old, he became Professor of Surgery at the University of Freiburg, Germany. In 1877 he moved to Heidelberg as Director of the new 122-bed surgical university hospital. As a general surgeon, he

was head of this hospital for 29 years (Fig. 2). He made this hospital flourish and become famous.

During the age of the emerging bacteriologic sciences, his main accomplishment was to initiate the operative therapy of abdominal organs (stomach, spleen, gallbladder, appendix, small and large intestine, and uterus) under the protection of antisepsis and asepsis. The operations for inguinal hernia and goiter (Fig. 3)—which up until then were also ventures of unjustifiable risk—became standard procedures.

In 1906 Czerny retired as Director of the

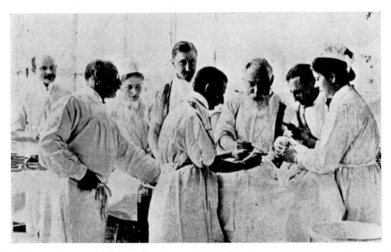

FIG. 3. Vincenz Czerny operating in the Academic Hospital of Heidelberg. (From p. 176 of *Heidelberger Chirurgie 1818–1968*, Springer-Verlag, Berlin, 1968. By permission.)

hospital and devoted his time and energy to the idea and development of his "Institute for Cancer Research." On October 13, 1916 he died—shortly before his 75th birthday.

Czerny was among the first of surgeons to realize that not only organ reconstruction, but also the function of personal appearance was sufficient motivation for a physician to operate upon a patient.

The operative procedure described herein was not concerned with the repair of lost parts—it was not even supposed to free a poor man from the blame of having led an immoral life. It dealt with the integration of his body image.

The operative risks (asepsis, anesthesia) had been reduced to such an extent that the ideas which had been present throughout the history of plastic surgery could now be realized.

Dr. Ursula Schmidt-Tintemann
Ismaninger Strasse 22
Munchen 8, Germany

TWO NEW METHODS OF RHINOPLASTY

JAMES ISRAEL, *Berlin, Germany*

(*Arch. f. Klin. chir., 53: 255–265, 1896.*)

Translated from the German by
DR. FRANK McDOWELL

Rhinoplasties done in recent times, using a compound skin-bone flap from the forehead, leave (as does every osteoplastic method) a deplorable result—bad scars of the forehead.

A case of saddle nose that I saw had been unsuccessfully operated upon in another place; there was such a scarred forehead. I was compelled to devise a new method of rhinoplasty with full preservation of the forehead. The process consisted of using a bone graft sawed off from the tibia to substitute for the lost bony skeleton of the nose. By this method, I obtained very satisfactory results in two men with saddle noses.

Another expedient was used successfully on a young woman who had had her nose almost completely destroyed by lupus and who wished her forehead to remain undisturbed. Here, I rebuilt the lost nose by a compound skin-bone flap from the ulnar side of the forearm, using the part of the bone situated along the edge of the ulna just under the skin.

BUILDING UP THE SADDLE NOSE WITH A FREE BONE GRAFT

Case I.

A 30-year-old man with a high-grade syphilitic saddle nose was operated upon in Vienna, having a plastic operation out of the forehead. He was sad, with so unfavorable a result that his condition after the operation was worse than before. Now he had not only the persistence of the retraction of the nose into the pyriform apertures, but he was even more disappointed about the uncommonly ugly lumped-up skin prominences on his forehead and in the grafted flap, which bedecked the saddling from the glabella downward. Under this unrealized build-up, his stump of a nose wasted away still more than before. Also, he had had a breadth of bone adherent to the forehead scar taken, which ruled out every possibility of a new rhinoplasty from the forehead (Fig. 1, *left*). In this situation, I got the idea that the lacking bony framework of the sunken nose might be restored through healing in place of a free bone graft from the tibia.

I made an incision down the dorsum of the nose, corresponding to the area of the saddle and some 2 cm in extent, and through this divided the subcutaneous tissue from the firm retracted scar underneath. This scar extended deep into the pyriform apertures, but through strong back and forth movements I mobilized the prominence of the nose until a normal profile was attained. Through this maneuver, the long cut over the saddle became transformed into a rhomboid; if these edges had been simply sutured, an insaddling would have occurred again. The cut edges had now to be mobilized sufficiently through undermining so that they could be closed without tension over the soon-to-be-grafted bone. To this end, I used elevators and a knife to separate the soft parts from the ascending proc-

Presented, as a lecture with illustrations, before the Free Society of Surgeons of Berlin.

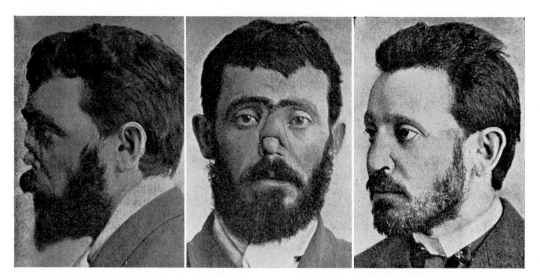

FIG. 1. *(left and center)* Case I, luetic saddle nose, before operation. *(right)* Result of one operation, free tibial bone graft to nose through a dorsal incision.

esses of the maxilla until, in spite of strong forward traction on the nasal dorsum, the incision did not gape.

However, after discontinuing the procedure, the soft parts of the nose sank back again at once and it became apparent that a firm scaffold would be required to keep them in the normal place.

To this end, I severed from one tibial edge a long bone spicule measuring 3 or 3.5 cm in length. For the reception of the sharp pointed end, I made a nice narrow tunnel in the subcutaneous tissues through the incision in the dorsum of the nose, using a narrow dressing forceps and a knife. After this, the piece of bone was introduced through the nasal incision and placed under the skin in its correct position. It was firmly clamped in the subcutaneous tissue in front of the nasal bones; and was between the inner and outer skin of the nasal tip (Fig. 2).

Immediately, the nose had the right projection; thereupon, the cut edges were sewed up over the new bony skeleton and the nostrils were firmly filled with iodoform gauze.

I was able to observe the patient 4 months after healing, when he came in

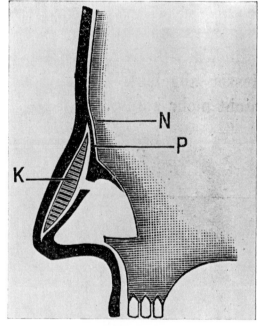

FIG. 2. Position of bone graft, *K,* in the nose in the patient shown in Figure 1.

for excision of the earlier mentioned out-of-shape forehead skin and some trimming of the flap on the nose. During this, there was an opportunity at two separate times for the eye to see the bare bone and I could recognize no difference

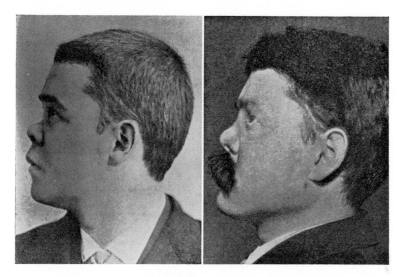

FIG. 3. Case II, before and after free tibial bone graft to nose.

from normal living bone. As the photograph (Fig. 1, *right*) shows, the cosmetic result corresponded to the demands.

Case II.

By the same method, I operated a second case of high-grade saddle nose in a 33-year-old man who, as a boy, had had a luetic exfoliation of the nasal bones, the hard palate, and gummatous ulceration of the frontal bone (Fig. 3, *left*). After a prior uranoplasty came the subcutaneous loosening and correction of the nose— then a bone graft from the tibia was done in the previously described manner. This made it possible to secure an after photograph (Fig. 3, *right*) corresponding to the before. In spite of the fact that here, also, the saddled area was completely loosened, the cosmetic result was not as good as in the first patient. In all cases of syphilitic destruction of the nasal bones in early childhood, there is considerable retardation of the growth of the nasal tip. As a consequence, even after my operation of a complete pulling forward and correction, out of it comes an organ which is always too small.

TOTAL RHINOPLASTY WITH A SKIN-BONE FLAP FROM THE FOREARM

A 19-year-old girl had had lupus of her nose and upper lip since the age of 12, which finally went on to full destruction of the nasal bones down to the adjacent parts (Fig. 4).

When seen, it lacked the cartilaginous and membranous septum, the lower half of the nasal dorsum, the tip, and most of the alae; there was a nasolabial defect nearly down to the vermilion border. The large defect and neighboring parts were interwoven with scars, partly as a residual of the lupus infection, partly from various cauteries which she herself had administered—using the sun's rays through a burning glass in her attempts to halt the spread of the lesion.

The patient wished a substitute nose to be made out of her arm, and was not willing to have any operation from her forehead. As it was not possible to get the necessary bone and skin flap out of the upper arm, however, I chose to use a substitute flap from the forearm—for here the ulnar edge was so near the skin surface that I could procure a compound

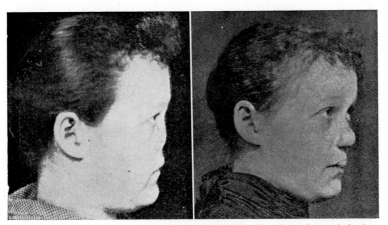

Fig. 4. Reconstruction of nose with compound skin-bone flap from forearm, in 6 stages.

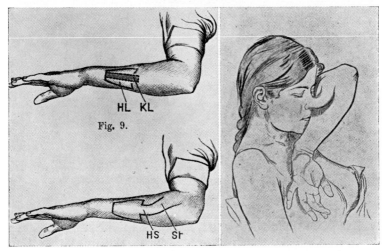

Fig. 5. Details of the operations in the patient shown in Figure 4.

flap with the bone graft organically bound to the skin.

The entire reconstruction required 6 stages. . . .

(Editor's note. Details of the 6 stages are rather tedious, but the procedure is depicted quite well in his illustrations, which are reproduced herewith (Fig. 5). The first stage was done on October 2, 1895, the last on November 29 of the same year. There were some problems with distal necrosis, requiring removal of the distal

end with that part of the bone, reimplantation, etc., but the end result was successful.)

. . . Without these two avoidable accidents, the building of a nose with a skin-bone flap from the forearm would not require longer than does the forehead rhinoplasty.

James Israel, M.D.
Jewish Hospital
Berlin

COMMENTARY: THE FIRST FREE BONE GRAFT TO THE NOSE

The history of bone transplantation is a checkered one and difficult to clarify. The earliest method consisted of moving the

bone in a compound flap with skin; one of the earliest descriptions of this was in 1864 by Ollier, who tried bringing a forehead

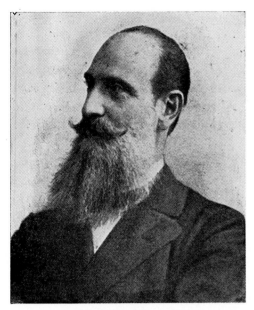

JAMES ISRAEL, M.D.
1848–1926

flap down to the nose with not only periosteum, but also some bone in it. In 1875, James Hardie described the curious operation of decorticating the little finger, and stuffing it into a prepared raw bed under the skin of a saddle nose; whereupon after 3 weeks he cut it off and allowed it to remain there. (This will be published later in this series.) In 1880, König boldly sawed out a considerable segment of the frontal bone, leaving it attached to the forehead skin, and rotated it down to the nose as a compound flap.

Perhaps the first description of successful free grafting of bone was by Sir James Macewen, the eminent surgeon of Glasgow who invented the osteotome (and nearly invented orthopedic surgery and neurosurgery, as well). In 1879, he had a young male patient with a defect in the humerus; strangely, he repaired it with a homograft of iliac bone chips from an adult; fortunately, he had to distract the fragments to get the chips in and there was enough bony contact and stress that solid union was obtained.

There is little doubt that the first free bone grafts to the nose were the ones described herewith by Israel. They were rarities in any location at that time, which reveals the temerity of this surgeon.

James Israel was born on Feb. 2, 1848 in Berlin, where he studied and received his doctorate in 1870. He remained for postgraduate work under von Langenbeck, then went to Vienna for further education, returning in 1872 to become an assistant physician in the Krankenhaus of the Berlin Jewish Community. A year or so later, he studied for a time in England and Scotland, returning again to become assistant chief of surgery in the Krankenhaus in 1875. In 1880, he became chief of the surgical department and gave his inaugural dissertation on Bright's disease of the kidneys. During the next few decades, he wrote more than 100 papers on diverse subjects, most of them surgical. One of his most famous papers was on actinomycosis in man; an organism (Israel's streptothrix) was named after him. He became known throughout Europe, however, for his work on surgical lesions of the kidney and he did much to elucidate the physiology and pathology of that organ. After a long and fruitful life in this field, he died in Berlin at the age of 78 on Feb. 2, 1926.

The various German biographical works consider him to be a pioneer in urological surgery; they list his main publications in that field, but do not mention this paper on bone grafting. Probably no one would be more surprised than Israel to find that today we are honoring him for this work on the nose, which he probably thought to be inconsequential. Thus it is as Blair said, "plastic surgery has been constructed out of the scraps and discards which other surgeons often believed to be unworthy of their more serious attentions."

—FRANK MCDOWELL

The photographs from the article were furnished by the National Library of Medicine, Bethesda, and the photograph of Dr. Israel was furnished by Dr. Eduard Schmid of Stuttgart.

CORRECTION, BY OPERATION, OF SOME NASAL DEFORMITIES AND DISFIGUREMENTS

DR. GEORGE H. MONKS, *Boston, Mass.*

(Boston Medical and Surgical Journal, *139:* 262, 1898)

It is not my intention to take up the time of the Society by reading a long paper which pretends to cover the correction of all possible deformities of the nose by operation. I propose simply to call your attention to a few of the ordinary deformities and disfigurements, and to briefly refer to some cases which illustrate the results obtained by certain operative procedures, some of which procedures are new and some old.

It is hardly necessary, I think, for me to dwell on the desirability of doing such operations. After considerable experience I have become convinced, as probably most of you have, that few patients suffer more of mental discomfort than the unfortunate possessors of some unsightly disfigurement on the face which attracts constant notice, few are more solicitous for any operation which promises relief, and none are more grateful for the slightest improvement in their condition.

VENOUS AND CAPILLARY CONGESTION OF THE NOSE

The first subject I shall speak of is what is known as "Red-nose" or "Toper's Nose."

One meets with all degrees of this form of passive hyperemia; but the variety which is permanent, and especially that kind which is associated with numerous visible and arborescent vessels, often reaching well back upon the alae, is usually very annoying to the person affected, especially if he be of a sensitive temperament, and often prevents his getting employment on account of a supposed alcoholic tendency.

In such cases much can be done in the way of treatment, by destroying the little vessels by *scarification* or *electrolysis;* but in order that the effects shall be permanent the treatment must extend over many sittings and must be conscientiously carried out.

To properly scarify such a nose, it should be first of all thoroughly cleansed with soap and hot water; then firmly squeezed between the thumb and finger of the left hand, and a few minims of a weak cocaine solution injected. When the part is no longer sensitive to pain, multiple incisions should be made in different directions all over the affected area with a small sharp knife (see Fig. 1). These cuts need not be very long but should all be deep enough to divide the superficial vessels, whose trunks may often be seen through the skin. If the patient will keep in the house for a few days afterwards, the whole of the reddened area may be thoroughly scarified at the first sitting, after which the surface may be covered with cotton and collodion and the escaping blood allowed to dry and form a crust under it. If the patient, however, cannot keep quiet for some days, only a few of the largest vessels should be divided at a sitting. In any case the operation will have to be repeated several times, before a satisfactory and permanent result is secured. Though there is

Presented at the meeting of the Massachusetts Medical Society on June 7, 1898.

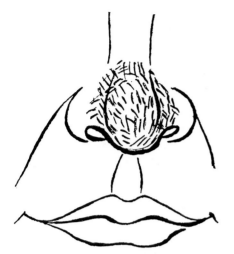

Fig. 1. Thorough scarification at the end of the nose.

reason to believe that the continuity is restored in many of the divided vessels, yet the contraction of the fibrous tissue which forms in all the little incisions will at least prevent the part from returning to its former condition of vascularity.

This congested condition at the tip of the nose can be treated equally well by electrolysis—indeed, some surgeons prefer it, and claim that by its use less scar results than is the case when scarification is used.

HYPERTROPHIC ACNE

This is a condition which is occasionally seen on the nose, and always interests the surgeon, though unfortunately few cases are induced to come to operation.

Some years ago a man with an enormous enlargement of the end and alae of his nose, due to one form of this condition, came to me, asking for an operation to relieve his deformity. He stated that he was unable to get anything to do in the way of work, as everybody thought him a drinker, which he certainly was not. The whole nose, but especially about the end of it and the alae, was greatly thickened, nodulated and reddened, with here and there acne pustules in all stages. All over this area little depressions or pits were to be seen, representing the openings of the sebaceous follicles, and from all of these long worms of sebum could be squeezed out. After thoroughly cleansing the parts, I split the skin and underlying tissue of the nose down the middle line for its entire length, from base to tip, turned back the two flaps to the sides and removed all the subcutaneous tissue I could get hold of. I then replaced the flaps and sewed them together. The alae, which projected like two small cherries from the sides of the nose, were also treated in this same way, and so much underlying tissue was cut away that the nose was considerably diminished in size. Although the result was not so perfect as one might wish, it showed at least a distinct improvement, and the man was apparently perfectly satisfied.

Some time after this operation I described it to one of my colleagues, and showed him the case. He seemed much interested, and was pleased when, some months later, a similar case came under his own charge. He operated upon the man by the procedure which I had employed. Imagine his disgust, however, when, soon after the operation, the flaps sloughed! I fancy he had been more radical in his operation than I should have dared to be, and did not leave enough tissue for his pedicles. In time, however, the dead flaps separated, and left the nose without any cutaneous covering, the raw surface granulated, and finally cicatrized; and the man was ultimately glad to possess a small, thin, white nose (even if it was nothing but the framework of a nose, covered with one enormous scar), in place of the large, reddish, nodulated organ which he formerly had, and he (who, by the way, thought that the sloughing process had been intended as a part of the operation) pronounced the result a complete success! Referring to the result of his operation, my colleague suggested that the best treatment for these cases was probably, after all, simply to pare them down with the knife to the desired size and shape, and leave the raw surface to granulate. I should seriously consider doing this very thing if another of these extreme cases should come to me, only I should certainly prefer to cover the raw surface with skin grafts rather than to leave it to granulate.

BIFID NOSE

This is a congenital condition, though a rare one. It would appear in these cases that during the developmental period of life the two halves of the nose fail to approach sufficiently near each other in front, and for this reason a long vertical depression remains in the middle line. This depression is permanent, and causes a very noticeable deformity. It of course belongs to that large group of malformations known as "defects in the median line of the body."

Some years ago I operated upon such a case. The patient, who was sent to me by Dr. Gilbert N. Jones, then of Gloucester, was a young girl of fourteen years (see Fig. 2), who had always been particularly sensitive about the deformity; her acquaintances having done their best that she should not forget it. I removed an elliptical piece of skin and underlying tissue from the depression, brought the two sides together, and united them with buried and superficial stitches. The result was very satisfactory, for instead of the peculiar double-pointed nose which attracted so much attention wherever she went, she now had a nose that was normal in appearance, except for a slight scar in the median line (see Fig. 2).

DEFORMITIES DUE TO OLD INJURY

We frequently meet with noses deformed by injury in which the displacement occurring at the time of the accident has been allowed to remain unreduced. The appearance of such injured noses naturally varies; they may be bent, twisted or depressed, or there may have been loss of substance. Probably the commonest form is that in which there is a certain deviation of the bridge to one side or the other. The upper or bony part of the bridge may deviate, or it may be straight while the lower or cartilaginous part may be deviated, or the entire nose may be pushed to one side or the other. Such conditions may be congenital, but they are far more frequently due to some blow or fall. While in certain cases the nasal bones are undoubtedly fractured, and perhaps also the septum, I think it probable, judging from many of the cases I have seen, that the cartilaginous part of the nose is quite frequently torn away from the nasal bones, for in many cases where the nose has been injured we later see a bunch, indicating probably a new bone formation, on one side of the nose at a point exactly where the bony and cartilaginous parts should join.

I have operated upon one such case by chiselling off the little bony hump through a small incision in the skin at one side of it. The patient expressed himself as pleased with the result. Although the procedure was satisfactory in this special case, I felt that it would not do in all cases, for one meets with many of them where the bony projections on the bridge are so large that they cannot be cut away without making very large incisions, and also running the risk of opening into the

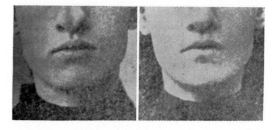

FIGURE 2

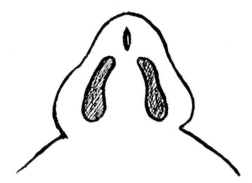

FIG. 3. Showing the incision just below the tip of the nose—being the opening of the tunnel leading upward to the area between the skin and the framework of the bridge of the nose.

nose and thus leaving a permanent hole through the bone.

In seeking to discover some means of fracturing the bony bridge of a nose without bruising or cutting the skin, I devised a method which has worked very well indeed. After the patient is under an anesthetic a small incision is made just beneath the tip of the nose, its axis being continuous with that of the columna (Fig. 3). Through this incision the points of a small pair of blunt-pointed scissors are inserted. It is now found that by opening and closing the scissors laterally so far as the limited size of the incision will allow and pushing them upwards the

points of the scissors can be made to travel in that direction, and a narrow pathway or, more properly speaking, a long flat tunnel is cut in the tissue between the skin and the bridge of the nose. This subcutaneous tunnel is continued well up to, and upon, the bony bridge (see Fig. 4). The projecting bony parts are then depressed, to any desired degree and extent, by a process to which I should like to call your special attention; for by its means the bony bridge of the nose can be fractured without leaving in the skin over the bridge any sign of injury except two or three minute punctures. Two little instruments (A and B, Fig. 4), besides a mallet, are necessary for this operation, each instrument being about two or three inches long. Instrument A has a flattened extremity at one end and a handle at the other. On one side of the flattened extremity the surface is roughened like a coarse file, and on the other side is a minute depression which receives the point of instrument B. Instrument B closely resembles a very sharp-pointed lead pencil.

Instrument A is inserted into the incision, just below the point of the nose, and is then pushed upwards along the subcutaneous tunnel already spoken of, until

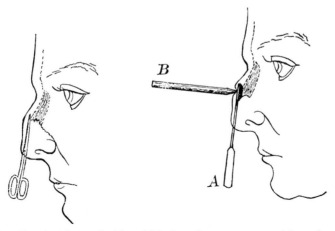

FIG. 4. (left) Showing the method by which the subcutaneous tunnel is made with the scissors. (right) Instrument A has been inserted into the subcutaneous tunnel until its roughened extremity rests upon the projecting bone. The point of Instrument B, having punctured the skin, is made to rest in the little depression on the back of Instrument A.

its roughened end is made to rest over the projecting part of the bony bridge which it is desired to fracture (as in Fig. 4). The point of the instrument B is then gently inserted through the skin into the little hole already referred to on the back of the flattened extremity of the instrument A. The two instruments, being then in the position shown in Fig. 4, are rigidly held, a few taps of the mallet on the end of the instrument B being sufficient to cause the fracture and depression desired at any point in the bony bridge. It may, in certain cases, be necessary to fracture the bone over a larger area. This of course can be easily accomplished by the same method.

After the operation has been completed there remain on the bridge of the nose where the bone has been fractured only a few minute punctures, which eventually cicatrize and are not noticed. This method of fracturing the bony bridge of the nose is of course only applicable to cases where there is undue prominence confined to a limited area on the bridge, and is not to be used in cases where there is deviation to one side or the other of the entire bony framework of the nose.

The method of tunnelling under the skin by means of scissors is one which I devised some years ago for other purposes than that mentioned here, and which I have found most useful in many cases.

SADDLE-BACK NOSE

Another kind of deformed nose is what is called "Depressed or Saddle-Back Nose." This may be due to injury or disease, and the operation selected for its relief naturally varies with the cause or the special deformity in each case.

One case of this kind, already reported at length,* and simply referred to here, was a young girl of sixteen, who, as a result of inherited disease, had a saddle-

* See Boston Medical and Surgical Journal, June 25, 1896.

back nose of such an extreme degree that the bridge of the nose was sunken to nearly the level of the cheeks, and was covered with a dense scar. The end of the nose was tipped up and the nostrils looked forwards. On account of her deformity she could get no employment. In this case, for certain reasons too many to be mentioned here, I thought it best to dissect off the scar over the depressed bridge, and, after freeing the tip and nostrils by a horizontal cut directly backwards through the lower part of the nose, I depressed them downwards into place, and then covered the gaping wound and the raw surface left by the removal of the scar with a flap from the left forearm. The result was satisfactory; the flap grew in place and covered both raw surface and gap. The tip of the nose faced forwards instead of upwards, and the nostrils faced downwards instead of forwards.

In another case, a young woman of twenty, with depressed nose from inherited disease, I inserted a platinum plate, which lifted up the bridge and gave perfect satisfaction until one day, many months after the operation, she was in sport peeping through a keyhole, when another girl gave her head a push, driving it against the door so violently that the end of the plate came out. This was of course followed by suppuration which necessitated the removal of the plate. In spite of this, however, the collapse of the nose was apparently not so marked as before the operation, and the patient declared that she thought the nose was firmer and that there was more bone in the bridge than before the plate was inserted. I did another operation on this nose, trimming a little here and there, and finally inserting a small bit of bone (from which the animal matter had been removed) which bone seemed to elevate the bridge somewhat, and which to this day—the operation was done three or four months ago—has given no trouble.

A young woman of twenty was referred

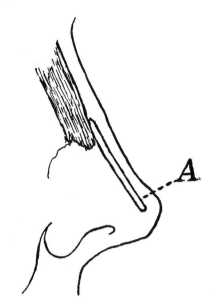

FIG. 5. Showing where the piece of celluloid should rest in order to restore the lower part of the bridge.

to me some time ago by Dr. Mahoney, of Medford. Two years previously she had a fall upon the ice, which had apparently caused a permanent depression of the cartilaginous bridge of the nose, giving rise to very unsightly depression in the lower part of the bridge, and a corresponding elevation of the tip of the nose. A celluloid piece (A, Fig. 5) was inserted through an incision below the tip, which

raised the bridge of the nose, so that the line of the entire bridge was nearly a straight one, and the patient was very well satisfied. The appearance of the nose after operation is well shown in Fig. 6.

The photographs from which Figure 6 was made are now in my possession.

In another case, a young lady, referred to me by Dr. E. H. Bradford, where there was a depression of the entire bridge, but especially of its upper part, I inserted a piece of celluloid high up on the bridge under the skin, having extended my subcutaneous tunnel higher upwards for that purpose. The operation was done several months ago, and the result has been an entirely satisfactory one. Not only is the depression, as seen in profile, far less marked than formerly, but the patient writes me that since operation she can breathe more freely through the nostrils than ever before.

DEPRESSION OF LOWER HALF OF NOSE

Occasionally one meets with cases where both the cartilaginous bridge and also the tip of the nose are collapsed. In such cases operative procedures are of no great avail; for unless some pretty extensive artificial framework is inserted under the skin there is nothing to support the parts. In one case of this kind where the

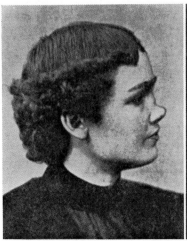
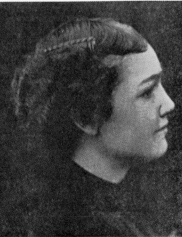

FIGURE 6.

tip of the nose and the cartilaginous bridge were greatly depressed as a result of disease, and the columna of the nose (that is, the narrow isthmus in the median line which connects the base of the nose with the tip) was wanting, I was able to supply a new columna from the skin of the arm, thus giving the man a somewhat more sightly organ, but I could not raise the tip and keep it in position.

The plan has been advocated, and put into operation in a few cases, of inserting a large artificial framework to overcome a collapsed condition of the nose. Judging from the reported cases I have seen, the good results have not been sufficiently lasting to lead us to hope much from the operation, for the apparatus, which it must be extremely difficult to cover up completely in the tissues, probably acts as a constant irritant, causing chronic suppuration and necrosis, necessitating its ultimate removal.

In conclusion I would say that, while many cases of deformed nose are so extreme that nothing can be done for them in the way of operation, there are many others in which a distinct *improvement* may be brought about, which, though not always entirely satisfactory to the surgeon, is almost invariably appreciated by the grateful patient.

George H. Monks, M.D.
Department of Surgery
Harvard Medical School
Boston, Mass.

EDITORIAL ADDENDUM

This is the most renowned of Dr. Monk's papers in the field of plastic surgery, and it is the reason for Dr. Goldwyn's biography of Monks (*cf*. page 467). The paper is concerned with a wide variety of lesions and deformities of the nose, and it illustrates superbly the genius of Monks as an innovator.

Under the title of "hypertrophic acne" he initiates the surgical treatment of rhinophyma, and within two paragraphs he brings it to that of the present day. Next, he initiates the treatment of bifid nose, and leaves little more that we can say today about a really severe case.

Monks was one of the first surgeons to be concerned with the twisted nose. Though the remedies he described would seem inadequate today, they were a start. His implants to the nose, and bone graft to the nose, were excellent examples of the early treatment of "saddle-back" nose.

The cumbersome glass plate processes used in those days made photography an extremely difficult and uncertain business. However, the esthetic eye of Monks perceived readily the necessity of comparing "before" and "after" views with the heads the same size, in the same position, and with the same lighting. How he must have delighted the editors of that day!

—Frank McDowell

ACKNOWLEDGMENT

The copies of the photographs in this article were kindly furnished by the historical section of the National Library of Medicine, Bethesda, Md.

And Then Came Joseph!

OPERATIVE REDUCTION OF THE SIZE OF A NOSE (RHINOMIOSIS)

JACQUES JOSEPH, M.D., *Berlin, Germany*

(Berlin Klinische Wochenschrift, 40: 882, 1898.)

Translated from the German by
DR. GUSTAVE AUFRICHT

Gentlemen: I take the liberty of presenting a new method of rhinoplasty. While the general purpose of rhinoplasty is to cover nasal defects to eliminate the effect of injuries and, especially, pathologic conditions, I was recently confronted with the task of transforming a perfectly healthy but (due to its size and shape) conspicuous nose into an inconspicuous nose. Briefly, the case was as follows:

The end of January this year, a 28-year-old landowner appeared in my office. He inquired whether I could make his nose smaller as he had heard that I had done some ear reductions. He related that his nose was the source of considerable annoyance. Wherever he went, everybody stared at him; often, he was the target of remarks or ridiculing gestures. On account of this he became melancholic, withdrew almost completely from social life, and had the earnest desire to be relieved from this deformity.

Gentlemen! I could not resist the impression that this otherwise highly intelligent gentleman, due to the peculiar characteristic of his nose, was in a deep psychic depression. Furthermore, I was convinced that the patient could not be helped otherwise but by a surgical reduction of his nose. Since my first ear reduction, I had occupied myself with the idea of how a large or otherwise conspicuous nose could be rendered inconspicuous. I

declared myself willing to carry out the operation.

Before I describe the surgical method, I wish to show these two plaster models (demonstration), how the nose was before the operation and how the same looked afterward.

Before operation: *1.* the dorsum was too long, and the tip was downward protruding; *2.* the nose was too far protruding from the face, and accordingly the nostrils were very large; *3.* there was an unattractive hump.

After operation: *1.* the nose is rather too short than too long; *2.* it protrudes the normal distance from the face and, accordingly, the nostrils are considerably smaller; *3.* with the hump removed, the nose is straight. If I am permitted to present some figures, I submit the following table.

TABLE I

	Before cm	Now cm	Difference cm
I. Distance from radix to furthest point of tip..............	6½	5½	1
II. Distance of foremost point of tip from the nasolabial fold.	4½	3½	1

Now I shall commence with the surgical method (but not without mentioning first that the day before the actual opera-

Presented before the Medical Society of Berlin, May 11, 1898.

tion, I performed an experimental operation on a cadaver—of course, on an entirely different shaped nose as a similar one could not be found—and it is my pleasant duty to express my warmest thanks to Prof. Waldeyer, for his friendly permission to use the cadaver material).

Gentlemen! For clarity's sake I wish to speak of the three phases of the operation.

Phase I. Excision of the excess skin not needed for the future nose, and reduction of the nostrils.

Phase II. Removal of the bony and cartilaginous nasal dome, as far as it was superfluous.

Phase III. Shortening of the nasal septum, for the purpose of raising the tip of the nose.

OPERATION

The first phase I carried out as follows. I made two straight incisions, beginning at the middle of the radix and proceeding symmetrically divergent to the nostrils. The upper part of the incisions reached (in depth) the nasal bone and the upper lateral cartilage; however, in their lower portion they went through the entire thickness of the alae. Similarly, through the full thickness of the alae, about ½ cm medially from the previous ones, two other incisions were made—converging to a point in the middle of the nose, about 1½ cm above the tip and saving the same. Afterward, the circumscribed area (representing an equilateral triangle with two downward extensions partly in the alae, including cartilage) was dissected from its base (Fig. 1).*

Now followed the second phase of the operation—the removal of the bony and cartilaginous nasal dome. For this purpose I undermined the remaining skin on the nasal bones and triangular cartilages (upper lateral cartilages) for about 1 cm. Then I set the chisel successively on both nasal bones, at the level of the future nose, and with a few strokes I severed the nasal bone. At the same level and extent I chiseled through the bony septum, thereby creating an upward directed open split (in the bone). I set the knife in this split and cut through simultaneously the protruding lower part of the nasal dorsum (not only the hump) (Fig. 1). Thereby both nasal

* In all Figures the excisions are indicated by shading.

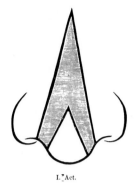

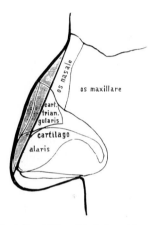

FIG. 1. (*above*) Phase I. (*below*) Phase II.

cavities were open from upward down, though on the upper part only two narrow slits were visible.

Henceforth the third phase of the operation consisted of a wedge-shaped horizontal excision from the lower part of the septum, the upper incision being through the quadrangular cartilage and the lower through the membranous septum (Fig. 2).

With this, the operation was actually finished and I began suturing. First I approximated the edges of the wedge excision from the septum (septal suture); following that, commencing at the radix nasi I closed the wound edges of the skin. The skin suture assumed the shape of an inverted Y. The operation took a little over one hour.

About the recovery there is not much to say. The healing was *per primam* and the patient was discharged from treatment in 13 days. No untoward symptoms affecting his general health have occurred so far.

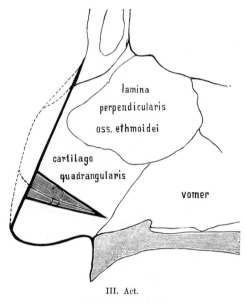

III. Act.

FIG. 2. Phase III.

The scars are linear and inconspicuous. I take the liberty to demonstrate the excised pieces. You can see the triangular piece of skin from the middle of the nose, about 2 cm wide. Furthermore, you see the resected nasal roof. The surface of it is slightly convex; inside, however, three ridges show clearly (the side walls and the septum, in between them two furrows covered with mucosa) representing beforehand the most anterior part of the nasal cavity. Thirdly, you see the wedge resected from the septum for the purpose of raising the tip of the nose (demonstration).

The psychologic effect of the operation is of utmost importance. The depressed attitude of the patient subsided completely. He is happy to move around unnoticed. His happiness in life has increased, his wife was glad to report; the patient who formerly avoided social contact now wishes to attend and give parties. In other words, he is happy over the result.

It would have been an extraordinary pleasure for me to present the patient, himself, today. Unfortunately he could

not be persuaded, but he was willing to present himself to the chairman and a few of our executive members. However, in order to demonstrate to the membership of our Society the best possible substitute in lieu of personal appearance, I had photographs* taken of the patient before and after the operation; from these, photo-engravings and slides were made (Fig. 3).† They offer a more life-like resemblance than the cadaver-like plaster models. Thanks to the courtesy of Prof. Lassar, who permitted me to use his magnificent projecting machine this evening, I am in the pleasant position of showing them in considerable enlargement.

As far as the literature is concerned, had I had the opportunity to address you 8 days before, I would have reported that in spite of diligent search of the complete literature I found not a single similar case written up. Today I cannot entirely insist upon this. Namely, at the end of the previous meeting of the Medical Society I showed the result of my operation to a surgeon from San Francisco, Dr. Rosenstirn, and he thought that he had seen something similar in the American literature. Dr. Rosenstirn then was so very kind as to study the American literature, as far as it was available here, and we found the mention of a few endonasal hump removals by Dr. Row‡ (partial nasal reduction actually, in one case, similar to mine) on account of psychic depression; a total reduction of a healthy nose was performed. However, the surgical method (as you'll soon see) was considerably different.

His case was as follows: This gentleman, with an important position in New York felt very

* The photos were taken by Mr. Guenther, Behrenstrasse No. 24.

† The sketches were prepared, based on the photos, by Mr. Weber the engraver of the periodical Berliner Klinische Wochenschrift, Address: Tempelhofer Berg 4.

‡ New York Medical Journal 1892, pp. 452 and 453.

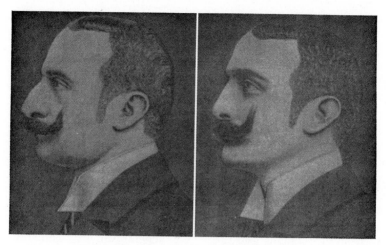

Fig. 3. The patient, before and after operation.

unhappy on account of his somewhat protruding nose. As you see, Gentlemen, this nose had only one fault, in contrast with the case I have operated on; it was neither too long, nor had a hump on it. The patient called on two doctors, who in turn consulted Prof. Robert Weir; the three agreed that in order to restore the patient's mental balance, surgical reduction of the nose should be tried. The operation was carried out by Robert Weir in the following manner.... (*Editorial note.* Joseph then describes Weir's case, as published.) ...

I take the liberty now to show you the end result of these four operations by projection (demonstration), and that Weir's patient had to exchange his somewhat prominent nose for a somewhat long nose.

Robert Weir's case and mine are similar in their indication and extent (after all Weir's case was also a rhinomiosis totalis). On the other hand, they differ considerably in the surgical method, and especially in the success, which in my case was achieved in a single operation, without any secondary correction.

Jacques Joseph, M.D.
Berlin

COMMENTARY BY DR. GUSTAVE AUFRICHT

It is a fascinating experience to read the report of the first rhinoplasty operation by a man who eventually became one of the world's foremost plastic surgeons and who developed the classic rhinoplastic methods. The fascination of this paper is even greater for me because of my personal contact with Joseph and because, after practicing plastic surgery for almost half a century, I still find Joseph's classic methods unsurpassed.

Joseph began originally as an orthopedic surgeon, but soon he became involved with the reduction of large, protruding ears. Apparently the rumor of this successful operation spread around, and one day a male patient appeared in his office, asking to have his unshapely large nose reduced.

Joseph describes the psychologic effect of the conspicuous nose and makes the fundamental observation that the rhinoplasty was performed *to make the patient inconspicuous.* After the operation he noted that the patient "is happy to move around unnoticed." Even today, 70 years later, one often hears the erroneous remark that rhinoplasty is an operation for vanity's sake. That is not true. Vanity is the desire to excel. The average rhinoplasty patient wishes to be relieved of a real or imagined conspicuousness of his nose.

Joseph used the name "Rhinomiosis" for the operation. He liked to coin technical terms, usually Greek and Latin (*e.g.* "Rhinoneoplastik" for nasal reconstruction, "Melomioplastik" for a face lift, or "Metopo-mioplastik" for wrinkles and frowns of the forehead).

The day before the operation, Joseph tried it on a cadaver. He was extremely thorough, and his analytical approach manifested itself in the exact nose measurements, made before and after operation. I always admired this exactness when he fashioned a skin flap. He would measure the defect and flap from every angle, and carefully study the effect of turning the pedicle. The flap fitted perfectly; it never had to be stretched to make up for shortages. His sense of form was that of an artist. I have never seen a better total nasal reconstruction, whether from the forehead or arm, than Joseph's.

Joseph had an ingenious and constructive mind and devised many instruments, some of them obsolete today. It was bewildering for a young surgeon to see that he had a special instrument for practically every step of a rhinoplasty. It almost seemed that one only had to have all those instruments and the operation was easy. He also devised, for "aseptic" suturing, a horseshoe-shaped double-pronged forceps. It was to thread the suture material without touching either the needle or the thread. He gave this method the fancy name "Apodactyle suture" (fingerless suture). This was to prevent stitch infections. Joseph did not use gloves, only three rubber fingers on each hand. He considered the sense of touch important in endonasal plastic work.

He did not wear cap or mask. Nevertheless, he observed accurate aseptic technique and had few complications. This was due to his extreme care and gentleness in handling tissues; he called it "biologic sense."

Joseph amassed a vast experience which he crystallized into definite methods. No operative step was ever haphazard, nor without careful consideration. One could sense his concentration during an operation, saying many times "it can be done this way or that way." He often uttered the word "so," when he accomplished a step.

Joseph has been accused of being secretive about his methods. To a certain extent this was true. On the other hand, one must realize that there was sharp rivalry at that time among some of his colleagues in Germany who jealously observed Joseph's meteoric rise in this new specialty. They were eager both to learn and to appropriate his methods under their own names. Some of the general surgeons thought that rhinoplasty was a very simple operation, and that was the reason Joseph was reluctant to show it. It was said that Prof. Axhausen, one of Germany's leading plastic surgeons, asked and received permission to observe Joseph's operation. He admitted afterward that while rhinoplasty was surgically simple it took Joseph's special talent to perform it successfully.

Joseph gave some courses to foreigners (mostly Americans) after World War I—for which he charged a considerable fee. These consisted of observing (without questions in the operating room) his operations. He also gave a few courses in the Anatomical Institute on well-dissected specimens. In the beginning I had to pay him also, but only a nominal fee (coming from a poor European country). After a couple of months he relinquished my tuition, which was a great favor. At that time it was customary to pay for knowledge and experience.

Joseph did not lose much time in reporting his first rhinoplasty. Within about three months after doing it he presented this, his only case, before the Medical Society of Berlin. Priority was (and apparently always will be) an important ambition of surgeons. It must have been a shock and disappointment when Joseph learned that his rhinoplasty was not the first one. Nevertheless, without doubt, it was his original operation. It is touching, and characteristic of his reasoning, that he insisted that in certain respects his operation was the first one, just the same. With exacting mind he took apart Weir's operation, step by step, and compared it with his own. Finally he came to the conclusion that the only similarities between the two operations were that they both were done to relieve the psychologic effect of a large, conspicuous nose—and that both noses were radically reduced in size (rhinomiosis totalis). Otherwise his surgical method was entirely different, he claimed, and he achieved a better result with a single operation than Weir did with four. There-fore, Joseph felt that his priority claim was valid.

Peculiarly, both patients were men.

I am sure that if Joseph read this paper 20 to 25 years later, he must have smiled. Compared with later refinements, this first operation (which he so jealously defended) was primitive and crude. Nevertheless, from an historical point of view, it clearly shows the characteristics and the germs of the genius—who became the world's unchallenged father of modern rhinoplastic surgery.

—GUSTAVE AUFRICHT

RECONSTRUCTION OF SADDLENOSE BY CARTILAGE OVERLAY

DR. VON MANGOLDT, *Dresden, Germany*

Excerpt from "Die Einpflanzung von Rippenknorpel in den Kehlkopf zur Heilung schwerer Stenosen und Defecte, und Heilung der Sattelnase durch Knorpelübertragung."

(Deutsche Gesell. f. chir., 29: 460, 1900)

Translated from the German by
DR. FRANK McDOWELL

The favorable experiences which I have had with transplanting costal cartilage to the larynx made me think of using the same technique in plastic operations. The idea that a piece of transplanted cartilage with perichondrium will become bow-shaped on the perichondrial side, when placed under the skin, seemed to me particularly valuable for plastic operations on the nose. There it may be necessary to straighten out a sunken bridge, or to relax nostrils (which have been pulled up by tongues of cartilage) to restore the normal vault.

Lately, I have had the opportunity of trying this out in two nose cases.

The first case was one of loss, through lupus, of all the soft nasal tissue and the replacement of the same by plastic surgical methods. The patient, now a 15-year-old girl, is still under treatment—so I will not report her case here.

The second patient I will present to you today—healed. He is a 16-year-old boy, Bruno M. His father suffers from tabes dorsalis. The boy was in good health in early life, but became ill in his sixth year with corneal ulcers which healed completely with residual scars.

At the age of 12 he suffered from ulcerations in his nose. From August 31 to October 20, 1898, he was in the Dresden Children's Hospital with luetic iritis, laryngitis, gumma of the palate, and fresh ulcers of the nose—for which he received therapy. Despite energetic treatment at this time, the vomer (and also, later, the *ossa nasalis*) collapsed and beginning in January, 1899, a typical saddlenose developed—with a sunken saddle between the bony and soft parts. This shortened the bridge, raised the nasal tip, and pulled on the nostrils—which were so sunken in on the sides that they were not supported on inhalation and flapped like sails on exhalation. This can be seen in the photographs I have brought (Fig. 1). After his discharge, the youth took potassium iodide and was ambulatory until his complete recovery—the nose being treated locally.

On June 21, 1899, a piece of costal cartilage with perichondrium (4 to 5 cm long, by 1 cm wide, by ½ cm thick) was removed from the right 7th costal area. A small incision was made then across the glabella, the skin undermined with a small Kocher's sound down to the nasal tip, and the cartilage graft inserted so that it would hold the tip forward; the small forehead wound was closed with sutures. In this manner the not-peri-

Presented at the first session of the Congress of the German Association of Surgeons on April 18, 1900.

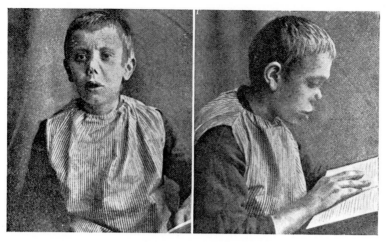

FIG. 1. Condition of Bruno M. when first seen.

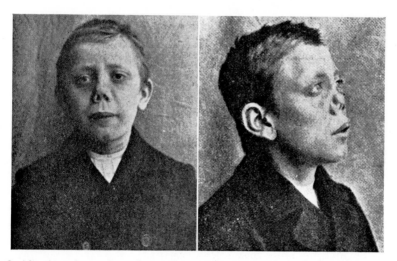

FIG. 2. After inserting a piece of rib cartilage from the glabella to the tip, and small pieces in both nostril walls.

chondrium-covered side of the cartilage was placed under the skin.

Two wide but thin cartilage tongues were then introduced into the nostril walls, through small incisions in both nasolabial folds. These small wounds were then closed with one suture each.

On the whole, these cartilages healed without complication and here are the photographs (Fig. 2).

Through the operations undertaken, the saddle and the loose nostrils were corrected. However, treatment for healing the nasal ulcers had resulted in a shortening of the bridge of the nose, which required a further correction. To achieve this, on November 28, 1899, I loosened the entire soft part of the nose plus the costal cartilage with an inverted-V incision from the glabella downward, and closed it as a Y after pulling everything downward. Thus the bridge of the nose was lengthened and a normal profile was achieved (Fig. 3). The in-

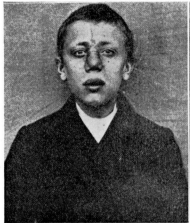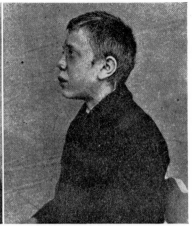

FIG. 3. Final result after the V-Y elongation.

cisions were closed with sutures of the finest thread.

On the basis of these experiences, I believe that costal cartilage will be valuable to use in some plastic operations, and

I would like to recommend the procedure to you.

Prof. Dr. F. von Mangoldt
Children's Hospital
Dresden, Germany

COMMENTARY BY THE EDITOR

This appears to be the first report of a cartilage transplant to the nose. Curiously, little is known about von Mangoldt; there is almost no record of him, other than this paper. Inquiries to the principal medical libraries in this country and to many sources in Europe failed to turn up a photograph of him, or anything more than a few tidbits of information.

Dr. Leo Clodius of Zurich found that the first section of this paper (not translated here), about curing stenoses and defects of the larynx with costal cartilage transplants, was published earlier as a separate essay (*Arch. f. klin. chir., 59: 928, 1899*). In this laryngeal work, von Mangoldt transplanted a piece of costal cartilage (3 cm × 1.5 cm) under the skin of the neck; when it was obvious, 8 months later, that it had not resorbed, he transferred the cartilage in a compound flap with the skin to the larynx. "In this paper of 1899, Dr. von Mangoldt also mentions that he had transplanted cartilage with perichondrium in rabbits

and, 9 months later, he demonstrated by intravascular injection the survival of the perichondrium by filling its blood-vessels. In humans, he also demonstrated the survival of costal cartilage 7 months after subcutaneous transplantation. He mentions, too, that in taking small sections of rib cartilage the piece of cartilage bends itself towards the perichondrium and that this remains after transplantation."

Prof. Dr. Dr. W. Bethmann of Leipzig also searched for material on von Mangoldt and writes as follows. "Unfortunately, all my searches in the likely places (our large libraries, the Institute for the History of Medicine in Berlin, the Dresden Archives) have proved fruitless. The work in which von Mangoldt achieved the free cartilage transplant stemmed from the Children's Hospital (Recovery Station) in Dresden. This institute was founded in 1834, became a state institution in 1918, and existed as such until 1945. In the bombings of 1945 it was completely demolished; at the same

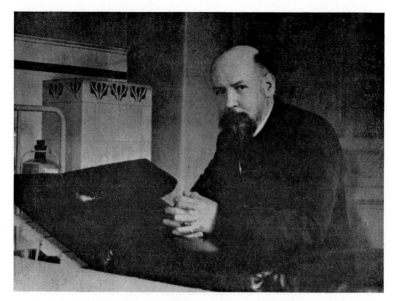

DR. FRIEDRICH VON MANGOLDT
1859–1909

time the papers in it were burned. A direct descendant of this institution does not exist today. In the Archives of the city of Dresden there are no records of von Mangoldt at this time; most of their records were also destroyed in the bombings of 1945. In addition, there is the possibility that records of von Mangoldt were destroyed by the fascists for racial reasons, so that his identity would forever be removed from the libraries. Unfortunately, I can give you no information about this."

Whereupon, Dr. Clodius continued his efforts to find out something more about this remarkable Prof. von Mangoldt, but the Swiss libraries contained no additional information. However, in searching the directories he found the present address in West Germany of a Dr. Burkhard von Mangold who formerly lived in Dresden. Dr. Clodius wrote him—on the chance that he might be a relative. And what a stroke of fortune this turned out to be! Dr. Burkhard von Mangold replied quickly, enclosing the photograph published herewith (which is the first time that a portrait of Prof. von Mangoldt has been published) and wrote as follows.

My grandfather, Dr. Friedrich "Fritz" von Mangoldt was the third son of Dr. Hans Carl Emil von Mangoldt, Professor of Political Sciences, and his wife, Luise Caroline von Lengerke. He was born in Göttingen on August 27, 1859, and died in Dresden on March 22, 1909. He was married to Anna Amalie Lampe, from Leipzig, and achieved many honors. His offices included "Counselor to the King of Saxony," "Chief Surgeon of the Karola Hospital in Dresden-Altstadt," and "Royal Saxonian Staff Physician to the Reserve Army." As far as I can remember, my grandfather died at the age of 49 from lymphangitis—due to a laceration which he sustained during a postmortem examination. The photograph was made shortly before his death.

Thus, the sun rose, shone, and set in this one paper—for von Mangoldt. But what a valuable contribution it was!

—*Frank McDowell*

The photographs from Dr. Mangoldt's article were furnished by the National Library of Medicine in Bethesda, Md.

NASAL REDUCTIONS

JACQUES JOSEPH, M.D., *Berlin, Germany*

(*Deutsche Med. Wchnschr., 30: 1095–1098, 1904.*)

Translated from the German by
DR. FRANK McDOWELL

Allow me, gentlemen, to report to you on the nasal reductions performed by me. There are 43 finished cases, 30 men and 13 women. All had deformities of the external nose; several had an inner deformity of the septum.

I have tabulated the defects (with practical nomenclature) in a manner indicating whether the whole nose or only part of the nose was involved, and I describe the corrective procedures as total or partial rhinomiosis...

The number of cases since my last publication (*Berl. klin. Wchnschr., 1902, No. 36*) has not only increased, but also new methods of treatment have been required—some of which are new operative methods and some of which are modifications of procedures previously used.

In changing the nasal shape, it is of first importance to remove the abnormal breadth of the nasal bones, which I have done 7 times (3 times unilaterally, 4 times bilaterally)—twice as a separate operation, and 4 times as part of a complete nasal reduction. I performed my first operation for narrowing the bony parts on August 18, 1901. The operation consisted of sawing through the frontal process of the upper jaw (Fig. 1, through the thick dotted line in the direction indicated). When the sidewall of the nose was freed from the upper jaw, light pressure with the thumb and index finger was all that was necessary to reposition it toward the midline.

The operation can be carried out so that there is no visible scar; namely, it can be performed inside the nose. A double-edged knife is inserted in the outermost border of the pyriform recess, exactly under the nasolabial fold, so that the tip lies on the outer edge of the upper jaw. This incision is enlarged sufficiently to allow the keyhole saw to be inserted. The notched parts of the saw must not be too long, to avoid injuring the ala of the nose. For greater con-

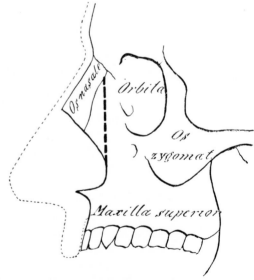

Die dicke punktierte Linie giebt die Richtung und Ausdehnung des zum Zwecke der Nasenverschmälerung auszuführenden Sägeschnitts an.
FIG. 1.

Presented before the 33rd Congress of the Deutschen Gesellschaft fur Chirurgie on April 7, 1904.

Fig. 2.

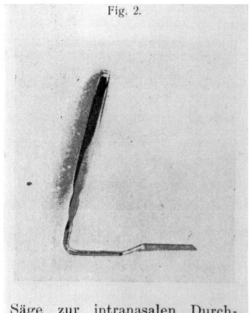

Säge zur intranasalen Durch-
trennung des Processus frontalis
des Oberkiefers.
(½ natürlicher Größe.)

venience, I lay the handle of the saw
under a corner at an approximate angle
of 70°. To enter the intranasal incision
easily, even when the nostrils are narrow, I make a second bayonet-like bend
in front of the teeth as a supplement.
This bend is toward the right for the left
nasal sidewall, and for the right nasal
sidewall it is to the left (Fig. 2). It is far
more practical to use a specially formed
saw for each side . . .

If the bony sidewalls are medially displaced, as indicated, so must they be
held in this state as they have a tendency
to return to their original position. For
this reason I use a nasal clamp (Fig.
3) . . . The nasal clamp is placed on the
nose and then screwed together as tightly
as is desired. If the clamp does not cling
correctly, especially where there is fatty
skin, one presses on the head and places
a band horizontally around the head to
hold the clamp in place. In this way we
make a very suitable substitute for the

otherwise necessary, but unpleasant,
plaster of paris bandage.

If an outside wound has been created,
the patients wear this nasal clamp after
the 10th day. If, however, the operation
has been performed intranasally, one
affixes the clamp immediately after the
subsidence of swelling—usually around
the 5th postoperative day. The clamp
must be worn until the tendency of the
nose to regress to the old position has
passed; this takes, on the average, 10
days . . .

Editorial note. Joseph goes on to describe the
removal of nasal humps, shortening the nose,
and the treatment of hanging columella. At this
time he was apparently doing most of his cases
intranasally, but was using open operation for
some.

As regards the question of danger from
these operations—in my 43 cases I have
had no case of death or injury, and may
thus state that this operation is not dangerous. Healing in all cases was unevent-

Fig. 3.

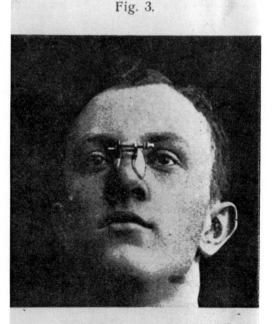

Nasenklemme (im Gebrauch).

ful; the scars became invisible after a time. I have asked a patient of mine who lives in Berlin to come to this gathering. You have, in your hands, preoperative photographs of her. I would like you to notice now that her nose is not prominent, that the scars are not apparent. I have also a number of photographs of other patients in which you can see the cosmetic results...

Dr. Jacques Joseph
Specialist in Orthopedic Surgery
Berlin

The photographs in this article were furnished through the kind assistance of the National Library of Medicine, History of Medicine Section, Bethesda, Md.

COMMENTARY BY THE EDITOR

With this additional paper of Joseph's, we conclude our series of classic reprints on rhinoplasty.

During the 6-year period since his first publication on rhinoplasty, it can be seen that Joseph made remarkable improvements of lasting value in the technique. His total number of cases for 6 years was small; perhaps the most difficult part of the whole thing was in convincing other doctors and the public that there was not something sinful *per se* about this kind of surgery. He was, of course, far ahead of his time.

For a man who did so much, remarkably little is known about Joseph. Only the scantiest references to the man and his life could be found; these are appended.

Joseph was born in Königsberg on September 6, 1865, took his first medical courses at some place in Berlin, but received his doctor's degree from the University of Leipzig in 1890. Afterwards, he did general practice in Berlin for a while, then became interested in orthopedic surgery and studied it at the J. Wolff Clinic. Coelst[4] states Joseph had a remarkable gift for drawing, which was in evidence from early childhood. Little by little he became interested in plastic surgery and, of course, reported his first rhinoplasty in 1898—just 8 years after he finished medical school. Later, he became interested in plastic surgery on other parts of the face and body and published numerous papers in the *Berliner Klinische Wochenschrift, Münchener Medizinische Wochenschrift,* and *Deutsche Medizinische Wochenschrift.*

In 1912, there appeared a chapter by him on rhinoplasty and otoplasty in the famed *Handbuch der Speziellen Chirurgie des Ohres und der Oberen Luftwege.* Coelst[4] states that during World War I "he directed the department of facial reconstruction, by order of the Prussian ministry." Fischer[5] notes, however, that he was chief of the section on facial plastic surgery in the ENT clinic of the Charité hospital in Berlin, where he was given the title of Professor in 1918.

Coelst[4] also made the following comments about him. "One of his finest char-

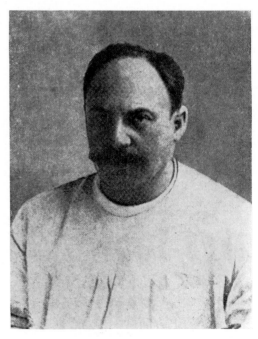

PROF. JACQUES JOSEPH
1865–1934

acteristics, it seems to me, was combining diverse operations to attain the same objective, but more artistically. Under a rude exterior he hid a generous soul and a sympathetic heart. An eccentric character toward the end of his life, he hated to be followed by a large number of assistants when he operated, and allowed only newcomers who were not antipathetic to him to approach. His greatest desire was a complete reconciliation among nations, which would permit all plastic surgeons to form an international society of plastic surgery."

In 1928, C. Kabitsch of Leipzig published the first edition of Joseph's great *Nasenplastik und Sonstige Gesichtsplastik*. This was followed by a second edition in 1931.

Fred[1] states that Joseph did his last rhinoplasty on January 12, 1934, in his own hospital on Wilmersdorfstrasse. The patient was 16-year-old Adolphine Schwarz, daughter of the owner of a celebrated restaurant in Munich. "After voluminous correspondence through the mail, she presented herself alone at the hospital at 11:30 A.M. on the morning of the operation. She was examined by Professor Joseph for the first time, photographed by Professor Joseph himself, and taken to the operating room at 1 P.M., in the fashionable two-story wooden Villa which served as his hospital. There were no doctors in the operating room other than Professor Joseph, but many nurses were in evidence. Little or no premedication was administered, and the patient stated she was 'wide awake' during the operation. The operating time was 2½ hours. The fee was reputed to be 4000 marks (equivalent to $1000). The patient remained in the hospital five days, and in Berlin for a total of two weeks."

There is a good deal of uncertainty about the manner of Joseph's death. He was Jewish, of course, and this was at a time when Hitler's brownshirts were undertaking the grossest persecutions of Jewish people. Fred[1] states (in 1957) that in February 1934 "the newspapers carried the tragic news that the incomparable Jacques Joseph . . . had blown the top of his head off with a revolver shot through the mouth." Coelst[4] wrote from Brussels in 1934, "His death dates from last February and was unexpected, in the hospital universally known for the master, where we met him and where he displayed his untiring activity." In 1944 Marino[3] wrote, "In March 1934, just a decade ago, Prof. Jacques Joseph died in Czechoslovakia at the age of 69." It is Safian's[2] understanding that it was Joseph's son-in-law who was shot at the Czechoslovakian border, while trying to flee Germany—and that this event precipitated a fatal coronary attack in Joseph. He notes that Joseph's widow reached San Francisco and lived for many years there. Those of us who attended the banquet of the annual meeting of the American Society of Plastic and Reconstructive Surgeons (at the Fairmont Hotel in San Francisco) in 1957 were privileged to see her and speak with her.

—*Frank McDowell*

REFERENCES

1. Fred, G. B.: Jacques Joseph's last rhinoplasty. Eye, Ear, Nose & Throat Month., *36:* 283–287, 1957.
2. Safian, J.: Personal recollections of Professor Jacques Joseph. Plast. & Reconstr. Surg., *46:* 175–177, 1970.
3. Marino, H.: J. Joseph (1865–1934). Prensa med. argent., *31:* 449–450, 1944.
4. Coelst, M.: Le Professeur Jacques Joseph. Rev. chir. plastique, *2:* 83–84, 1934.
5. Fischer, I.: *Biographisches Lexikon der Hervorragenden Ärzte der letzten Funfzig Jahre*, p. 722. Urban & Schwarzenberg, München, 1962.

PUBLICATIONS BY DR. JOSEPH

1. Operative reduction of the size of a nose (rhinomiosis). Berl. klin. Wchnschr., *40:* 882, 1898.
2. About some further nasal reductions. Berl. klin. Wchnschr., p. 851, 1902.
3. Nasal reductions. Deutsche med. Wchnschr., *30:* 1095–1098, 1904.
4. Intranasal hump removal. Berl. klin. Wchnschr., p. 650–653, 1904.
5. More about nasal reductions. Munchen. med. Wchnschr., *52:* 1489–1490, 1905.
6. Treatise on rhinoplasty. Berl. klin. Wchnschr., *44:* 470, 1907.
7. Correction of twisted nose. Deutsche med. Wchnschr., *49:* 203, 1907.
8. Nasal corrections. Verhandl. d. Deutsch. Gesellsch. Natursforscher und ärtzte in Konigsberg, 1910.

9. On artificial nose plastic. Verhandl. d. deutsch. Gesell. f. chir., *4:* 82, 1912.

10. Treatise on total rhinoplasty. Munch. med. Wchnschr., *51:* 705, 1914.

11. Principles of building out the face, especially by rhinoplasty. Beitr. z. Anat., Phys., Path., Ohres., *13:* 244, 1919.

12. Treatise on total and partial rhinoplasty, espe-cially on technic of free skin transplantation. Berl. klin. Wchnschr., p. 678, 1922.

13. Corrective nasal plastic. In *Handbuch der Spe-ziellen Chirurgie*. Edited by Katz and Blumen-feld. C. Kabitsch, Leipzig, 1922.

14. *Nasenplastik und Sonstige Gesichtsplastik*. C. Kabitsch Co., Leipzig (First Edition, 1928, Sec-ond Edition, 1931).

SECTION III

The Origins of Cleft Lip Repairs

The first paper in this section describes some early re-pairs in Colonial America, but more importantly it re-views world developments in this field up to the end of the 18th century.

HARELIP REPAIR IN COLONIAL AMERICA

A REVIEW OF 18TH CENTURY AND EARLIER SURGICAL TECHNIQUES*

BLAIR O. ROGERS†

New York, New York

On Friday, September 1, 1770, a young child of Roxbury, Massachusetts, having been left alone, unfortunately fell into a tub of hot beer and was scalded to death.[1] This local mishap, reported in the Boston Evening Post, was followed by several other choice news items which included the following:

> A few Weeks since the Operation for the Hare-Lip was performed to great Perfection on a young Man in Milton near Brush-Hill; and a Child in Boston has received as much Bene-fit from the Operation as the Case would admit of, by Mr. HALL, Surgeon to the 14th. Regiment. . . . The Impression these unhappy Sights are apt to make on married Women, should be an Inducement to have this Defect in Nature rectified early in Life, as there are numerous Instances of the Mother's Affection having impressed her Offspring with the like Deformity.[1]

This reference to a harelip operation, twice performed successfully in 1770 in Colonial America, is only one of several other descriptions of harelip repair which were reported or advertised in Colonial newspapers, including those of a certain "Dr." Lawrence Stork (from Germany) and an equally mysterious "Dr." Anthony Yeldall (apparently from Philadelphia).

On May 22, 1775, in a Philadelphia paper,[2] the following advertisement by "Dr." Anthony Yeldall with four testimonials from satisfied patients could be read:

> For the benefit of others, be it made public, that I John Dunbar, of the City of Phila-delphia, had a daughter with the deformity of a Hare-lip; I had it cut by a surgeon, but it broke open; I had it cut again and it broke open again; I then applied to Dr. YELDALL, who, to my satisfaction, did the operation in one minute, by the watch, and compleated the cure in four days.
>
> JOHN DUNBAR
>
> None need dispair, having the above mentioned deformity, for let them be ever so large or frightful, or have been cut ever so often before, they will be done in one minute, and the cure compleated in four days, or nothing will be required.
>
> Poor people may have them done GRATIS."

The following advertisement appeared in a New London, Connecticut, news-paper on March 29, 1780:

> DOCT. Lawrence Stork, From Germany, Informs the Public, That he undertakes to cure the following disorders incident to the human body, viz. Loss of hearing—loss of sight—

Read at the Section on Historical Medicine, The New York Academy of Medicine, November 27, 1963.

* The historical research described in this paper was supported by a grant from the Association for the Aid of Crippled Children, New York, New York.

† Assistant Professor of Clinical Surgery (Plastic Surgery), School of Medicine, New York University; Institute of Reconstructive Plastic Surgery, N. Y. U. Medical Center.

cancers—hair-lips—the falling sickness, and all kinds of fits whatever—likewise cholics—fevers—all sorts of wens—all breaches of the body—fever-sores—broken bones—and in general all disorders of the human body, whether internal or external. He also informs those who live at a distance, that by sending their urine in a phial, with the age of the person, he can give them ease. And he farther informs, that if he makes no cure, he expects no pay. He may be seen at Mr. Jacob Fink's in New-London. Feb. 28, 1780.[3]

The apparently successful repair of harelips by these three gentlemen, begs the question, therefore, as to their medical and surgical qualifications. What do we know of these three pioneering spirits whose surgery predated the earliest reconstructive surgical operations which have been officially recorded in the medical literature[4] of the post colonial period following the Revolutionary War?

Of the three men, only Mr. Charles Hall seems to have been legitimately registered in Johnston's *Roll of Commissioned Officers in the Medical Service of the British Army.*[5] Mr. Hall was apparently a British regimental medical officer, assigned to the 14th Foot Regiment, whose post was in the Boston, Massachusetts area just prior to the American Revolution. His last military assignment placed him on the staff in Jamaica on December 25, 1782. He was placed on half pay on December 25, 1783, after having served in the American War of Independence, and died in 1805. His birth date and formal medical education are both unknown.[6]

As far as the credentials of "Dr." Stork and "Dr." Yeldall are concerned, none of the routine references[7, 8] consulted, nor any other ancillary material have revealed even the slightest smidgen of information about these two gentlemen. Whether they were legitimately trained physicians or surgeons, or whether they could be classified by the circumstantial evidence of their newspaper advertisements in the realm of quacks, mountebanks, charlatans, itinerant medicasters, etc., remains an unsolved mystery. By checking with Guerra's[9] *American Medical Bibliography (1639–1783)*, however, it is interesting to trace their meanderings in more detail[10] up and down the Middle Atlantic and the New England States, between the years 1761 to 1780 for Dr. Stork, "Surgeon and Oculist to Her Royal Highness the Princess of Wales,"[11] and between the years 1771 to 1781 for Dr. Yeldall, who according to a 1771 copy of the Boston Evening Post,[12] ". . . sells medicines from a stage; his harangue, odd tricks of his Merry Andrew, and activity of his little boy diverts the people."

In all fairness to these two bold "surgeons," it might be emphasized that it was not uncommon for physicians and surgeons of this period, such as the illustrious Dr. Benjamin Rush,[13] to take out advertisements and to announce their activities in the local newspapers. Gordon,[14] in his book *Aesculapius Comes to the Colonies* reminds us:

Today when only quacks advertise their healing prowess to the public, one is amused upon reading the ads and testimonials offered by legitimate physicians in Colonial times.

Dr. Benjamin Rush, in the same newspaper which carried an announcement by Dr. Yeldall, advertised: ". . . At the Request of a number of his Fellow Citizens . . . eight Lectures on such parts of Chemistry . . . in the College of this city".

Among the subjects included in his lectures were those dealing with:

. . . the manufactories of glass and porcelane. . . of the causes of meteors, fire, damps, etc. . . . of the art of alchemy, or the Philosophers stone. Of the causes of earthquakes and volcanos . . . [and] of wines, beer, etc.[13]

That Dr. Rush was not adverse to making a little profit on these homey subjects is revealed in the final paragraph of his advertisement when he stated that:

These Lectures will begin on Tuesday the 10th of January, at six o'clock in the evening, and will be continued three times a week until the whole are delivered. Tickets at One Guinea each may be had of Mr. John Dunlap, Mr. Robert Aitken, and at the London Coffee-house.

In view of Dr. Yeldall's apparent success, as verified by the testimonial of John Dunbar,[2] one must ask oneself, "Just exactly what surgical technique did Yeldall or Stork use?" Did they use hairlip pins (fig. 9) with the figure-of-8 suture which was probably the most commonly employed technique of the mid- and late 18th century, or were they decades ahead of their surgical colleagues if, as mountebanks, they employed true knotted "interrupted" sutures to close the cleft, as alluded to by Heister,[15] the founder of scientific surgery in Germany. Heister (1683 to 1758) described the methods they might have used in his *Chirurgie*, the most popular surgical work of the 18th century. In the 1743 English translation, Heister recounts:

. . . VIII. Many German Quacks and Mountebanks frequently retain the Lips of the Wound together by strong Thread passed through them instead of Needles, after which they tie the Ends of the Thread in the same manner as we directed for the knotted Suture in Part I, Book 1 Chap. VI No. III. They observed the same Order in tying the Threads as other Surgeons do in making the Ligature about the Needles, making no Difference in their other Dressings, and the Remainder of the Cure; at last they cut the middle Thread on the third or fourth Day, as they do the uppermost upon the fifth, and the lowermost on the sixth or seventh Day; and thus they frequently succeed, and perform good Cures, though in an awkward manner, and by obtuse and unfit Instruments, especially when the Fissure is but small, for when it is large this method will hardly succeed.[15]

This 18th century controversy on the use of harelip pins with the figure-of-8 suture *versus* "threads" or interrupted sutures placed in the edges of the cleft lips, is a fascinating one.

If Drs. Yeldall and Stork, in Colonial America, really did employ the technique of knotted interrupted suturing in harelip repair as described so colorfully by Heister, and if, by inference, of course, they abandoned the use of costly and cumbersome harelip pins or needles which were usually made of expensive silver or gold with or without movable steel points, then they were probably, despite their sale of "antivenereal sugar plums"[16] and cures for blindness,[17] a half century or more ahead of many of their legitimately trained surgical colleagues, some of whom[18, 19] had not yet even in 1879 or 1880 given up the use of harelip pins one century later.

As so frequently happens in the development of an interest in historical medicine one then finds oneself asking questions: "But when did surgical repair of the harelip first take place." With this question as a starting point in the always fascinating game of historical detective work, it was no great surprise to uncover another reference to repair of the harelip deformity[20] in Colonial America.

Matthew Wilson (1734 to 1790), a minister and a physician as well a native of Chester County, Pennsylvania, who practiced medicine in Lewes, Delaware, wrote an unpublished compendium of medicine from 1756 to 1787 called the *Therapeutic Alphabet*, in which a method of harelip repair is rather completely described in the quaint vernacular of that period.[20] Although there is no evidence that Dr. Wilson had obtained a medical degree, his contributions were profound enough for him to have been cited in Thacher's *American Medical Biography*.[7] Dr. Wilson referred alphabetically to the deformity as follows:

Labium Leporinum: Hare Lip. See Lagocheilos.

Lagocheilos: Hare Lip. Is a Deformity in which ye Lip is divided by Chasms or Fissures. See Lab. Leporin. The Operation should be omitted, untill ye Child has some Reason to suffer it to be done. On we see Van Swieten, Sharp [⁶⁵]. It is pretty common for ye Roof of ye Mouth to admit of Reunion. Fissures of ye Palate often close in some years. Separate ye Lip from ye upper Jaw; divide ye Frenulum we connects it to ye Gums. If ye Dentes Incisorii too much projected, cut ym out in Infants. Cut off ye callous Lips wt Scissors ye whole length, but take Care to make ye Wound in Straight Lines. Then bring ye two Lips of ye wound exactly together, & pass a couple of pins, one pretty near ye Top & ye other as near ye bottome, thro' middle of both edges of it, & secure ym in yt Situation by twisting a Piece of Wax'd thread, across & round ye pins 7 or 8 times. Then cut off ye points, lay a small Bolster of Plaster under ym, to prevent their Scratching. Wn only ye lower Part of ye Hare Lip can be brought into Contact, one Pin is Sufficient. The practice of bolstering ye Cheek upward does more injury to ye Patient, yn good to ye Wound. Dress superficially as often as is Necessary for Cleanliness. In 8 or 9 Days ye parts generally are found united, yn gently extract the Pins & apply dry Lint and Adhesive Plaster. This method may be useful in some Fistulae &c. Silver Pins & Steel Points suit ye Pomp of ye Great, but common Pins Answer ye End fully as well. See Cullen on Copper.

Lagostoma: The Upper Lip divided. See Lagocheilos.

Obviously, Dr. Wilson preferred harelip pins, and if incisor teeth projected too far into the region of his repair, he cut them out. This, of course, was neither a new, a brutal nor an uncommon surgical measure for this era, nor was it uncommon when Pierre Franco[21] recommended approximately the same procedure two centuries earlier. One may then wonder just how far back in medical history can surgical repair of the harelip be traced?

HARELIP REPAIR PRIOR TO THE 18TH CENTURY

Harelip apparently attracted very little attention among ancient medical writers. No mention of its existence or its surgical repair can be found in either the Ebers[22] or the Edwin Smith[23] papyri or in the writings[24] of Hippocrates (460 to 375 B.C.). Celsus (25 B.C. to 50 A.D.), who lived during the reign of Augustus Caesar, although often given credit for first mentioning harelip, in reality did not, but only described the treatment of lip fissures or cracks in the lip.[25, 26]

Celsus, however, was one of the first to use cautery for the treatment of wounds of the skin, reducing their margins to a state of rawness which then apparently healed by "second intention" and, probably, by considerable scarring. Thus, he predated the use of cautery or the hot iron which Arab surgeons subsequently employed so routinely, centuries later.

Galen[27] (130 to 200 A.D.) did not concern himself with harelip repair, but he may have been one of the first to use catgut in surgery.

Antyllus[28] (*ca.* 250 A.D), although describing methods to improve the loss of tissue substance and deforming scars by use of relaxing incisions, made no mention of harelip According to Morse,[29] however, Chinese surgeons[30] may possibly be the first who mentioned or performed surgical repair of the harelip. Whether this surgery only involved cautery or more refined techniques is not explained by Morse, who merely states:

In the Chin Dynasty (229–317 A.D.) there was a surgeon who did plastic surgery for harelip. In the Tang Dynasty (618–901 AD) another surgeon, Fang Kan, was designated as "the doctor of lips' repair" from which he obtained considerable repute.

Paulus Aegineta[31] (625 to 690 A.D.), who did not refer to harelip, is often thought to be the major link between the Eastern medical and surgical learning of Hindu and Arab schools of medicine, and the ever increasing numbers of Western medical and surgical scholars during this era. In his medical works, he was interested, however, in the prevention of another more common affliction of the face, wrinkles, for which he recommended a troche or lozenge made of ivory shavings, bruised fish gelatin (ichthyocolla) and male frankincense.

Albucasis[32] (936 to 1013 A.D.), the greatest surgeon of the Arabian School from Cordoba in Spain, did not use the hot iron or cautery to abrade the edges of the harelip, despite statements by Velpeau to the contrary. Cautery, however, was a special feature of Arabian surgery, Arab surgeons having literally set aside any more frequent use of the knife, which had been employed by earlier surgeons such as Antyllus, in favor of the use of cautery.[33] Albucasis employed cauterization only for *fissures des lèvres* or fissures of the lips,[32] known as *chouquouq eckchifah* in Arabic. He did recommend, however, the use of needles and sutures for certain wounds of the lips, nose and ears. According to Garrison[33] it was not until Saliceto[34] (1201 to 1277 A.D.) of Bologna that the use of the knife in surgery was reintroduced into Western medicine.

The Saxon surgeons of pre-Norman Britain,[35] known archaically as "leeches," may very well have been the first to specifically describe the repair of harelip in Europe. In the *Leech-book of Bald*, thought by manuscript experts to be written about 950 A.D., the operation is simply but rationally described:

For hair lip, pound mastic very small, add the white of an egg, and mingle as thou dost vermillion, cut with a knife *the false edges of the lip*, sew fast with silk, then smear without and within with the salve, ere the silk rot. If it draw together, arrange it with the hand; anoint again soon.[35]

Harelip repair was not described[36] by Roger of Salerno (*c.* 12th century) in his *Practica chirurgiae* (*c.* 1180 A.D.), nor by his famous pupil, Roland of Parma (*c.* early 13th century), nor by Saliceto[34] of Bologna (1201 to 1277 A.D.), nor by Lanfranchi[37] of Milan (? to 1315 A.D.) nor by Henri de Mondeville[38] ((?) 1260 to 1320 A.D.).

Jehan Yperman (1295 to 1351 A.D.), apparently the first Flemish authority on surgery in the Low Countries during the 14th century, and a pupil of Lanfranchi, wrote specifically not only of unilateral harelip but of the bilateral harelip as well, and to him one might historically assign the first fully documented description of harelip and its surgical repair[39] which can be attributed to a specific author. Yperman freshened the borders of the cleft with a bistouri, the narrow-bladed knife used by surgeons of this period. The cleft margins were then sutured with a triangular needle armed with a twisted wax suture ("cousez-les à l'aide d'une aiguille triangulaire") and reinforced with a long harelip needle passed through the lips some distance from the edges of the cleft, in order to make for a more accurate approximation of the internal and external wound edges. The latter needle was held in place with a wrap-around figure-of-8 suture or thread. Yperman mentions that some surgeons of the period did not suture the harelip but treated it merely by bringing its edges together with long needles. Others apparently made relaxing incisions [editor: externally?] (fig. 4) in the cheeks to close very wide clefts, but Yperman did not advise their use because the facial disfigurement which resulted might "compromise the reputation of the surgeon."

Yperman referred to the deformity as a "notched-mouth" (*sarte monde*). Until the 14th century, at least in Anglo-Saxon Britain, it was known as *hari*lip.[35] There is still a translator's controversy, not yet settled, as to whether Albucasis' reference to fissures of the lips, [which are called] *poils*[32] in the French translation, or *chara* in Arabic, or *pili* in Latin, also implies *hari*lip, or, because of its plural form, *poils*, *pili*, and the ambiguous phrase following it, "et cela surtout aux lévres des enfants" [tr.—which occur chiefly (?) on the lips of infants], merely refers to cracks or chaps or fissures of the lips which during this era, because of their thin slitlike quality, might have resembled *hairs*.

The first English use of the word *hare* in context with *hare*lip, as contrasted to the word *hair* in *hair*lip, probably occurred in Johnson's translation (51) of Ambroise Paré's first original use of the term *bec-de-lièvre* (tr.—lip of the hare).

Guy de Chauliac[40] ((?) 1298 to 1368), one of the most famous surgeons of the Middle Ages, did not describe harelip, nor its treatment *per se*. He merely recommended, as did Roger of Salerno, a salve or walnut oil application for fissures or small cracks of the lips, (*fendilleures des lèvres*), and if these were unsuccessful, he referred to Albucasis' use of cautery. De Chauliac's frequent reliance upon salves and cautery prompted Garrison[33] to make the following comment:

> In spite of his wide experience, Guy de Chauliac was on the whole a reactionary in the important matter of the treatment of wounds, and threw back the progress of surgery for some six centuries by giving his personal weight to the doctrine that the healing of a wound must be accomplished by the surgeon's interference—salves, plasters and other meddling— rather than by the healing power of nature.

Castiglioni[41] also agrees with Garrison's assessment of de Chauliac. It now seems that de Chauliac's long forgotten contemporary, Jehan Yperman, was much the better surgeon in many respects.

John of Arderne[42] (1307 to 1380), the first to revive the art of surgery in

England, does not mention harelip in his book. Although he condescendingly looked down upon the barbers who also practiced surgery during the early 14th century, he still placed some reliance upon spells and charms,[43] and being skilled in leechcraft, he must have been aware of the old Saxon methods of suturing "hair-lips." In subsequent centuries, the barber-surgeons whom John of Arderne and others despised so vehemently, were possibly the one group who passed on from generation to generation the skill for repairing harelip.[15] In his highly readable *Surgeons All*, Graham[43] states:

"The Barber-Surgeons' Company at this time had many individual members who did all they could to discourage quackery, but as a company the Barber-Surgeons found it politic to deal with charlatans. All who presented themselves to the Masters of the Company were examined, and even those with a minimum of knowledge of the prescribed subjects were given some sort of temporary license to practise . . . The licenses were often limited ones, and would state that the reformed quack was to practise only couching for cataract . . . or whatever particular operation was that the man had previously practised outside the profession. Two other operations, belonging properly to plastic surgery, were practised almost exclusively by quacks within or without the shelter of the Barber-Surgeon's Company—namely, the operations for harelip and for wryneck."

Heinrich von Pfolsprundt, a Bavarian Army surgeon, who lived about the year 1460 when his *Buch der Bundth-Ertznei*[44] was written, described harelip and its treatment. His book is usually considered the first work of early German surgery; in it he also described plastic surgical techniques, *e.g*, rhinoplasty, probably learned from one of the Brancas, itinerant Sicilian surgeons of the early 15th century.[45-46] For harelip repair Pfolsprundt used either a razor or a scissors to make the harelip wound margins somewhat higher than the apex of the cleft itself, and he recommended that sutures be placed through the entire thickness of the lip. At the end of the operation, he applied a plaster containing red healing salve to the entire wound area, and then he dressed the wound twice every day, giving his patients strengthening wound drinks (*wundtrangk*) which other surgeons such as de Mondeville, the teacher of Guy de Chauliac, were accustomed to use. According to Pfolsprundt, the repair was completed and the lip wound entirely healed in 3 weeks' time.

Charaf ed-Din (*ca.* 1465), the author of the first Turkish surgical manuscript,[47] carried on traditions in the 15th century described five centuries earlier by Albucasis. Some medical historians, who first inspected the figure showing cauterization of a lip fissure, believed that Turkish surgeons used this technique (fig. 1) for repair of harelip. But Huard and Grmek[47] have recently emphasized that the figure actually represents a fissure of the *lower* lip, not the upper. The frequent occurrence of fissures or cracks in the lips of infants was probably as much a problem to Turkish surgeons as it was to surgeons of previous centuries (see Celsus). No direct reference to the treatment of harelip can be found in this fascinating Turkish manuscript.

Hieronymus Brunschwig (*c.* 1450 to 1533), an Alsatian Army surgeon from Strassburg, in his surgical treatise[48] which dealt chiefly with treatment of gunshot wounds, also described harelip repair. He advised that the patient being

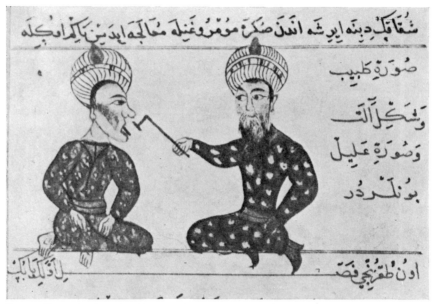

FIG. 1. Cauterization of a fissure (chap or crack) of the lower lip. (From an illustrated manuscript of the Turkish surgeon, Charaf ed-Din[47] written in 1465 A.D.)

operated upon either lie upon a table to which he was fastened down with three hand towels, [this was a surgical era three centuries prior to the invention of anesthesia] or that he sit on a table to which he was fastened in a similar manner. The freshening of the wound or cleft edges was made with a scissors, and their union was performed by use of an interrupted waxed silk suture, which by drawing blood was known as a *bloody* suture, or in wider clefts, by use of a pinching clasp dressing (Zwickhafft) or a self retaining clasp (Selphafften). Over the wound he then applied a thick, melted powder of eggshell chalk and an eggpaste. He then described a rather complicated dressing which he also attributed to Roger of Salerno, in which a long bandage with two ends was so placed that the middle of the bandage lay directly over the wound; then each half of the bandage was wound back and forth like a cross over the wound, around the head and neck and under the arms for fixation.

Hans von Gersdorff (*ca.* 1500), another Alsatian Army surgeon, whose *Feldtbuch der Wund-Artzney* (*Field Book of Wound Surgery*) contained illustrations of surgical procedures and instruments in use in the early 16th century, referred (perhaps mistakenly) to cautery instruments for treating harelip which were direct copies of those seen in Albucasis' *Al-Tasrif*. As an alternative to cautery, he suggested that "a knife is equally good."[49]

Pierre Franco (1500 to 1561), a Huguenot surgeon from the Provence, and a pupil of Ambroise Paré, recommended that the harelip edges be cut either with a knife or a scissors or adjusted with a cautery.[21] Following cauterization, and only after the scab fell off or was loosened by applying fresh butter, he recommended the dry suture technique (fig. 2), or the use of agglutinative plaster dressings (*em-*

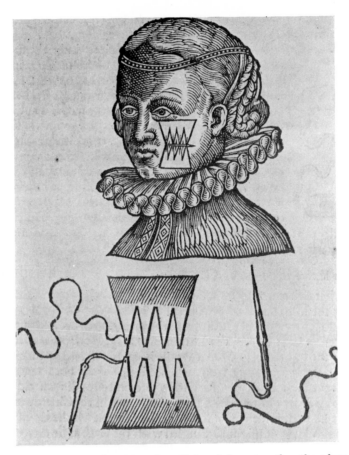

Fig. 2. Method of using a dry suture to splint and draw together the edges of a cheek wound, as described by Ambroise Paré. (From Johnson's translation of Parés "Workes."[51] Illustration is a good copy of Paré's original woodcut.)

plastre) to bring the edges together. He also employed the method of uniting the cleft lip edges with an untwisted or interrupted suture placed in the middle of the defect followed by the application of two or three unthreaded harelip pins or needles placed through the wound margins and then wound about, probably in a figure-of-8 fashion, with threads or suture material. In double harelip, with protrusion of the premaxilla, he suggested that superfluous portions of the pre-maxilla "which were not necessary" should be cut away with a bone scissors or saw to allow for better closure.

Ambroise Paré (1510 to 1590), one of the greatest surgical figures of the Renaissance and undoubtedly its finest surgeon, might well have been the first surgeon to include an illustration[50] of the repaired harelip in his surgical works (fig. 3). In an English translation of his works,[51] in describing the treatment of wounds of the cheek, which includes a section on harelip repair (fig. 3), Paré advised:

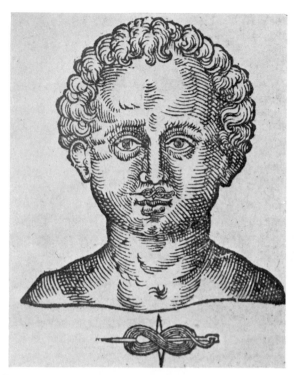

FIG. 3. "The figure of the suture fit for cloven or hare lips: as also the dilineation of the Needle about whose ends the thred is wrapped over and under, to and again." (Legend from Johnson's translation of Pare's "Workes."[51] Illustration is a good copy of Pare's original woodcut.)

Seeing a wound of the cheek seems to require a suture, it must have a dry suture (as they term it) lest that the scar should become deformed. For that deformity is very grievous to many, as to women who are highly pleased with their beauties. Therefore you shall spread two peeces of new cloath of an indifferent fineness, and proportionable bigness with this insuing medicine. . . . [An old medical formula for an agglutinative mixture to be applied to the dressing is included here] Apply the peeces of cloth spread with this on each side of the wound one, some fingers breadth asunder, and let it alone till it be hard dryed to the skin. Then you shall so draw them together with your needle and thred, that the flesh by their sticking may also follow, and be mutually adjoined, as you may see it here exprest. [see Fig. 2] The wound shall be agglutinated by this means, together with the use of fit medicines, pledgets, ligatures. But all the ligatures and stayes which shall be used for that purpose must be fastened to the Patients night-lap.

But when the wound is great and deep, and the lips thereof are much distant the one from the other, there can be no use of such a dry suture. Wherefore you must use a three or four square needle (that so it may the more readily and easily enter into the flesh) being thred with a waxed thred; and with this you must thrust through the lips of the wound, and leave the needle sticking in the wound, then wrap the thred to and again over the ends thereof eight or ten times, just after that manner which women use to fasten a needle with thred in it, upon their sleeves, or Tailors to their hats or caps, that they may not lose them.

The needle thus fastened, shall be there untill the perfect agglutination of the wound; this kind of suture is used in the wounds of the lips, as also in hare-lips, for so we commonly call lips which are cleft from the first conformation in the wombe by the error of the forming faculty. But such a suture will help nothing to agglutination, if there lye or remain any skin between the lips of the wound; Wherefore you shall cut away whatsoever thereof shall be there, otherwise you must expect no union. Other kind of sutures are of no great use in wounds of these parts, for out of the necessity of eating and speaking, they are in perpetuall motion; wherefore a third would cut the flesh; for which reason you shall take up much flesh with such Needles mentioned in this last described kind of Suture as this following figure shewes. [fig. 3]

Paré is especially remembered because of his abandonment of the use of cautery and of boiling oil in the treatment of wounds; he was thus largely responsible for the gradual abolition of the cauterization methods employed by the Arabian surgeons, who themselves had probably learned of them from their apparent origin among Hindu surgeons of the 6th or 7th century B.C., where they were described in the Sushruta Samhita.[43, 52] Ambroise Paré, like his best known pupil, Pierre Franco, was also a Huguenot; Garrison[33] states that he was the only Protestant spared by a Royal Mandate from the St. Bartholomew Day massacre.

His faith in the healing power of nature is summed up in the famous inscription on his statue, a famous remark he has said to have made after being congratulated on his cure of a very difficult case. Je le pansay, Dieu le guarit' (I treated him, but God cured him).

Jacques Guillemeau (1550 to 1613), a pupil of Ambroise Paré, who probably wrote the best book on ophthalmology during the Renaissance, also discussed harelip in his general surgical works[53] published in 1612. His illustrations for harelip repair and for wounds of the cheek (fig. 4), were almost identical to those previously found in the works of Paré.[50] Guillemeau recommended the use of a curved knife inserted into the most superior margins of the cleft near the nostril border and drawn in a downward direction to freshen the cleft edges prior to the insertion of one or two harelip needles, secured in place by a figure-of-8 wrap-around suture. Two needles rather than one were considered more appropriate for wider clefts. Guillemeau cut off the points of the needles to blunt them at the end of the operation and coated their tips with plaster. In order to better approximate the cleft margins, when a very wide cleft made this impossible, he recommended the use of two, half-moon shaped, full-thickness relaxation incisions (fig. 4) made in the cheeks without penetrating into the mouth, just lateral to the nasolabial folds. The facial disfigurement probably caused by these incisions had already been referred to 2½ centuries earlier by Yperman.[39]

Hieronymus Fabricius ab Aquapendente (1537 to 1619), a pupil of Fallopius and Harvey's teacher in Padua, was not only a famous anatomist and physiologist, but a great surgeon of his time as well.[54] He advised the use of buccal mucosa or tissue from the gums in closing either the harelip or the margins of other wound defects of the lips. If the cleft lip was too wide, Fabricius used an agglutinative bandage to bring the edges of the cleft together or to relieve any tension on the cleft margins before he started the freshening of these margins, followed by the insertion of flexible needles whose ends he turned up after having inserted them. According to Periat,[55] if the cleft was too wide, Fabricius actually tried to bring the edges together with sutures after the agglutinative bandage had been applied, apparently by inserting sutures in the middle of, or between the separate arms of the bandage itself.

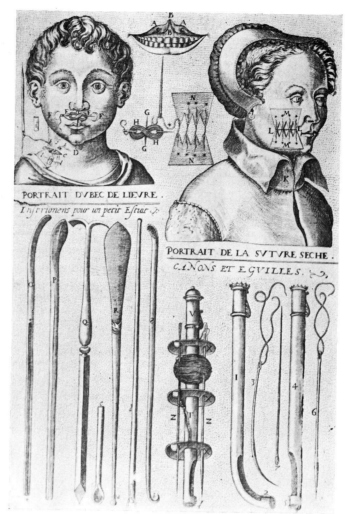

FIG. 4. Illustrations from Guillemeau,[53] in the year 1612, demonstrating the use of a dry suture for closing a cheek wound, and semicircular or crescentic external relaxation incisions in the cheek tissue (*upper left, F*) to relieve tension on the harelip closure.

Gaspare Tagliacozzi (1545 to 1599), in addition to his description of rhinoplasty, also described the treatment of harelips, both single and double, in his classical text, *De curtorum chirurgia*[45] published in 1597:

. . . First we will begin with the Hare-lip, because this is the most simple evil, and easiest to cure. If both Lips be such, the same method of cure must be used for both. . . . Let the Artist therefore take up that part of the Lip, which must be excoriated, in his Left Hand, and then take off the Skin equally with a very sharp Knife, till the Blood comes to the very Angle of the *Hiatus*, and then he must smoothe the Wound. This Operation may also be done very quickly and safely with a pair of Scissors. The same must be done on the other side. Then we must draw the parts together with his Hand, and stitch them. We must observe this, not to take our stitches superficially, but through all. The Artist must therefore pass his Needle straight thorow the Lip from the outside inwards, and on the other side he must pass the Needle from the inside outwards. He must tie the threads and fasten the ends, and then cut them off. He must take his stitches not too near the edges of the Wound, but at a good distance, lest the hold should brake. The number of the stitches is best defined by the amplitude of the Wound. After stitching is done, some compresses, dipped in Whites of Eggs and Rosewater, must be applied both to the inside and outside of the Wound. Then a thin, soft, and even Roller of about three Fingers breadth, dipped in *Posca*, must be brought along obliquely above the Ears, and must be tied tightly behind the Head. A piece of Linen Cloth also, dipped in mild *Posca*, must be applied to the inside of the Lip, to defend it likewise from Fluxion. Within a day or two the compresses must be removed, and conglutinants must be applied. The outside may have such things applied to it, as mentioned before in the cure of the curt nose, as with Lint and *unguentum* ex cerussa, and a Plaister of *ceratum ex cerussa* applied over it.[56] (Translation By Alexander Read).

With Tagliacozzi's description which appeared at the end of the 16th century, the next century and a half saw numerous minor technical improvements which will be dealt with in a more comprehensive review paper.[10]

Needless to say, however, there were some fascinating technics described, some of which, such as a head cap[57] for relieving tension on the lip repair itself, would do justice to many of the devices now being experimented with by our modern colleagues in holding orthodontic appliances in place in the cleft lip-cleft palate infant.

To catch the flavor of the 17th century and the first half of the 18th century, just prior to the surgery of Dr. Matthew Wilson[20] of Delaware and Mr. Charles Hall of Boston,[1] a few chronologic facts and quotations are now included for the curious reader:

1600

Oberon. "Now, until the break of day,
       Through this house each fairy stray.
       To the best bride-bed will we,
       Which by us shall blessed be;
       And the issue there create
       Ever shall be fortunate.
       So shall all the couples three
       Ever true in loving be;
       And the blots of Nature's hand
       Shall not in their issue stand:
       Never mole, hare-lip, nor scar,
       Nor mark prodigious, such as are
       Despised in nativity,
       Shall upon their children be."
(From the final scene, Act Fifth, *A Midsommer nights dreame*. Written by William Shakespeare)

1674

Hendrik van Roonhuyze (1622–1672), a skillful surgeon from Amsterdam, was one of the first to recommend operating upon the harelip patient soon after birth.[58] A careful translation of his work reveals that he actually implied and suggested the operation could be safe and successful, if done when the infant was

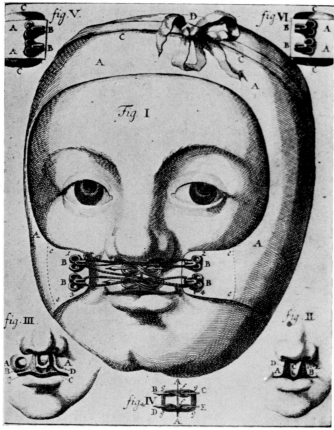

FIG. 5. An ingenious head cap devised by Hofmann[57] in 1686 to relieve tension along the harelip repair by means of a simple system of clasps, around which threads were drawn and tensed, depending upon the discretion of the surgeon, and the amount of cheek-bolstering required.

3 to 4 months old, but if performed prior to this period, however, Roonhuyze felt that the chances for success were markedly reduced.

1686

Several decades later, Johan Philip Hofman (fig. 5) in a thesis on harelip,[57] provided the surgical world with one of the first illustrations of a head cap with clasped edges in the lip region, which apparently served the same purpose as a dry suture or agglutinative bandage, with the possible exception that this clasp-suture or dry suture was attached to the supportive cap itself, but not to the patient's own cheek skin.

1693

In the fourth edition of one of the early textbooks of surgery in English by a native Englishman, James Cooke of Warwick (1614 to 1688), advised the following:

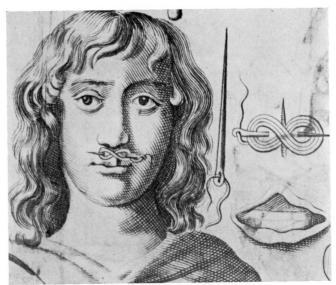

FIG. 6. An illustration in an early textbook of surgery published in England in 1676 by James Cooke,[60] showing the use of the harelip pin with the method of "... winding the threed about, as Taylors do when they stick them on their Skirts."[60]

The Lip is sometimes much cleft, shewing two or three Teeth of the upper Jaw, sometimes less, and sometimes 'tis double cleft, there remaining only a piece between both, which unless it be callous, it need not be taken away. . . .

They are usually caus'd by some Frights and strong Fancies, which are usually the cause of monstrous Births.

'Tis more dangerous to perform upon a grown than young person, though happily perform'd on some of 28 years of age. [fig. 6.] The younger children are when cut, 'tis the better, yea while Infants, unless they be sick or weak. It's more fitly done in Summer than Winter, in Spring than Fall.[59]

. . . To operate in, choose a very clear place, and put the Child in the Lap of a discreet person, and let one stand behind to hold the Head, the Child's Hands being ty'd down, and if possible keep it from Sleep for ten or twelve hours before the Operation, that it may be disposed to sleep presently after. For it have ready a glass of Wine or Cordial, in case of fainting upon the loss of Blood. Let there be also at hand a Bason of lukewarm Water, a couple of Sponges, Pledgets, Boulsters and Bands; Incision Knife, sharp Scissors, cutting Pincers, five or six Needles three angled, threaded with crimson Silk. [fig. 7] *Observe*, if there be great deformity, consider what to do, lest you make it worse than it was. If it stick unto the Gums, which sometimes it doth, 'tis to be divided from them, putting Lint, etc. betwixt: after when fit, cut both sides of the Hair-Lip with Scissors, so much as is needful; after pass through a Needle or two as there may be occasion, leaving them in, winding the thread about, as Taylors do when they stick them on their Skirts: anoint the Lips first, and wound, with Spanish *Balsam*, or any other. This may be strengthen'd with a dry stitch. Of this see Pareus, Scultet. & c.

1701

In keeping with the general French attitude that early operations were hazardous and uncalled for, Le Clerc[62] strongly advises that the operation should not:

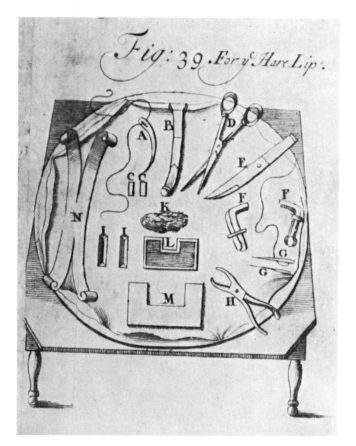

FIG. 7. A surgical table containing most of the instruments considered essential for harelip repair in the early 18th century (1712) by Dionis.[61] *A*, curved needle threaded; *B*, small Pipe to aid in passing the needle; *C*, bolsters around which sutures were tied; *D*, harelip scissors to freshen cleft edges; *E*, incision knife; *F*, lip pincers for hemostasis; *G*, harelip pins or straight needles to be left in place; *H*, pincers to cut off sharp ends of harelip pins; *I*, bolsters to lay under needle ends to protect underlying lip tissue; *K*, pledget covered with white Balsam of Peru to lay on the repaired lip closure; *L*, plaster cut to fit upper lip and entire area of surgical closure; *M*, bolster cut to fit over the plaster (*L*); *N*, head-lip bandage with four ends to support the dressing of balsamed pledget (*K*), plaster (*L*) and bolster (*M*).

. . . be practis'd upon old nor scorbutic Persons, nor upon young Children, by reason that their continual Crying would hinder the Re-union. But if any are desirous that it should be done to these last, they are to be kept from taking any Rest for a long time; to the end that they may fall asleep after the Operation, which is thus effected: . . . If the Lip sticks to the Gums, it is to be separated with an Incision-Knife, without hurting 'em; then the Hare-Lip must be cut a little about the Edges with Scissors, [fig. 8], that it may more easily re-unite, the Edges being held for that Purpose with a Pair of Pincers, whilst the Servant who supports the Patient's Head, presseth his Cheeks forwards to bring together the sides of the Hare-Lip.

. . . After the Lips are wash'd with war Wine, the Points of the Needles must be cut off, small Bolsters being laid under their Ends; then the Wound is to be drest with a little Pledgit arm'd with some proper Balsam, putting at the same time under the Gum a Linnen

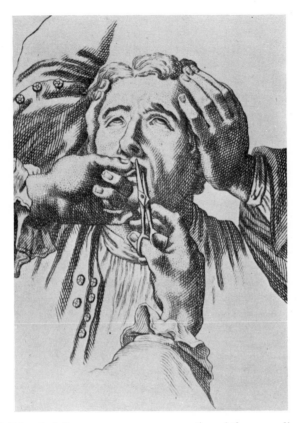

FIG. 8. The left hand of the surgeon grasps one portion of the upper lip, as he cuts the cleft margins to freshen them with a scissors held in his right hand. The patient's head is firmly held by a surgical aide. (From an illustration in 1748 in a book on surgery by de Garengeot.[63]

Rag steep'd in some desiccative Liquor, lest the Lip shou'd stick to the Gum, if it be necessar to keep 'em apart.

   . . . The Patient must be drest three Days after; and it is requisite at the first time only to untwist half the Needle, loosening the middle Thread if there be three; to which purpose a Servant is to thrust the Cheeks somewhat foreward. On the eighth Day the middle Needle may be taken off, if it be a young Infant; Nevertheless the Needles must not be remov'd till it appears that Sides are well join'd; neither must they be left too long, because the Holes would scarce be brought to close.

By the middle of the 18th century, refinements in harelip repair, which did not yet include abandonment of the need for harelip pins, however, resulted in the following appearance, typical of patients who had recently undergone surgery (fig. 9).

Thus, to end this brief review, and to bring it up to the Colonial period, we include a final quotation from Sharp,[65] whose book was referred to by the Reverend Dr. Matthew Wilson[20] in 1756 to 1787. The quotation gives us some idea of the follow-up care of a patient repaired by the techniques just outlined:

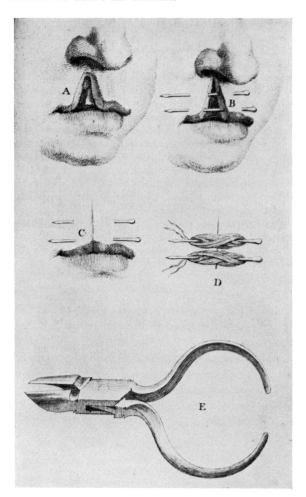

FIG. 9. Illustrations of harelip repair in common practice in Europe and apparently in Colonial America (see description by Matthew Wilson,[20] in the middle of the 18th century. "*A*, a hare-lip . . . In the division may be observed a tooth, which usually projects in this manner in those cases where the jaw-bone is divided as well as the lip. This tooth, with so much of the jawbone as is protruberant, must be taken off previous to the operation; and the lip largely severed from the gum . . . *E*, an instrument called a nail-nipper, which I have found extremely useful in taking off a bit of the jaw-bone, as mentioned in letter *A*." (Illustration and legend from LeDran,[64] published in 1749.)

   . . . You first with a Knife separate the Lip from the Upper Jaw, by dividing the Fraenulum between it and the Gums; and if the Dentes Incisorii project, as is usual in Infants, they must be cut with the same Knife; then with a thin pair of straight Scissars take off the callous Edges of the Fissure the whole Length of it, observing the Rule of making the new Wound in straight Lines, because the Sides of it can never be made to correspond without this Caution.

   The two Lips of the Wound being brought exactly together, you pass a couple of Pins, one pretty near the Top, and the other as near the Bottom, thro' the Middle of both Edges of it, and secure them in that Situation by twisting a Piece of waxed Thread cross and round the Pins seven or eight times; you must then cut off the Points, and lay a small Bolster of

Plaister underneath them to prevent their scratching: But when the lower Part only of the Hare Lip can be brought into Contact, it will not be proper to use more than one Pin.

The Pins I employ are made three fourths of their lengths of Silver, and the other Part towards the Point, of Steel; the Silver Pin is not quite so offensive to a Wound as a Brass or Steel one; but a Steel Point is necessary for their easier Penetration, which indeed makes them pass so readily, that there is no need of any Instrument to assist in pushing them thro'. The Practice of bolstering the Cheeks forward does little or no Service to the Wound, and is very uneasy to the Patient; wherefore I would not advise the Use of it. The Manner of dressing will be to remove the Applications which are quite superficial, as often only as is necessary for Cleanliness. The Method I would recommend, is to desist the three first Days, and afterwards to do it every Day, or every other Day: I do not think it at all requisite to dress between the Jaw and Lip where the Fraenulum was wounded, there being no Danger that an inconvenient Adhesion should ensue. In about eight or nine Days, the Parts are usually united, and in Children much sooner, when you must gently cut the Threads, and draw out the Pins, applying upon the Orifices a Piece of Plaister and dry Lint. It will be proper in order to withdraw the Pins more easily, to dab the Ligatures and Pins with warm Water, and also moisten them with sweet Oil, two or three Days before you remove them, which will wash off the coagulated Blood, that would otherwise fasten them so hard to the Ligature as to make Extraction painful.

SUMMARY

The surgical details of harelip repair, traced as far back as the Saxon surgeons of pre-Norman Britain and described in their *Leech-book of Bald* (*c.* 950 A.D.), were apparently known eight centuries later, with additional refinements, to their English, German and American heirs who practiced surgery in Colonial America. One of them, a minister-physician, Matthew Wilson, formerly a native of Chester County, Pennsylvania, who practised in Lewes, Delaware, described the operation in detail in his unpublished compendium *Therapeutic Alphabet* written between the years 1756 to 1787.

REFERENCES

1. From *The Boston Evening-Post*. Printed by Thomas Fleet, at the Heart & Crown, in Cornhill, Boston. No. 1824, page 3, Sept. 10, 1770.
2. From *Dunlap's Pennsylvania Packet Or, The General Advertiser*. Printed by John Dunlap, at the Newest-Printing-Office in Market-Street, Philadelphia. No. 187, page 1, May 22, 1775.
3. From *The Connecticut Gazette, and The Universal Intelligencer*. Printed by Timothy Green near the Court House, New London. No. 855, page 4, March 29, 1780.
4. SMITH, H. H.: A System of Operative Surgery: Based Upon the Practice of Surgeons in the United States: With a Bibliographical Index and Historical Record of Many of Their Operations, During a Period of Two Hundred and Thirty-Four Years. 2nd Ed. J. B. Lippincott and Co., Philadelphia, Vol. I., 1856.
5. JOHNSTON, W.: Roll of Commissioned Officers in the Medical Service of the British Army Who Served on Full Pay Within the Period Between the Accession of George II and the Formation of the Royal Army Medical Corps 20 June 1727 to 23 June 1898. The University Press, Aberdeen, page 30, 1917.
6. Personal communication from Mr. W. R. Le Fanu, Librarian, Royal College of Surgeons of England, Lincoln's Inn Fields, London.
7. THACHER, J.: American Medical Biography: Or Memoirs of Eminent Physicians Who Have Flourished in America. Richardson & Lord and Cotton & Barnard, Boston, 1828.
8. WILLIAMS, S. W.: American Medical Biography: Or, Memoirs of Eminent Physicians, Embracing Principally Those Who Have Died Since the Publication of Dr. Thacher's Work on the Same Subject. L. Merriam and Co., Greenfield, Mass., 1845.
9. GUERRA, F.: American Medical Bibliography 1639–1783. Lathrop C. Harper Inc., New York, 1962.
10. ROGERS, B. O.: Harelip repair prior to Mirault: A comprehensive review of the history of harelip surgery. (in preparation).

11. From *The Pennsylvania Gazette*. Printed by B. Franklin and H. Meredith, at the New Printing-Office near the Market, Philadelphia. No. 1714, Oct. 29, 1761.
12. From *The Boston Evening-Post*. Printed by Thomas Fleet, at the Heart & Crown, in Cornhill, Boston. No. 1876, Sept. 9, 1771.
13. From *The Pennsylvania Journal; and the Weekly Advertiser*. Printed and Sold by William and Thomas Bradford, at the Corner of Front and Market-Streets, Philadelphia. No. 1674, page 4, Jan. 4, 1775.
14. GORDON, M. B.: Aesculapius Comes To the Colonies: The Story of the Early Days of Medicine in the Thirteen Original Colonies. Ventnor Publishers, Inc., Ventnor, N. J., page 381, 1949.
15. HEISTER, L.: A General System of Surgery in Three Parts. W. Innys at the West-End of St. Paul's, etc., London, page 452, 1743.
16. From *The Pennsylvania Evening Post*. Printed by Benjamin Towne, in Front-Street, near the London Coffee-House, Philadelphia. No. 655, March 20, 1780.
17. From *The New-York Mercury: Containing the freshest Advices Foreign and Domestick*. Printed by Hugh Gaine, at his Printing-Office on Hunter's Key, next door to Mr. Walton's storehouse. No. 545, Jan. 10, 1763.
18. MASON, F.: On the Surgery of the Face. Lindsay and Blakiston, Philadelphia, page 102, 1879.
19. WHEELER, W. I.: On the Operative Treatment of Harelip. J. Falconer, Dublin, 1880.
20. FRIEDBERG, S. A.: Laryngology and otology in colonial times. Ann. Med. History, 1: 86, 1917.
21. FRANCO, P.: Traité des Hernies. ... Thibauld Payon, Lyon, 1561.
22. BREASTED, J. H.: The Edwin Smith Surgical Papyrus: Published in Facsimile and Hieroglyphic Transliteration with Translation and Commentary in Two Volumes. The University of Chicago Press, Chicago, Illinois, 1930.
23. BRYAN, C. P.: The Papyrus Ebers: Translated from the German Version. D. Appleton and Co., N. Y., 1931.
24. LITTRÉ, M. P. E.: Oeuvres Complètes d'Hippocrate. J. B. Baillière, Paris, 1839–1861.
25. COLLIER, G. F.: A Translation of the Eight Books of Aulus Aurelius Cornelius Celsus on Medicine. Longman & Co., London, 1840.
26. SPENCER, W. G.: Celsus: De Medicina: With an English Translation by W. G. Spencer. Harvard University Press, Cambridge, Mass., 1938.
27. KÜHN, C. G.: Opera omnia. . . . C. Cnobloch, Leipzig, 1821–1833.
28. BUSSEMAKER, AND DAREMBERG. Oeuvres d'Oribase, texte grec. . . . Imprimerie nationale, Paris, 1851–1876.
29. MORSE, W. R.: Chinese Medicine. Paul B. Hoeber, Inc., New York, page 129, 1934.
30. WONG, K. C. AND WU, L. T.: History of Chinese Medicine. Tientsin Press, Tientsin, 1932.
31. ADAMS, F.: The Medical Works of Paulus Aegineta. . . . J. Welsh; Treuttel, Würtz, & Co. London 1834.
32. LECLERC, L.: La Chirurgie d'Abulcasis. J. B. Baillière, Paris, page 27, 1861.
33. GARRISON, F. H.: An Introduction to the History of Medicine. 4th ed. W. B. Saunders Co., Philadelphia, 1929.
34. PIFTEAU, P.: Chirurgie de Guillaume de Salicet: Achevée en 1275. Imprimerie Saint-Cyprien, Toulouse, 1898.
35. COCKAYNE, T. O.: Leechdoms, Wortcunning and Starcraft of Early England, Being a Collection of Documents, For the Most Part Never Before Printed, Illustrating the History of Science in This Country Before the Norman Conquest. Longman, Green, Longman, Roberts, and Green, London, page 57, 1865.
36. DAREMBERG, C. V.: Glossulae quatuor magistrorum super chirurgiam Rogerii et Rolandi. J. B. Baillière, Paris, 1854.
37. HALLE, J.: A most excellent and learned woorke of Chirurgerie, called Chirurgia parva Lanfranci, Lanfranke of Mylayne. . . . Imprinted at London in Flete streate, nyghy unto saint Dunstones churche, by Thomas Marshe, 1565.
38. PAGEL, J. L.: Die Chirurgie des Heinrich de Mondeville. A. Hirschwald, Berlin, 1892.
39. CAROLUS, J. M. F.: La Chirurgie de Maître Jean Yperman. . . . F. and E. Gyselynck, Gand, 1854.
40. NICAISE, E.: La Grande Chirurgie de Guy de Chauliac. Alcan, Paris, 1890.
41. CASTIGLIONI, A.: A History of Medicine. 2nd Ed. Alfred A. Knopf, New York, 1958.
42. POWER, D. (tr.): De arte phisicale et de cirurgia by John of Arderne. John Bale, London, 1922.
43. GRAHAM, H.: Surgeons All. Philosophical Library, New York, 1957.
44. VON PFOLSPRUNDT, H.: Buch der Bündth-Ertznei. Edited by H. Haeser and A. Middeldorpf. George Reimer, Berlin, 1868.
45. GNUDI, M. T. AND WEBSTER, J. P.: The Life and Times of Gaspare Tagliacozzi: Surgeon of Bologna. . . . Herbert Reichner, New York, 1950.
46. LEONARDO, R. A.: History of Surgery. Froben Press, New York, 1943.

47. HUARD, P. AND GRMEK, M. D.: Le Premier Manuscrit Chirurgical Turc Rédigé par Charaf ed-Din (1465) et Illustré de 140 Miniatures. Les Editions Roger Dacosta, Paris, 1960.
48. BRUNSCHWIG, H.: Die ist das Buch der Cirurgia: Hautwirckung der wund Artz. H. Schönsperger, Augsburg, 1497.
49. VON GERSDORFF, H.: Feldtbuch der Wund-Artzney . . . sampt vilen Instrumenten der Chirurgey vss. dem Albucasi contrafayt. . . . Hans Schotten, Strasszburg, 1540.
50. PARÉ, A.: Les Oeuvres de M. Ambroise Paré. G. Buon, Paris, 1575.
51. JOHNSON, T.: The Workes of that Famous Chirurgion Ambrose Parey: Translated out of Latine and Compared with the French by Tho. Johnson. Printed by Richard Cotes, and Willi Du-gard, and are to be sold by John Clarke, entring into Mercers Chappell, London, 1649.
52. BHISHAGRATNA, K. K. L.: An English Translation of the Sushruta Samhita, Based on Original Sanskrit Text. 3 Vols. Bose, Calcutta, 1907–1916.
53. GUILLEMEAU, J.: Les Oeuvres de Chirurgie. Che Nicolas Buon, au Mont sainct Hilaire, à l'Image sainct Claude, Paris, 1612.
54. FABRITIO, GIROLAMO, d'AQUAPENDENTE.: L'opere Chirugiche. Gioseffo Longhi, Bologna 1678.
55. PERIAT, H. H.: Recherches Historiques sur L'Operation du Bec-de-Lièvre. Thése de Faculté de Médecine de Paris, No. 74, 1857.
56. READ, A.: Chirurgorum comes: or, The whole practice of chirurgery. . . . Jones, London, 1687.
57. HOFMANN, J. P.: De labiis leporinis: von Hasen-Scharten. J. B. Bergmann, Heidelbergae, 1686.
58. VAN ROONHUYSE, H.: Historischer Heil-Curen in zwey Theile verfassete Anmerckungen. . . . Michael und Johann Friederich Endtern, Nürnberg, 1674.
59. COOKE, J.: Mellificium Chirurgiae: or, the Marrow of Chirurgery. With the Anatomy of Human Bodies. 4th Ed. Printed for W. Marshall at the BIBLE in Newgate-street, London, 1693, page 195.
60. COOKE, J.: Mellificium Chirurgiae: . . . Chirurgery Much Enlarged. . . . To which is now added Anatomy. . . . Printed by J. D. for Benj. Shirley, and are to be sold at his Shop under the Dial of St. Dunstan's Church in Fleetstreet, London, 1676.
61. DION [DIONIS, P.]: Of the Hare-Lip: Taken from Fig. 39. of Dion. in Bibliotheca Anatomica, Medica, Chirurgica, etc. Vol. II, pages 293–295 and Fig. 39. Printed by John Nutt; and Sold by W. Lewis in Russelstreet, Covent-Garden. London, 1712.
62. LeCLERC, M.: C. G.: The Compleat Surgeon: or, the Whole Art of SURGERY explain'd in a most Familiar Method. 3rd Ed. Printed for W. Freeman, J. Walthoe, T. Goodwin, M. Wotton and R. Parker, London, page 258, 1701.
63. DE GARENGEOT, R. J. C.: Traité des Operations de Chirurgie. . . . 3rd Ed. Chez Cavelier près la Fontaine Saint Severin, au Lys d'or, Paris, Vol. III: 16, 1748.
64. LeDRAN: The Operations in Surgery of Mons. Le Dran: Transl. by Thomas Gataker, Surgeon: With Remarks, Plates of the Operations, and a Sett of Instruments by William Cheselden, Esq. Printed for C. Hitch in Pater-noster-Row, and R. Dodsley in Pall-Mall, London, page 450, 1749.
65. SHARP, S.: A Treatise on the Operations of Surgery. 8th Ed. J. and R. Tonson, London, page 198, 1761.

THE CURE OF CLEFT LIPS IN 1561

PIERRE FRANCO, *Orange, France*

(From Nicaise, Edouard: *Chirurgie de Pierre Franco, de Turriers en Provence, Composée en 1561*)

Translated from the French by
MARY McDOWELL

First it is necessary to cut the edges so that they can be adjusted, one to the other, with a razor or scissors or other suitable instrument, or they can be actually cauterized. While making the cut to join them together one can, if he wishes, apply splints to dull the pain—leaving them in place then for two or 3 days.

If one uses a hot cautery, it is best to wait until the eschar comes off (one can accelerate this by applying fresh butter or similar substances) before rejoining the edges to stick them together; otherwise one would work in vain (they wouldn't stick together unless the eschar had come off first).

This done, one must join the edges to each other, as one and well united; this can be done by proceeding in the following way.

A dressing is made with two pieces of cloth in a triangle, of a size according to the person. (This method is quite appropriate and causes less pain. With this there is also not such a big scar because there is no needle in the flesh; this is most desirable, particularly in the face and especially in girls.)

When the eschar has fallen off one applies the above-named bandages, which are then covered by a plaster containing *pul. sang. drac. thuris, masticis,* and *farinae volatil, molend. picis,* in equal parts, incorporated in egg albumen. The plaster is put on each piece, which is then applied to one part of the lip, not too near the edge of the ulcer (about a finger breadth away), so as not to hinder the application of medicines for healing the flesh and to stick the edges together. After they are glued firmly on the skin, it is necessary to fold each piece of cloth before you sew. Then they are sewn, one to the other, holding the points close to each other so the cloth edges are approximated—using the hands to help hold them together, or using a forceps if necessary (if the edges are too far apart).

ANOTHER METHOD

First, having made the cut as explained above, with the instruments mentioned, it is necessary to immediately apply a hollow needle carrying a thread*—as one does to other wounds, so that the threaded needle will take hold of the lip in such a way as to grasp the tissues well (by taking hold of the skin on one side and the tissues below the skin on the other). After this one can insert two or 3 needles across as the case requires, then make two or 3 turns around them with the thread, but not more, so that the thread does not hinder the application of the medicine which is to stick the parts together. It is necessary that the wound edges touch in all parts; to make this easier, one can use forceps (as we have suggested). When the edges are too far apart to be joined, they pull away so that the needles cut

* *Editorial note.* Swaged-on needles preceded needles with eyes in medieval French surgery.

This material was kindly made available to us by Mr. Richard Wolfe, Rare Books Librarian of the Francis A. Countway Library of Medicine, Boston.

the flesh; then the edges separate and can't stick together, and it becomes necessary to rejoin them as before.

When the edges are initially too far apart, as I have seen several times, so that one can't bring them together by any means, it is necessary to cut each lip segment inside lengthwise and across to rejoin them, guarding as much as possible against movement by the muscles. Always, when it is necessary, one should so cut them rather than leave the segments apart, for of the two this is better.

Be careful about cutting the skin outside, because there the lip can be elongated (which I have done several times). Then after having applied the needles, it is necessary to put on clips to hold the whole thing together.

To do this, one obtains little pieces of wood in the form of a square, about the size of a finger, one or two at the most, according to the size of the patient, and the length of the cleft lip. These wood squares are dressed with fine linen and put over the two cheeks (one on each side), straight to the cleft lip, and sewn to a cap which comes just to the middle of the cheek. Then a bandage, large enough to go behind the occiput or neck and under the ears, is used to bring the two blocks up to the middle of the cheek near the cap. Then we also have another bandage which is attached to the first by the two ends under the ears, which we pass under the head. When this is accomplished, it is necessary to pass and put behind this clip two batons, one on each side. These are as big as a finger and about one foot long, according to the size of the patient. They are dressed with something soft, especially below where they are attached together at the two ends. With one of them one can tighten the ligatures over the chin and (with the other) on the forehead, quite firmly. Now the batons push the wood clips toward the front, and the clips push the flesh. By this means the edges of the lip are held together. They must be left like this until they can heal solidly.

This is a good operation, suitable and unusual. Before applying the splints on the lip, it is necessary to put a wet oxycratum dressing on. The splints are put over that. Otherwise the needles would not grip and would become tangled with the splints, which would be difficult to remove. Besides, the oxycratum relieves the pain.

ANOTHER KIND CALLED DENTS DE LIEVRE

(Double Cleft Lip with Middle Teeth Outside the Mouth)

This kind of cleft lip is commonly called *dents de lievre* because at the front of the maxilla, in place of the incisor teeth, there are teeth which come outside the mouth—sometimes only one, other times two, most often more. The maxilla is split in two and the *dents de lievre* go right in front of the length of the palate, which is also cleft on each side. Between these two clefts in the middle is the part of the maxilla in which the teeth are driven, which is often so far forward that the mouth cannot cover it—an infamous thing and ugly to see.

CURE FOR DENTS DE LIEVRE

To extirpate this turpitude, we must first proceed in the manner described above, except when the teeth and maxillary segment are outside and cannot be covered by the mouth. There is no danger of cutting too much or that which serves no purpose, so one uses cutting forceps, or a saw or other instrument suitable for this—leaving the flesh which is over these teeth, if there is any, as it helps when sewing to the two other parts (on each side). And if there is such a distance between these lips that one cannot bring them together, it will be necessary to use dissections in the mouth similar to those in the preceding case—and proceed with the remainder of the closure as we have described.

Pierre Franco
Orange, France

COMMENTARY BY THE EDITOR

As the light of the Renaissance melted the darkness of a thousand years, the figures of two great French surgeons emerged—Pierre Franco and Ambroise Paré. They were colleagues and rivals according to the preponderance of the evidence, not student and teacher as some have suggested.

Now, in the middle of the 16th century, the time had come for the first printing of a book on surgery (the Gutenberg Bible had appeared in 1455). The one to seize the opportunity was Franco, whose *Petit Traité, etc.*[1] was printed in Lyons in 1556. It was a small book covering much of what was known about all kinds of surgery up to that date—and it contained one great pearl, the first description of a suprapubic cystotomy (for stone, in a 10-year-old child). It is for this that Franco is best known.

In 1561 Franco published his *Grand Traité, etc.*[2] a book of about 560 pages—a few of which constitute this Classic Reprint. This book was to be a standard reference work for the next 200 years; it went through 5 editions. (The first book to be published by Paré was his *Dix Livres, etc.*[3]—a small book of 10 chapters—in 1564. In it he more or less copied, without credit, the sections of Franco's book on lithotomy and cystotomy. However, Paré acknowledged this later in his 1575 *Oeuvres*,[4] wherein he also acknowledged that he had learned the operation of *debridement* from Franco.)

We do not know much about Franco. He was born, probably about 1500, in Tur-riers—a small town in Provence near the lower Alps. Mettler[5] says he was a member of the class of itinerant lithotomists and ocular operators which had grown up in medieval Europe—where operations upon the eye and inguinal, scrotal, and perineal areas were not usually performed by those who devoted their attention to other aspects of surgery. (These latter "surgeons" comprised the "Confraternity of Surgeons" in each larger city; they conducted examinations in Latin and did operations of a more aristocratic nature.)

Malgaigne[6] noted that the group below the town barbers was the wandering surgeons, composed of two classes: "(1) the fellow barbers who went from town to town selling and administering drugs and antidotes they had in their boxes, and (2) the itinerant *inciseurs* for stone, herniers, couchers of cataracts, bonesetters, and toothpullers. Some had followed a master long enough to have learned his methods, but others called themselves *inciseurs* without any prior apprenticeship and by virtue of their boldness alone . . . Franco, that great *inciseur* of the sixteenth century, indignantly set himself up against these wretches (saying):

'Who are responsible for this part of surgery being so despised, who being ignorant and knowing it, nevertheless without any fear of God or of men undertake to treat all sorts of curable and incurable ailments, as long as they can attract the money of poor simple people; who seduce and enchant by their lies and good words, to the great harm of poor patients who often are brought to death by such swindlers.' "

Malgaigne continues, "they (inciseurs) had no fixed home, but went from one place to another, hunting operations to do, and they had still another cause for this nomadic life, which earned them the insulting name of tramps. As Franco correctly remarked, the faults of the physician and the apothecary were excused; 'the surgeon who does not play this role is also excused not at all. But if what we have undertaken does not always succeed as happily as wished, we lack any support when they call us murderers and executioners, and often enough are constrained to take to the fields.' "

Malgaigne concludes, "The name of surgeon has fascinated; no one wanted to see surgery except in the little Confraternity of Paris, and they have totally neglected those two other great classes of practitioners, the barbers and the inciseurs. But, if we have shown that for the periods before the sixteenth century the highest of those three classes had no greater merit than the others to the science and, consequently, to the history, we can even add that for the period which would follow, the barbers and the inciseurs would really be the renovators of French surgery; it was from their midst that would come those two great surgical celebrities of the sixteenth century, Franco and A. Paré."

At the height of his career, Franco, a Huguenot, was driven from his native France in a frenzied mass persecution of Protestants (known as the Waldensian massacres). He went to Switzerland where he practiced for some years in the employ of the lords of Berne and of Lausanne. In the last years of his life he returned to France to practice in the small city of Orange. The date and place of his death are unknown.

A few years after the publications of Franco and Paré, the great Italian surgeon Tagliacozzi brought forth his famous work on rhinoplasty. For this innovation he was roundly criticized by Paré and Fallopius—and the ecclesiastics pronounced such operations as meddling with the handiwork of God. As a result, plastic surgery fell into disrepute and was almost abandoned for the next 150 years.

—*Frank McDowell, M.D.*

REFERENCES

1. Franco, Pierre: *Petit traité contenant une des parties principalles de chirurgie laquelle les chirurgiens hernières exercent.* Lyons, 1556.

2. Franco, Pierre: *Traité des hernies contenant une ample déclaration de toutes leurs espèces & autres excellentes parties de la chirurgie, assavoir de la pierre, des cataractes des yeux, & autres maladies, desquelles comme la cure est perilleuse, aussi est elle de peu d'hommes bien exercée.* Thibauld Payon, Lyons, 1561. (Edited and reprinted later under the following title. Nicaise, Edouard: *Chirurgie de Pierre Franco, de Turriers, en Provence, Composée en 1561.* Nouvelle edition. Paris, Felix Alcan, Editeur, 1895.)

3. Paré, Ambroise: *Dix livres de la chirurgie.* Jean le Royer, Paris, 1564.

4. Paré, Ambroise: *Les Oeuvres de M. Ambroise Paré.* G. Buon, Paris, 1575.

5. Mettler, C. C.: *History of Medicine.* Blakiston Co., Philadelpha, 1947.

6. Malgaigne, J. F.: *Surgery and Ambroise Paré* (the 1840 edition translated from the French and edited by W. B. Hamby), University of Oklahoma Press, Norman, 1965.

After the Renaissance

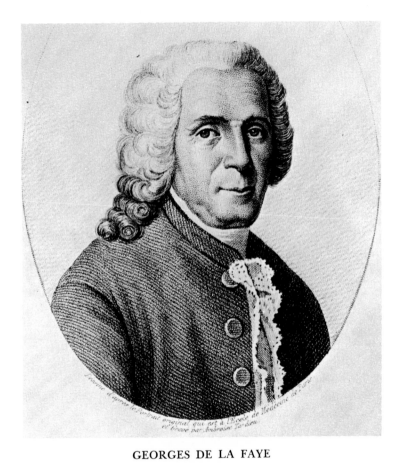

GEORGES DE LA FAYE

1699–1781

(Courtesy of the Boston Medical Library
in The Countway Library of Medicine)

OBSERVATIONS ON THE CLEFT LIP

GEORGES DE LA FAYE, M.D., *Paris, France*

(Memoires de l'Academie Royale de Chirurgie, 1: 605, 1743)

Translated from the French by
MARY McDOWELL

In 1733 I saw a 4-year-old child, born with an unusual kind of cleft lip. The upper lip, all the arch of the palate, and even the uvula were divided in two; each edge of the upper lip formed, toward the lower part, a mound which was distended when the child laughed. Figure 3 shows the two mounds when the child was laughing, and Figure 1 shows them when the child was tranquil.

The borders of the lip surrounded these mounds and terminated at the alae of the nose. A little bridle (or rather a little string) attached each part of the lip to the gum near the border of the division of the maxillary bone inter-

nally. Thus the two parts of the lip had a considerable space between them; it seemed like 12 cords when the child was tranquil, like 6 when he laughed or cried.

In the middle of this space one could see part of the maxillary bone, from which emerged two incisor teeth surrounded by their sockets and covered by their gums. This part, which was isolated and loose, formed in comparison with the rest of the jaw a projection of about 5 lines which I would call an osseous eminence. A little round piece of flesh, attached toward the end of the nose and which seemed to be the part which was lost from the lip, hung in front of this eminence. This kind of pimple of flesh considerably augmented the deformity of the child, especially when he opened his mouth. (This is shown in Figure 2.)

The two spaces between the osseous eminence and the two parts of the lip separated the maxillary bone into 3 parts anteriorly, and became a space which divided into two parts all the osseous arch of the palate, the velum, and the uvula. This space allowed one to see into the nose and see the nasal septum, which separated all the arch of the palate into two parts. One can judge by this description that not only was this infant quite deformed, but that he had been raised with great difficulty and he could not form articulate sounds.

When I interrogated the mother

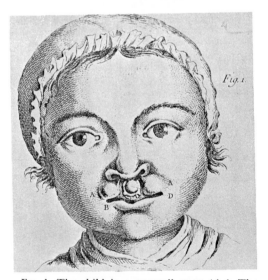

FIG. 1. The child in a tranquil state. (*A,A.* The two mounds.) Note the round piece of flesh attached to the end of the nose; behind it is the bony eminence, the portion of the maxillary bone in which were set the two incisors.

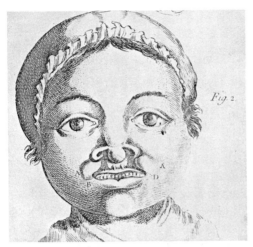

FIG. 2. The child with his mouth open. The bony eminence seems larger than in the preceding illustration.

about her pregnancy, she said she had been frightened at the sight of the head of a deer; but the slight resemblance between the head of this animal and a harelip does not favor the conjecture that this might cause such a deformity by malformation of the fetus; this sentiment was attributed to the imagination of the mother.

Manget, Anton de Heydes, Henr. Volglnadius, Bartholin, Nuck, and Job. Ludov. Hannemannus have described this kind of cleft lip. Daniel Ludovic, Van-Horne, and Franco have said something about the manner of repairing it.

Ludovic reported that he operated on a child who had this defect with an osseous eminence, to procure for him the ability to nurse —and he had to apply the actual cautery to stop the hemorrhaging. This operation done at such a young age was, as you can imagine, not too successful.

The two others (Van-Horne and Franco) preferred to cut the osseous eminence with sharp nippers, of the kind one sees in the figure in the Arcenal de Chirurgie de Scultet, and to correct the rest of the deformity in the same way one does an ordinary cleft lip. That which is different is very difficult—*hic casus sane difficilis est,* says Van-Horne.

The approbation of M. De la Peyronie, to whom I had communicated the plan of the operation I proposed to use on this patient, reassured me. First, I used general remedies on this infant. (Several authors pretend that this precaution is useless, but at least it does not harm the patient.)

OPERATION

On May 13, 1733 I did the operation in the following manner—in the presence of M. De la Peyronie,* and of Messieurs Petit,† Malaval, Morand,‡ Pibrac, Verdier, Caumont, Houstet, *etc.*

I separated with a lancet the round piece of flesh (Figs. 1–3) from the osseous eminence which I cut with a scissors (which had very long blades and were made like a watchmaker's chisel). I cut the round piece of flesh (*D*) to the right and to the left to give it an angle. Then I divided the two bridles which attached the two parts of the lip

---

EDITORIAL NOTES

* François de la Peyronie (1678–1747), whose name has come down to us in "Peyronie's Disease." He was named Chief Surgeon to the Hôpital de la Charité and Second Royal Surgeon in 1717, and he was appointed Principal Surgeon to Louis XV in 1736. Peyronie then obtained civil rights for surgeons equivalent to those long in effect for university physicians. Later he converted his castle to a hospital when he moved to the palace of Versailles —where he died on April 24, 1747.

† Jean Louis Petit (1674–1750), whose name has come down to us in "Petit's triangle" and "Petit's hernia." With Peyronie, he was a founder of the French Academy of Surgery. Petit wrote the first authoritative book on diseases of the nose and paranasal sinuses. He was the first to describe osteomalacia, and he performed the first successful operation for mastoiditis (in 1736).

‡ Sauveur François Morand (1697–1773) was Principal Surgeon at Les Invalides. In 1730 he succeeded Peyronie as Surgeon-in-Chief at the Hôpital de la Charité. He was a member of the academies of science at Petersburg, Stockholm, Bologna, Florence, and Rouen—and was Professor of Anatomy at the French Academy of Sciences. Morand wrote a book on *Surgery of the Skin,* and was the first to describe cleidocranial dysostosis (in 1766).

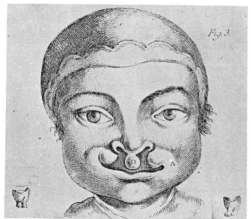

Fig. 3. The child laughing. The two mounds are larger and farther apart than in the first two figures. (*left inset*) The bony eminence separated from the jaw, with the two incisors attached thereto. It is shown in life size, as seen from the interior. (*right inset*) The same bony eminence, seen from the anterior view.

to the gums, and which prevented me from uniting the parts.

When I cut around the edge of these parts, the artery bled profusely. This did not embarrass me, because after the hemorrhage the parts were united; I sutured them with the help of an aide, who brought the two edges together.

I inserted two pins as close as I could to the internal membrane of the lip, to help the union of the interior part. The first was passed near the nose and I wound it around with a band made of two or 3 strands of silk, under the round piece of flesh (which it was not possible to traverse). I passed the second pin very near to the lower edge of the lip, and wound it around with another band of silk (to be able to later take away the silks and the two pins separately). The pins I used were the German ones—flexible, long, and slender; they are better for this purpose than pins of gold, silver, or steel (and better than those one calls "larding pins").

DISCUSSION

When the separation of the two parts of the lip is very wide, Celsus, Guillemeau, Thevenin, *etc.* advise (to facilitate the closure) that one make an incision on each cheek in the form of a cross. Some others prefer, in such a case, to make incisions inside the mouth. However, the incisions in the cheeks produce a deformity from their scars which I think useless (when they could be inside the mouth). If the skin is stretched as much as possible, one can bring the two parts of the lip together. If one encounters some obstacle, it will be the nose—and this obstacle will not be removed by making incisions in the cheek or in the mouth.

If the two parts of the lip on which I am operating have so much space between them that I fear the stress on the pins, then it is necessary for the dressing to help the pins to resist. It is often on this that the success of the operation depends. I cross two linen bandages under the nose, applying the ends (which are covered with the plaster of Andrew of the Cross) to the cheeks to hold them together.

To prevent the cheeks from becoming detached from the plaster, and to diminish the effect of the action of the muscles of the lips, I put two thick compresses on each cheek—which I make firm with a small bandage which I fasten in this way.

I apply the middle to the nape of the neck, making the ends go behind and in front of each compress, and cross them under the nose. I again pass the ends over the compresses and attach them to a bonnet, which I have adjusted on the head of the baby. As the movement of the lower jaw can cause some disturbance, I also apply a bandage under the chin, of which I attach the ends on the bonnet; this permits the jaw to go down only enough to take bouillon or jelly.

Some authors like to use a plaque of lead to fasten the lip, if the subject has no teeth behind the place where the lip parts are brought together. If this plaque was of any use, I would have em-

ployed it after I had cut out the anterior part of the jaw (in the patient of
whom I speak). But the length of the
pins I used to make the suture kept me
from resorting to this method. The two
ends of these pins were supported by
the ends of the two lateral parts of the
jaw (of which I had cut out the middle).

POSTOPERATIVE COURSE

The child, who had fallen asleep during the operation, woke up then and
passed a peaceful night. A slight fever
the next morning obliged me to bleed
him. I observed that his fear and cries
did not cause much movement, because
the bandage held everything in place.

I lifted the bandage the second day
and found that the round piece of flesh
had escaped from under the thread, and
I could not readjust it. I applied a dressing similar to the first one, which I did
not remove until the fourth day.

The seventh day I dressed this child
for the third time and I pulled out the
lower pin, which was wobbly. Two days
later I removed the second one and
found the lip perfectly united—but as
the union was not solid enough to resist
movement of the parts, I put back the
same dressing for several days. I found
the wound which I had made in cutting
the osseous eminence was perfectly
healed.

To appreciate the success of the operation and the good result, see Figure 4.
Compare this to Figures 1, 2, and 3
(which show the patient preopera-
tively). The alae of the nose in Figure 4
are much less widespread. Under the
nose one no longer sees a continuation
of the lip traversing to the middle by a
scar; the upper lip, in spite of the gap
in the maxillary bone, is level with the
lower lip. On this lip there is still a very
small cleft (Fig. 4) which is the result,

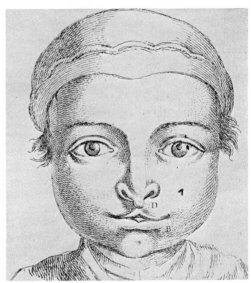

FIG. 4. The child after the repair had healed. The
central round piece of flesh has not united with the
lip and now is very much smaller than it appeared
in Figures 1–3.

not of a faulty union, but because I
could not cut close enough to the
mounds (Figs. 1–3). (These mounds are
semicircular and it is necessary to cut
into them if one wishes to unite the lip
without leaving any cleft.)

The child is now infinitely less deformed than it was before the operation; one can look at him without a
shock. This is not the only advantage.
He talks distinctly, though a little
through the nose—a defect he would
not have if his palate were entirely
closed.

I saw him 4 years after the operation,
and the space in the arch of the palate
was already diminishing. Consequently
there is hope that, little by little, the
bones will come together and close the
space. Perhaps nature itself has already
made the closure.

A SECOND CASE

Some time after this operation, a
young boy of 15 years who had a cleft
lip came to me with his father. This

cleft was less deforming than that of which I have spoken. The maxillary bones were not at all lacking, but the nose was very large; a round piece of flesh was attached near the end and seemed to be part of the lip, covering the two incisors imperfectly. All the arch of the palate was divided, and the distance from one part of the lip to the other was very large.

The father of this young boy told me that his wife, who was now dead, had been, in her imagination, frightened by the sight of a lion. (This does not throw any more light on the cause and origin of this kind of deformity than the tale told me by the mother of the first child.)

Although I had read in Juncker* that these clefts where the lip is split in two places can almost never be healed (*duobus in locis quando fissum est labium, vix unquam malum curatur,* says he) the success of my operation on the 4-year-old child was so perfect that I did not doubt I could correct the deformity of this boy by a similar operation. I did it in the presence of Messieurs Verdier, Caumont, Houstet, and Debiat.

The Operation

I did not remove any of the jaw, because none projected. I cut the borders of each part of the lip beyond the circumference of each mound. Then I cut an acute angle.

I put the first pin through not only

* *Editorial note.* Johann Juncker (1679–1759) was Professor of Medicine at the University of Halle (Germany). He helped to spread Stahl's theories of phlogiston and animistic medicine, and published a well-known textbook of chemistry. Juncker was the originator of policlinics in Germany, and he published the book *Conspectus Chemiae Theoretica-Practicae* in Latin—the probable source of the above quotation.

the border of the round piece to form the two parts of the lip, but also through the round piece of flesh to fill in the angular space between the two parts, after I brought them together. I applied a dressing similar to that described in the first operation.

Postoperative Course

I bled this boy several times after the operation, and repeated the bleeding the next day because he had a fever. I made him lie on his back so that the mucous which flowed out of his nose onto the bandage in great quantities could come out of his mouth.

The fifth day after the operation I had left everything in good shape and was counting on removing the pins the next day, but an accident of the father ruined in one instant the success of the operation. Some tobacco fell on the bed of his son and made him sneeze violently 15 or 20 times.

On removing the dressing next day I found a trouble I had not anticipated. One of the pins was buried, the other held only on one side. They had been torn away from the places where I had put them, and they had carried some of the substance of the lip to the right side. The two parts of the lip, which I had approximated exactly with the round piece of flesh, were separated and they remained united only in the lower part. As the lip and the round piece of flesh were swollen and suppurating, I put off the repair until the next day. I flattered myself that I could procure the reunion of the two parts of the lip to the round piece of flesh without cutting them again.

I fastened two points with interrupted sutures which held the lateral parts of the lip to the round piece of flesh (and not the lower parts). To supply what these two points of suture could not do, I used two adhesive plasters—large on one side and narrow on the other. I applied the larger part on the cheeks, and in the same way the narrow part near each commissure—to which was attached a cord made of several strands of waxed silk. I passed the two lower cords under the lips and tied them together. Then I tied the two superior cords and attached them to the cap—so that in pulling on the plasters he would raise the lower cords which brought together, by means of the round piece of flesh, the part of the lip which the suture had not reunited. By this kind of suture I obtained the advantage of dressing the wound without undoing anything.

I applied the rest of the dressing the same as I had done with the 4-year-old child. Twenty days later the lip was all perfectly healed; the scar was in the shape of a Y.

The deformity of this young boy is so well corrected that it is almost impossible to tell now that he has had an operation. . . .

Georges de la Faye, M.D.
Royal Academy of Surgery
Paris, France

Editorial note. The *Journal* is grateful to Mr. Richard Wolfe, Rare Books Librarian, Francis Countway Library of Medicine, Boston, for making this paper available to us.

COMMENTARY BY THE EDITOR

The paper by de la Faye appeared 200 years after the operation described by Pierre Franco, the medieval barber surgeon—about half way between Franco's time and our time. De la Faye's descriptions are of double cleft lips, in contrast to the more simple single cleft lip described by Franco—but it is surprising that so little progress had been made in two centuries. However, plastic surgery was awakening—after the long sleep engendered by the church's condemnation of Tagliacozzi and (by implication) all plastic surgical procedures.

Georges de la Faye was born on October 10, 1699 in Faubourg du Roule, where his father was a surgeon. After the death of his father, and when he was 15 or 16 years of age, Faye became apprenticed to his uncle who was surgeon-major in the military hospital of Berg-St. Vinox. He remained there 3 years, then returned to Paris to become a student of de la Peyronie's in the Hôpital de la Charité. From 1720 to 1730 he served

as an intern at the Hotel Dieu, and in 1731 he became a teacher of surgery at that hospital. Later he served in the French army, then became a member of the Royal Academy of Surgery.

In 1739, de la Faye published his famous *Principes de Chirurgie,* a handbook that was reprinted in Paris in 1744, 1747, 1757, and 1761; a German translation (by Suberling) was published in Strasbourg in 1751, again in Berlin in 1758; an Italian translation was brought out in Venice in 1751, a Spanish translation in Madrid in 1761, a Swedish translation in Stockholm in 1763. Some 30 years after his death the book was published again in Paris, in 1811. We are reading here a surgical author second to none in his time.

In 1742, the esteem of his colleagues at the Royal Academy was evident when they elected him as the "royal demonstrator of operations," to serve as a substitute for de Garengeot. De la Faye succeeded the latter in 1757—but before that, in 1751, he was made vice-director of the Royal Academy of Surgery, a post which he held for a long time. Some years before his death, which occurred on August 17, 1781, he gave his collection of instruments, apparatus, *etc.,* to his beloved Academy.

Curiously, de la Faye was puzzled by the presence of a tooth-bearing premaxilla in the double cleft in his first patient; he attempted to solve that problem by excising the offending bone and bringing the two lateral segments of the lip together behind the prolabium—not an easy task. In his second case he was more circumspect and he attached the lateral segments to the prolabium, using the latter as the central portion of the repaired lip. His description of all this was in Volume I of one of the earliest surgical journals extant. The portion of his article reproduced here (in translation) stops at the end of his second case report, but the original goes on to describe several other cleft lip repairs during the early 1700s in the Paris area—including one by de la Peyronie, done at Compiegne.

By de la Faye's time surgery, even plastic surgery, had come in out of the streets and become a respectable occupation—one suitable for gentlemen who wore powdered wigs and ruffles and had portraits made. Moreover, the elite knew each other, then as now, and on occasion they watched one another operate.

—Frank McDowell, M.D.

HOW A PATIENT EXPERIENCED A CLEFT LIP
OPERATION IN 1763

AARNE E. RINTALA, M.D.

Helsinki, Finland

Although we know of cleft lip surgery being done in China as early as the fourth century A.D.,[7] and in Europe in the tenth century, its history proper does not begin until the fourteenth century.[2] All these descriptions of cleft lip operations are, without exception, from the surgeon's point of view.

Before the development of anesthesia and antiseptics, the patient experienced the operation quite differently from nowadays. As I have not found any report on this operation from the patient's point of view in the literature, I submit the following very lively description from the eighteenth century.

THE PATIENT

The writer of the description, Thomas Ragwaldinpoika (Ragwaldson) was born on December 6, 1774, the eighth child of a farmer at Tyrvää, about 70 miles from Turku (then the Finnish capital of the kingdom of Sweden-Finland). Although he had none of the advantages of the higher education of that time, he was unable during his whole life to do physical work and lived modestly (often on charity and local aid for the poor). He became the most important Finnish lay psalm writer of his time.[3]

Lay psalms were, as the name suggests, occasional verses printed on loose sheets. Generally they dealt with topical events, and thus corresponded to some extent to modern newspapers. About 700 lay psalms were published in the Finnish language between 1636 and 1810; of these, Thomas Ragwaldinpoika wrote 140 known psalms between 1760 and 1793. Most of his work is religious in content, and is marked throughout by the fervent piety which influenced his childhood home.

Thomas had a unilateral cleft lip and palate, and he was otherwise sickly. In

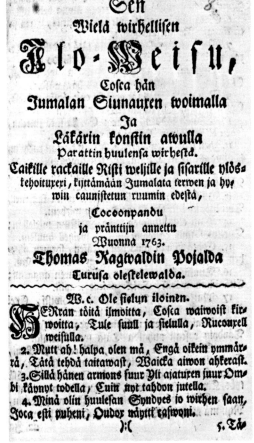

FIG. 1. Original title page of Thomas Ragwaldson's ballad *Psalm of Praise of the Still-Deformed.*

From the Plastic Surgery Service of the Finnish Red Cross Hospital.

214

the opening psalm of his first publication [4] he describes himself as follows:

1. Hail to God, Thou great Creator!
   With Thy counsel Thou hast sought me
   From my Life's start, Thou my Spirit
   Hast protected mercifully.

2. To this Vale of Tears Thou broughtst me,
   Marked with a Deformity;
   Which I bear upon my Body,
   On my Face for all to see.

3. But another flaw lies hidden
   In the roofing of my Mouth,
   Which confuses my Speech sadly,
   Cuts me off from other Folk.

4. Thus my voice doth not sound clearly
   In the Ear of other Folk;
   Nor come Words from my Lips rightly,
   Though my Meaning is right clear.

5. When I came into this poor World
   Borne of Parents kind and good,
   God gave them a heavy burden
   They must bear with Fortitude.

6. They were caused a deal of trouble
   On behalf of their poor Child;
   For my Mother's milk I could not
   Drink for my Deformity.

7. Other Nourishment they gave me
   Such as animals provide,
   While I lay there in my Cradle;
   Cared for me as best they could.

Thomas's brief description contains almost all the handicaps caused by a cleft lip and palate—cosmetic defect, speech difficulty (open nasality), and inability to suck.

THE CLEFT LIP OPERATION

Thomas describes his preoperative fears and trials, the operation itself, the after-care, and his own gratitude in a lay psalm of 50 verses[5] that appeared in 1763 (Fig. 1). The following are the first 38 verses (the last part is not of medical interest).

1. Work of God I sing to Thee, Who healed my Deformity,
   Come with Psalms and Soul of Joy, Pray and sing to Him on high.

2. But ah! poor thing that I am, Nor do rightly understand,
   How to do this skilfully, Though I try most manfully.

3. For his mercy great, if aught, Lies beyond the Power of Thought,
   What in fact to me befell, Herewithall I would fain tell.

4. For when born, in my poor Lip, From the first there was a slip,
   Which prevented me to talk, Strangely seemed my Face at fault.

5. Oftentimes for my sad Flaw, I did try to find a Cure,
   But it was not yet the day, When God's help was given to me.

6. For this thought I with me bore, And it was a burden sore,
   That the Pain I could not stand, It would leave me quite unmann'd.

7. It was also in my mind, When a cure I tried to find,
   That God's Will it could not be, Since at birth 'twas given to me.

8. Till at last God gave me strength, Broke the bonds of fear at length,
   So that being afraid of Pain, Seemed no surprise again.

9. In my Conscience I found Peace, in my Heart a sweet Release,
   For the Preacher of the Word, Strengthened me to trust my Lord.

10. To a Doctor I did go, My Deformity to show,
    And he vowed to me he would, Do for me all that he could.

11. And I did myself prepare, Called to Jesus in my Prayer,
    That He who had suffered so, Might help me in my Trouble now.

12. At God's Mass, upon my knee, Did I make my humble Plea,
    And indeed I was assured, Of help coming from the Lord.

13. In the month of April sweet, On the Sixteenth day of it,
Did the Doctor me attend, My Deformity to mend.

14. Put before me then a Chair, And I sat me gladly there;
Held my Face and with knife-tip, Cut into my deformed Lip.

15. Soon I held my Eyes closed tight, And my Hands with all their might,
On my Heart together pressed, Fingers twisted in Distress.

16. Felt a sharp and dreadful Pain, Felt the agony again,
So my Flesh shivers and shakes, All my Body the pain takes.

17. But within with Jesu's strength, Helpen was my Mind at length,
So no sound from me was heard, Not a cry nor yet a word.

18. Though the Blood from me did pour, From my Veins came more and more.
I was in a sorry plight, and I was a gory sight.

19. For my Shirt, my Clothes, my Breast, Every part of me was messed,
With the stream of warm red Blood, Running down me like a Flood.

20. But the good God's mercy too, Helped me in my Plight anew,
And the hardest Pain he tempered, His Son's suffering remembered.

21. And when my poor Gums were cut, Where the Doctor's knife was put,
Then did I remember Jesus, With his Wounds that came to save us.

22. And when the Scissors cut away, Skin from flesh of lip that day,
I remembered how He bore, Many a harsh blow so sore.

23. When the needles sharply pricked, And my lip together stitched,
I remembered then the Spear, That did pierce our Lord so dear.

24. Pierced the side and through the heart, Of our Saviour, Jesus Christ,
In these thoughts I did attain, Sweet relief from all my pain.

25. Lo! See how God's mighty strength, Gave me comfort now at length,
So that my Head did not swoon, Nor my Heart stop beating soon.

26. When I saw before me next, How the Blood upon my Breast
In a kind of Jelly set, Then with dreadful fear I sweat.

27. When the Doctor's work was ceased, From his task he was released,
Then at last I oped my Eyes, And my hands did clean and dry,

28. Wiped the sweat from off my brow, that from pain did start and flow,
And my Shirt too did I change, Cleaned the blood from every place.

29. 'Twas with weary toil that day, From my chair I went away,
Went to lie upon my Bed, On my Pillow laid my head.

30. Now I was a prisoner, Bound up like a poor slave there,
Not a piece of bread to eat, For two weeks no taste of meat.

31. The while the Doctor came to see me, Several times that he could see,
How my poor lips they did look; At last from me the needles took.

32. The first he took upon the Tuesday, The second he removed on Wednesday,
The third he took on Friday then, Ah! I could really feel the pain,

33. For that they had rusted fast, To the flesh had stuck at last,
So I was changed in feature, Pale I was, a sorry creature.

34. Yea, it was a dreadful thing, How the needles they did sting,
When the Doctor pulled them out; Then I suffered without doubt.

35. But all thanks to God I sing, Who created Everything;
From the pain He me relieved, and from my Deformity;

36. And a good Physician gave, Doctor Odenadt the grave,
Blessings to his potent Salves, To his Ointments and his Balms.

37. Thus the mercy of the Lord, To man's work He doth afford,
Let us honour Him most high, Who gives help to the needy.

38. So my suffering and sorrow, Were relieved for the morrow,
Jesus, of Physicians best, To Thee be my thanks addressed.

DISCUSSION

Evidently, Thomas had been long aware of the possibility of an operation but, understandably, had lacked the courage to have it for fear of the pain. Between the lines one may read that his was not the first operation of its kind in the neighborhood.

Another difficulty for him was the uncertainty as to whether it was morally right to correct a deformity given by the Creator. This idea was still deep-rooted at that time. About 160 years earlier in Italy the body of Tagliocozzi was dug up from its consecrated grave and transferred to an unknown place, because his rhinoplasties were considered by certain ecclesiastics to insult the works of "the Creator." In the middle of the eighteenth century, just before the operation under discussion, the Cathedral Chapter of Turku had urged the clergy, in two circularized letters, to stress this matter particularly. The final decision to operate required consultation with both the doctor and the priest, then the administration of Holy Communion.

The mode of operation appears to have been more or less that described by Johan Yperman in the fourteenth century.[2] Our patient's own report of his operation of April 16, 1763 is vivid enough to require no comment. Immobilization and liquid nourishment were part of the postoperative care.

The truth of the line from the Finnish national anthem, "Our country is poor, and will so remain, if gold you desire," is shown by the fact that the surgeon did not have at his disposal the commonly used gilded or silver cleft lip needles—which did not rust, caused less

tissue reaction, and were removed less painfully. Another Finnish "plastic surgeon"[6] of the eighteenth century also complained of the lack of gold needles.

The patient's overwhelming gratitude because he married a bride 10 years younger than himself less than two years later suggests that the operation was "successful" (by the yardstick of the times). True, the marriage was broken off later because of the wife's infidelity —and the wife was condemned to pay a fine or, if unable to pay, to two weeks' imprisonment on bread and water.[3] However, Thomas did not lose heart; he married again, two years later in 1777. From these two marriages he had 9 children. There is no record of possible anomalies in the children, but it is congruous with the high child mortality of the times that only two of them lived to become adults. Six months after his second wife died in childbirth, in 1788, Thomas married for a third time. He lived until March 14, 1804, when he died of urinary stone disease—at the age of almost 80 years.

THE SURGEON

Dr. Gerhard Odenadt, Surgeon of the Turku Royal Dragoon Guards regiment, performed the operation. He was born in Malmö (in Southern Sweden) on June 2, 1722. He studied surgery in Sweden, in Finland, and in Copenhagen from 1740 to 1756, and medicine at Turku Academy in Finland from 1753 to 1755.[7]

Odenadt was a colorful and highly respected citizen, as shown by his receiving the title of "assessor" in 1781.[8] He disagreed vehemently, even in the columns of natural scientific publications, with his long-time adversary, Dr. J. Haartman,[9, 10] Professor of Medicine at Turku Academy and the first superintendent of the Turku Provincial Hospital. In criticizing Haartman's recommendation of medical compresses for hemorrhage, Odenadt said: "One should not resort to methods that in case of accident may cost the patient his health and his life if the hand of an experienced surgeon does not intervene." In those days of blood-letting, this shows good scientific observation and a surgical way of thought.

Odenadt ends his list of qualifications, written by himself[7] on May 24, 1776, with the words: ". . . I am 54 years old and during the 32 years that I have practiced surgery and medicine I have contributed to the life and health of many a person and citizen and to their worldly success, depending on them." He died in Turku of a stroke on December 27, 1786, and he was buried on the church's "south side with all the bells ringing four times." [8]

EPILOGUE

Thomas Ragwaldinpoika's description clearly shows the almost unbelievable stress under which patients were operated on before the days of anesthesia and antiseptics. At the same time it describes the characteristic features of cleft lip and palate patients. Defective appearance and speech, combined with normal intelligence, caused the patient to seek compensation or employment from other sources [11]—in this case from creative intellectual work.

According to the experts, the artistic value of Thomas Ragwaldinpoika's verse is relatively slight. Along with his other work, however, it shows the talent of an ordinary man who lacked almost all the external qualifications for success.

Aarne E. Rintala, M.D.
Merikatu 5 A 11
00140 Helsinki 14, Finland

ACKNOWLEDGMENT

I sincerely thank Mr. Philip Binham, M.A., for his most successful translation from the ancient Finnish language of this very difficult verse text.

REFERENCES

1. Boo Chai, K.: An ancient Chinese text on a cleft lip. Plast. & Reconstr. Surg., *38:* 89, 1966.
2. Rogers, B. O.: Harelip repair in colonial America. A review of 18th century and earlier techniques. Plast. & Reconstr. Surg., *34:* 142, 1964.
3. Raittila, P.: *Tuomas Ragvaldinpoika.* Tyrvään Kirjapaino Oy, Vammala, 1949.
4. Ragwaldinpoika, T.: *Psalm of one burdened by deformity and the cross of suffering from childhood and youth onward* (Finnish). C. J. Frenckel, Turku, 1760. Helsinki University Library, Pipp. 971, main series 1753–62, 17.
5. Ragwaldinpoika, T.: *Psalm of Praise of the Still-Deformed* (Finnish). C. J. Frenckel, Turku, 1763. Helsinki University Library, Pipp. 1047, main series 1763–64, 8–9.
6. Hjelt, O. E.: *The History of the Swedish and Finnish Health Organization,* II, p. 280 (Swedish). Helsingfors Centraltryckeri, Helsinki, 1892.
7. Odenadt, G.: Schedule of qualifications. State Archives of Finland, Militaria II, Nr. 122.
8. The history books of the Swedish Church in Finland, Turku. Turku Provincial Archives.
9. Odenadt, G.: Remarks on the article "Common means of arresting hemorrhages in Finland" (Swedish). Svenska Mercurius, p. 794, June 1757.
10. Haartman, J.: Letter on account of Mr. Surgeon Odenath's remarks on the common means of arresting hemorrhages in Finland (Swedish). Svenska Mercurius, p. 835, Jan. 1758.
11. Skoog, T.: A head from ancient Corinth. Scand. J. Plast. & Reconstr. Surg., *3:* 49, 1969.

DU BEC-DE-LIÈVRE

(New method for the harelip operation)

DR. J. F. MALGAIGNE, *Paris, France*

(J. de Chir. de Paris, 2: 1–6, 1844)

Translated from the French by
DR. ROBERT H. IVY

Today I have again had occasion to remark how operative medicine, so rich in procedures and maneuvers, becomes poor and miserly when it is a question of reporting results. Concerning harelip, for example, the young surgeon, called upon to perform his first operation in the simplest case, will be perfectly informed on the choice of instruments, on the way to produce the raw edges, on the method of approximation of the pins—but of what he can promise as the result of all his care, the hope he can give the patient, he finds nothing. In other words, most of the books expose him to a cruel deception in letting him believe that he will easily conquer the deformity.

MY FIRST CASE

The first time I operated on a harelip the patient was a 7- to 8-year-old only daughter of parents who had not wished to have the operation performed earlier, in order not to overlook all chances of success. It must be believed, therefore, that I proceeded with the greatest of caution. On the 4th day, after removal of all the pins, I was pained to see that the free border of the lip was separated by a notch of two to 3 mm.

A consultation was held: it was presumed that the restless child had talked or cried too soon, and it was decided to reoperate. For even this slight notch I used two pins, one of which was placed right on the border of the lip. I took care to introduce this last pin very obliquely, from below upward for the left side of the cleft and to make it emerge in the opposite way on the right side. Under these conditions the notch was notably diminished, but a disagreeable trace was left.

SOME SECOND THOUGHTS

This first experience gave me much to think about. Accustomed to look upon this operation as of little import, I had followed casually the results of the operations that I had witnessed by the master surgeons—more interested, as most students are, in following the operative technique than in checking the results. I, too, was disposed in that respect to accept the word of the operators. However, after my double attempt, I no longer dared trust the classic procedure.

I then tried the elliptical freshening and I still had a notch. Once, after paring by the ordinary method, I made on each raw edge a little horizontal incision near the mucocutaneous border, with the object of turning down the two little resulting flaps; and this was also a loss of effort.

Presented at the Société de Chirurgie de Paris on December 20, 1843.

Meanwhile, I had undertaken the service at Bicêtre, and in reviewing the numerous pensioners of the establishment I noticed two or 3 among them who had been operated on for harelip by some of the best-known surgeons of Paris—some of them quite recently. Not having encountered a single one of those successes described in the books as being so easy and ordinary, I reached the sad conclusion that with all the resources of the art, a more or less severe harelip could well be transformed into one infinitely less severe; but to eradicate it completely was practically impossible.

Before going any further, it is well to add that at the time of my first communication before the Société de Chirurgie, one of my colleagues considered it advisable to point out that my assertion was too absolute. He announced that he personally had seen several complete successes. This occasion was a suitable one to judge the question, so each of the members present was invited to tell in turn what he had learned from his own experience. The testimony of all these witnesses put the number of complete successes at not more than 5 or 6, while the failures reached the neighborhood of 60. The majority, therefore, had been constantly as unfortunate as myself.

M. Nelaton, among others, after having twice tried the usual procedure had resorted in 3 cases to the elliptic incisions, and he had been satisfied with neither method. M. Guersant, with a personal experience of 25 to 30 operations, had never been able to deprive one of his patients of the inevitable notch.

Returning to the cause of this difficulty, it is easy to convince oneself that it is, on the one hand, due to the nature of the congenital lesion, and on the other hand to the operative procedure itself. Louis has attempted to demonstrate that in harelip there is no loss of substance. Evidently all his argumentation is but a play of words; there has not been an ablation of substance, but there has been an atrophy, and through

one cause or another a defect of development, which for the surgeon amounts to the same thing. This atrophy in simple harelip is especially marked near the two prominent angles at the borders of the cleft; if one tries to bring them together prior to an operation, one will note that these angles are not cut squarely as in an accidental section, but they are rounded in such a way that the most exact attempt at approximation cannot reproduce the free border of the lip—but leaves a very visible notch. (For double harelip the atrophy is still more striking; generally, the median lobe of the lip is shorter than the other sections, and it cannot contribute to reconstruction of the labial border; the median notch is, therefore, much deeper than in unilateral cases.)

THE CLASSIC OPERATION

Is the present operation thought out with a view of remedying this loss of substance (or, if one prefers, this diminution of substance)? In no way. Far from it, the preparation of the raw edges with scissors or bistoury directly causes a further loss of substance and thus commences by increasing the deformity. The idea behind this technique is to destroy the roundness of the angles and to make them almost square—a vain hope, which deep reflection should dispel.

Draw on a compress or on a piece of paper a harelip with the ordinary separation, then prepare the borders according to the accustomed procedure. If you remove only just what is necessary for the freshening, you allow half the roundness of the angles to remain. If the excision is carried out further, the freshened borders of the cleft form an angle, with the border of the lip becoming more obtuse according to the extent of the excision. Now try to approximate the two cut edges of the lip. You will see that they do not come horizontally toward one another, but that each one is forced to rise a little—in such a way that after they are brought together, the restored labial border necessarily describes an obtuse angle, often surmounted by a notch.

No doubt one might say that these things are easy to figure on an inert piece of cloth or paper, but the more flexible living tissues accommodate themselves much better to the necessary traction exerted on them—and experience proves that with the help of slight pressure one is able to force the two lateral halves more horizontally toward one another. Yes, this is true; but experience also proves that when this pressure is removed, they resume of their own accord the oblique direction by virtue of which they together describe an obtuse angle; and in the living, there is another unfavorable element to be taken into account—the retraction of the scar, which draws the top of the angle of the labial border up nearer and nearer to the nostril.

All of these difficulties increase when the harelip is double, and the complication becomes so much the more evident. This is too clear to require further comment.

A NEW OPERATION

One must, therefore, by necessity either change the character of the deformity to suit the operation (which is not even proposable) or else change the form of the operation to suit the deformity. What should be the basis for the new operation?

Because the harelip consists primarily of an absence of substance, and this absence of substance involves more particularly the labial border, instead of increasing the loss of tissue (as does the ordinary procedure) one must preserve as much of it as possible—by borrowing as needed from the neighboring parts. And if this extra tissue could be taken from the part that the paring requires to be discarded, the benefit would be gained without risk (and if I am permitted to use the expression, without expenditure of funds). In a word, the freshening of the harelip should only be done by cutting from the skin a few parings—and it is the utilization of these lost cuttings that constitutes the new method. I say *method,* with the understanding that the harelip operation which is now classified as *cheilorrhaphy* becomes so transformed that it enters the classification of *cheiloplasty.* Instead of becoming a seam it adds a piece.

As to the method of execution, nothing is more simple. Instead of cutting from below upward, one cuts from above downward—and one saves, near the labial border on each side, a little flap turned down by the paring, to be used in the repair according to need.

One will gain a more exact idea by reading the following.

CASE REPORT

A man named Maréchal, aged 23 years, cabinet maker, rue de Charenton 57, a robust and well-built individual, entered my service at the Hôpital Saint-Antoine on December 5, 1842 for treatment of a congenital cleft lip. The upper lip presented, on the left side and 6 to 7 mm from the median line, a cleft which involved three-quarters of its height. (The upper quarter exhibited a sort of rosy scar extending up into the nostril, which resembled an incomplete division. The edges of the cleft likewise showed this rose-colored character.)

The edges of the cleft were much separated below, and each became continuous with the free border of the lip by a very rounded angle. The gap exposed to view a partly erupted left lateral incisor tooth, and a still more unsightly space resulting from the loss of the central incisor. The two lips had a remarkable thickness, which increased still more near the edges of the cleft (as though the absence of the teeth at this point had favored the hypertrophy of the lip).

Attempts at approximating the two portions of the lip with my fingers resulted in forcing the edges into the gap at this point, and the marked notch thus produced at the border of the lip demonstrated the difficulties its restoration would involve if the ordinary procedure were attempted. (It is important, also, to note here the existence of a frequent enough condition that most authors have not taken into consideration. The red and mucous border of the lip did not continue as far as the solution of continuity, as would have existed, for example, following an accidental section; but it turned up toward the nostril, following the rounded angle of the lip cleft, and gradually diminishing in breadth lost itself finally in the rosy tissue of the cicatrix mentioned.)

The patient ate and drank without trouble. The only difficulty he had was in the enunciation of labial consonants.

He was operated on December 12, 1842, in the following manner.

Operation

The patient was seated on a chair facing the light, the surgeon standing in front of him. With the first cut of the scissors I divided the frenum of the lip, which had too low an attachment. With a second cut I prolonged the cleft of the lip above, as far as the lower edge of the nostril. Then, placing myself at the left of the patient (to allow the scissors to cut from above downward), I proceeded with the paring—keeping in the same incision that I had just made and continuing to within two mm of the free border of the lip.

The paring proceeded as promptly and as easily as by the ordinary method, and I did not encroach on the tissues any more or less. However, I took great care to keep along on each side in a parallel manner to the rounded angles joining the cleft lip to the labial border, so the flaps would be equally thick throughout and I would arrive at the lip border at a point where it was still horizontal. To accomplish this, two cuts of the scissors were necessary on each side, one which reached as far as the angle, the other which passed around this angle—in such a way that the wound to be reunited was composed of 3 sections, first in a vertical direction, then more and more oblique, then the raw surface of the little flaps which remained hanging from each

side and which again had a different direction. Following the application of the first pin (which I placed at the lower end of the cutaneous part of the lip), the reunion was exact; as the little flaps were only attached by a very thin pedicle, their being turned down and brought together face-to-face presented not the slightest difficulty.

The lip being at the same time very high and thick, I added two other pins above the first, after which I occupied myself with my flaps. They offered much more material than was needed to fill the defect in the lip. I, therefore, took my time in trimming them with scissors in such a way as to keep just what I judged desirable and to give the shape which pleased me best. I joined them with two points of interrupted suture in front; a third posteriorly; and I regarded the operation as finished when, giving it a last look, I perceived that the edge of one of the little flaps extended perhaps a half mm beyond the other. This would have spoiled the evenness of the scar, so I passed a miniature (insect) pin from one flap into the other, carrying it less into the too prominent edge and more in the other to bring them exactly to the same level.

After cutting the points of all my pins, with no other bandage or apparatus, I sent the patient back to his bed. I simply advised him to avoid all movement of the lips, and I fed him only on soups.

The second day a slight swelling appeared around the pins; the following day this had disappeared. At the left of the miniature pin the epidermis appeared raised by a droplet of pus, so I pricked it with the point of a needle. On the 4th day I removed the pins and the interrupted sutures. The 6th day the figure-of-eight ligatures came away, leaving a complete

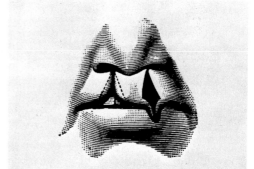

FIG. 1. The procedure of Clémot-Malgaigne. (*Editorial note.* There was no illustration in this classic article by Malgaigne; the drawing was published later in a book by Broca.)

rosy and tender scar, about one to two mm broad.

The succeeding days the wound became covered with little yellowish crusts, which when detached showed it to be more and more solid and narrow. The patient having a desire to leave the hospital on December 26, I made a sketch of the restored lip and noted the following details.

"The scar of the union is linear above; but in approaching the mucous border of the lip at the point where the first pin was placed, it becomes all at once two mm wide. From this point it bifurcates like an inverted V—circumscribing a little firm, fleshy, rosy tubercle, in which it is impossible to recognize any traces of the real cicatrix. (One must have been witness to the operation to know that this tubercle is precisely the result of the approximation of the two little floating flaps, that the apparent bifurcation of the scar is the point at which these flaps were turned down, and that the true scar is to be found right in the middle of the tubercle.) The lip is fuller and thicker on the side of the operation than on the other. When the mouth is closed, the lip appears as regular as if there had been, instead of a harelip, only an incision united by first intention. When the mouth is open, the greater thickness of the lip strikes the eyes—and all the more so because the prominence is not the result of pressure from behind by the incisor teeth."

DISCUSSION

I presented this patient on December 27 to the Société de Chirurgie which was impressed by the beauty of the result.

One point I particularly emphasize should be noted, and that is the absence of visible scar on all the mucosa of the lip—a phenomenon unheard of up to now in the history of harelip, and all the more interesting because of its involvement in a much more general question.

I had written in my *Anatomie Chirurgicale,* after Travers and M. Reybard, that the divided intestinal mucosa is not capable of an immediate reunion; indirect experiments have demonstrated

to me since, not only that it reunites marvellously well, but that after a certain time has elapsed it is impossible to find the traces of the scar. A similar thing is observed in the conjunctiva. And it now seems that the lips participate equally well in this curious property. I propose to investigate what happens in this respect to other mucous membranes, and to what extent this reunion without scar could be formulated into a general law.

I have only a few more observations to add. Working on a simple harelip, I have kept only enough tissue from my flaps to avoid notching; the little tubercle which I mentioned does not make a disagreeable prominence, and I have kept it in reserve in the event of a longitudinal retraction of the scar (which after the unexpected aspect of the reunion, today hardly seems probable). But if one were dealing with a double harelip, it is easily understandable how one could, for the creation of a median tubercle, take advantage of these two floating flaps which will always offer more than the necessary amount of substance.

I employ scissors, which I regard as preferable in every way to the bistoury.

It appears needless to tell how to handle the various complications of harelip. All reduces itself to this one point: trim from above downward the two lateral portions of the lip; the others, if there are any, should be cut in the ordinary manner.

The only criticism that has been made of the new operation bears on the difficulty of cutting from above downward. I am only able to reply that I have encountered no difficulty of any sort. Nevertheless, with a view to avoiding this, M. Monod has proposed making with scissors two little transverse incisions near the free border of the lip.

which would then permit operation of the instrument from below upward. The two little flaps left below would suffice to fill the notch, and there would be no further need to trim them afterward. M. Huguier proposes to make use of the bistoury, penetrating with one cut of the point near the labial border and proceeding then from below upward to the top of the harelip. These modifications are ingenious and could no doubt be tried successfully. However, I have already said that the scissors appeared to me to be more convenient than the bistoury; and as to the procedure of M. Monod, I prefer to trim my flaps after the placement of the first pin. I am more sure then of the amount of material absolutely necessary, and more in control of the situation.

I have added several interrupted sutures in addition to the classic pins. This appears to me essential for obtaining an exact union. It is in large part to the absence of these little sutures that one can attribute, in my opinion, the visible scar which follows the ordinary operation. In contrast to the precautions recommended by most surgeons, I have placed my trust in my sutures—without bandage, without apparatus, with no other dressing. This has been justified by the results, and that is all I wish to say at this time—this simplification being no more than the application of a much more general rule of conduct, all the motives and applications of which I intend to expose elsewhere.*

J. F. Malgaigne, M.D.
Faculté de Médécine
Paris, France

* The new method had been communicated and discussed at the Société de Chirurgie, and this report had already gone to the printer, when I learned from M. Roux that a very similar idea had been described to him by M. Clémot, of Rochefort—which he himself had employed in two patients, after which he returned to the ordinary method, in which he finds the advantage of greater speed.

The idea of M. Clémot has never been published as far as I know.

Aside from M. Roux, it has not been brought to the attention of any of the surgeons of Paris. The Journal de Chirurgie would cordially welcome any communications that M. Clémot would wish to address to it in this subject.

COMMENTARY BY THE EDITOR

There are 3 things of interest in this presentation.

(1) The paper was carefully and beautifully translated from the French by Dr. Robert H. Ivy, in his 90th year.

(2) The operation described was the first departure from a straight-line closure (or V-closure). It was time for a little finesse to be introduced into cleft lip repair, to make it something more artistic than the gross closing of a hole. Malgaigne perceived that a whistling defect was the almost inevitable sequel to a straight-line closure, due to the linear contracture of a straight scar—and he thought of something to do to prevent it.

(3) The life and career of Joseph-François Malgaigne are interesting. He was born of humble stock with meager resources in the village of Charmes, in 1806, but he rose to become one of the great scholars in the history of surgery.

Motivated by inspired teaching in his early years, Malgaigne began the study of medicine in Nancy at the age of 15. Four years later he had finished his courses and assumed the duties of sanitation officer at Nancy. At 21 years of age he was appointed extern in the Hospitals of Paris, and at the end of the year he won a prize for his thesis. Hard pressed for finances, he entered the

Val-de-Grâce military school of surgery, where he won several honors. His first major treatise was in 1830, *A New Theory of Vision.*

After spending a few months with an ambulance corps in the war between Poland and Russia, he returned to Paris and became associated with the St. Louis Hospital and la Charité. In 1834 he wrote his famous *Manuel de Medécine Opératoire,* which passed through 7 editions and 5 translations, one of them Arabic. In 1838 he published the two-volume treatise *Surgical Anatomy and Experimental Surgery,* and in 1840 he published a translation from Latin into modern French of *The Works of Ambroise Paré,* a 3-volume work which is still the standard reference source for this material. (Malgaigne was well schooled in Latin and Greek, and he became self-taught in Hebrew so that he could better understand the early books of the Bible.)

In 1843 he started his *Journal de Chirurgie,* and the article reproduced herewith (in translation) appeared in its second volume. In 1847 the name of this journal was

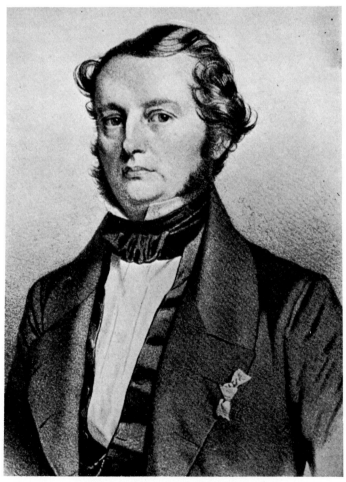

JOSEPH-FRANÇOIS MALGAIGNE
(1806–1865)
(From Garrison, F. H.: *History of Medicine,* 2nd Ed. W. B. Saunders Co., Philadelphia, 1917.)

changed to the *Revue medico-chirurgicale de Paris*; Malgaigne continued to edit it for many years.

In 1847–1855 his two-volume *Treatise on Fractures and Luxations* appeared; this became the standard work in this field for many years and it was later translated into English and published in Philadelphia.

The founder of our National Library of Medicine, Dr. John Shaw Billings, had the following to say about our subject. "Malgaigne was the greatest surgical historian and critic which the world has yet seen, a brilliant speaker and writer, whose native genius, joined to incessant labor, brought about a new mode of judging of the merits of surgical procedures—the mode of statistical comparison joined to experiment. He was not a great operator, and although he made some improvement in the art, such as his hooks for the treatment of fractures of the patella, his suggestion of suprathyroid laryngotomy, *etc.*, these are of small importance as compared with his work of exploding errors, exposing fallacies in reasoning, and bringing to bear upon the work of the present day the light of the experience of the past, of which his treatise on fractures and dislocations affords many excellent examples. The reports of his speeches in the Bulletins of the Academy of Medicine are among the most delightful reading in surgical literature."

—*Frank McDowell, M.D.*

LETTRE SUR L'OPÉRATION DU BEC-DE-LIEVRE

(Letter on Operation for Harelip)

DR. G. MIRAULT, *Paris, France*

(*Journal de Chirurgie, Par M. Malgaigne, September* [2: 257–265] *1844*)

Translated from the French by
DR. ROBERT H. IVY

To Professor Malgaigne

My dear and very honored colleague:

This work, which has been collected for a long time, would perhaps never have seen daylight if I had not become aware (in the *Bulletin de Therapeutique* for February, 1844) of your new harelip operation.* I have applauded, like many others no doubt, your ingenious discovery and I was preparing to inform you of the result of my trial of it when, reflecting on the numerous cases of harelip operated by me, I decided to extend my report on the subject. . . .

I will divide this communication into 4 sections. In the *first,* I will speak of the reconstruction of the median lobule of the upper lip; in the *second,* of the methods for reuniting the borders of the cleft; in the *third,* the treatment of bilateral harelip; in the *fourth,* I will seek to resolve the controversial question of the proper age for performance of the operation.†

I. RECONSTRUCTION OF THE MEDIAN LOBULE OF THE UPPER LIP

I state without hesitation that all that has been done prior to your work to obtain this important result has been marked with the stigma of frustration.

* See J. Chir. (Malgaigne), January, 1844.
† *Note by editor of PRS. The* third *and* fourth sections were published later (J. Chir., *3:* 5–20, 1845) and will not be reproduced here.

The lowest point of fixation, in which the harelip pin follows at first an ascending direction and then descends to describe a curve, admittedly produces a certain prominence of the lip border; but this prominence, which results from a temporary distortion of the tissues, disappears as soon as the pin has been withdrawn.

Making facing concave incisions on either side of the cleft, as proposed by M. Husson, Jr., seemed at first to solve the problem; but this was only one more theoretical view which experimentation on cadavers and clinical practice do not confirm (*cf.* operations by Malgaigne and Nelaton cited in J. Chir., Jan. 1844). . . . After this latest attempt, one sees, nevertheless, the formation of the notch which has always been deplored by surgeons.

Your method, my clever colleague, through a new proposal has overcome the difficulty. However, I wish to tell you that the operation through which you have obtained such a good result appears to me to be susceptible to being made more perfect.

First, you freshened the borders of the lip cleft by scissors from above downward. One can readily understand that this was easy in your patient whose cleft involved only ¾ of the lip; but if the cleft had extended high into the nostril, as nearly always happens, the projection of the nose would have prevented extension of the incision that high and the freshening would have had to be made separately by two incisions.

Then, as I have observed, the two flaps that you intend to use for construction of the median lobule, and that you are obliged to fashion separately, are difficult to fit together by their raw surfaces. In spite of the 3 points of interrupted suture which hold them together, a space tends to appear at their outer angles. It is doubtful whether they reproduce perfectly the median prominence of the upper lip.

In the two cases which follow, my savant colleague, I have introduced a variation of your method. Please decide whether I am right or wrong. Your judgment will always bear great weight with me.

Case 1. Single harelip, complicated by cleft of hard and soft palate; reconstruction of the median lobule of the upper lip by a variation of the method of M. Malgaigne.

Rosalie Bellanger, 15 years old, entered the Hotel Dieu in Angers on June 17, 1844, with a congenital harelip on the right side (Fig. 1). . . .*

Operation

After having severed with the bistoury the adhesion uniting the upper part of the left side of the cleft lip to the maxilla, I controlled this left side by seizing it by its midportion with thumb and index finger. With scissors I then cut into its lower part, by an oblique section from above downward and outward, a flap 6 to 8 mm in length. This flap, suspended at the border of the lip, was everted by an assistant and I completed the freshening of the tissues by another section, approximately vertical. To explain bet-

*By an error of the engraver, the illustration has been reversed so that it presents the cleft on the left side when it really existed on the right. All the other details being exact, it is only necessary to inform the reader of this transformation.

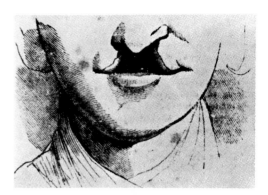

Fig. 1

ter . . . the cut which formed the flap commenced at the superior part of the rounded angle of this side of the lip and then extended in a direction toward the oral commissure, then approached closer and closer the border of the natural opening of the mouth; the pedicle was narrow, which permitted the flap to be turned downward and thus facilitated the cutting of the vertical part.

I proceeded in the same manner on the right (medial) side of the cleft, and then commenced to attach the borders of the cleft by applying the pin and the twisted ligature at the lower end of the vertical section—that is, at its point of junction with the oblique part of the flap. Two other points of pin-ligature closure were made above the first, to complete the reunion of the vertical part.

There still remained the reconstruction of the median lobule. I attempted, as did M. Malgaigne, to bring face-to-face by their freshened borders the two little flaps. . . . In fact, I brought them together after turning them downward, but they adapted themselves badly to each other near their attachment to the lip, where a little gap formed which would have been difficult to eliminate with a suture. While I was considering the best means of obtaining an even coaptation, the two little flaps by chance fell one upon the other, imbricating themselves. In this position they imitated very well the lobular prominence of the lip, except it was a little too marked.

Then an idea came to me. At the moment when I was getting ready to put it into execution, however, I heard the assistants expressing the idea of removing the greater part of the medial flap and applying on the raw surface thus made available, the upper or raw surface of the flap of the left (lateral) side. Then the remade median lobule was perfect and all that was necessary was to fix this flap by a fourth point of pin and twisted ligature.

Sufficient for the dressing was a pledget of lint covered with ointment, held in place by a bandage attached to the bonnet of the patient.

At 48 hours I removed the lowest pin which fixed the lobule, and also the two uppermost ones. I thought it best to leave the one in place at the junction of the vertical and oblique incisions, and I did not remove it until the end of 96 hours. At this time the pin had not cut into the flesh and the union of the entire lip was complete. After removal of the pins the parts were kept covered by a supportive bandage until the 10th day.

On June 30th Rosalie was in very satisfactory condition. Her mouth and nose had their natural conformation, and there remained from her deformity only a scar which, no doubt with time, would become less and less apparent (Fig. 2).

The modifications I have brought to your method, my dear colleague, in the operation on Rosalie, have resulted, if I am not mistaken, in a simpler and more perfect lobule—but I make haste to add, I have operated according to your concepts. To you belongs the idea of utilizing the mucous pad from the border of the lip cleft for reproduction of the median lobule. . .

Case 2. Single harelip, complicated by cleft of hard and soft palate; re-establishment of the lobule of the upper lip by the new procedure.

Réné Lelièvre of Baugé, 15 years of age, was born with a left harelip, accompanied by a cleft of the hard and soft palate. At 6 months of age, he was operated on unsuccessfully in his home town. · · · On examination at this time, the separation of the edges of the cleft was two cm wide at its upper end . . . and 3 cm wide below. . . Réné's intelligence was better developed than is usually the case in rural inhabitants.

Operation (August 13, 1844, at 2 P.M.)

(1) On the right and left sides I cut the two mucous bands that bound each border of the cleft to the corresponding maxillary bone.

(2) On the right, with one cut of the scissors obliquely from within out and from above down, on the inferior part of the lip and beneath its rounded angle, I cut (at the expense of this angle) a little flap which was suspended from the lip by a sort of pedicle; then it was turned outward by an assistant. By a vertical cut, I now freshened from below upward the whole extent of the border of the cleft.

(3) On the left, I resected the entire border of the lip cleft in all its height, and in the usual manner. . . .

For closure, I applied the first pin at the level of the angle formed by the two parts of the right border of the cleft. Then I placed two other pins above, toward the nostril. It remained to adjust the little flap for reconstruction of the median lobule; a fourth pin, directed from below upward and from within outward, sufficed for that.

One will understand that a place was reserved for this flap at the left inferior border of the cleft, beneath the first point of closure, as a consequence of the excessive length of this border over that of the right side. Four hours after the operation I applied the bandage supporting the two sides of the lip.

That night the patient had only a short nap.

On August 15 the dressing was renewed and the wound was found to be closed at all points. The two upper pins were removed and were replaced by strips of court plaster.

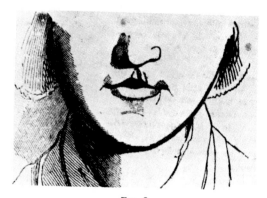

FIG. 2

On the 8th postoperative day, the restoration of the lip was complete. At the middle of the lip there was a little prominence, which imitated closely the natural appearance of the median lobule. At the same time, however, the nose was not as perfect. The ala and the nostril opening of the left side were less correct than on the right, and the tip of the nose was slightly deviated to the left. . . .

In this case (cleft on the left side), I fashioned only one flap, made on the right side. . . . You will see later (*Ed. note:* in the next paper) that in another circumstance, and with the objective of establishing a comparison between these two methods, I have substituted for this single rectilinear cut of one of the sides of the cleft a double angular cut—more capable, perhaps, of adapting itself to the configuration of the other side of the fissure (the one which carries the flap destined to form the median lobule of the lip).

II. METHODS OF UNITING THE BORDERS OF THE CLEFT

The twisted ligature and pin,* the bandage holding the two sides of the lip together, and the adhesives are the means employed at present to bring about immediate union of divided parts. All 3 are not equally effective—but because they can be applied simultaneously and promptly and give mutual support it

would be irrational to repudiate one or the other and not allow their combined support to contribute to the success of the treatment.

Today there is no surgeon who, intrigued by the fine theories of Louis, would trust to the bandage alone for maintenance of the edges of the wound. At the beginning one can, if need be, limit himself to the pin and ligature; but then the pins would have to withstand the contraction of the muscles and the retractility of the tissues, with much more risk of cutting into the latter.

Thus, at operation the ligature and the bandage are used; then, when some or all of the pins are removed, the bandage and the adhesives are relied on. Finally, a little later, the adhesives are used to support the scar whose organization is still very imperfect and which, until about the 10th day, is apt to yield or spread and may even disrupt.

I find, my dear colleague, that our authors, as far as the twisted ligature is concerned, express themselves in a manner too absolute on the time at which the pins should be withdrawn. . . . The conduct of the surgeon should depend on the circumstances. . . .

(Editorial note, by editor of PRS. Mirault then goes on to describe in great detail all varieties of his usage of the various modalities of fixation, and illustrates them with 3 more case reports. Later, in 1857, in a communication to the Society of Surgery of Paris, Mirault announced that he had abandoned the use of harelip pins and figure-of-8 ligatures and would henceforth rely on conventional interrupted sutures for this purpose.)

Germanicus Mirault, M.D.
Hotel Dieu
Angers, France

---

* *Explanatory note to modern readers, by Dr. Ivy.* The harelip pins referred to were in universal use at that time and came in various sizes. A twisted figure-of-8 (entortillé) ligature was passed around the two exposed ends of the inserted pin, thus binding the edges of the wound together. Some surgeons continued to use these pins as late as about 1900, and I personally have encountered several patients in whom they had been used. Mirault employs the word *suture* throughout this article when describing the twisted threads over the two ends of a pin. In my translation I have changed this to *ligature,* because in English a *suture* goes through tissue and a *ligature* goes around tissue. *R.H.I.*

ACKNOWLEDGMENT

The *Journal* is grateful to Dr. John Blake of the National Library of Medicine, Bethesda, Md., for a copy of this article and the illustrations.

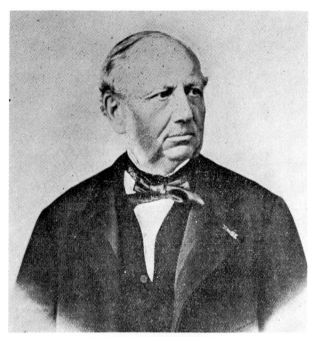

GERMANICUS MIRAULT, M.D.
1796–1879

COMMENTARY BY DR. ROBERT H. IVY

Germanicus Mirault was born at Angers, capital of the Department of Maine-et-Loire in the west of France, on March 1, 1796. His father and grandfather were renowned surgeons, his father's practice being almost exclusively limited to ophthalmology. This had considerable influence on the future of his son.

Germanicus started his medical studies in 1814 under his father. Upon his father's death soon afterward, he proceeded to Paris to complete his medical education—and some of it was under Malgaigne. In 1817 he served as extern, and later as intern first class, of the Hospitals of Paris.

In 1823, after having presented a thesis on keratitis, which long remained a classic, Mirault returned to Angers. There he began a series of successes which were destined to bring him into the front rank of medical circles. In 1836 he arrived at the most enviable situation for a surgeon—he was made Professor of the Outpatient Clinics and Surgeon-in-Chief of the Hospitals of Angers.

During his long career Mirault published many papers on diverse surgical subjects, particularly on diseases of the eyes. He had inherited the paternal aptitude in this respect and he achieved a place among the leading oculists of the time without, however, limiting himself absolutely to this specialty. He possessed a high degree of dexterity; no one knew how to extract a cataract more gracefully; no one could more happily apply the procedures of facial repair.

He was not only a fine operator but also a superb clinician and teacher, a professor of the greatest merit. Those who were chosen as interns for his service regarded this as the greatest honor obtainable in Angers. Mirault was of a generation of medical men of integrity, ones against whom the reproach of indelicacy could never be lodged, ones who recognized as their supreme guidelines conscience and duty.

Many are the poor who benefited from his unselfishness and generosity. As an example, on his retirement he turned over permanently to the poor of the hospital the annuity he was to receive in recognition of the 38 years of services he had rendered.

In 1825, at the age of 29 years, Mirault was named corresponding member of the Academy of Medicine and of the Society of Surgery of Paris. Later, the same honor was extended to him by the medical societies of Geneva, Marseilles, Liège, *etc.* The Society of Medicine of Angers was happy and proud to count him among its most active members. Rather than seek public honors, he went out of his way to avoid them. However, he could not refuse to receive from the hand of the President of France, in 1850, the Cross of the Legion of Honor; this was awarded for his care of the seriously injured in a major bridge accident.

Mirault wished to devote his entire time to the practice of his profession and he refused to accept the position of dean of his School of Medicine, which was offered to him in 1860. Seven years later, at the age of 71, he retired as professor and surgeon-in-chief—and he had the rare wisdom to bid adieu at the same time to his surgical practice. However, 3 years later, during the war of 1870 at the call of his unhappy country, he entered the ambulance service for several months with the title of Vice-President of the Committee for Relief.

Dr. Mirault then survived 8 more years in glorious retirement and passed away on January 19, 1879.

Robert H. Ivy, M.D., D.Sc.

EPILOGUE BY THE EDITOR

On March 1, 1968, in his 87th year, Dr. Ivy wrote to me—"We arrived home from Florida yesterday in a snowstorm. I enclose the material on Mirault. . . . What to do about illustrations of Mirault's methods creates a dilemma, because there is no satisfactory picture furnished by him showing what he actually did. . . . So, on close consideration, *mon tres honore confrere,* I find the Mirault matter to be not a question of a mere translation of a French article into English. It requires explanatory notes."

Enclosed was the crisp, bright translation and notes you have just read.

F. McD.

A MODIFICATION OF THE HARELIP OPERATION

WERNER H. HAGEDORN, M.D., *Magdeburg, Germany*

(*Centralbl. f. Chirurgie, 11: 756, 1884*)

Translated from the German by
KITTY DABNEY

Regarding harelip operations in young children, a crease or unevenness on the vermilion can be avoided with the operative procedure König described (Deutsche Zeitschr. f. Chir., *19:* 11). He not only joined the edge of the vermilion, but he also brought in a wider piece of the lip for closure. However, healing by primary intention was hampered, because there is a weak spot where the sutures meet.

To avoid this disadvantage, Hagedorn* operates in the following manner.

First (Fig. 1), with a sharp knife he makes incision *3–4–2* on the narrow lateral side of the lip; the beginning of *3–4* runs parallel to the vermilion. On the wider medial side, he then makes the incision 4_1–3_1–2_1. Finally, on both sides the scissor incisions *5–4* and 5_1–4_1 are made approximately where the vermilion becomes slanted.

There has never been a contracture after this procedure, but usually a small protuberance will result which seems to correspond to the middle of the upper lip. (A precise first suturing will not in itself hurt anything.)

Lately Hagedorn has modified the plan of the incisions in the following simple and practical way—which he mainly recommends now (Fig. 3).

First, on the narrow lateral side of the lip and with a pointed knife, he makes incision *1–2*, then incision *3–4*, parallel to the lip edge. Last, incision *1–5* is made obliquely through the lip edge (with scissors). On the wider medial side, he makes with a knife incisions 4_1–1_1–5_1, and then 2_1–3_1, so that points 1_1 and 3_1 will fall together on the rim of the lip edge. Thus one sees that lines *3–4* and *4–1;* and 4_1–1_1, are all the same length; thus the closure can be effected in the easiest way.

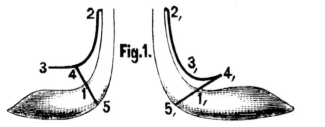

Fig.1.   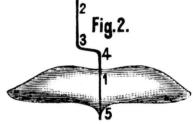 **Fig.2.**

Closure is illustrated in Figure 2; first, point 3_1 on the medial side is attached to corner *3* on the lateral side.

The result is also shown in Figure 2.

* *Editorial note.* Although this paper was written in the third person, the evidence indicates that Hagedorn himself wrote it. Not a few of the *Herr Professors* of that day sometimes wrote in this diffident manner, apparently trying to impress the reader with either their great modesty or great objectivity.

To lay the wound edges together better, it is expedient to somewhat round out corner *e* with scissors. Closure is as in Figure 2—so that again right angle point *3* of the medial side comes to lie in corner *3* of the lateral side.

The protuberance on the lip edge becomes proportionately larger as one spares more of the lip by making the incision through it more oblique; it be-

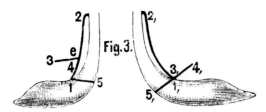

Fig. 3.

comes smaller or disappears entirely when one almost, or completely, cuts vertically through the lip edge.

In easier cases, because one can place incision 4_1–1_1–5_1 more outwardly on the medial side, one can make both halves of the lip the same size. Then the protuberance can be brought to the exact center of the lip, as occurs in the normal condition.

DOUBLE CLEFT LIP

This modification is also advantageous in the double cleft lip and palate, with a protruding intermaxillary bone.

Following König's procedure, Hagedorn had 3 such cases this year; each was repaired in one stage.

Both lateral sides are incised as described for one lateral side of a single harelip. First (Fig. 4) one incises 2–1–4 then a_1–1_1, then 2–3 through the lip edge; on the other side, 2_1–1_1–4_1, then o_1–1_1, then 2_1–3_1.

The midsection is cut with scissors a–4, o–4_1; then 1–a and 1–o are cut into a point, so that corners a and o will match angles a_1 and o_1, and the side sections can be joined together. The closure is shown in Figure 5.

An appropriate protuberance results at the exact center of the so-formed upper lip.

Case 1

The first patient, a strong 6-month-old child (A.J.), was operated on as described above on April 2, 1884. Previously, the subperiosteal vomer had been released (according to the method of Bardeleben) and bent backward. Healing was *per primam*. The considerable tension did not disturb the wound.

Case 2

The second patient, 7-day-old P.P., was operated likewise in one stage on June 7. However, here the tension was so great that Hagedorn found it necessary to insert a mattress suture; then he secured the suture with an adhesive plaster dressing (see Centralbl. f. Chir., *9:* 718). Otherwise, the thread would have cut through between the two arms of the suture. Healing was *per primam*, in any case. The mattress suture served a double purpose here; first, it fixed the intermaxillary bone, then it eliminated the tension of the soft parts.

Case 3

The third case was 5-day-old F.H., operated on May 27 in the same way—also with the use of the adhesive plaster and mattress suture. The patient was discharged after 7 days, as healing by first intention seemed perfect. This healing was confirmed later.

Hagedorn had never operated before on such young children, but had postponed these operations. Therefore, during the first 21 years he had only two cases so young, which he operated in two stages. However, these patients died later.

Hagedorn shows the attachment of

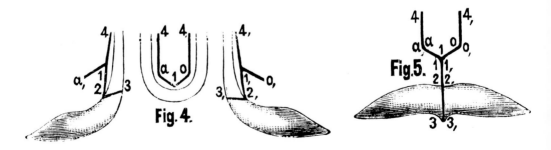

Fig. 4.

Fig. 5.

the adhesive plaster dressing which prevents the thread from cutting through.

After these 3 consecutive cases of double cleft lip and cleft palate, which healed *per priman*, Hagedorn concludes that for this malformation this early operation of setting back the intermaxillary bone, with immediate joining of the soft parts on each side, is not only warranted but is preferable to the two-stage operation.

He recommends his modifications of the direction of the incision in the lip, and of the closure—as these seem important to him.

Werner H. Hagedorn, M.D.
Magdeburger Krankenhause
Magdeburg, Germany

Editorial note. Following the above 1884 paper, a number of surgeons adopted the first method described by Hagedorn but the second method did not achieve popularity, possibly because most persons could not understand it. Hagedorn favored the second method, so he published the following paper in 1892 in an attempt to clarify his earlier confusing description.

OPERATION FOR HARELIP WITH A ZIGZAG SUTURE

(*Centralbl. f. Chirurgie, 19: 281, 1892*)

At the meeting of the German Natural Scientists and Physicians in Magdeburg in 1884, two modifications of the harelip operation were presented.[*] The purpose of these modifications was to avoid the weak spot (established by König's [†] experiences) where the freshened angles of the flaps meet.

The direction of the incisions described first therein became later the only ones to be published in textbooks of surgery, and to become well known.

Even so, I still think the second modification is better; I recommended it highly at that time and since then I have practiced and improved on it with great success. At first glance, this second method seems complicated, and therefore it did not attract more attention (especially because the drawings were defective and not clear). Yet, this method is easy and simple to do if one follows the directions and the description exactly. These follow.[‡]

[*] Centralblatt fur Chirurgie, 1884. No. 45
[†] König's Chirurgie, Aufl. 4, Bd. I., p. 315.
[‡] Incidentally, I'd like to mention that I use

OPERATIVE TECHNIQUE

First, one determines how wide the freshening and the joining of both cleft edges will be (*i.e.* points *1* and *1₁* in Figure 1). With the lip held very tight, a narrow pointed knife is inserted at point *1* through the lip edge, and the entire lip edge is separated upward to the nostril. In so doing, the incision is exactly on the border of the vermilion and remains so up to point 2. Thus, with incisions *1–2* and *1₁–2₁* on either side, the lip edge is separated; the free nasal wing is always held with a clamp forceps (one lets this hang down freely).

The width of the freshening will depend upon the direction in which the knife is held while the tissue is separated. Because the margins are thin and usually atrophic, it is easy to make the freshening too narrow. Therefore the knife must not be held perpendicular to the lip edge, but obliquely—so that more mucosa is separated and the wound edge is wide enough.

Now one must turn to the lateral side and plan transverse incision *3–4*. One confirms point

only my fingers and no instruments to hold and stretch the lip (just as would be done with gut sutures), because the thin lips of small children are easily injured by instruments. The lip and the finger must be well dried with sterile gauze. A small dry piece of this gauze placed between the lip and the finger helps to maintain a firm grip.

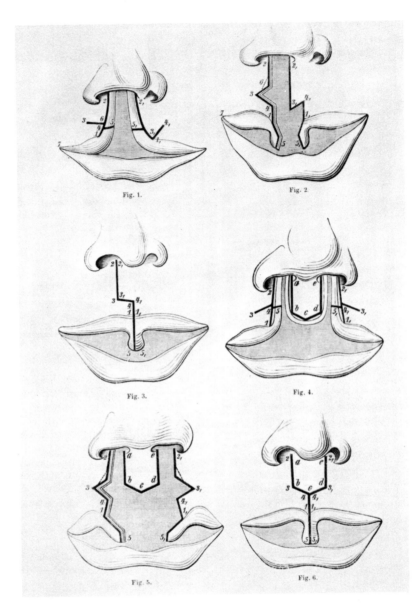

Fig. 1. Fig. 2. Fig. 3. Fig. 4. Fig. 5. Fig. 6.

4 on the freshened lip, by dividing the entire freshening line (*1–2*) into 3 or 4 approximately equal parts, so that length *1–4* equals a 4th or a 3rd part of *1–2*.* The direction of *3–4* parallels the lip edge (*7–1*) (Fig. 2). The confirmed point *4* is marked by a puncture with the point of the knife. One then pushes the sharp knife through the tight lip at point *3*, to make incision *3–4* up to point *4*. So that this incision will be as long as *1–4*, and no longer, one first

---

* The determination of point *4*, and thus the decision whether line *1–4* should amount to a 4th part or a 3rd part of line *1–2* (*i.e.* whether it should be shorter or longer) will be limited by the size of the lip defect and by the tension anticipated to be pro-

duced by the suture. Where there will be little or no tension, line *1–4* can be longer; but where there will be considerable or great tension, line *1–4* must be shorter. A long *1–4* line increases the tension; a short *1–4* line decreases the tension. The length of line *1–4* is equal to the measurement that is needed to increase the height of the lip at the expense of its width; it is from this point of the face that the length of line *1–4* is determined (and thus also the length of *3–4* and *4_1–1_1*) as the three incisions (*1–4*, *3–4*, and *4_1–1_1*) must all be of equal length.

makes it somewhat shorter. When the lip is very tight the proportions are easily changed, but it is very difficult to adjust incision $3–4$ if it is too long. However, if incision $3–4$ is made somewhat shorter, it is then easy to work accurately from point 3 on up and to lengthen the incision until it equals $1–4$.

Now we return to the medial side to make incision $4_1–1_1$, which must be the same length as $1–4$ (also $= 3–4$). The direction of incision $4_1–1_1$ conforms approximately to the midpoint of the stretched corner of the lip by 1_1. The pointed knife is inserted at point 4_1 on the tight upper lip, and incision $4_1–1_1$ is completed. One first makes this incision somewhat shorter, and then easily and accurately lengthens it with an incision at 4_1 until the exact length $4_1–1_1 = 4–1 = 3–4$ is attained. Finally, with scissors one cuts off the remaining piece of lip edge at points 5 and 5_1, leaving $\frac{1}{2}$ cm. To make suturing easier, corner 6 on the lateral side is also cut off with the scissors (Fig. 2).

If one follows this description and this exact sequence, the procedure presents no difficulties and is easy to perform. The correct sequence is necessary, and it cannot be disregarded entirely: (1) freshening the lip edges $1–2$ and $1_1–2_1$; (2) transverse incision $3–4$ on the lateral side; (3) oblique incision $4_1–1_1$ on the medial side, ʀ actly the same length as incisions $3–4 = 1–4 = 4_1–1_1$. Finally, excision of the long lip edges at points 5 and 5_1. The wound edges will then match each other exactly. They will fit exactly at their notches and angles, and create a true zigzag line (thus the name "zigzag suture," as the edges must match each other exactly; incisions $3–4 = 3_1–4_1 = 4–1 = 4_1–1_1$ must all be the same size).

DISCUSSION

With this zigzag line, as with no other operation, one can avoid the weak point described by König.

Great tension of the wound edges must be avoided in this operation, as in any other procedure. This is done best by making side incisions in the cheeks, close under the nasal wings; but this is seldom required. Of course, the mucosa of the upper lip, where it attaches to the upper jaw, must be separated.

At closure, using a deep suture, one

must necessarily first attach lateral angle 4 to medial angle 4_1, rather than medial angle 3_1 to lateral corner 3 (Fig. 3).

At the very end, the two remaining pieces of lip are joined together, and thus a protuberance is created (the more of each lip edge that is left behind, the larger will be the protuberance). If one wants to avoid a protuberance, one takes off almost all of the lip edges and separates them not at points 5 and 5_1, but closer to 1 and 1_1.

Even though this protuberance (when it is large) diminishes the first cosmetic impression, it does guarantee a more certain joining of the lip edge. The protuberance itself will disappear spontaneously in a few weeks, and then leave only a small, natural bump (through which each contracture will be bent).

In only one of my many operations did the suture separate, and no cause could be found for this. Only the outer lip edge remained joined—and it was so long that it lay over the wide cleft like a narrow bridge—but it held. From this bridge the cleft unexpectedly healed upward and it gradually contracted, so the result was mediocre (which I never would have thought possible). The parents were so satisfied with this result, however, that they did not want any further improvement.

The protuberance of the remnants of the lip margin is even more important in the bilateral cleft lip, as it is always exactly in the middle of the upper lip; at the same time, it forms a reliable closure. The larger the remnant of the lip edge is, the more any separation of the two sides is prevented. Thus, the protuberance will be larger but the tension of the suture will be lessened.

In the case of a bilateral cleft lip, each side is handled in exactly the same way as the lateral side in a single cleft. The middle piece is cut to conform to the wound, as seen in Figure 1. Also, the wound edges come together well here and produce a good result, even when a true zigzag suture cannot be used.

Werner H. Hagedorn, M.D.
Magdeburger Krankenhause
Magdeburg, Germany

COMMENTARY BY THE EDITOR

Hagedorn was the inventor of the square flap for the closure of unilateral cleft lips, but beyond that little has been recorded about him. He was born on July 2, 1831 in Eichsfeld, Germany, and did postgraduate medical work in Berlin where he was an assistant to Johannes Müller for two years. Following this he studied under Bernhard von Langenbeck, and during 1854 he wrote a dissertation *"De forcipe Schoelleriana obstetrica."*

In 1855 he went to Magdeburg where he worked the remainder of his life in the Magdeburger Krankenhause, first as an assistant, and from 1863 onward as Director of the Surgical Division. In addition to the articles reprinted herewith, Hagedorn published several articles in Langenbeck's *Arch. f. klin. chir.* (Volumes 18, 26, 28, and 29) and in the *Verhandlungen der Deutschen Gesell. f. Chir.* (in the years 1875–77–80–81–82–83). He died on June 20, 1894.

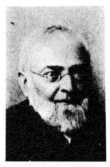

WERNER H. HAGEDORN, M.D.
1831–1894

The Sequelae

For the developments in cleft lip operations after 1892, the reader is referred to the standard textbooks on the subject (especially to Washio's chapter in Stark's book) and to a review article by McDowell.[2]

For a while a profusion of flaps—triangular flaps, square flaps, round flaps, zigzag flaps, *etc.*—from either or both sides, were advocated by various surgeons. As the procedures became more complicated, the complications increased; constant change and confusion reigned.

Sir William Fergusson and his pupil, William Rose,[3] brought order out of this chaos, by demonstrating that they could obtain results far better than the prevailing ones by doing a simple V-closure under general anesthesia, concentrating on precision cutting and accurate approximation in layers with fine sutures. This accurate V-excision technique dominated the field from about 1900 to 1930.

Noting that longitudinal contracture of the straight scars tended to produce whistling deformities, however, Blair and Brown[4] revived the Mirault triangular flap repair in 1930. But they used a much larger flap, one depicted in 1852 in Smith's[5] book—one that Mirault would scarcely have recognized. Later the triangular flap was markedly reduced in size, to about halfway between Mirault's flap and Smith's flap, by Brown and McDowell;[6] they also introduced a precision method of marking, one that could consistently be duplicated. The triangular flap repair dominated the world scene from about 1930 to about 1955.

In 1938, Veau[7] introduced a rather poorly described operation in which the anterior palate was closed along with the lip. Several surgeons in Britain and on the continent adopted it, claiming that it was nearly impossible for them to close the labial fornix unless it and the anterior palate were closed before the lip was closed. Along with other features, the Veau operation used a small triangular flap from under the alar base, fitted into a cut in the columella—a feature of Millard's later operation.

In the late 1940's LeMesurier[8] revived the Hagedorn square-flap operation—and for a time it became quite popular. The marking technique for it was vague, however, so Tennison[9] (in 1952) published a method of marking the patient by using a bent wire.

In 1959 Randall[10] published a triangular flap method in which he created an opening for the flap on the medial side by making an incision similar to that used by Hagedorn and LeMesurier on the medial side.

In 1957 and 1964 Millard[11,12] published his "rotation-advancement" operation, taking a triangular flap from high on the lateral side, under the alar base, and insetting it into an incision on the side of the columella. For the past 15 years or so, it has probably been the most popular method of repair—especially for partial clefts or the narrower complete clefts.

Throughout the last 200 years there have been two great problems with cleft lip operations. (*1*) Most any superb surgeon can attain a far better result with any of the described methods than a clumsy or careless surgeon can obtain with that or any other method. Precision of execution is just as important as design, perhaps more so. (*2*) With the patient's growth for a period of 15 to 20 years, distortions increase after any method of repair (or after no repair, for that matter). Then everyone tends to become discouraged with the method of repair most recently in vogue—and is anxious "to try" any new method that comes along.

Meanwhile, there is an all-encompassing, enormous, incredible dearth of published photographs of patients which show them soon after birth with a wide single cleft, and then also show them 15 to 20 years later (after no further surgery on the lip) with an acceptable result—after any known method of repair. *That is the final critical test.* We should not be even moderately satisfied until someone can pass it.

—FRANK MCDOWELL, M.D.

REFERENCES

1. Stark, R. B.: *Cleft Palate.* Hoeber Med. Division, Harper & Row, New York, 1968.
2. McDowell, F.: Late results after long-term growth in cleft lip repairs. Plast. & Reconstr. Surg., *38:* 444, 1966.
3. Rose, W.: *On Harelip and Cleft Palate.* H. K. Lewis & Co., Ltd., London, 1891.
4. Blair, V. P., and Brown, J. B.: Mirault operation for single harelip. Surg. Gynec. & Obst., *51:* 81, 1930.
5. Smith, H. H.: *Operative Surgery.* Lippincott, Grambo, and Co., Philadelphia, 1852.
6. Brown, J. B., and McDowell, F.: Simplified design for repair of single cleft lips. Surg. Gynec. & Obst., *80:* 12, 1945.
7. Veau, V.: *Bec-de-Lièvre.* Masson et Cie, Paris, 1938.
8. LeMesurier, A. B.: A method of cutting and suturing the lip in the treatment of complete unilateral clefts. Plast. & Reconstr. Surg., *4:* 1, 1949.
9. Tennison, C. W.: Repair of unilateral cleft lip by stencil method. Plast. & Reconstr. Surg., *9:* 115, 1952.
10. Randall, P.: A triangular flap operation for the primary repair of unilateral clefts of the lip. Plast. & Reconstr. Surg., *23:* 331, 1959.
11. Millard, D. R.: Primary camouflage in unilateral harelip. In *Trans. First Internat. Cong. Plast. Surg.,* Edited by T. Skoog, p. 162. Williams & Wilkins Co., Baltimore, 1957.
12. Millard, D. R.: Refinements in rotation-advancement cleft lip technique. Plast. & Reconstr. Surg., *33:* 26, 1964.

Apparently the flap that Mirault was using was one of vermilion only (the type that Malgaigne was using when Mirault left Paris). Later, the great Claude Bernard[1] (a renowned Parisian surgeon, whom the physiologists like from the columellar side, from both sides, double flaps, triple flaps, zig-zag Ws or Zs, flaps thrown across the upper part of the cleft near or in the nostril floor, flaps across the midsection of the lip, and so on. Some repre-

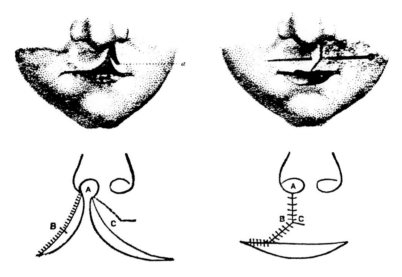

FIG. 1. Modifications of the Mirault operation. *above,* full-thickness lip flap containing skin and vermilion (From Bernard, C., and Huette, B.: *Medicine operatoire.* J. B. Bailliere et Fils, Paris, 1850.) *below,* the reverse flap, or Owen's operation, with displaced mouth.

to claim because of his avocation) was attracted by the flap idea. He came to use a much larger flap of skin and full-thickness of the lip from the cleft side; when he published this in 1850, he modestly designated it "the Mirault operation" (Fig. 1, *above*).

Predictably, a short while later someone had to try a flap from the columellar side; this unfortunate experiment was known as the Owen[2] (of England) operation. (The mouth tended to end up not under the nose; see Figure 1, *below*.)

While Hagedorn was experimenting with a square flap during the last half of the 19th century, others were trying nearly every conceivable type of flap — round, rectangular, from the alar side, sentative samples of these are shown in Figure 2.

The next step was also inevitable. From this frenzy of complicated flaps came chaos when operating on older children and adults sitting up without anesthesia. The designs were overly meticulous (*i.e.* unduly fussy) while the actual cutting was crude and gross, the sutures few. Toward the end of the 19th century, Fergusson of England refined the whole procedure by performing repairs in young children supine under general anesthesia. His pupil, William Rose,[3] carried this work forward by precision cutting and fine suturing in layers. To concentrate on refinements in execution, he returned to the simple V-excision design (Fig.

240

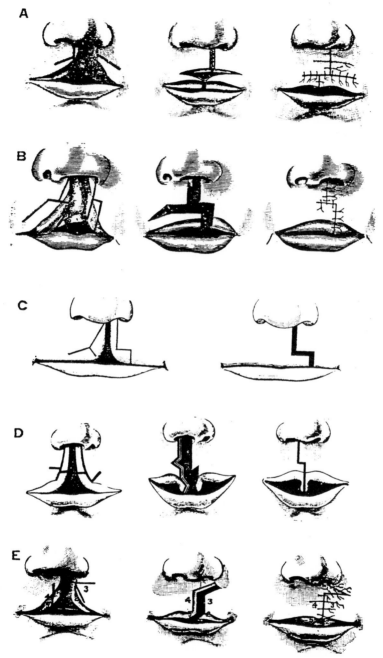

FIG. 2. Examples of complicated geometrical flap designs used on the continent during the latter half of the 19th century. *A*, König's method of freshening and suture. *B*, Maas' method — vivifying (*left*), wound (*center*), suture (*right*). *C*, Simon's method. *D*, Hagedorn's method of freshening and suture. *E*, Giraldès' method of freshening and suture. ("Maas Method" from Esmarch, F., and Kowalzig, J.: *Surgical Technic*. The MacMillan Company, New York, 1901. The other illustrations are from Bryant, J. D.: *Operative Surgery*. D. Appleton & Co., New York, 1899.)

3), with the lines bowed outward to give a little extra length. The results of this, published in his book in 1891, were so far superior to those obtained by others using the snatch and drag execution of complicated designs, that the V-excision operation dominated cleft lip repairs for the next 30 years.

In the late 1920's, however, these patients were growing up and Blair and Brown became dissatisfied with the late results from these V-excision repairs — even when they had been done with the greatest of care. In the complete clefts the resultant noses were bad, the lip was usually pulled up at the scar line, and most of these lips ended up tight and retruded. To obtain better noses, they decided the nostril base on the cleft side would have to be freed from the maxilla and rotated farther inward towards the columella; also, they thought more tissue was needed in the lower part of the lip to get it out in front of the lower lip. They worked out a triangular flap operation to accomplish these things, used it for some time, then found that it resembled a similar one for partial clefts shown in Henry Hollingsworth Smith's[5] 1852 book. Smith's operation had been copied from Claude Bernard,[1] who attributed it to Mirault. Thus when Blair and Brown published their paper[4] in 1930, they entitled it the "Mirault Operation for Single Harelip." The results shown in that paper, and in their presentations before various surgical groups, were so much better than any others that had been seen (particularly with regard to the noses and the forward protrusion of the lips) that this operation (Fig. 4) soon became the standard sought around the world.

In 1938, Victor Veau[6] of Paris pub-

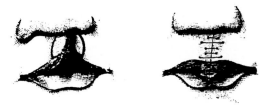

FIG. 3. Rose's return to the V-excision operation, with refinements in application. *A*, author's method of preparing edges of cleft, showing semilunar incision as far as red margin of lip and oblique upward cut on either side to form the prolabium. *B*, flaps in position and the nostrils symmetrical. The *wide stitch lines* represent the position of the wire sutures, the *narrow* those of the catgut. (From Rose, W. *On Harelip and Cleft Palate*. H. K. Lewis & Co., Ltd., London, 1891.)

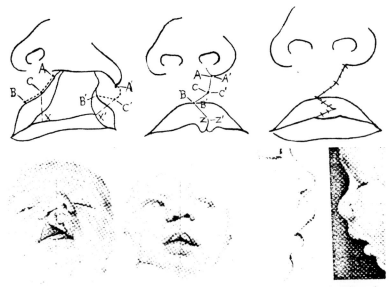

FIG. 4. The Blair-Brown operation of 1930, in which the surgeons used a half-length triangular flap and calipered markings to produce the first really satisfactory nostril repairs in total clefts that the world had seen. For the first time, great emphasis was laid upon thrusting the lower part of the upper lip forward and getting the entire upper lip in advance of the lower lip to avoid the "harelip look" of the last 2000 years. (From Blair, V. P., and Brown, J. B.: Mirault operation for single harelip. Surg. Gynec. & Obst., *51:* 81, 1930.)

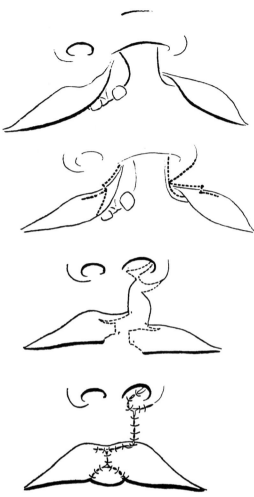

FIG. 5. The Veau operation of 1938, closing the anterior palate and lip simultaneously, with a "3-piece vermilion." (From Veau, V.: *Bec-de-Lièvre*. Masson & Cie, Paris, 1938.)

lished his operation, which consisted of closure of the anterior palate along with the lip. The operation, a rather ephemeral one (Fig. 5), entailed separation of the red from the white on both sides, incisions rather than excisions, and construction of the new vermilion from 3 separate flaps (which often led to lumps). It became quite popular for a time with some English plastic surgeons and their disciples, but it never achieved widespread popularity in America. It did feature a small triangular flap from up near the columella on the medial side, which was fitted across the cleft into a spread incision under the ala—an idea which has persisted in some respects in Millard's later operation (Fig. 9).

In working with the so-called "Mirault" triangular flap operation in the early 1940's, Brown and McDowell[7] found that the originally described half-length flap was too large after the child had grown, and that much smaller flaps gave better results. They also worked out a simplified design for consistently marking out the same small triangular flap procedure on all sorts of lips (Fig. 6); this operation then achieved considerable popularity for some years.

In the late 1940's LeMesurier[8] published a revival of the Hagedorn oper-

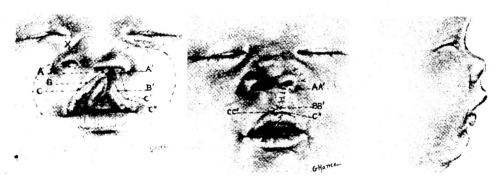

FIG. 6. The Brown-McDowell operation of 1945, in which the surgeons used a much smaller triangular flap, a simplified and repeatable method of marking applicable to all varieties of clefts, and a mucosal shift to thrust the upper lip farther forward. (From Brown, J. B., and McDowell, F.: Simplified design for repair of single cleft lips. Surg. Gynec. & Obst., *80:* 12, 1945.)

ation, with some variations (Fig. 7). Although his marking technique was difficult to duplicate, his surgery was done with great precision and he demonstrated some very good early results. Predictably, his operation was quickly adopted by a number of surgeons and used for some years. A principle prem-

ise of the operation was that the square flap would push the center of the prolabium downward to give a "cupid's bow" effect.

The vague marking technique of the Hagedorn-LeMesurier operation was improved in 1952 when Tennison[9] published a method of imprinting the design on the lip with a bent piece of wire (Fig. 8).

In 1955, Millard[10] first published his "rotation advancement" operation, which interdigitated triangular flaps across the nostril floor to build up a sill (Fig. 9). Millard's execution of this was superb, particularly in partial clefts, so his operation[11] has attracted quite a large current following.

In the late 1950's and early 1960's, there was considerable interest in primary bone grafting across the alveolar cleft under various types of lip repairs, a procedure popularized by Schmid[12] of Stuttgart, Germany. There has been some question as to how often these grafts take, and whether or not successful bone grafts act as a bridle to hinder growth expansion of the alveolar arch.

In 1965, Randall[13] published a preliminary lip adhesion operation which could be used in unilateral or bilateral complete cleft lips to convert them into partial cleft lips. It was his feeling that "although this adds an operative pro-

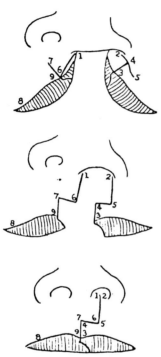

FIG. 7. The LeMesurier-Hagedorn operation of the late 1940's, with a square flap. (From Le-Mesurier, A. B.: Quadrilateral Mirault flap operation. Plast. & Reconstr. Surg., 16: 422, 1955.)

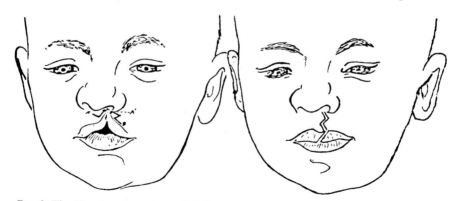

FIG. 8. The Tennison operation, which is essentially a repeatable method of marking out a square flap operation with a bent wire. (From Tennison, C. W.: Repair of unilateral cleft lip by stencil method. Plast. & Reconstr. Surg., 9: 115, 1952.)

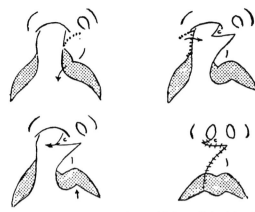

FIG. 9. Millard operation, with interdigitation of small triangular flaps at and near the nostril floor. (From Millard, D. R., Jr.: Primary camouflage in unilateral hare lip. In *Transactions of the First International Congress of Plastic Surgery*, edited by T. Skoog, p. 162. The Williams & Wilkins Co., Baltimore, 1957.)

cedure to the usual lip repair, it makes the definitive closure simpler and easier." He also thought the definitive closures were better when done in this manner.

There has been surprisingly little published on the primary repair of bilateral cleft lips, and astonishingly few papers show the results of these repairs after 15 or more years.

The history of the first 2,000 years of cleft lip repairs is that every surgeon doing them comes to feel there is something lacking when he views his results after 15 years of growth. As a result, he may adopt the newest procedure extant and become, for a while, enamored with his early results from it — forgetting, for the moment, that he was equally pleased 15 years ago with the early results from the operation he has just discarded.

Perhaps editors should be more reticent about publishing early results, especially of new designs for cleft lip repairs, and insist that authors show at least a few results after 10 years or more of growth.[14]

—Frank McDowell

REFERENCES

1. Bernard, C., and Huette, B.: *Médecine opératoire*. J. B. Balliere et fils, Paris, 1850.
2. Owen, E.: *Cleft Palate and Hare Lip*. W. T. Keener Co., Chicago, 1904.
3. Rose, W.: *On Harelip and Cleft Palate*. H. K. Lewis & Co., Ltd., London, 1891.
4. Blair, V. P., and Brown, J. B.: Mirault operation for single harelip. Surg., Gynec., & Obst., *51:* 81, 1930.
5. Smith, H. H.: *Operative Surgery*. Lippincott, Grambo & Co., Philadelphia, 1852.
6. Veau, V.: *Bec-de-Lièvre*. Masson & Cie, Paris, 1938.
7. Brown, J. B., and McDowell, F.: Simplified design for repair of single cleft lips. Surg., Gynec. & Obst., *80:* 12, 1945.
8. LeMesurier, A. B.: A method of cutting and suturing the lip in the treatment of complete unilateral clefts. Plast. & Reconstr. Surg., *4:* 1, 1949.
9. Tennison, C. W.: Repair of unilateral cleft lip by stencil method. Plast. & Reconstr. Surg., *9:* 115, 1952.
10. Millard, D. R.: Primary camouflage in unilateral harelip. In *Transactions of the First International Congress of Plastic Surgery*, p. 162. Williams & Wilkins Co., Baltimore, 1957.
11. Millard, D. R.: Refinements in rotation-advancement cleft lip technique. Plast. & Reconstr. Surg., *33:* 26, 1964.
12. Schmid, E.: Die Osteoplastik bei Lippen-Kiefer-Gaumenspalten. Arch. klin. Chir., *295:* 876, 1960.
13. Randall, P.: A lip adhesion operation in cleft lip surgery. Plast. & Reconstr. Surg., *35:* 371, 1965.
14. McDowell, F.: Late results after long-term growth in cleft lip repairs. Plast. & Reconstr. Surg., *38:* 444, 1966.

SECTION IV

The Origins of
Cleft Palate Repairs

CLEFT PALATE SURGERY PRIOR TO 1816

BLAIR O. ROGERS,* M.D.

New York, N.Y.

It happened to me at Paris to have a Chanon of Saint Anton, who had a certaine disease in his mouth, by the which he lost the pellet of his mouth, whereby he became dumbe, and that drinke which he ever dranke, he did avoyde the most part of it at his nose.

—*Peter Lowe, 1612*[1]

It happeneth often that part of the bone of the Palat, either by gunshot, or Lues Venerea is removed, so that the Patient cannot pronounce his words distinctly, but obscurely and snuffling.

—*James Cooke, 1648*[2]

Sometimes indeed some Member or other is wanting in Children when they born, or is after eaten off by Venereal Distempers ... Sometimes the small Bone in the Roof of the Mouth falls as in the Pox, and then the Patients Meat comes out of his Nose.

—*de la Vauguion, 1699*[3]

Let us be quite frank in discussing the history of cleft palate surgery! Its development was held back for many centuries because physicians and surgeons believed that most palate defects were the direct result of syphilitic infection. This destructive disease was known to our ancestors by a variety of names, including the pox, the great pox, the French pox, the Spanish disorder, the Neapolitan or Italian Disease, the disease of Espanola, the Polish disease, Morbus Gal-

Presented before the Annual Meeting of the American Association of Plastic Surgeons, Cleveland, April 28, 1966.

* Supported in part by National Institutes of Health Grant DE-01244 (New York University Cleft Palate Program).

† Attending Surgeon, Plastic Surgery Department, Manhattan Eye, Ear and Throat Hospital, New York City; Assistant Professor of Clinical Surgery (Plastic Surgery), Institute of Reconstructive Plastic Surgery, New York University School of Medicine.

licus, mal franzoso and malum francicum. A quick glance at these terms reveals that the French came out second best in the battle of terminology. Good,[4] in his popular early 19th century book, *The Study of Medicine*, described this inelegant disease as ". . . a gift to Europe from the French nation."

National feelings being what they are and, it seems, always were, it is not surprising to find that the etymologic skirmishes over which nation deserved the honor of going down in history as the fountainhead of syphilis were matched by equally heated passions in surgical controversies as well. Germans and Frenchmen were charging each other with the crime of surgical plagiarism 150 years ago; it was suggested that Roux[5] of Paris knowingly took credit in 1819 for first devising a successful closure of the soft palate, an operation performed 3 years earlier in 1816 by von Graefe, of Berlin.[6]

As venturesome as these original cases may have been, however, the inquisitive surgeon must certainly ask himself why such a simple operation had not been performed prior to 150 years ago, when one considers the much greater antiquity of harelip repair. An unknown Chinese surgeon, for example, in approximately 390 A.D. successfully closed the cleft lip of a poor, 18-year-old farmer boy, Wei Yang-Chi, who subsequently did not let his repaired deformity prevent him from becoming the governor general of six Chinese provinces.[7] Nor were Saxon surgeons of pre-Norman Britain[8] timid when faced with harelips, which they sewed ". . . fast with silk," at or before 950 A.D.

What factors, therefore, discouraged early surgeons such as Yperman, Franco, Paré and others from closing cleft palates centuries before von Graefe? Certainly palatal clefts existed for thousands of years before the year 1816. An Egyptian mummy of the pre-Christian era, for example, had a demonstrable cleft palate.[9]

After many months of research in the Rare Book Room of the New York Academy of Medicine, an answer to the above question has gradually been uncovered, namely, that surgeons prior to 1816 thought, and perhaps rightfully so, that most palate defects were the result of syphilitic infection, until proven otherwise, and, to a lesser degree, that they were also caused by other suppurating and/or destructive disorders such as scurvy, tuberculosis, and severe den-

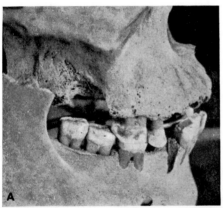

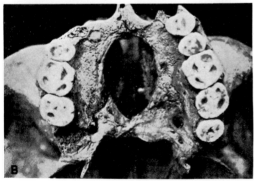

FIG. 1.*A*, skull from the Middle Empire of Ancient Egypt (2445 to 1731 B.C.), showing a large destruction of the maxilla and alveolus in the right upper molar region. *B,* ancient Peruvian skull (c. 1st century A.D.), showing evidence of a large palate perforation. The entire premaxilla is missing, suggesting the previous existence of a bilateral cleft palate and lip. (From Thoma, K. H.: Oral diseases of ancient nations and tribes. J. Allied Dent. Soc., *12:* 327, 1917.[16])

tal and alveolar abscesses or decay (fig. 1*A*). The general belief of surgeons in a syphilitic etiology is well summarized in the case history and comments of John Stephenson, the Canadian medical student, who described in his 1820 graduation thesis, *De Velosynthesi,*[10] the successful repair of his own cleft velum by Roux, in 1819, as follows:

> That the voice is affected by the nasal cavities and soft palate is shown by the fact that mine resembled that of a venereal patient who has suffered the partial or complete loss of his palate. . . .
>
> It may be asked why the British surgeons never spoke to me about such an operation. The answer is that all my medical friends suspected that my trouble was syphilitic; they had not examined my throat and so the condition of my soft palate was unknown. . . .[10]

Taking a cue from Stephenson's thesis, and tracing the chronology of man's awareness of syphilis in as parallel a manner as history permits, together with his awareness of "the palate" and its disorders, I shall attempt now to sketch briefly the gradual evolution of knowledge in syphilology, oral pathology, palatal anatomy, physiology and surgery which, all too slowly, finally led to von Graefe's pioneering operation performed only 150 years ago.

Prehistoric Era

Ricord, a great French syphilographer, claimed that the first line of Genesis really should be: "In the beginning, God created the heavens, the earth, man and venereal disease," [11] implying that most venereal diseases probably existed everywhere since the dawn of time.

Presumably, luetic crania and long bones have been identified in material from Neolithic France, Stone Age Japan, Neolithic Indo-China (Annam),[12] and prehistoric Argentina, Peru, Mexico, Arizona, New Mexico, Alabama and Illinois.[13]

A bitter controversy, however, which has by no means been settled, still rages over the "true" origin of syphilis.[14] Many still believe that the sailors of Columbus brought syphilis back from the New World on their return from America in 1493.

Prior to the voyages of Columbus, during the Middle Ages and earlier (see Sushruta), an obscure disease smoldered in various districts of Europe, Asia Minor and Asia. This disease apparently broke out in epidemic form at the end of the 15th century in Europe and received a variety of names, including the Pox and the French disease or Morbus Gallicus. It was only recognized as being of venereal origin long after it had ravaged thousands of victims in most European countries.[15]

In brief summary, therefore, with the existence of syphilis probably dating from prehistoric times, a search must first be directed toward our long dead surgical forbearers, the ancient Egyptians, Indians and Greeks.

Pre-Christian Era

Although no syphilitic diseases of the bones or teeth were demonstrated in an exhaustive study of Egyptian mummies, one case of cleft palate was conclusively demonstrated.[9] In addition, severe alveolar decay (fig. 1A) was already in evidence[16] in a skull from the Middle Empire of Ancient Egypt (2445 to 1731 B.C.). Interestingly, the earliest evidence of a simple retentive dental prosthesis was found at Gizeh, dating from the end of the Old Empire (c. 2500 B.C.). It was made of gold wire, linked together the lower left second and third molars, and had been woven around their gingival margins.[17] Thus began man's earliest attempts at intraoral prostheses.

Sushruta (c. 6th century B.C.) may have been the first to describe the upper jaw anatomically, including the palate (Talu), and alveolar processes (Udakhula).[18] He also described nine different diseases and/or tumors of the palate and its adjacent structures, including the tonsils, apparently none of which were congenital in origin.[18] There still seems to exist some confusion as to whether some of these diseases affected the tonsils or the uvula. Thus, what has been interpreted by some translators as a tonsillectomy, is considered by others as a uvulotomy.[18, 19] In one translation, Sushruta wrote: "By means of forceps between thumb and finger, drawing the uvula forward, the physician may cut it with a sickle-shaped knife above the top of the tongue."[19]

He also described a venereal disease (Upadansá), which bears a very close resemblance to syphilis, of which there were five distinct clinical types or phases. In its most severe form, ". . . the penile organ cracks, the ulcers or cancers become infested with parasites and death comes in to put a stop to the suffering of its wretched victim."[18] He also recommended nonsurgical treatment of palatal and/or uvular disorders (oil applications and fomentations), thus initiating the next 2400-year-old history of applying to the palate, soft palate and especially to the uvula, an incredible galaxy of preparations which included such questionable items as red copper scales, ox gall, pounded pepper powder, assafetida and one particularly ornithologic tidbit consisting of salt preserved nestling swallow, burned and crumbled into a powdered ash and administered as a draught (see Celsus).[20]

The Hippocratic Collection, as it is known, reveals that Hippocrates (c. 460 to 355 B.C.) and/or his followers were among the first to understand the mechanism of speech, stating that:

> . . . the tongue articulates and by its movement coming in contact with the palate and the teeth, renders the sound distinct.
>
> . . . Among those individuals whose heads are long shaped, some have thick necks, strong members and bones; others have strongly arched palates, their teeth are disposed irregularly, crowding one on the other and they are molested by headaches and otorrhea.[17]

Hippocrates also practiced uvulotomy, advising:

> It is very dangerous to cut off or scarify enlarged uvulae while they are red and large, for inflammations and hemorrhages supervene; but one should try to reduce such swellings by some other means at this season. When the whole of it is converted into an abscess, which is called uva, or when the extremity of the variety called columella is larger and round, but the upper part thinner, at this time it will be safe to operate.[21]

In book II of De Morbis he recommends: "When the uvula alone is inflamed seize it with the finger and press it up against the palate and cut off the end."[22]

Hippocrates also described two types of

intraoral necrosis, resembling syphilitic destruction, one of which involved the palatal bone. He wrote: ". . . in cases where the bones of the palate have exfoliated, the nose sinks in its middle but in those in which the sloughing is about the teeth, the ridge is flattened." [16]

Hippocrates also wrote of an apparently destructive, suppurative inflammation of the palate which was characterized by swelling in the form of a localized tumor. When the necrotic tissue fell away, the patient ate foods or took soup by introducing them through a gouged or grooved eating instrument, the use of which was continued until healing resulted.[23]

In none of Hippocrates' writings, however, is there any mention of congenital cleft palates.[21, 23, 24]

Asclepiades of Bithynia (c. 124 to 40 B.C.) scarified the palate and the tonsils with an instrument to treat very severe, unresponsive cases of quinsy sore throat, known to the Greeks as angina [anchonē].[25]

25 B.C. to 1000 A.D.

Celsus (25 B.C. to 50 A.D.) prescribed a specific medication for a disorder of the uvula and/or the genitalia. His description of the disorder suggests either a herpetic and/or secondary infection of both areas, but could equally implicate a venereal disease of the same two loci. He recommended:

> . . . the pastil of Andron for inflammation of the uvula, and for the genitals when foul, and even when affected by canker [septic or gangrenous inflammation]. It contains oak-galls, blacking, and myrrh . . . aristolochia and split alum . . . pomegranate-heads . . . compounded with raisin wine.[20]

For noninflammatory disorders of the uvula, his indications for uvulotomy were similar to, but slightly more detailed than, those of Hippocrates.[20]

No mention of palatal clefts or fissures, however, can be detected in Celsus' writings.

In the 1st century A.D., in Peru, a palatal defect of unknown origin [syphilis?] existed in some poor victim. Figure 1B reveals his skull with a large perforation of the hard palate. Interestingly, the premaxilla is entirely absent, which suggests that the patient

might also have suffered from a double cleft lip.[16]

Galen (c. 129 to 200) does not mention clefts of the palate in any of his voluminous writings.[26] He recommended operating upon the uvula only when this organ had assumed the physical characteristics of leather.

Oribasius (325 to 403) was one of the first to recommend caution in excising the uvula by taking care not to cut it off entirely, but to leave some portion remaining.[27] Without some remnant of uvula, he warned that the voice would be altered, and air inspired into the lungs would be too cold. Aurelianus Caelius (c. 5th century A.D.) improved upon the handiwork of Asclepiades by additionally scarifying the tongue and the soft palate to supposedly facilitate drainage in cases of severe quinsy.[25]

Paulus Aegineta (625 to 690) called the uvula ". . . the quill or plectrum of the organ of speech," frequently the seat of catarrhal inflammation flowing down from the head. He used the staphylotomus, a scalpel, to cut off portions of the elongated uvula. Burning caustics to necrose an uvular swelling were placed in a spoon-shaped staphylocaustos, into which the uvula was dipped. From the description which follows, pity the poor patient!

> The medicine must neither be of too liquid a consistence, lest it run down from the uva improperly, and burn the adjoining parts (and, therefore, we direct the patient not to swallow during the whole operation of burning), nor very hard, that it may soon act upon the uva. . . . During the whole time of its action the patient must sit with his head bent forwards, in order that the saliva which is melted down with the portions of the medicine may flow from the mouth. The part becomes dead [black] in one hour, and falls off about the third or fourth day.[28]

He was also not averse to using a little metaphysical nonsense:

> But a thread of a sea-purple colour which has been bound round the neck of a viper, and strangled her, has wonderful effects as an amulet in relieving affections of the [uvula] . . . as Galen testifies.[28]

With the death of Paul of Aegina, the great period of Greco-Roman medicine came to an end. In this same century, however, the rise of Islam dominated all medical thought, but most Arab physicians and surgeons merely repeated the therapies described by their Greek predecessors.

Johannes Mesuë, or John of Damascus (777 or 780 to 857), a Christian who directed the Arab hospital at Bagdad, probably first mentioned the combined use of "true" or hot burning cautery with surgery. He advised excising uvulas with a gold *bistouri* [a narrow bladed knife], heated to redness in a fire.[25] Hot cautery was a special feature of Arabian surgery, Arab surgeons having literally set aside the more customary Greco-Roman use of the knife.

Rhazes (865 to 925) shrank "relaxed" uvulae in spoons filled with alum.[25]

Albucasis (936 to 1013) made no mention of cleft palates and, in general, preferred caustics to knives in treating uvular disorders. In his therapy for patients who refused surgery (and who can blame them in this era of red hot cautery irons, and perhaps even cross eyed Arab surgeons, since "squint" or strabismus had been considered a mark of beauty in some Arab cultures) Albucasis cauterized with quicklime! Patients were advised to use profuse "spitting but no swallowing" for fear of gravely damaging deeper structures.[29]

Eleventh to Fifteenth Centuries, A.D.

Neither Roger of Palermo nor Roland of Parma described cleft palates, but Roger (*c.* 12th century A.D.) probably introduced the scissors to cut off portions of elongated uvulae.[25]

William of Saliceto (1210 to 1277), who literally reintroduced use of the knife in surgery, also employed cauterization with the hot iron, thrust down through a protective elderwood tube toward the elongated uvula.[25] Lanfranchi of Milan (? to 1315) made no mention of cleft palate although he recognized the function of the uvula and palate in speech mechanisms. He wrote:

...& than above this instrument [mouth] is uvula that is the palet of the mouth & helpith for to make soun/ For the wynd that cometh of the lungis reboundith agens the palet & makith the more soun ... If the palet be recchid along, & if

it be so long that it lie upon the tunge, than thou muste kutte awei as miche therof as thee thinkith good, so that it be nomore than it shulde be; & be war that thou kutte not to myche therof, for ther mighte come greet perel therof: as his vois mighte be apeirid the while he lyvede, & contynuely coughinge, & his lungis mighte be the worse therfore & also his piys [chest]. & therfore it is greet perel for to kutte a mannes palet.[30]

Jehan Yperman (1295 to 1351), the Flemish surgeon who was apparently the first to describe cleft lip repair in detail,[8, 31] did not describe cleft palates.

Bartolomeo da Montagnana (? *c.* 1460), who dissected at least 14 cadavers,[32] apparently learned little from his anatomical dissections, for he believed that the uvula lay in direct continuity with the scalp. How otherwise could one explain his treating swollen uvulae by exerting strong traction on the vertex, and pulling the patient's hair in an upward direction after first bracing himself by placing his knees or feet on the patient's shoulders.[25]

Of some chronologic interest from this period is the 500-year-old skull of a female from southern Hungary with a cleft lip. It shows a rudimentary premaxilla and an incomplete cleavage of the right alveolar process, but no cleft of the palate.[33]

Charaf ed-Din (*c.* 1465), a famous Turkish surgeon, advised cautery (fig. 2*A* and *B*), apparently unshielded by a protective tube, for alveolar abscesses and fistulae. No mention of cleft palate can be found in his beautifully illustrated surgical text.[34] In 1497, Brunschwig (*c.* 1450 to 1533) demonstrated his rather primitive knowledge of oral anatomy, in the following simple Middle English translation:

There be V partis of y mouth y lyppys/ tethe/ tonge/ rowfe/ and uvula/ y whiche is a lytelle deme hanginge in y throte lyke the skinne ... a for sayth y is ordeyned to take the ayre and to make it apte. The upper pte of y mouth is named the rowf/ y is covered with a panycle/ y taketh his begynnynge on the foynnerparte of y mawe or stomacke.[35, 36]

Brunschwig, although describing cleft lip repair, made no mention of cleft palates.

At the close of the 15th century, the first classical descriptions of buccopharyn-

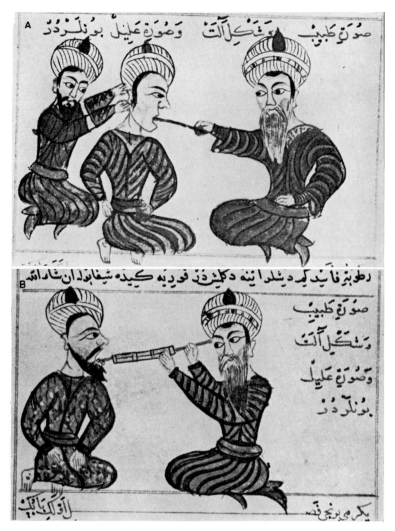

FIG. 2.*A,* old Turkish method of treating alveolar abscesses and fistulae by cauterizing them with a hot, burning iron (*c.* 1465 A.D.). *B,* old Turkish method of treating pyorrheic gingivitis by cauterizing the affected area with a hot cautery iron thrust down through a protective sleeve or tube to prevent injury to the surrounding tissues from the heat of the burning iron (*c.* 1465 A.D.). (From Huard, P., and Grmek, M. D.: *Le premier manuscrit chirurgical turc rédigé par Charat ed-Din (1465) et illustré de 140 miniatures,* pp. 27, 106. Editions Roger Dacosta, Paris, 1960.[34])

geal syphilis appeared, approximately half a century before the first unmistakable reference to cleft palates of congenital origin by Franco[37] in 1556. The syphilis seen at this period was usually a very acute disease, and its final tertiary and often terminal stage (fig. 3) made its appearance remarkably early.[38]

Tertiary lesions damaged the buccophar-

ynx severely, and destruction of the soft palate did not stay long unnoticed.

Thus, in 1498, Leonicenus (1428 to 1524), describing the great pandemic of syphilis, stated that in many syphilitics the mouth became covered with ulcers called *aptha.*[39] Jacob of Catania soon thereafter spoke of buccopharyngeal ulcers which at times perforated the palate and appeared

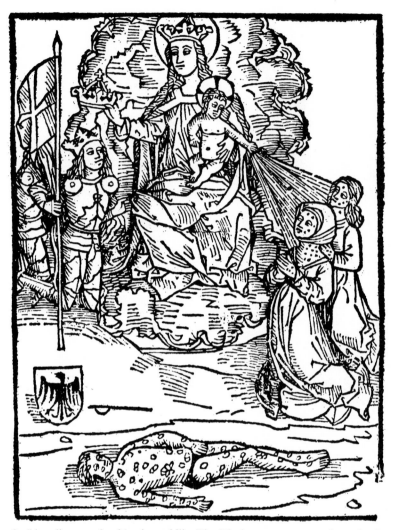

FIG. 3. "An allegory of epidemic syphilis. The Virgin crowns a crusader, who kneels by her side. The Holy Child casts forth the scourge of syphilis on mankind. Two suppliant women are covered with the syphilitic rash, as also is the corpse in the foreground." (From Grünspeck, J.: *Tractatus de pestilentiali scorra*, Augsburg, 1496. In *A Short History of Medicine*, Ed. 2, by Singer, C., and Underwood, E. A., p. 108. Oxford University Press, New York, 1962.[15])

concurrently with the dissemination of skin eruptions (figs. 4 and 5).[38]

Sixteenth Century

Giovanni da Vigo (1460 to 1525), in 1514, despite warnings of the ancients to the contrary, excised the uvula in its entirety and claimed no harmful effects.[38, 40]

Ulrich von Hutten (1488 to 1523), in 1519, told of the cure of his own syphilitic infection with guaiac or Holy Wood recently imported from the New World. He described its typical symptoms as follows:

In everyone, the throat, the tongue, and the palate were affected with ulcers and a great amount of saliva flowed from the mouth which emitted a repulsive odor. The lips were evidently affected by the acrid humours of this cavity. In some people, the ulcerous process seemed to extend the whole length of the throat, so that the

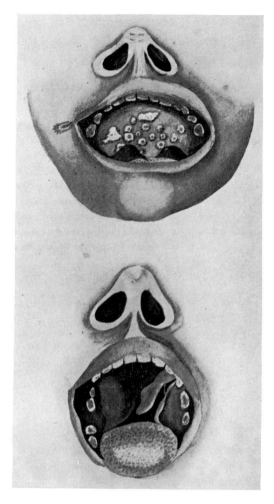

FIG. 4. (*upper figure*). Typical syphilitic ulcers of the throat, drawn by the artist several days after their first appearance. (*lower figure*). Destruction of the palate and uvula due to syphilis. The left side of the palate is missing and the uvular remant is hanging on a small muscular attachment to the alveolus. The right side of the palate is withdrawn posteriorly and seems attached only along its lateral alveolar margins. (From Martens, F. G.: *Tableaux des symptômes de la maladie vénérienne.* Baumgärtner, Leipzig, 1804?)

disturbed stomach did not crave any nourishment. I have seen some, who had not yet been carried away by death, who spit out real pus and ended by being soffocated by their disease.[41]

In 1530, Fracastorius (1483 to 1553) first suggested the name "syphilis" for the disease in a poem entitled "Syphilis, sive morbus Gallicus," [42] referring specifically to pharyn-

geal syphilides, their ravaging effects on the voice and a local remedy for the mouth ulcers, in the following passages:

> ... When on the vocal parts his Rage was spent,
> Imperfect sounds, for tuneful Speech was sent ...

> The Mass of Humours now dissolved within,
> To purge themselves by Spittle shall begin
> Till you with wonder at your feet shall see,
> A tide of Filth, and bless the Remedy.
> For Ulcers that shall then the Mouth offend,
> Boil Flowers that Privet and Pomgranets send.[43]

In 1549[44] and subsequently in 1561,[45] Ambroise Paré (1510 to 1590), whose perilous life as a Huguenot mirrored this fascinating period in history,[46] spoke rather deferentially of the palate in his brief anatomical studies. Perhaps, as a true Frenchman and a gourmet, he could not avoid the emphasis he placed upon it as an organ primarily concerned with eating "hard, acrid and sharp meats," rather than with speech mechanisms.

> The Palat ... is nothing else but the upper part of the mouth bounded with the teeth gums and upper Jaw. In which place the coat common to the whole mouth, is made rough with divers wrincles, that the meats put up and down between the tongue and the Palat might be broken and chawed more easily by that inequality and roughness.[45, 47]

He made up for this indifference, however, in later works, primarily in describing palate obturators in 1564, and the causes of palatal perforations in 1575.

For Paré, the uvula was more important for speech, being:

> ... a fleshy and spongy body, in shape like a pine apple ... so to diffuse the fuliginous vapour sent forth in breathing, that it may be dispersed over all the mouth, that resounding from thence it may be articulate, and by the motion of the tongue distinguished and formed into a certain voice. Which use is not small, when we see by experience that such as have this particle cut away, or eaten, or corrupted by any accident, have not only their voyce vitiated and depraved, but speak ill-favouredly, and, as they say, through the nose.[45, 47]

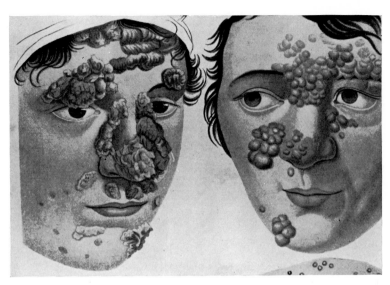

FIG. 5. Two types of extensive skin infections with syphilis from the early 1800's. *Left,* syphilis pustulosa crustacea (La syphilide pustuleuse crustacée of Alibert). *Right,* syphilis pustulosa racemiformis (La syphilide pustuleuse en grappe of Alibert). (From Froriep, R.: Chirurgische Kupfertafeln. Landes-Industrie-Comptoir, Weimar, Plates CCXXXI and CCXXXII, 1820–1847.)

Despite the supporters of Amatus Lusitanus as the "inventor of the obturator," [17] Paré was familiar with palatal obturators as early as 1537 to 1539, since he had observed their use many times ". . . in the battels fought beyond the Alps." [47, 48] The only battles he experienced beyond the Alps were in Savoy and Piedmont,[46] where he was an army surgeon in the Turin area from 1537 to 1539. It is, of course, possible that both Paré and Amatus Lusitanus learned of obturators from unknown Italians who fashioned them, but this is mere conjecture. Amatus Lusitanus, for example, moved from Antwerp to Northern Italy for the first time in 1540.

Jacques Houllier (? to 1562) was undoubtedly the first to propose suture of palate perforations undoubtedly caused by syphilis; this disease is implicated by his recommendation of guaiac therapy in treating the palatal discharge.[49, 50]

A free translation (by the author) from the Latin of 1552 reads:

In some [persons] the soft palate, as the result of a corrosive discharge, is perforated at the root of the tongue. The body should be purged [enemata], [the patient] bled, and a gargle of guaiac and milk decoction prescribed, with local applications of *aqua alchymistarum* made of gall nuts, malicorio and rose [water].

It is then advisable to take a very long needle, curved at its end and perforated [with an eye] at its sharp point, by means of which a thread of waxed silk can be brought to the place requiring stitching: it should be mentioned that if the first union of the wound edges tears apart, it can be once again resutured. If in consequence of this treatment a complete integrity [of the soft palate] has not been achieved, then the region can be occluded with wax or a sponge, and the patient can thereafter live comfortably.[50]

Houllier was apparently not afraid of syphilitic palates, as his surgical predecessors probably were, but experience taught him that primary repair of these palate defects was not always successful. His mention of the use of wax or sponge to plug palate perforations suggests that those primitive obturators were already in use by the mid-16th century, when buccopharyngeal syphilitic ulcers and palatal perforations were more prevalent and more easily recognizable.

Pierre Franco (*c.* 1505 to 1579), the other great Huguenot surgeon of this period,[51] was probably the "first" to emphasize the congenital origin of cleft palate in his famous 1556 text whose chapter was entitled "Des bouches ou levres fendues de nativité, ou autrement." [37] Franco wrote:

Cleft lips are sometimes congenital, through a defect of nature. At times they are caused by an accident which befalls them. Furthermore, they are sometimes cleft without a cleft of the jaw or palate, sometimes the cleft is only slight, and at times the cleft is as long and wide as the lip.[37, 51]

In 1561, he further elaborated:

Those who have cleft palates are more difficult to cure: and they always speak through the nose. If the palate is only slightly cleft, and if it can be plugged with cotton, the patient will speak more clearly, or perhaps even as well as if there were no cleft; or better, a plate of silver or lead can be applied by some means and retained there . . . Such procedures are used in some patients who have had "la grosse verolle" [syphilis] in which they have lost part of their palate.[52]

Interestingly, in bilateral cleft lip cases, when the premaxilla or its teeth projected too far out, making lip closure too difficult, Franco remedied this by cutting off the superfluous teeth or premaxilla with a saw and pliers. He apparently made no attempts, however, to close palatal defects by surgery.

Amatus Lusitanus (1511 to 1568), in fleeing from his residence in Ancona in 1555, lost the manuscript of his *Centuria V,* which was subsequently first published in 1560.[53] He can probably be credited, nevertheless, with first describing very briefly in 1560 (4 years before Paré's 1564 text) a "true" palatal obturator which restored speech by means of a gold plate held in place with a sponge.

In 1564, Paré described his small obturators which he termed *couvercles,*[54] but in a

later text of 1575 he changed the terminology to *obturateur,* probably using this word for the first time in medical history.[48] He made no mention of the congenital causes of palate defects, as did Franco, but referred only to those resulting from gunshot trauma or caused by "Lues Venerea." He remedied these by (fig. 6):

. . . filling the cavitie of the Palat with a plate of gold or silver, a little bigger than the cavitie it self is. But it must bee as thick as a French Crown, and made like unto a dish in figure; and on the upper side, which shall bee towards the brain, a little sponge must bee fastened, which, when it is moistened with the moisture distilling from the brain, will becom more swoln, and puffed up; so that it will fill the concavitie of the Palat, that the artificial Palat cannot fall down, but stand fast and firm, as if it stood of it self. This is the true figure of those instruments, whose certain use I have observed not by once or twice, but my manifold trials in the battels fought beyond the Alps.[47, 48]

The inventive Paré also described artificial gold or silver enameled eyes, an artificial nose with or without an upper lip and copious mustache attached, artificial bone or ivory teeth, artificial "glewed . . . paper" or leather ears, ". . . shadowed or counterfeited by som Painter, that thereby . . . resemble the color of a natural Ear," and a wooden instrument to improve speech for those with a loss of some or a great part of the anterior tongue.[47, 48]

Paré also removed uvular portions with a ligature instrument invented by Castellanus. The patient had to tolerate the ligation thread hanging out of his mouth for several days. Every day the thread was "twitched harder" than the previous day, until the

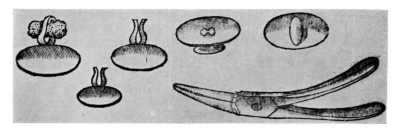

Fig. 6. The palatal obturators and their sponge or metal retention devices, as illustrated in Paré,[47] 1575. (From Gibson, T.: The prostheses of Ambroise Paré. Brit. J. Plast. Surg., *8:* 3, 1955.)

devascularized portion of the uvula fell off.[47, 48]

Jacques Guillemeau (1550 to 1613) has caused medical historians much grief, because, without mentioning specific Greek authors by name, he implied in 1598 that these ancients knew something of palatal obturators, having given them the Greek name, *hyperoe*.[55] A careful and exhaustive scrutiny of the Greco-Roman literature, however, fails to uncover these "unknown Greeks," perhaps known only to the imagination of Guillemeau.

Fabricius Hildanus (1560 to 1634) described an uvula which was so hypertrophied that it almost filled a patient's entire mouth, and touched the teeth! The patient was sent home to die, having been judged inoperable.[56] It is difficult to learn, despite the number of texts consulted, why persons living in these earlier centuries suffered so greatly from uvular inflammation and elongation, which we rarely see today. How, for example, can one explain the case of Peter Lowe (c. 1550 to 1612), who wrote in 1596:

> Sometime it hangeth so long that it falleth on the tongue, and so grieveth the sicke, that sometime he is constrained to put his finger in his mouth to helpe the over-going of the meate. ... Sometime it groweth to such bignesse that it filleth the throat, and causeth the sicke to suffocate, if it be not quickly cut.[57]

Fabricius of Aquapendente (1533 to 1619), in 1619, was probably the first to mention that many newborn infants with cleft palates were unable to suck and frequently died as a result.[58]

Seventeenth Century

The 17th century was, in general, a very uninspired period as far as palatal or uvular surgery was concerned. But here and there a few interesting operations and concepts were developed.

John Banester (1533 to 1610) was one of the first to implicate dental decay as causing or associated with "corruption" of the palatal bones and "rarity of the flesh" [palatal and alveolar ulcers].[59] One can certainly sympathize with these early surgeons who probably preferred not to operate on the palate or even in the depths of the oral cavity for fear of

the complications which might result from such conditions as syphilis, dental decay, scurvy, scrofula and tuberculosis—all of which would result in an unsuccessful closure of any palatal defect, no matter how small.

Zacutus Lusitanus (1575 to 1642) recalled that not every syphilitic palatal ulceration terminated in an incurable perforation defect which could be remedied only by an obturator. He described a case which, following guaiac therapy, underwent a spontaneous cure of the perforation; healing marginal tissues apparently gradually filled in the fissure completely.[60]

Paul Barbette seems to have studied very little of the anatomy in which he professed to be an expert; he thought very little of the oral cavity. One cannot understand why anyone would have taken the time to translate his unscholarly but amusing drivel from Low Dutch into the English which follows:

> The *Gums* offer nothing worthy a particular consideration. *The Palate* consists of a sensible Membrane common to the Stomack, which hath its rise from the Dura Mater. The *Uvula* is a long little Body, it hath two ligaments, and as many Muscles, but very little.[61]

Hendrik van Roonhuyse (1622 to 1672), author of the best description of cleft lip repair in the 17th century, also seemed less fearful of incising the palatal region than his contemporaries, although he never attempted to repair a congenital cleft palate. He described several cases of necrosis that required incision and drainage of the hard palate; following surgery, he advised washing the draining palate twice daily with a mixture of gin (or brandy) and spirits of vitriol until the affected area was healed by the formation of smooth mucosal walls which eventually covered the exposed palatal bones.[62]

Richard Wiseman (1622 to 1676)[63] recommended the temporary use of obturators until spontaneous closure of palatal perforations occurred.

Wiseman also spoke of filling in palatal defects with a paste made of mastic, sandarac, gum guaiac, myrrh and other ingredients, but gave no instructions as to how this palatal paste was held in place.[63]

Eighteenth Century

With the onset of the 18th century, especially in France (where the few palatal operations and obturators that did exist had been developed almost exclusively during the previous 2½ centuries), a bolder surgical approach to the palatal region began to take shape.

Thus, in approximately 1706, André Myrrhen[64] actually lengthened the soft palate, by a technique not described, in order to compensate for a completely destroyed uvula, causing no damage to the patient's speech! It seems a shame, nevertheless, that Myrrhen, by a little inductive reasoning, did not come to the conclusion that any cleft soft palate could have been just as easily closed by his elongation technique.

In 1710, Pierre Dionis (? to 1718) described only one palate operation, using thin iron cautery instruments to stop the further progression of palatal "caries," some of which were the results of syphilis.[65]

In 1717, Manne cut the velum in order to expose large nasal polyps. In his extensive description of the procedure, however, he made no mention of resuturing the soft palate.[66]

In 1718, Lorenz Heister (1683 to 1758) first specifically mentioned scurvy as a cause of palatal ulcers "which not only destroy the adjacent fleshy Parts, but also erode and extend themselves into the Bones of the Nose."[67, 68] Like van Roonhuyse, he helped to separate carious palatal bones from healthy bony tissue by applications of *Mel. Rosar.* acidulated with *Spiritus Vitrioli.* His sense of oral hygiene was perhaps far advanced for this age of "stinking breaths," when he advised that a patient be provided with two obturators:

... that after one has been wore a Day, it may be extracted, washed, and dried against the next Day, to prevent the imbibed Humours from putrifying and smelling.[68]

de Garengeot (1688 to 1759), in 1723, described a patient of Petit (1674 to 1750) whose nasal polyps were so large that their obstruction of his breathing and swallowing endangered his life. In order to save his life, Petit "began with cutting the Vale of the Mouth in two places, that he might more easily touch the Ligament of the *Polypus.*"[69] When removed, the polypoid mass was as big as a fist. de Garengeot did not state whether the surgically divided velum was resutured.

In 1728, Fauchard (1678 to 1761) minutely described five different obturators of a very sophisticated design, some with movable wings which, moved by screws, and each covered with soft sponges, could fill in most palatal perforations, no matter how irregular their margins.[70]

In 1751, Ingram, a surgeon and "man-midwife" on the island of Barbados, described several cases which give us a good idea of the magnitude of dental caries and their effects on the palatal region in the mid-18th century. One lady from Surinam had severe dental caries which had ulcerated and eaten through one-third of her tongue; her upper jaw and palate "were overspread with a fleshy Substance, which discharged a sanious putrid Ichor, of a foetid Stench almost too much to be withstood."[71] Some of her maxilla was lost when Ingram extracted her rotten molars. Dental hygiene, therefore, had apparently not progressed very far beyond its Egyptian level 4200 years earlier (fig. 1).

Another patient suffered from a violent scurvy; following intensive local therapy, the removal of carious teeth and the application of washes consisting of red wine, tincture of myrrh and tincture of dragon's blood [?]:

He continued in this Method [local applications] for near a Fortnight, when one Morning he came to me with Part of his Jaw, and the two Teeth in his Hand, having removed them himself in the Night as he lay in Bed.[71]

Warner, in 1754, still had to resort to hot cauterization to control severe arterial bleeding in a patient from whom he excised a tumor of the entire roof of the mouth. He used "a curved Knife, such as Gardeners make use of in pruning Trees."[72]

Matthew Wilson (1734 to 1790), a minister and physician who practiced medicine in Lewes, Delaware, wrote an unpublished compendium of medicine[73] from 1756 to 1787 called the *Therapeutic Alphabet.* He makes us aware that our Colonial American ancestors were familiar with cleft palate in 1756 when he defined:

Aphonia—Is a deprav'd Voice and the same wt Paraphonia. This may be from many Causes. If from Cold see Catarrhus. If from a Fright see Hysteria. If from Lues Venerea, see Scorbutis. If from any other Cause, remove the Cause. But if from ill-configuration of the Parts, it seems incurable . . .

Palate Diseased—See Hypostaphyle . . .

Hypostaphyle—Is a Prolapse or Production of ye Palate wn it is either relax'd, inflamed, ulcerated, incrassated, attenuated or forked. V. Scorbutis. Blow Allum or Nitre on it. Wash Acid Elixir, Honey, etc.[73]

In 1757, Bourdet improved palatal obturators by fixing them, not to the palate itself or inside the nose, but by means of lateral clasps fitted to the teeth.[74] Bourdet attributed many palatal and maxillary defects to dental caries, venereal vices, scurvy and erosions due to the improper use of mercury in treating syphilis!

One of the earliest pathologic illustrations of a bilateral cleft lip and palate to appear in the literature was reported by Christopher Trew, in 1757, in a newborn infant who died 6 weeks after birth[75] (fig. 7).

In 1766, Siebold (1736 to 1807) first drew attention to specific speech defects in a 3-year-old child with a soft palate cleft who poorly pronounced the letters "z," "b," "s" and "r" and many others. Siebold deplored the fact that there was as yet no surgical procedure known to him which could correct such soft palate defects.[76]

Yet, in this same year, 1766, Robert described the earlier work of Le Monnier, a dentist from Rouen, who successfully operated upon a child with a complete palatal cleft extending from the velum to the incisors. Le Monnier first placed a few sutures along the two edges of the cleft to approximate them and then freshened them with the "actual" or hot cautery. An inflammation resulted which terminated in suppuration and was then followed by the union of the two edges of the "artificially created wound" with a complete cure of the child.[77] Contrary to the opinion of many of his colleagues, Le Monnier also succeeded in filling

in palatal "holes" for which obturators were normally used. His technique consisted in stimulating an inflammation by means of light [scratchings?] or irritations. As the resultant inflammation became more severe, more "humours" [pus?] were produced. The fissure then gradually closed by the application of successive layers of "mucous" to the area.

According to Dorrance[78] [but unverified by this author because of an inability to uncover these references], Eustache, of Beziers in September, 1779:

. . . proposed to the old Academy of Surgery of Paris suture of vela that had been split for the extraction of nasal polyps after the method of Manne. He also called attention to the difficulties in deglutition and speech in these subjects and in cases of congenital absence of the velum. Four years later, Eustache described his operation for suturing the split velum and added that this method could be applied in cases of congenital split of the velum. In 1784, Dubois, reporting to the same Academy, disapproved of Eustache's procedure for split vela and spoke of it as being impracticable.[78]

Nothing more was heard from either Le Monnier or from Eustache, and one can only wonder whether Eustache took his own advice and successfully closed soft palate defects 37 years before von Graefe.

Soon after the end of the American Revolutionary War, "Mr. Clabeau," a dentist, advertised in the February 24, 1784, edition of the *Pennsylvania Gazette* that he could fix "obturatures artificial palate." [79] One year later, in 1785, Josiah Flagg, Jr. (1763 to 1816), an oral surgeon, demonstrated his skill by advertising in handbills or broadsides (fig. 8). In these he informed the public that he ". . . sews up hare lips and fixes gold roofs and palates, greatly assisting the pronunciation and the swallow." [79] Thus, together with Clabeau and Flagg, several surgeons and dentists of the Colonial, Revolutionary and Postrevolutionary periods in America, including Drs. Wilson, Hall, Yeldall and Stork,[8] might have been as familiar with palatal obturators and their uses as they were with the cleft lip operation.

In 1797, Desault (1744 to 1795) advised that simple, contused, transverse and ragged

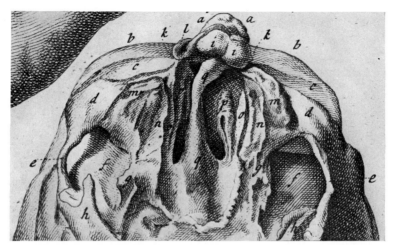

FIG. 7. One of the first illustrations in the medical literature (1757) of a specimen with a bilateral harelip, and palatal defect, taken from an infant who died 6 weeks after birth. (From Trew, C. I.: Sistens plura exempla palati deficientis. Obs. 103. Nova acta physico-med., pp. 445–447, 1757.[75])

edged wounds of the velum would reunite if the parts are kept ". . . at rest by means of a plate of lead or silver fixed to the teeth, and touching the bleeding vessels with hot cautery if hemorrhage from the wound edges continued unchecked." [80]

In 1798, Desault and his editor Bichat wrote of "nature's closure" of palate [alveolar?] clefts following a cleft lip repair as follows:

In the harelip a double fissure is not the most unfavourable complication which art has to overcome. . . . The fissure of the palatine arch varies in extent and in size. Sometimes limited to the maxillary bones, it always unites after the operation; but frequently occupying the palate bones, it crosses the velum palati, and then examples of union are not so commonly observed. In general, Desault has observed, whatever was the form of the fissure, that as a consequence of the operation, there was constantly, if not an exact union, at least a very sensible approximation. If the direct cause of this phenomenon escapes our researches, we are at least certain that the re-establishment of the lip in its natural state is the disposing cause. From thence this consequence may be drawn, that the operation should be more speedily performed, in proportion as the symptoms resulting from the fissure of the palate are more pressing. . . .The approximation of this fissure is more or less slow. It is only by degrees that nature reestablishes the regular conformation which she had originally neglected. Still there are cases in

which she departs from this rule, and where, more rapid in her progress, she effects speedily the union of the bones.[81]

Perhaps Desault's findings in many ways support or complement those of Schweckendiek[82] and others, who 150 years later have drawn attention to the favorable diminution in size of, or partial, gradual closure of hard palate defects following simple primary closure of the soft palate.

Desault was a devoted propounder of extraoral bandage compression in cases of bilateral cleft lip, in order to establish a more normal alveolar arch alignment, and thus facilitate cleft closure "by nature's means." He was also one of the first to advise against Pierre Franco's custom of excising a portion or all of the projecting premaxilla in order to facilitate lip closure, stating that:

a cavity more or less considerable, constantly results, and then the two united portions of the lip are in want of a favourable point of support at the place of their contact.[81]

As an interesting sidelight on this lusty age, in the daily life of some or perhaps even many Parisians with loose teeth, foul gums, stinking breaths and infrequent baths, Desault advised that in preparing a child for the harelip operation one should: "comb carefully the head of the child . . . to put in

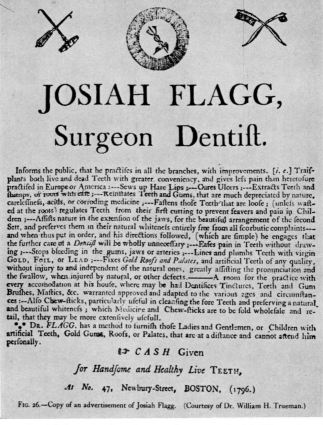

FIG. 8. Broadside of the early American oral surgeon, Josiah Flagg, Jr., advertising that he "Fixes Gold Roofs and Palates" and "Sews up Hare Lips." (From Taylor, J. A.: *History of Dentistry*. Lea & Febiger, Philadelphia, p. 72, 1922.)

his hair a little gray ointment, lest being troubled with vermin, he might derange his dressing." [81] In this age of no anesthesia whatsoever, Desault told of a patient of Benjamin Bell (1749 to 1806) who stressed that the side of his lip which was cut with a knife was more painful than the side which had been cut with a scissors![81]

Nineteenth Century

According to Velpeau, Dupuytren (1777 to 1835) and Delpech (1777 to 1832) offered nothing new to palate surgery except that both still resorted, as did Velpeau, to the centuries-old Arabian custom of cauterizing small holes in the velum.[83]

In 1813, Colombe is said to have sutured a split velum in a cadaver, but he failed to persuade a patient to submit to the operation in 1815.[78] Roux stated that Itard, a physician in Holland, suggested the suture of a split velum to a girl who consulted him several years prior to 1819, but the operation was not carried out because a more prominent surgeon advised against it.[5]

Thus, in this second decade of the 19th century, with little fanfare and no inkling of the change it would make in the daily miserable lives of thousands of cleft palate victims, within a 3-year-period, von Graefe[84] in 1816 and Roux[5] in 1819 simply undid the harmful and indifferent effects of 4300 previous years of unintentional ignorance, superstition, surgical timidity and "the venereal taint" by introducing, each in his own manner, a simple closure of the congenitally cleft soft palate (Fig. 9).

The subsequent history of the rapid im-

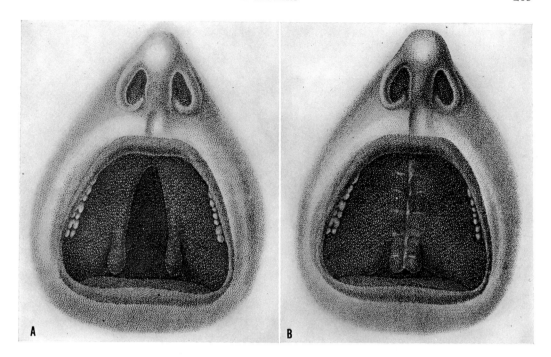

FIG. 9. Illustrations from the first article by von Graefe which demonstrated the pre- and postoperative appearance of a patient with a congenital cleft of the soft palate. (From von Graefe, C.: Die Gaumennath, ein neuentdecktes Mittel gegen angeborene Fehler der Sprache. J. Chir. u. Augenh., *1:* 1, 1820.[6])

provements in surgery of the congenitally cleft soft and hard palate and the telling of it is yet another fascinating story which, however, must wait for this writer to recover his literary breath and his weary eyesight flecked with rare-book dust.

Summary

A brief chronologic survey of the history of early surgery of the palate and the uvula reveals that prior to 1816 most surgeons preferred not to operate upon palate defects because, until proven otherwise, and despite the congenital origin of some of them, the majority of palate perforations were thought to be caused by syphilis. The poor quality of palatal tissues surrounding any perforation or fissure was complicated either by the possible presence of active or temporarily dormant syphilis, or by pathologic changes secondary to severe dental and alveolar decay, scurvy, scrofula, or tuberculosis, in a fair proportion of patients. This would help to easily explain the timidity of most surgeons prior to 1816, only 150 years ago, and/or their inability to devise any successful, simple closure of congenital defects of the soft and hard palate.

Acknowledgments. The author wishes to express his deep and sincere appreciation to Mlle. Magdeleine Blachère d'Amoreux for her dedicated endeavours and for her translations of many of the cited articles from their original French into English; to Miss Pauline Porowski for her generous readiness to always help in the secretarial chores of compiling and readying such a paper for publication; and to the warm and friendly help given to him by the staff of the Malloch Rare Book Room of The New York Academy of Medicine, including Miss Gertrude L. Annan, Mrs. Alice D. Weaver, Miss Bettina Thrall, Mrs. Nancy B. Willey and Mrs. Laveda Lewis.

Some of the photographs and illustrations in this article (figs. 1, 4, 7, 8 and 9) have been provided from material available at The New York Academy of Medicine and printed with the permission of its Library.

Blair O. Rogers, M.D.
875 Fifth Avenue
New York, New York 10021

REFERENCES

1. Lowe, P.: *A Discourse of the Whole Art of Chyrurgerie*... Ed. 2, p. 207. Thomas Purfoot, London, 1612.
2. Cooke, J.: *Mellificium Chirurgiae: Or the Marrow of Many good Authours wherein is briefly and faithfully handle the arts of Chyrurgery, in its foure parts*... p. 376. Printed at London for Samuel Cartwright, at the sign of the Hand and Bible in Duck-Lane, London, 1648.
3. de La Vauguion: *A Compleat Body of Chirurgical Operations Containing The Whole Practice of Surgery*... p. 354. Printed for Henry Bonwick in St. Paul's Church Yard, T. Goodwin, M. Wotton, B. Took in Fleetstreet, and S. Manship in Cornhil, London, 1699.
4. Good, J. M.: *The Study of Medicine,* Ed. 2, Vol. III, p. 374. Baldwin, Cradock and Joy, London, 1825.
5. Roux, [P. J.] Observation sur une division congénitale du voile du palais et de la luette, guérie au moyen d'une opération analogue à celle du bec-de-lièvre. J. Univ. Sc. Méd., *15:* 356, 1819.
6. von Graefe, C.: Die Gaumennath, ein neuentdecktes Mittel gegen angeborene Fehler der Sprache. J. Chir. u. Augenh., *1:* 1, 1820.
7. Khoo, B. C.: An ancient Chinese text on a cleft lip. Plast. & Reconstruct. Surg., *38:* 89, 1966.
8. Rogers, B. O.: Harelip repair in colonial America: A review of 18th century and earlier surgical techniques. Plast. & Reconstruct. Surg., *34:* 142, 1964.
9. Smith, G. E., and Dawson, W. R.: *Egyptian Mummies.* p. 157. George Allen & Unwin, Ltd., London, 1924.
10. Francis, W. W.: Repair of cleft palate by Philibert Roux in 1819: A translation of John Stephenson's *De Velosynthesi.* J. Hist. Med. & Allied Sc., *18:* 209, 1963.
11. Buret, F.: *Syphilis in Ancient and Prehistoric Times,* Vol. I, p. 156. F. A. Davis Company, Philadelphia, 1891.
12. Krogman, W. M.: The pathologies of pre- and protohistoric man. Ciba Sympos., *2:* 442, 1940.
13. Krogman, W. M.: Medical practices and diseases of the aboriginal American Indians. Ciba Sympos., *1:* 14, 1939.
14. Weisman, A. I.: Syphilis: Was it endemic in Pre-Columbian America or was it brought here from Europe? Bull. New York Acad. Med., *42:* 284, 1966.
15. Singer, C., and Underwood, E. A.: *A Short History of Medicine,* Ed. 2, p. 108. Oxford University Press, New York, 1962.
16. Thoma, K. H.: Oral diseases of ancient nations and tribes. J. Allied Dent. Soc., *12:* 327, 1917.

17. Weinberger, B. W.: *An Introduction to the History of Dentistry.* Vol I., p. 390. C. V. Mosby Company, St. Louis, 1948.
18. Bhishagratna, K. K.: *An English Translation of The Sushruta Samhita Based on Original Sanskrit Text.* Ed. 2, Vol. II, pp. 81, 106, 469. The Chowkhamba Sanskrit Series Office, Varanasi-1, India, 1963.
19. Wright, J.: *The Nose and Throat in Medical History,* p. 20. Lewis S. Matthews & Co., St. Louis, 1904.
20. Spencer, W. G.: *Celsus: De Medicina.* Harvard University Press, Cambridge, Mass., 1938.
21. Adams, F.: *The Genuine Works of Hippocrates.* p. 55, The Williams & Wilkins Co., Baltimore, 1939.
22. Wright, J.: *A History of Laryngology and Rhinology,* Ed. 2, p. 52. Lea & Febiger, Philadelphia, 1914.
23. Chaveau, C.: *Histoire des Maladies du Pharynx,* Vol. I, p. 137. J. B. Ballière et Fils, Paris, 1901.
24. Jones, W. H. S., and Withington, E. T.: *Hippocrates.* Vol. I–IV. Harvard University Press, Cambridge, Mass., 1923–1931.
25. Sprengel, K.: *Histoire de la Médecine, Depuis son Origine jusqu'au Dix-Nevième Siècle,* Vol. 8, pp. 338–408. Chez Deterville, Libraire, Paris, 1820.
26. Kühn, C. G.: *Opera omnia*... [by Galen]. C. Cnobloch, Leipzig, 1821–1833.
27. Oribasius: *Oribasii Sardiani Collectorum Medicinalium*... p. 298. Apud Bernardinum Turrisanum, via Iacobaea, sub officina Aldina, Paris, 1555.
28. Adams, F.: *The Medical Works of Paulus Aegineta*... Vol. I, p. 457, Vol. II, p. 298. J. Welsh, Treuttel, Würtz, & Co., London 1834.
29. Leclerc, L.: *La Chirurgie d'Abulcasis.* J. B. Baillière, Paris, 1861.
30. Fleischhacker, R. V.: *Lanfrank's "Science of Cirurgie."* Early English Text Society, Original Series, 102, p. 261. Kegan Paul, Trench, Trübner & Co., London, 1894.
31. Carolus, J. M. F.: *La Chirurgie de Maître Jean Yperman.*... F. and E. Gyselynck, Gand, 1854.
32. Castiglioni, A.: *A History of Medicine,* Ed. 2, Alfred A. Knopf Inc., New York, 1958.
33. Berndorfer, A.: A 500-year-old skull with cleft lip. Brit. J. Plast. Surg., *15:* 123, 1962.
34. Huard, P., and Grmek, M. D.: *Le Premier Manuscrit Chirurgical Turc Rédigé par Charaf ed-Din (1465) et Illustré de 140 Miniatures,* pp. 27, 106. Editions Roger Dacosta, Paris, 1960.
35. Brunschwig, H.: *Die ist das Buch der Cirurgia: Hautwirckung der wund Artz.* H. Schönsperger, Augsburg, 1497.
36. Brunschwig, H.: *The noble experyence of the vertuous handy warke of surgeri.*... Imprynted at London in Southwarke by Petrus Treueris, 1525.

37. Franco, P.: *Petit Traite Contenant une des Parties Principalles de Chirurgie*. Antoine Vincent, Lyon, 1556.

38. Chaveau, C.: *Histoire des Maladies du Pharynx*, Vol. 2, p. 292–308. J. B. Ballière et Fils, Paris, 1902.

39. Leonicenus, N.: *Libellus de epidemia, quam vulgo morbum Gallicum vocant*. In domo Aldi Manutii, Venetiis, 1497.

40. da Vigo, G.: *Practica in arte chirurgica copiosae* .... edited by Stephanu Guillireti, Book II, Ch. 15, pp. 37–38. Herculem Bononiense, Roma, 1514.

41. von Hutten, U.: *De guaiaci medicina et morbo Gallico*.... In aedibus Ioannis Scheffer, Mogutiae, 1519.

42. Fracastorius, H.: *Syphilis, sive morbus gallicus*. Johann Bebel, Basel, 1536.

43. Tate, N. [translator]: *Syphilis, or, A Poetical History of the French Disease*, pp. 26, 55. Printed for *Jacob Tonson*, at the *Judge's Head* in *Chancery-lane* near Fleetstreet, London, 1686.

44. Paré, A.: *Briefve Collection de Ladministration Anatomique...*, p. 47. En la boutique de Guillaume Cavellat ... devant le colège de Cambray, Paris, 1549.

45. Paré, A.: *Anatomie Universelle du Corps humain*.... Iehan le Royer, Paris, 1561.

46. Paget, A.: *Ambroise Paré and His Times: 1510–1590*. G. P. Putnam's Sons, New York, 1899.

47. Johnson, T.: *The Workes of that Famous Chirurgion Ambrose Parey*. Richard Cotes, and Willi Du-gard, London, 1649.

48. Paré, A.: *Les Oeuvres de M. Ambroise Paré*. Chez Gabriel Buon, Paris, 1575.

49. Gurlt, E. J.: *Geschichte der Chirurgie und ihrer Ausübung*, Vol. II, p. 671. A. Hirschwald, Berlin, 1898.

50. Hollerii [Stempai] I.: *Omnio Opera practica*. De morbis internis. Singulares aliquot Hollerii observationes, quae ad consilia curandi pertinent. In Book I, p. 573. Excudebat Iacobus Stoer, Coloniae Allobrogum, Observation IV, 1623.

51. Barsky, A. J.: Pierre Franco, father of cleft lip surgery: his life and times. Brit. J. Plast. Surg., *17*: 53, 1964.

52. Franco, P.: *Traité des Hernies*. Thibauld Payan, Lyon, 1561.

53. Lusitani, A.: *Curationum Medicinalium*.... *Tomus Secundus, Continens Centurias Tres, Quintam videlicet* ... curatio 14, p. 39. Apud Vincentium Valgrisium, Venetiis, 1556.

54. Paré, A.:*Dix Livres de la Chirurgie* ... p. 211. Iean le Royer, Paris, 1564.

55. Guillemeau, J.: *Les Oeuvres de Chirurgie* ... p. 138. Chez Nicolas de Lovvain Marchant, Paris, 1598.

56. Fabricius Hildanus, G.: *Opera quae extant omnia*... Ed. 2, Sumpt. Ioan. Ludovici Dufour, Francofurti ad Maenum, 1682.

57. Lowe, P.: *A Discourse of the Whole Art of Chyrurgerie* ... Thomas Purfoot, London, 1596.

58. Fabricius ab Aquapendente, H.: De Chirurgicis Operationibus. In *Operationes Chirurgicae In duas Partes divisae* ... p. 34. Apud Paulum Megliettum, Venetiis, 1619.

59. Banester, J.: *A Treatise of Chirurgerie: Briefly comprehending the generall and particular curation of Ulcers* ... p. 63. Thomas Harper, London, 1633.

60. Lusitanus, Z.: *Praxis historiaum*.... *Accessit Praxis medica admiranda*... Editio novissima.... Sumpt. Ioannis Antonii Huguetan, Lugduni, 1644.

61. Barbette, P.: *The Chirurgical and Anatomical Works of Paul Barbette* ... p. 278. J. Darby, London, 1672.

62. van Roonhuyse, H.: *Historischer Heil-Curen in zwey Theile verfassete Anmerckungen* ... p. 26. Michael und Johann Friederich Endtern, Nürnberg, 1674.

63. Wiseman, R.: *Severall Chirurgicall Treatises*. R. Royston and B. Took ... St. Paul's Churchyard, London, 1676.

64. Myrrhen, A.: Uvulae, ab ortu, defectum resarciunt vicinae partes, sine incommodo. In *Bibliotheca Chirurgica*, [edited by J. J. Mangeti]. p. 352. Gabrielis de Tournes & Filiorum, Genevae, 1721.

65. Dionis, P.: Of the Chirurgical operations of the palate. In *Bibliotheca Anatomica, Medica, Chirurgica*. Vol. I, p. 394. 1711.

66. Manne, L. F.: *Dissertation au sujet d'un polype extraordinaire, qui occupait la narine droite*. Charles Giroud, Avignon, 1747.

67. Heister, L.: *Chirurgie, in welcher alles, was zur Wund-Artzney gehöret, nach der neuesten und besten Art*. J. Hoffman, Nürnberg, 1718.

68. Heister, L.: *A General System of Surgery in Three Parts*, p. 468. W. Innys, London, 1743.

69. de Garengeot, R. J. C.: *A Treatise of Chirurgical Operations* ... p. 332. Thomas Woodward, London, 1723.

70. Fauchard, P.: *Le Chirurgien Dentiste, ou Traité des Dents*, Vol. II, p. 285. J. Mariette, Paris, 1728.

71. Ingram, D.: *Practical Cases and Observations in Surgery*.... Printed for J. Clarke, under the Royal-Exchange, London, 1751.

72. Warner, J.: *Cases in Surgery with Remarks*.... Printed for J. and R. Tonson and S. Draper in the Strand, London, 1754.

73. Friedberg, S. A.: Laryngology and otology in colonial times. Ann. Med. Hist., *1*: 86, 1917.

74. Bourdet, B.: *Recherches et observations sur toutes les parties de l'art du dentiste*. J. T. Hérissant, Paris, 1757.

75. Trew, C. I.: Sistens plura exempla palati deficientis. Obs. 103. Nova acta physico-med., pp. 445–447, 1757.

76. Siebold, K. K.: Ein in zwey Theile bis an das Gaumenbein gespaltenes Zäpfchen. In

Chirurgisches Tagebuch, obs. XII, p. 32. E. C. Grattenauer Nürnberg, 1792.

77. Robert: *Traité des principaux objets de médecine, avec un sommaire de la plûpart des Theses soutenues aux Ecoles de Paris, depuis 1762 jusqu'en 1764,* Vol. I, p. 8. Chez Lacombe, Paris, 1766.

78. Dorrance, G. M.: *The Operative Story of Cleft Palate,* p. 3. W. B. Saunders Company, Philadelphia, 1933.

79. Weinberger, B. W.: *An Introduction to the History of Dentistry in America,* Vol. II, pp. 51, 159, 193. C. V. Mosby Company, St. Louis, 1948.

80. Turnbull, W.: *A Treatise on Chirurgical Diseases, and on the Operations Required in Their Treatment from the French of Messrs.*

Chopart and Desault, Vol. 1, p. 457. W. J. & J. Richardson, London, 1797.

81. Smith, E. D.: *The Surgical Works or Statement of the Doctrine and Practice of P. J. Desault by Xavier Bichat,* p. 148. Thomas Dobson, Philadelphia, 1814.

82. Schweckendiek, W.: Die Ergebnisse der Kieferbildung und die Sprache nach der primäen Veloplastik. Arch. Ohren-usw. Heilk. u. Z. Hals.-usw. Heilk., *180:* 541, 1962.

83. Velpeau, A. A. L. M.: *New Elements of Operative Surgery,* Vol. I, p. 652. Henry G. Langley, New York, 1845.

84. von Graefe, C. F.: Kurze Nachrichten und Auszuge. J. Pract. Arznek. u. Wundarzk., *44:* 116, 1817.

OBSERVATION ON A CONGENITAL DIVISION OF THE SOFT PALATE AND THE UVULA CURED BY MEANS OF AN OPERATION SIMILAR TO THAT FOR A HARE-LIP

PHILIBERT ROUX, M.D., *Paris, France*

(*Journal Universel des Sciences Médicales, 16: 356, 1819*)

Translated from the French by

DR. DANIEL MOREL-FATIO

Editorial Note*

A few years ago M. Itard was consulted by the family of a young Dutch woman suffering from this congenital malformation, of which there are plenty of examples. He proposed attempting to join the two parts together with stitches. The operation was not carried out, as a distinguished surgeon of the capital considered that it would not be successful. The following operation performed by M. Roux, however, was a complete success. Our readers will certainly be interested to learn the following details, pronounced in front of one of the learned societies of Paris.

It is the case of a young man, suffering from a congenital malformation completely dividing the soft palate and the uvula. The voice was affected, as it normally is in such a case. The two edges of the division could easily be brought together; the mouth was big, and the posterior part of the mouth was almost insensitive. The patient strongly desired to be cured of this annoying infirmity. All conditions were met for the success of the skillful surgeon's judicious undertaking.

The patient was suitably placed so that the parts to be operated on were visible, and the mouth would be open as wide as possible. M. Roux passed 3 wax-threaded loops, using a curved needle placed in a handle. Then he drew together the wax-threaded loops so as to bring together the two edges of the division, and thus evaluate exactly the extent of the loss of substance that he would have to inflict upon them. Half a line of the soft palate and of the uvula was taken out with great dexterity; the ligatures were drawn tight and the wax-threaded loops cut close to the knots.

Immediately after the operation, the voice returned almost to normal—with hardly any change. The patient was put on a strict diet for 3 days; complete silence was enforced. In a few days the two parts had come together completely, but the two lips of the uvula were not completely touching. One of them was lower than the other, and M. Roux proposed his cutting it.

Although without danger for the patient's life, the operation corrected a malformation in an organ whose integrity is vital for normal swallowing and speech. It must be considered amongst those successful innovations which have increased the field of the curative art. It would be wrong to call attention only to operations which endanger the life of patients.

Philibert J. Roux, M.D.
Faculté de Médecine
Université de Paris
Paris, France

* By the editor of the *Journal Universel des Sciences Médicales,* 1819.

From the Hôpital de la Charité, and the Faculté de Médecine of the Université de Paris.

COMMENTARY BY DR. McDOWELL

This article by Roux is generally considered to be the first description of a successful surgical closure of a congenitally cleft palate. The description of this operation from the patient's point of view begins on page 271.

Some writers have referred, from time to time, to a possibly earlier paper on this subject by one Monsieur Robert of Paris. It is in a volume, now exceedingly rare, which was made available to the Journal through the courtesy of Dr. John Blake of the National Library of Medicine. It follows in its entirety (translated by Mary McDowell).

TREATISE ON THE PRINCIPAL AIMS OF MEDICINE, WITH A SUMMARY OF MOST OF THE THESES PRESENTED AT THE SCHOOLS OF PARIS FROM 1762 TO 1764. *By M. Robert, Regent of the Faculty of Medicine of Paris. First Volume. Lacombe, Bookseller, Quai de Conti, Paris. Pp. 8–9.*

First Observation

A child had a palate cleft extending from the velum to the incisor teeth; M. le Monnier, a very capable dentist (of Rouen), succeeded in reuniting the two edges of the cleft. First, he put in several stitches to hold the edges together, then he freshened them with a sharp instrument. This caused an inflammation which suppurated. It was followed by union of the two edges of the artificial wound and the child was perfectly healed.

The same dentist has succeeded, contrary to the opinion of many practitioners of this art, in stopping up holes in the palate for which one usually uses obturators. His art consists of lightly irritating the edges of the wound, causing an inflammation. The action then becomes more lively and the humours flow through the area with more abundance. Finally, the different layers of mucous membrane apply themselves successively until the hole is successfully closed.

BIOGRAPHICAL SKETCH OF ROUX, BY DR. MOREL-FATIO

Philibert Joseph Roux, Professor at the Paris Faculty of Medicine, Surgeon-in-Chief at the Charité and at the Hôtel-Dieu, Member of the Royal Academy of Medicine and Member of the Institute, was born at Auxerre (Yonne) on April 26, 1780.

He came from a family of surgeons; his father was surgeon to the Hôtel-Dieu of that town. At the Military School in Auxerre, Roux led a light, joyful, and carefree student life; he was a frank and spontaneous lad. At the age of 14 years he entered his father's surgical department and 1½ years later (in 1796) he left for the military hospital of Aix-la-Chapelle—with his bag on his back.

By 1797 he was in Paris, where he became the favorite student of the great Bichat and worked daily for 4 years with him. Roux was the only other contributor to Bichat's famous work on descriptive anatomy. At the age of 22, after Bichat's death, Roux was put in charge of an amphitheater for the teaching of Anatomy and of Surgical Medicine.

In 1802, while working on his thesis, Roux took the competitive examination for Surgeon-in-Chief to the famous Hôtel-Dieu—but Dupuytren won this

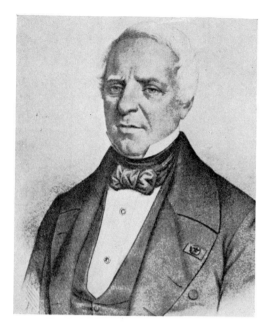

PHILIBERT J. ROUX
1780–1854

coveted position. In 1810, Roux became the Second Surgeon in the Charité—
in Boyer's department (whose daughter he had just married).

From this, he climbed steadily, little-by-little, until he reached his pinnacle
of glory. Roux became full professor in the Faculty of Medicine, then Surgeon-
in-Chief at la Pitié. In 1835, he succeeded Dupuytren as Surgeon to the Hôtel-
Dieu. Later he became President of the Academy of Medicine, then of the
Academy of Sciences. These successes brought him many enemies, of course,
who succeeded (at times) by false insinuations in breaking the confidence his
students and the people had in him.

Roused to indignation by the unfair rumors, Roux reacted. His good-hearted-
ness, his friendliness towards everyone, and his undeniable skill as a surgeon
brought him back both respect and favor. He remained for 20 years at the
Hôtel-Dieu, where his superiority became universally recognized.

At the age of 74, Roux began to write a huge clinical work entitled *Forty
Years of Surgical Practice,* which was to contain all the observations that he had
jotted down since 1811. Unfortunately, he died of a cerebral hemorrhage on
March 23, 1854—before the work was finished.

His researches and publications concerned a considerable number of subjects—his operation for cataract, the treatment of aneurysms, repair of the
ruptured female perineum (1832), treatment of wounds caused by fire-arms, and
treatment for bladder stones; in 1847 he suggested the administration of ether
per rectum for anesthesia. But Roux will stand out as a great pioneer in plastic
surgery. He devoted the first volume of his *Forty Years* to this favorite subject,
and dedicated it to W. Lawrence of St. Bartholomew's Hospital (showing his
debt to the London surgeons who taught him in 1814).

The 1819 paper on closure of the cleft palate is, of course, the backbone of his work and his principal claim to fame. This paper aroused much envy; Richerand was among those who violently attacked him. They questioned the role of Roux as inventor of this operation, noting that as early as 1817 von Graefe (of Berlin) had attempted it without success. This is verifiable, but it is also true that Roux was quite unaware of this attempt and first found out about it after the publication of his own successful effort.

Of the 3 great French surgeons of the first half of the 19th Century—Boyer, Dupuytren, and Roux—the latter was, without doubt, the most skillful, ingenious, and enterprising. It was he, also, who most closely embodied the spirit of plastic surgery.

Daniel Morel-Fatio, M.D.
4 Place de Mexico
Paris 16, France

REPAIR OF CLEFT PALATE BY PHILIBERT ROUX IN 1819

(De Velosynthesi)

DR. JOHN STEPHENSON, Montreal, Canada

(A Graduation Thesis in Surgery, Submitted to the University of Edinburgh, August 1, 1820. Printed by P. Neill, Edinburgh, 1820.)

Translated from the Latin by
DR. WILLIAM W. FRANCIS

INTRODUCTORY NOTE BY DR. LLOYD G. STEVENSON

John Stephenson (1797–1842) of Montreal was the first patient to be operated on for cleft palate by the famous Paris surgeon Philibert Roux in 1819. Stephenson described his own case, and the successful operation, in his graduation thesis at Edinburgh the following year, 1820. He named the operation with the expressive term *velosynthesis,* but Roux in his own account of the procedure (published in 1825) preferred the term *staphyloraphie.* Though the operation had been attempted by others, it was Roux's publication which brought it into current surgical use.

Stephenson subsequently became a leading surgeon in his native city and was the principal founder of the Montreal Medical Institution, out of which the Medical Faculty at McGill University developed. He was a prime mover in the establishment of the University, lectured on anatomy and surgery from 1823, and was appointed the first professor of anatomy in 1832.

AUTHOR'S FOREWORD

In publishing this, my first essay, with the consent of the University and to obtain the doctor's degree, I take the opportunity of expressing my humble thanks and of showing my appreciation of the place which has produced such famous men of science. A stranger, now about to leave Scotland and the most learned University in Europe, which has taught me so much, I should be seriously neglecting my duty to you if I failed to describe this case hitherto unreported in surgical or medical literature. I offer it, therefore, as a small token of my great gratitude to you.

The report will be authentic for the subject is one which I perhaps am best qualified to discuss, since I am myself the patient. The absence of any writings on the subject adds to the difficulties of my thesis, but I have received most helpful notes from Dr. Roux, who led aberrant nature back into her proper course.

> He conceived and executed the whole work;
> He could mingle practice and theory.
> *La Harpe.*

This translation is reproduced, by permission, from the *Journal of the History of Medicine and Allied Sciences.*

MY HISTORY FROM BIRTH TO THE TIME
OF THE OPERATION

Some account must be given of myself and of any disabilities before the operation. It will also serve to show my qualifications. I was born at Montreal, a city of North America, in January* [1797] on the coldest night of many years. I was healthy and fat at birth, but my mother noticed that though she had abundant milk not only did I not thrive but I soon began to lose weight, and that the milk flowed from my nostrils and wet the whole bed.

A doctor summoned by my father made a cursory examination of the fauces and said the trouble was a fissure, the result of inflammation and ulceration caused by the intensely cold weather. In this he was wrong. For, in the first place, I know of cases in Scotland and France, countries warmer than Canada. Secondly, in my adolescence others, as well as I, most carefully examined my fauces and could see no loss of substance of the soft palate. Part of the velum would certainly have been eroded if there had been any ulceration, as the physician said. Thirdly, though formerly an excellent army surgeon, he was at that time old and feeble, and had pronounced the disease incurable after the most cursory inspection. Indeed, all the least authors, ancient and modern, have made the same mistake. Fourthly, one of my brothers was born with a cleft uvula.

But in my case the soft palate as well as the uvula was involved in a vertical fissure of the whole median raphe. The two halves, habitually retracted by the continuous muscular action, presented a huge triangular opening with unobstructed communication between the pharynx and buccal cavity, and with the two halves of the uvula at the angles of the triangle whose apex was at the poste-

* He fails to give the year (1797) and, consequently, his age (22) at the time of operation.

rior junction of the palate bones. There was no fissure of the lip nor any other associated deformity. When my mother saw me gradually failing, she tried to discover some way of feeding me. Finally, she found that if she held me upright I rejected little or no milk, and thereafter I improved and gained in weight. But indeed she had trouble nursing me:

A pensive anguish pining at the heart,
That noble wish, that never cloyed desire
Which, selfish love disdaining, seeks alone
To bless the dearer object of its flame.
                                        Thomson.

For several years of my childhood I was not very robust, but became perfectly strong after the age of puberty. So late was I in learning to speak that my relations feared I would never acquire that faculty, and it was some years before I could say certain words distinctly. I always pronounced $/th/$ like $/s/$. As I grew up, the adjacent parts tended to close the defect, and by speaking slowly I articulated better. Thanks to the nasal quality of the language I used to speak French more clearly than English. Nature is kind and trying to correct her mistakes, did her best to improve my unpleasant voice by contracting as strongly as possible the muscles of the nasopharynx. That the voice is affected by the nasal cavities and soft palate is shown by the fact that mine resembled that of a venereal patient who has suffered the partial or complete loss of his palate.

I seemed to speak through my nose. I believe that the nasal sound was due to faulty vibration of the air in its passage from lungs to nares, because the fissure prevented the soft palate from functioning, and, moreover, I could speak more clearly with my head bent back. All but my intimate friends had difficulty in understanding me. It was only when I had a cold in my head that my voice seemed different, though I could not describe the change; at other times it never sounded unpleasant to me, though if any one else's voice sounded nasal, I was immediately aware of its unpleasantness.

When I grew up, I had no trouble in eating or drinking with my body erect; it was only when I leaned forward that anything came through my nose. I was never able to drink from a spring lying down as boys often do. And there were more unpleasant difficulties. The worst was vomiting, when the stomach contents would be expelled through my nose. I could not blow up a bladder nor play a pipe or any wind instrument, unless I closed my nostrils with my fingers. In my youth, without much professional experience, I had never heard of any way of curing my defect, nor have I ever found any light thrown upon it in medical literature.

I used to think there might be a way to repair the damage, but even so I never dreamed that any operation could be as successful as the one I am about to describe. There was scant hope that such a congenital defect and its disabilities could be cured in a few days. Fearing that trouble was permanent, I bore it patiently.

"J'ai nourri mes chagrins sans les manifester."
Voltaire.

It may be asked why the British surgeons never spoke to me about such an operation. The answer is that all my medical friends suspected that my trouble was syphilitic; they had not examined my throat and so the condition of my soft palate was unknown.

"Tendresse dangereuse, autant comme importune."
Corneille.

When in Paris in 1819 pursuing my professional studies, I was talking one day to Dr. Roux, most famous of French surgeons, about something quite unrelated to my affection. He suddenly took notice of the harshness of my voice and, rightly dropping his politeness, enquired if I had ever had a syphilitic ulceration of the palate, for there were no external signs of the disease; whereupon I showed him the lesion and explained it all.

He immediately thought it operable and spoke to me of the possibility. In favour of the operation was the fact that certain movements of the fauces, as in holding the breath, would almost close the fissure. I weighed the possibilities and promised that he should operate on my velum, but since I was about to leave France and make a long journey, I would put it off till my return to France the next year.

Meanwhile, my medical friends persuaded me to have the fissure treated without delay. And so, after due consideration, I yielded; for, in the first place, Dr. Roux having suggested the procedure would do his best. Secondly, I had nothing to lose, but if it turned out well everything to gain. Thirdly, if the operation was not entirely successful, another might be advisable and a whole year would not have to lapse before the attempt. And fourthly, many hazards, such as war, might interfere with my returning to Paris, and with this skillful surgeon earning another well-merited laurel.

So two days later I again saw Dr. Roux and told him I wanted the operation done. I wasted no time before getting through with it, for it was done the next day.

No one had ever thought about the procedure; complete fissure of the soft palate had always been considered incurable, and the afflicted were doomed to endure this deformity and its consequences. Dr. Roux believed it could be cured by using the hare-lip suture and keeping the parts immobile for some days. The operation lasted nearly an hour and needed all his skill and all my endurance for its successful performance. I suffered less from the pain than from the irritation and tickling caused by the introduction of the needles, a sensation that would run up to the ear like the pain of toothache. This would seem to show that, in some people at least, the fauces are not very sensitive.

ACCOUNT OF THE OPERATION

It was carried out on the 28th of last September (1819) shortly after 4 p.m. I adopted a sitting position which seemed best to facilitate breathing and the flow of blood out of the mouth and to get as much as possible of the very necessary light.

Three interrupted *sutures*, stout enough to avoid laceration of the tissues, as far as possible, were introduced with two surgical needles alternately from behind forwards, each suture being thus drawn three times. Since fingers are too short to do the work at such depth, and the needles were rendered slippery by the constant flow of saliva, use was made of a stylus-like instrument (*porte-aiguille* in French) with what we call in English a slider to grasp the needles.

Before the edges were freshened the sutures were put in place in order to see whether the fissure could be closed. It would have been unfortunate to do the cutting to no purpose, for then the defect would only have been enlarged. The edges were thereupon cut with forceps and a guarded scalpel. The sutures were separately tied and severed.

The ligatures had been placed in position before the incision not only to see that the fissure could be closed, but also because the oozing of blood from the freshened edges, especially in the next stage, would have been troublesome both to the operator and to me. The union seemed to be as firm as skill could make it, and nature's healing inflammation would perfect the cure.

The halves of the uvula were not sutured, so I still have two uvulas. Immediately after the operation I gratified a certainly unwise, but perhaps pardonable, curiosity by pronouncing a few words for Dr. Roux and the others. All agreed that there was a great change in my voice.

AFTER HISTORY OF THE SUCCESSFUL OPERATION

There was little pain but some feeling of tension the first two nights. Respiration was difficult, as I had to keep my mouth closed thereby increasing the painful tension, and for 4 days I breathed entirely through the nose. For 29 hours I had no food or drink, then only a little bouillon conveyed into my oesophagus with a spoon. No solid food for 4 days.

After 72 hours, the middle suture was taken out, and union seemed firm. Dr. Roux wanted to remove the superior one, but another physician* and I persuaded him to leave the other sutures. (1) Success depended entirely on adhesive inflammation and union. (2) There were no analogous cases with which to compare ours. (3) The muscular action of these parts is very strong. Nevertheless I now think that all the sutures should have been cut at that time, or at any rate the superior section along with the median. What relief from painful tension the cutting of a suture afforded. The velum thereupon acquired its motility and elasticity.

Eighty-four hours after the operation the other two sutures, the superior and inferior, were cut in the presence of Dr. Boyer. We were delighted to find the *synthesis* firm. I was now free to talk, and the next day I took some solid food, chewing it carefully. The parts gradually strengthened and on October 11, at Dr. Roux's request, I had the honor of reading a report of my case before the Royal Institute of Paris.

The next day I left Paris and after a long journey by land and sea without any harm, I reached Edinburgh. All my medical friends said that my voice was

* Holmes? [*i.e.* Andrew F. Holmes (1797–1860), M.D. Edin. 1819, afterwards Professor of Medicine at McGill, and first Dean of its Medical Faculty].

now more distinct, stronger, and more normal.

I, myself, noticed a change in my voice but could not define its nature. It must be confessed that some of the nasal quality is still present. Old habit and the above-mentioned muscular contraction were too much for me. The repaired instrument is not yet fulfilling its proper duties nor giving the help it should to my vocal faculty. Who can deny the all-importance of habit? . . .

Many disabilities I have got rid of: I can now drink perfectly well in a horizontal position; can play on hitherto noiseless wind instruments, and have lost that very disagreeable habit, when vomiting, of expelling stomach contents through my nose. I learned this in October last, when crossing from Ostend to Dover on the 22nd day after the operation; though I was seasick and vomiting, nothing entered my nose. This also proved that the union was a solid *synthesis* for, as all surgeons know, vomiting throws the velum into violent motion. For a time I could not whistle. Sometimes the *uvula* would give rise to an irritation and cough, or there would be a pain running up to the ear, something like a toothache, and possibly a sequel to the operation. I am no longer thus affected.

COMMENTS ON THE OPERATION

Although the operation, considering the circumstances and the haste, was very well carried out by Dr. Roux, I would respectfully suggest some modifications. The chief trouble was caused by the instrument called a *slider;* its handling was so difficult that one needle was broken and another had to be introduced. If the edges of the instrument are closed by a *cochlea,* I think this disadvantage will be avoided. When at my suggestion the edges were thus opened and closed, the parts of the instrument did not shake.

Secondly, since muscular action is intense in the velum, and the sutures, as in my case, are so prone to lacerate the tissue that Dr. Roux had difficulty removing these deeply buried ligatures, especially the last one, I would make the following suggestion. Gum elastic, light at the back, thicker in front, should be placed between the velum and the sutures and then the threads should be tied over the elastic as in the suture called quilled [quilted?] in English, when the edges of the fissure have been tightly joined together without anything intervening. Other materials may perhaps be substituted for gum elastic.

It is of great importance that the ligature be fine but widely spaced so as not to lacerate the tissue nor to excite the sometimes dreaded suppuration. The sutures should enclose as much of the velum as possible. Let the patient drink and eat as little as possible, or even let him take his nourishment through a tube or the skin of an eel introduced into the oesophagus (as John Hunter recommended in certain cases).

But there are many disadvantages and in some cases danger in these methods; therefore I would advise my own method, described above, if feeding is particularly difficult. Absolute silence should be observed in all cases and this is easy in adults. Other regimen is rarely necessary unless there be complications, such as convulsions in children, when the treatment is then adapted to each case. . . .

MOST SUITABLE AGE FOR OPERATION

The operation is not possible in childhood. In the first place the child is too restless for the operation to be done without danger. Secondly, I think, from my own experience, that a child would suffocate if its nasal cavities filled with mucus; if my nose had been obstructed at the time, I am sure that the sutures could hardly have remained in place. Thirdly;

children are liable to *tetanus* and other complications after any wounds; certainly they would be very liable to such symptoms after operation on a sensitive part. Fourthly, children cannot avoid crying, and the crying caused by more or less acute pain and tension will perhaps entail a less successful result. Lastly, the age of choice is, in my opinion, between the 4th and 6th year, when the child is less sensitive than before and less powerful than later. In any case I strongly advise that the operation be done before puberty to avoid all the disadvantages of habit.

ON THE FREQUENCY OF THE CONDITION

Although not very common, my deformity is not rare; several cases being recorded in medical literature. In the great Boerhaave's lectures reported by his distinguished pupil Haller, vol. I, section 70, one case of fissure of the velum is described. The deformity, I believe, was in the velum, for it is in the section on diseases and deformities of the velum, and he says that the child could not drink, eat, or speak unless his head was retracted and his nostrils closed with the fingers. Light is thus thrown on the cause of the muscular contraction in adults so affected.

Dr. Roux saw one case before mine and Dr. Dupuytren, the Paris surgeon, saw another a few weeks before my operation, but without any thought of suturing or other measures. My friend Lizars, extramural professor of anatomy and physiology at Edinburgh, had a case

(which I saw) with the fissure extending through upper lip, hard and soft palate, and uvula.

I know of two cases in Canada, but with cleft uvula only, one in a friend of mine, the other in my brother. My friend stuttered a little and some people thought this was caused by the fissure; but many without this deformity stutter, and others with it pronounce their words distinctly. My brother spoke perfectly clearly. All my other relations were born without any deformities. In the Edinburgh Infirmary at present there is a case of syphilitic fissure extending through the velum.

Believing that this new operation needs a name, I suggest *Velosynthesis,* a term derived from both Greek and Latin.

John Stephenson, M.D.
Montreal, Canada

ACKNOWLEDGMENT

We wish to thank the editor of the *Journal of the History of Medicine and Allied Sciences* for permission to reprint this translation by Dr. Francis and the introduction by Dr. Lloyd Stevenson.

EDITORIAL NOTE

This is one of the rare instances, perhaps the only one, in which the first successful performance of an operation is described in separate papers by the surgeon and by the patient. It is for this unique reason that Stephenson's thesis is included in this series.

For additional fascinating material pertaining to Stephenson and this operation, the reader is referred to A. B. Wallace's masterful treatment in the *British Journal of Plastic Surgery (19: 1, 1966).*

Because John Stephenson (the author), William W. Francis (the translator), and Lloyd Stevenson (writer of the introduction) were all important to McGill University, the editor has asked Dr. Martin Entin for a word on these men.

COMMENTARY BY DR. MARTIN ENTIN

It is heartening to reflect that while James McGill spent only two years at the University of Glasgow before he emigrated to Montreal, his experiences in this short period of time became so ingrained in his

sinews that when the time came to make his will, he left most of his estate for the establishment of an "Institution of Higher Learning." (This has been true of educational endeavors in all periods of our history; it is private individuals, not "the Establishment," who usually act as patrons and founders of educational institutions at all levels.)

McGill died in 1813 and one of the colleges of the future McGill University was established by Royal Charter in 1821, but there was no active teaching in the ensuing years. To meet the deadline of the bequest, it was necessary to start "active educational work" and this was done when the four founding members of the Montreal Medical Institutions were "engrafted" upon inactive McGill College as its Medical Faculty, on June 29, 1829. One of these was John Stephenson, who then became University Registrar in 1833. It was the act of these four that saved McGill's legacy from reverting back to his estate, and assured the development of the medical school and the university. Thus the surgical repair done by Philibert Roux bore lasting fruit in a manner which no one could have predicted.

I knew Dr. W. W. Francis, the translator, throughout my medical undergraduate and postgraduate years at McGill, where he was Professor of Medical History. Uncle Willie, as we affectionately called him, was a wonderful scholar, a bibliophile, and a second cousin to William Osler. He became custodian of the Osler Library even before it arrived at McGill, the institution to which Osler willed it. His annotations in the catalogue of the Osler Library (in pencil, in longhand) comprise some priceless vignettes; each is probably of more interest than the original entry in the catalogue— however rare the volume might be. Some day I will write a personal tribute to Dr. Francis; I considered him my friend, notwithstanding "the generation gap."

The other work of love (besides the Osler Library) that Dr. Francis left behind was this translation of Stephenson's thesis. Francis translated it from Latin with painstak-

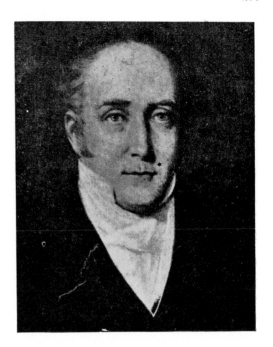

DR. JOHN STEPHENSON
1797–1842

First patient to have had his cleft palate successfully repaired. Principal founder of McGill University and its medical school. (Courtesy, Osler Library of McGill University. Obtained by Dr. Entin.)

ing accuracy but, because he did not live long enough to put the final polish on it, it was not published during his lifetime. This is a reflection of his search for accuracy; there were two or three translations of words on the specific surgical technique which did not completely satisfy Dr. Francis.

Lloyd Stevenson followed Francis as Professor of Medical History and Librarian of the Osler Library at McGill. It was while he was in this position that he was responsible for the first publication of this translation. Subsequently, he left to take the Chair vacated by John Fulton at Yale University. Currently, he is Director of the Institute of the History of Medicine at Johns Hopkins University.

—*Martin A. Entin*

Journal

der

practischen Heilkunde

herausgegeben

von

C. W. Hufeland,

Königl. Preufs. Staatsrath, Ritter des rothen Adler.
Ordens dritter Klasse, wirkl. Leibarzt, erstem Arzt
der Charité, Mitglied der Academie der
Wissenschaften etc.

und

J. Ch. F. Harles,

Geh. Hofrath, ordentlichem öffentlichen Lehrer der
Klinik auf der Universität zu Erlangen, ordentlichem
Mitglied der Königl. Baierschen Academie der
Wissenschaften etc.

Grau, Freund, ist alle Theorie,
Doch grün des Lebens goldner Baum.
Göthe.

I. Stück. Januar.

Berlin 1817.
Im Verlag der Realschulbuchhandlung.

(left) Title page of the January 1817 issue of the Journal of Practical Therapeutics. Goethe's couplet is marked. (right) Within the brackets is the paragraph relating Graefe's presentation before the Association on December 27, 1816. It is written in the third person. (Courtesy, Prof. Schuchardt.)

Translated from the German by
PROF. KARL SCHUCHARDT

"Gray, friend, is every theory,
But green is the golden tree of life."
Goethe.

Dec. 27, 1817

Geheimrath Graefe spoke about the clefts of the soft palate, which could be congenital or acquired. He had tried several times in vain to cure the evil or to replace it artificially until finally, in the case of a cleft so extremely severe that it reached to the bone, he conceived the idea to unite it by suture and by an artificially caused inflammation. For this purpose he invented special needles and needle holders. With these he made a suture which, in conjunction with spreading it with *Acidum Muriaticum* and *Tinctura Cantharidum* (which latter he preferred for the excitement of the plastic process), achieved such perfect healing of the cleft that the person afterwards could swallow quite well and speak distinctly.

COMMENTARY BY THE EDITOR

The short paragraph reproduced here became a *cause célèbre* in European surgical circles during the first part of the 19th century.

When Roux published his more complete account in 1819 (of the repair of John Stephenson's cleft palate) he assumed (as did most readers) that this was the first report of a successful closure. But he awakened a sleeping tiger.

Graefe had presented his case most casually in a few words before the biweekly meeting of the Medical-Surgical Society of Berlin some 3 years before. This resulted in the subsequent publication of this untitled paragraph, but Graefe had not bothered to write a paper on his feat. Though he appeared to have little interest in this procedure at the time, apparently deeming it of no importance (which seems to be a general and continuing fate of plastic surgical procedures), it now became the chief concern of his life. He busied himself doing as many more cases as possible and wrote a long treatise on the subject in 1820 (which will be excerpted in the next paper).

Nothing seemed so important to Von Graefe, at this point, as establishing this priority; Roux responded in kind. It became a matter of national honor when many surgeons in Europe had to choose whether to side with the French or the German. The matter will never be settled, of course; many priority claims aren't.

Let this be a lesson to the reader. If you believe that you have originated a useful procedure, don't sit on your duff. Write a proper paper describing it in some detail, prepare proper illustrations, give it a proper title, and submit it to a proper scientific journal! Otherwise it may be lost and you may later find yourself spending most of your energies trying to recoup that which you so casually tossed away.

—*Frank McDowell!*

THE PALATE SUTURE

A Newly Discovered Method to Correct Congenital Speech Defects

DR. CARL FERDINAND VON GRAEFE, *Berlin*

(*J. der Chirurgie und Augenheilkunde, 1: 1, 1820*)

Translated from the German by
DR. HANS MAY

Our voice is produced by air which is driven from the lungs through the larynx; it becomes clearer when the air reflects upon the dome of the palate, the nasal cavities, and the sinuses. Articulation becomes complete by proper movement of the lips, tongue, and the soft palate. Distortion and anomalies of the voice can be caused by defects and dysfunction of any of these structures. In my opinion, the most important of these voice-forming and voice-influencing structures is the soft palate. In defects of the other structures the patient is able to overcome the handicap completely or to a certain degree (the ventriloquist doesn't need the function of the lips at all) but the slightest defect of the soft palate causes a speech derangement which increases with the extent of the cleft.

It is strange that thus far anomalies of the soft palate and their influence on voice and articulation have been mentioned only in passing—only in connection with clefts of the hard palate and through-and-through clefts. No author in Germany, France, England, or Italy has singled out the anomalies of the soft palate. It is impossible that rarity of the lesion is the reason. I, myself, have had occasion to observe soft palate clefts without cleft of the hard palate in 5 individuals.

The consequences resulting from those clefts depend upon the length and width of the same. In short and narrow clefts, phonation is impaired, but not to such a degree that speech is not understandable; it becomes so in wide clefts; regurgitation of the food through the nose may then also be present. All this becomes worse in soft and hard palate, through-and-through, clefts.

I will show a complete cleft of the soft palate, by means of a drawing which I had made of an individual in whom I obtained a complete surgical closure of the cleft.

Before going into details of his technique, Graefe describes the various means by which attempts have been made to overcome the handicaps resulting from these clefts, *i.e.* clefts of the soft and hard palate, lip clefts, and through-and-through clefts. Clefts of the soft palate alone had never been treated before. In through-and-through clefts, some physicians recommended closure of the lip cleft, hoping that after such an operation the cleft of the hard and soft palate would narrow. Others endeavored to bring this about by additional outside pressure, using clamps placed upon the cheeks at the level of the lateral jaw parts. Others expected much from scarifying the cleft edges.

Editorial note. This was the first article in the first issue of this journal, which was founded and edited by Graefe and Walther. It is some 54 pages in length and could not be reproduced in its entirety here. Instead, Dr. May has given us a free and clear translation of the most important parts—interspersing them with his abstracts of the remainder. This will be far more interesting to the reader than a literal translation of this much-too-long article.

From experience, all these measures proved to be unsatisfactory and therefore expert wound physicians gave them up—particularly as clefts tend to become narrower with the passing of time without any therapy (through growth of the bones). One now aims at perfecting closure of the clefts of the hard palate by insertion of obturators but, so far as speech is concerned, they are of advantage only in clefts of the hard palate. In clefts of the hard and soft palate, the speech cannot be improved by such means. They are, nevertheless, recommendable because they prevent regurgitation of food through the nose. One may be inclined to construct obturators which can be fastened to the hard palate and have posteriorly a moveable plate, which rests upon the cleft soft palate. But such a contraption is not recommended, as its action is not voluntary.

I considered restoration of the integrity of the cleft soft palate as the only way to obtain a normal voice, and this can be accomplished only by suturing. I foresaw formidable difficulties such as the sutures cutting through the mucous membrane, life-endangering inflammation, the wound edges not forming adhesions (because of the productivity of mucous), difficulty of inserting needles because of gagging, the whole procedure causing a constriction of the pharynx and impairing swallowing, *etc.*

How the author solved these problems is now described in detail. First, there is a detailed, 11-page description of the author's special instruments, which contributed essentially to the success of the procedure.

The first one is called a uranotome, and was designed as a punch to scarify the edges of the cleft. It consists of a straight or curved chisel, within a brass cylinder; the chisel can be released by a spring and its edge hits a wooden board, which is attached to this instrument.

The palate needle differs from ordinary needles inasmuch as it is not a half curve, but U-shaped. It has 3 cutting edges and a strong eye, so that the needle holder cannot bend or break it.

The palate needle holder consists of two parts. The part which grasps the needle is made of steel and these surfaces are grooved to afford a firmer hold on the needle. The middle part consists of two smaller and two larger rings, which are connected by small steel bars; these are the locking device of the needle holder. The handles are made of wood.

There is also a detailed description of ligature screws (cylindric screw-mother and a screw-head) made of silver. The screw holder differs from an ordinary needle holder, inasmuch as the grasping part is at right angles to the handles.

The sutures consist of waxed cotton.

TECHNIQUE OF THE OPERATION

(As to the age at which to operate, the author refers to former publications of his.)

Separation of Epidermis from Cleft Edge.

This can be done in one of two ways: mechanically or chemically. The mechanical way is performed as follows: The patient is seated on a chair in a bright light and leans his head against the chest of an orderly, who grasps firmly the temporal regions of the patient and the forehead. The operator, who is seated in front of the patient, inserts now the uranotome through the cleft in such a way that the wooden platform comes to lie against the nasal side of the palate and the edge of the chisel upon the cleft edge. If, after checking the position of the instrument, it is found to be correct, the chisel is now punched hard against the board to cut a narrow strip of the cleft edge off. The latter is now hanging down. By continuing the same procedure, it is finally cut off completely. The curved part on the anterior side of the cleft is cut loose by using a gauge chisel. After each punch the patient rinses his mouth with cold water to stop the bleeding. According to the patient's statement, this procedure causes very little pain.

The second way to scarify the cleft edges is by touching the same with chemicals—such as concentrated hydrochloric or sulfuric acid, or with the caustic stick. One must then wait until all necrotic tissue has become detached and granulation tissue is visible, before one can plan the operation.

I am inclined to prefer the chemical scarification because it causes much more inflammatory reaction, resulting in broader wound surfaces from swelling and better adhesions of the same after suturing. I use the uranotome whenever the cleft edges are unequal and differ in width. Otherwise, I touch the edges once daily with concentrated sulfuric acid until a scar has formed. After the latter has been thrown off, the raw surface is touched with diluted hydrochloric acid. One then must wait until the granulations are pink and the cleft edges thick and reddish colored.

Insertion of Sutures.

Depending upon the length of the cleft, about 4 to 5 stitches are required. It is advisable to let the patient rest and relax between the insertion of each suture. Retractors and tongue depressors are not necessary; they only crowd the operating field, cause gagging, and prevent the patient from opening his mouth widely.

Then follows a detailed description of each needle and how it is grasped in the needle holder and inserted.

Closure.

This is done by threading both ends of each suture through the cylindric mother-screw of the ligature screws.

The author then describes in great detail and by means of drawings the various steps which are necessary to tighten the sutures and to fasten them with the ligature screws.

The threads are left long and attached to one cheek with adhesive strips.

AFTER TREATMENT

This must first be directed toward relief of the patient's discomfort; secondly it must include local care of the wound and dietary measures; thirdly, it must keep the sutures constantly tight.

Due to excessive secretion of mucous, and difficulty in swallowing from swelling and tightness of the velum, the patient feels nauseated and coughs. Coughing may become convulsive and dangerously close to suffocation. To relieve this condition, mechanical cleansing is done by frequently wiping the palate with applicators—every 15 minutes day and night—and using mouth washes of cold water. Since this procedure weakens the patient considerably (from lack of rest). I have prescribed belladonna in later cases.

General Support and Local Care.

Due to difficulty in swallowing, the patient's general condition soon becomes impaired. To counteract this, the patient, from the beginning, must be given a proper liquid and semi-liquid diet consisting of egg yolk in strong wine, egg yolk in milk, and strong coffee. Also recommended are washing the face and body with wine and aromatic solutions. The healing process is locally stimulated by increasing the inflammation, without increasing the production of mucous. This is accomplished by application of hydrochloric acid or naphtha—or a solution of equal parts of *Tinctura Euphorbii, Tinctura Cantharidum,* and *Tinctura Myrrhae*—to the suture line. In one case I touched the suture line with a small hot iron, but I am not inclined to recommend this procedure as yet.

Keeping the Sutures Tight.

This is as important as the dynamic support in the healing process. The sutures become slack in 12 to 24 hours after the operation, due to their cutting into the wound edges. (One sees some of the ligature screws hanging loose and the wound edges slightly relaxed.) This must be counteracted by removing the small screw heads, tightening the threads, and fastening the screw heads again.

The final phases of treatment are concerned with removal of the sutures and improvement of speech.

So far as the former is concerned, it will be noticed that some of the sutures have cut through already on the third postoperative day (latest, by the fifth) due to the softness of the velar tissue and also from the constant mechanical tightening. Those which are completely loose are simply removed. Others are cut free with a pair of Cowper's scissors.

Immediately after removal of the sutures one must further the process of cicatrization of the injured area. This differs, according to whether the operation was a total failure or a partial or complete success. In the first case, the cleft reappears. The patient can now take house diet, since he is able to swallow. He should irrigate his mouth with red wine; the sore areas are painted with a mixture of rose honey, beeswax, and *Tinctura of Myrrhae, t.i.d.* Under this treatment, complete cicatrization is accomplished within 8—or at the latest—10 days. In all cases, the resulting cleft seemed to be narrower than before the operation; in some cases speech was rather clearer. Thus the operation is recommendable, even if a total failure may be anticipated.

In cases of partial organic union, one must see to it that there will be a firm cicatrization of the united area. One must avoid the local application of strongly irritant drugs to the separated wound edges. Recommended are gentle mouth washes with red wine; the above mentioned mixtures are applied to the united areas *q.i.d.* The patient is not permitted to talk or chew. Diet is liquid.

After all areas have healed, measures for reclosure of the open part can be considered and the treatment will depend upon the length of the remaining cleft. In clefts not more than 4 mm long, closure can be accomplished merely by applying hydrochloric acid to the separated wound edges. In longer clefts, resuturing of the cleft edges, after removal of the epidermis from the edges, is necessary. This is done 3 to 4 weeks after complete cicatrization. (By that time the patient has completely recovered, and the velum has stretched and is apt to give more easily when re-sutured.)

If under the most favorable circumstances the cleft remains closed, then the only local treatment necessary is that recommended for partial recurrence of the cleft—until cicatrization is complete.

The patient is now instructed to speak properly. This is difficult to achieve in the beginning. Speech may even be worse than before the operation, because of postoperative tightness of the velum. However, according to my experience, the velum becomes more elastic after several weeks and the patient regains his speech, but by no means clarity of articulation. As he was used to impairment of his speech, he has difficulty in overcoming it unless he is properly instructed. My advice is to let the patient repeat after the instructor single letters (later, syllables); finally, he is instructed in clear articulation.

I devised this operation in 1816 and performed it on 4 individuals. The operation was fully successful in only one patient. If I had had more experience, I might not have advised and performed the operation in patients like the one who had a wide cleft of his hard and soft palates, another who was an anemic, frail individual, and another who was cachectic.

The circumstances under which the

operation was successfully performed were entirely different. One was a female patient of robust constitution, whose skin color was florid, and who had no history of previous illness. In this case the cleft edges had been denuded chemically. There was a small hole in the upper wound angle after healing. This was closed according to the method described above. This case was demonstrated before eminent physicians and students.

SUMMARY

Palate suture is not a dangerous treatment. The operation causes more discomfort than pain. It can be attempted even under unfavorable circumstances, because if unsuccessful it does not increase the difficulty. One can almost be sure of the success of the palate suture in cases where the cleft is not unduly wide, the mucous membrane of the cleft edges is thick, and the patient is a healthy, strong individual.

The author realizes the various difficulties connected with his method but does not know of any better way to overcome them than by publicizing the technique in great detail. He hopes that since a path has been opened difficult hurdles have been taken, and the success of this operation has been demonstrated beyond any doubt. This publication may stimulate all physicians to make attempts to perfect this endeavor which is only in the developing stage, but of eminent importance.

Carl Ferdinand von Graefe, M.D.
Clinical Professor of Surgery, II Clinic
University of Berlin

ADDENDUM BY THE AUTHOR

Just after the galley proofs had been finished, I found in the *Constitutionel* (Vendredi, 22 October 1819, No. 296, p. 3) that Roux in Paris had successfully performed a palate suture a short time ago. This operation was advertised in said journal as an operation never performed before.

This remark could hardly come from this physician, who is well read in the medical literature. The first palate suture was successfully performed by me in the spring of 1816. It was demonstrated to Herr Staatsrath Hufeland, die Herrn Geheimenräthe Rudolphi und Richter, Herr Professor Bernstein, die Herrn Doctoren Boehm, Jüngken, Michaelis, and several others.

In the year 1816—to be precise, on December 27th—I delivered a paper about this operative procedure before the Medical-Surgical Society of Berlin, and also demonstrated my instruments.

In 1817 and 1818 I gave lectures about the technique of the palate suture to a large audience. In 1817 one can find printed references to my technique in Volume 44 of Hufeland's *Journal der Practischen Heilkunde,* page 116. News of my operation must have reached Paris by traveling young physicians, as there is a lively exchange of students between the medical schools of Berlin and Paris.

In addition, the Paris journals of medicine frequently include excerpts from Hufeland's Journal and it must be strongly assumed that my operation—performed by me for the first time in the spring of 1816—has become generally known in France within the last 3 to 4 years. Its existence could not have remained unknown to Herr Roux.

—*C.F.G.*

BEITRAGE ZUR GAUMENNATH

(Contributions on Suture of the Palate)

DR. J. F. DIEFFENBACH, *Berlin, Germany*

(*Litt. Ann. d. ges. Heilk., 4: 145, 1826*)

Translated from the German by
DR. EDUARD SCHMID

Amongst surgical operations, next to cataract operation and artificial formation of a pupil, suture of the palate is one of the most sensible and most interesting. Thus the attention which this procedure has gained in most countries since its inventor, Gräfe, published it has been quite large and it has been, almost without exception, readily accepted by physicians and surgeons. However . . . at the present time it is still associated with so many difficulties . . . and the number of successes is so much smaller than the number of failures, that entire countries can hardly demonstrate a few examples in whom the outcome was completely favorable.

During the few years which have elapsed since suture of the palate first became known, the original surgical method reported by Gräfe has been modified several times—in part by Gräfe, himself, and in part by his successors in Germany, France, and England. Thus, everybody who has theoretically or practically concerned himself with this problem has designed a modification. . . .

I, also, would like to contribute something regarding this matter. . . . In my opinion, the first step (*i.e.,* sharp dissection of the margin of the cleft) is not difficult and I believe that it should be preferred to chemical means which produce inflammation. . . .

However, all these difficulties and unpleasant situations which have been reported to occur with surgical procedures for the correction of cleft palate, particularly during the third stage (*i.e.,* tying the knot), can be avoided if a material is used for approximation which is almost as soft and pliable as a waxed suture and which merely turned on itself, provides the necessary durability. Such a material is *purified lead* which has been shaped into a wire . . . However, first of all I would like to describe the instruments which I found to be necessary for this surgical procedure (Plate I).

1. *Forceps.* The grooves on the inner aspect of the tip should not run transversely, as is usually the case, but should pursue a longitudinal course, next to one another.

2. *A narrow pointed bistoury* with a long handle, similar to the cataract knife of Richter.

3. *Palate needles,* 7 lines long, which are scarcely curved from the tip to the middle and which are triple-edged with a broader area on the concave side and two smaller side areas. Thus the needle does not only cut on the two sides, but also on the back. . . . The needles must be made of finest steel, the workmanship must be particularly good, and the thread must cut deeply enough.

4. *Lead wire* of moderate thickness. The lead must have been purified as much as possible from tin and other components which would decrease its pliability. Only then does the wire have the correct degree of pliability and can be

---

Editorial note. Dieffenbach had an extremely busy mind, as well as busy hands, and he wrote many articles on cleft palate repair during the first years of this operation. Near the end of this article he describes, for the first time, a rational plan for uranoplasty—closure of the cleft in a hard palate. His plan was used successfully by another surgeon a few years later.

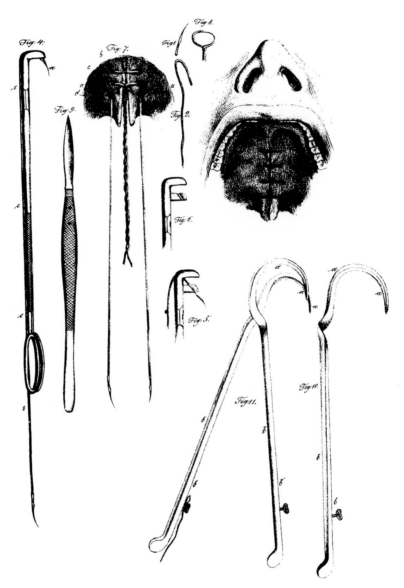

PLATE I

Figure 1, palate needle. Figure 2, ligature with screwed-on needle. Figure 4, closed needle holder with needle and ligature. Figures 5 and 6, grasping the needle in the needle holder. Figure 7, a cleft palate being approximated by ligatures. Figure 8, the ligature after completion of the knot in the velum. Figure 9, the knife for debridement of the margin. Figure 10, palate forceps for approximating the velum without sutures. Figure 11, the simple forceps for one-half of the velum. (Courtesy, John Crerar Library, Chicago.)

readily screwed into the thread of the needle, with which it firmly connects.

5. *Pliers* which are long, thin, and with corrugated handles....

The operation is carried out in three steps, in the following manner.

First stage. Freshening up the margins of the cleft.... The velum is put under tension and it is perforated with the tip of the knife at the most inferior angle and a small strip is removed from one side of the velum along the entire length of the cleft. The incision is extended to beyond the angle of the cleft and it meets the incision on the opposite side.

Second stage. Insertion of the ligatures. After the needles have been firmly screwed to the wire ends (which are two spans in length) the posterior third of the first is inserted into the notch of the forceps in such a manner that the tip looks toward the arms of the forceps. . . . The tip of the needle holder is inserted into the cleft and this is perforated from a posterior to an anterior direction . . . the needle with the trailing lead ligature is pulled out through the mouth. It is pulled out until the needle which is attached to the other end of the suture has arrived in the cleft. Now the second needle is grabbed in the manner just described, the opposite side of the velum is perforated, and the needle with the wire is once again advanced until both needles hang equally outside the mouth. . . .

Third stage. Tying the knots. One starts to close the sutures by twisting the ends on themselves outside the mouth. The turns gradually push forward to the soft palate whose margins approximate one another more and more, and finally are in close contact with one another. It is suitable, toward the end of the turning, to hold the ligatures close to the velum with the tip of the needle holder to avoid unnecessary strain on the soft palate. . . .

Even after successful operations, the patient must not be allowed to talk for a few days after surgery; he is allowed to eat only thin soup.

(*Editor's note.* At this point, Dieffenbach describes at great length a case in which he split the palate to remove an enormous malignant tumor of the nasopharynx—probably a malignant mixed salivary gland tumor—and his subsequent closure of the surgical cleft in the palate.)

In conclusion, I would like to make a few remarks regarding congenital cleft of the hard palate, which either occurs by itself or in association with the same condition of the velum; it is a lesion which hitherto could not be treated.

If at the same time the upper lip is split once or several times, the cleft, after operation of the harelip, is most likely to close where it runs through the alveolar process. This is particularly true when the operation is carried out during earliest childhood. If, however, the velum is also split, it is possible to approximate the margins to one another but closure of the cleft in the hard palate never occurs. . . . It has been unsuccessfully attempted to effect closure of the bony gap by frequent scarification of the margins. The soft cover of the palate has also been dissected bilaterally and pulled over the cleft, but this has also never been successful.

Numerous clinical aids have been suggested. Autenrieth recommends that a steel brace be worn on the head to make persistent pressure on both sides of the upper jaw. This is certainly effective if the patient is still very young, when the growth of the bone reinforces the pressure. However, I believe that this purpose can be better achieved by using a one-half inch wide ring of rubber resin which, in the stretched position, is put around the alveolar process inside the lips like a closed elastic band. Posteriorly, where the ring transversely crosses the palate it may be interrupted and the ends may be brought in connection with a palate plate. In very small children, one could initially use a very thin and narrow rubber ring; mechanically, at least, this would have a stronger action than the circular muscle of the mouth.

Several attempts to surgically close the bony gap with the soft cover of the palate have been unsuccessful. However, it might be possible by an operation on the bone of the palate to approximate the bones to one another and thus also the margins of the velum. After incising the soft cover, the palatine bones would have to be cut with a saw along the alveolar process in a curved line from the posterior margin in an anterior direction up to close to the cleft. After this, the freshened medial cleft margins would have to be pulled together by a gold or lead wire. The bone would have an adequate blood supply from its superior attachment; one could also expect later closure of the lateral opening, particularly if one provided some help to nature. After successful healing, suture of the palate would still have to be carried out.

A few animal experiments which I have carried out in reference to this subject appear to promise a somewhat favorable result. Small burr holes in the roof of the palate which were 3 or 4 lines in diameter soon closed once again, particularly if the soft cover of the palate was not incised crosswise but only in a simple manner and was carefully separated from the bone and, after the burr hole had been performed,

was once again pulled over the opening. . . . A piece of bone which was reinserted and which was once again covered with skin produced an elevation of the palate at this point; exfoliation did not occur.

In one dog, a long cleft which was two lines wide, and which had been made with a fine saw throughout the entire length of the cover of the palate, closed. . . .

> *J. F. Dieffenbach, M.D.*
> *General Practitioner*
> *Berlin*

UEBER DAS GAUMENSEGEL DES MENSCHEN UND DER SAUGETHIERE

(On the Soft Palate of Human Beings and of Mammals)

DR. J. F. DIEFFENBACH, *Berlin, Germany*

(*Litt. Ann. d. ges. Heilk., 4: 298, 1826*)

Translated from the German by
DR. EDUARD SCHMID

Editorial note. In this extensive study, Dieffenbach describes in detail the anatomy and movements of the soft palate in humans. He then describes the comparative anatomy of the velum, noting that it first appears in whales, that it appears in no lower animals, and that without exception all mammals have a velum. In the course of this, he describes the soft palates in a large variety of mammals—including mice, horses, camels, and various apes. Finally, as a curious afterthought to this mammoth and erudite study, he appends an unsuccessful (but intriguing) case report of a palate repair. It was in this report that lateral relaxation incisions were first described. This "appendage" follows.

A 40-year-old male patient had, in previous years, lost a significant part of his soft palate from syphilis. Thus a wide opening in the middle of the velum permitted a free view of the posterior part of his pharynx. This opening was more than 1¼ inches in diameter, almost 1½ inches in length. . . .

As this man had been cured for a number of years by correct treatment with mercury, and as since that time he had been entirely healthy, I did not decline to carry out this operation. I was concerned only about the large width of the opening. . . .

Excision of the margin was very easy. . . . The minimal hemorrhage ceased soon after gargling with cold water. At first the supe-

rior, then the middle, and finally the inferior ligature were placed. The suture points had been placed exactly opposite one another; thus, after the sutures were tightened by turning, the wound margins were perfectly approximated. Subsequent to this, they were cut off and the short ends were bent in an upward direction.

However, palpation of the velum with a finger indicated that it was under such tension that it almost threatened to tear. Indeed, I already noticed a tear in the middle of the right semi-velum. The fact that the tear occurred at this point, and not at the point of transection, was probably due to the higher coarseness and strength of the margins. To release this tension, and to ascertain the success of the operation, I transected the anterior mucosa of the velum and the muscle fibers of the *constrictor isthmi faucium* at both sides of the approximated cleft, using an oblique cut with the knife which ascended in a lateral direction. The unpleasant sensation of tension immediately subsided. The patient was advised to keep as quiet as possible. For a period, he was forbidden to eat and to drink; he was requested to allow his saliva to drain from the mouth. . . .

On the fourth day the inferior ligature had transected the margin. On the fifth day I removed the other two ligatures. The approximation held until the sixth day. On the seventh day the margins in this area separated once again and only an area 3 to 4 lines in width remained approximated during the subsequent days. . . . Nevertheless, the opening is somewhat smaller and this is the basis for the hope of this man for a second operation, which he intends to have during the summer.

J. F. Dieffenbach, M.D.
General Practitioner
Berlin

COMMENTARY BY DR. EDUARD SCHMID

Goldwyn has drawn a vital picture of the life of Johann Friedrich Dieffenbach and his extensive surgical and research accomplishments, particularly with regard to plastic surgery (Plast. & Reconstr. Surg., *42:* 18, 1968). With regard to the Classic Reprints herein, I would like to supplement Dieffenbach's statements.

The old authors, even Dieffenbach and his contemporaries, still regarded the uvula as an important organ which, amongst other things, kept the lungs free of dust, warmed the air, and had a considerable pathogenetic function. In the opinion of Hippocrates, it was dangerous to resect a severely swollen uvula. Branding irons were used, and so were caustic agents and the sliding loops which they constructed. Astringent gargling fluid and paintings with diluted hydrochloric acid (perhaps mixed with equal parts of honey) were prescribed to invigorate a relaxed uvula; elder and malvae tea and other agents were prescribed, conversely, to relax the uvula.

Dieffenbach reported that he observed prolongation of the uvula frequently in his practice, and that he had cured many cases with significant respiratory symptoms by cutting off the uvula. He felt that this operation was also a means to combat early tuberculosis of the trachea.

Dieffenbach, the successor of Gräfe at the Charité, translated Roux's article ("Mémoires sur la Staphyloraphie," Paris 1822) and instead of cotton sutures he introduced a wire suture of non-oxidated, non-aged lead, which was as pure as possible. His suture, probably a precursor of Veau's wire suture, was undoubtedly an advance. However, it produced severe, painful tension which may have threatened the suture line in the sutured soft palate—particularly in patients with broad clefts. This changed with Dieffenbach's introduction of the lateral relaxation incision.

Though surgeons then did not as yet know suture closure in layers, the sutures were removed on the 5th and 6th days—after testing the suture line with an impaled painting brush; this was much too early.

Dieffenbach also carried out the first attempt of total reconstruction of an almost completely absent soft palate from the buccal mucosa. This attempt failed, and a repetition of this operation, which was planned, did not take place.

Closure of the hard palate was also associated with major difficulties. Osteotomy of the palatine plates, which is advocated in this article, was first used in patients by Wutzer (1834). As this operation was performed at that time only in adolescents, growth disorders were not produced as yet.

One might also mention an attempt at closing a cleft of the hard palate by Krimer (1824), who sutured mucosal flaps which were pedicled on the margins.

Dieffenbach was an excellent observer. He had observed the stimulating effect of plates which bridged residual defects, and of obturators. He also noted that, in the course of time, this stimulating effect (in combination with the use of Cantharides-tincture) produced closure of residual openings as wide as a finger.

Thorough as he was, Dieffenbach extensively studied the anatomical structures, including their comparative anatomy and their variations, to be able to arrive at conclusions on the basis of their functional effects; he investigated also the problem of the development of cleft formation in embryos. With his friend Kleeberg, from Königsberg, he arrived at correct concepts regarding the time of cleft development, as well as its character as an inhibition-malformation of the palatine processes which had failed to unite.

Later, he also observed the favorable effect of staphylorraphy on decreased hearing. He was convinced that he had cured patients who were deaf.

Eduard Schmid, M.D.
Stuttgart, Germany

SUTURE OF THE PALATE

NATHAN SMITH, M.D., *New Haven, Conn.*

(*Am. M. Rev.*, 3: 396, 1826)

The effect of suture of the lip in partially closing the fissure of the palate, when this deformity exists together with hare-lip, some time since suggested to me the propriety of applying the suture, when the operation is performed at an early period, directly to the palate itself.

Every one must have observed that, when in early infancy the suture of the lip is properly made, the gentle pressure which the lip, then more straight than natural, exerts upon the cleft portions of the jaw, has a tendency gradually to approximate them, for at this time the bones of the face being yet in part cartilaginous, readily yield to little force.

Something more than a year since, in the state of Maine, a case occurred to me in which I judged it proper to attempt the more perfect closure of the palate by sutures applied directly to that part itself. I reflected that the parts must at that period (infancy) be so soft as to offer but little resistance to the needle, and so yielding as to be brought, with little force, in close contact with each other. It ap-

peared to me, also, that the closure of the lip would be much more complete by thus bringing the sides of the jaw into their natural situation with respect to each other.

The operation was accomplished with less difficulty than I had anticipated. The margins of the palate were pared with the knife, and a ligature of suitable size, with a needle very much curved, was carried through on one side, a sufficient distance from the margin, and brought back through the opposite. Two threads were employed in this manner, and the parts were brought into contact with very little difficulty. I have not since seen the patient but have reason to believe that the operation was perfectly effectual.

I have since seen an account of a similar operation performed by an English surgeon.

Nathan Smith, M.D.
Professor of Surgery
Yale College
New Haven, Conn.

STAPHYLORAPHE, OR PALATE-SUTURE, SUCCESSFULLY PERFORMED*

ALEXANDER H. STEVENS, M.D., *New York, N.Y.*

(*North Am. Med. & Surg. J.*, 3: 233–238, 1827)

Mr. Thomas Pearsall, aged 25 years, of Greene County, New York applied to me in September, 1826 for advice respecting a machine he wished to have fitted for a congenital division of the palate.

The division extended from about the

* From the Department of Surgery, College of Physicians and Surgeons.

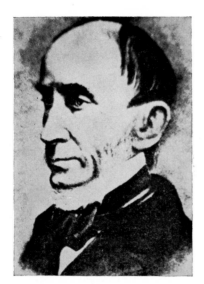

FIG. 1. Alexander Hodgon Stevens, M.D. (1789–1869). (From Packard, Francis R.: *History of Medicine in the United States*. Hafner Publishing Co., New York, 1963.)

anterior part of the palatine bones directly backwards in the median line, through the *velum pendulum palati* and uvula. The retraction of the parts left an opening like an inverted V, with a rounded top or, perhaps, more like the Greek letter Ω; but in the space between the palatine bones, the soft parts projected a little on each side towards the median line.

I proposed to him an operation for uniting the divided parts, which appeared to be rather separated than wanting. He assented to this and having, by my advice, arranged his affairs and provided himself with a person to attend to his wants, he agreed not to speak or swallow anything whatsoever for 4 days. I performed the operation in the following manner.

The patient being seated near a window, and his head thrown back and supported by an assistant standing behind, I interposed a handkerchief, tightly rolled up, between the molar teeth of the right side, and depressing the tongue with the left hand, introduced with the right hand a curved needle, armed with a thread, passed through an opening near its point. The head of the needle formed a small screw, and was received into a straight cylinder of iron, furnished with a female screw for the purpose. The needle was passed through the lower part of the velum pendulum, opposite the base of the uvula, and on the left side, about one-sixth of an inch from the edge. The shaft was now unscrewed, and the needle brought out. The two ends of the thread were then held back at the angle of the mouth, and two other ligatures were introduced in a similar manner, and then also on the opposite side. With a hawk's-bill forceps, I now seized the anterior part of the divided palate and inserting a cataract knife about one line anterior to the division, pared off a thin slice of the membrane on each side. One end of each of the ligatures was next tied to one end of the corresponding ligature on the opposite side, and the knot was then drawn through and divided. The lower ligature was then drawn with a surgeon's knot and a single knot upon it; next, the middle and, lastly, the upper one; and the ends of each cut closely.

The operation lasted nearly one hour, time being given, in the intervals of introducing the threads, for the patient to rest and recover from the efforts to vomit, which were occasioned by them, and also for the bleeding to cease. The patient, by request, went to bed to prevent hunger, and did not speak or swallow anything for 4 days, only wetting his mouth with cold water.

At the expiration of the fourth day, I removed the threads, and found the parts perfectly united. On the morning of the fifth day, when I visited him, I found he had already taken a bowl of rye mush and milk; no separation of the parts had taken place. An astringent gargle was prescribed. In the afternoon he ate several pies, and began to speak freely, but not with much improvement in his articulation. Supposing it might proceed from the division of the uvula, the parts of which hung like a swallow's tail from the end of the velum pendulum, I removed one of them. The inflammation soon subsided, and on the tenth day, he came to take leave, being about to return home. The parts were entirely united, and the inflammation scarcely perceptible. The voice was materially improved but far from being perfect. He felt that the air did not go so much up into his nose as before the operation, or on the first days after it; and that the palate was not so tightly stretched across his mouth as before. Indeed, it was evidently getting further back than it was at first, in consequence of its yielding.

This young man was operated upon in the presence of Dr. E. G. Ludlow, of this city, and was visited in the progress of his case by Dr. Hodge, of Philadelphia, and Dr. Kissam of this city.

I am not aware that this operation has been attempted before in this country; the author of it is Mr. Roux, of Paris; he first performed it upon a Mr. Stephens, a medical gentleman of Canada. Mr. R. states that the speech was corrected as soon as the ligatures were applied. It was not so in Mr. Pearsall's case. Mr. R. does not enter into the particular mode of tying the ligatures.

Mr. Alcock of London has also performed the operation but did not succeed in effecting union on the first trial, except at the lower part of the soft palate; and was obliged to repeat the operation 5 or 6 times, with threads and with needles, owing, as I conceive, to his applying a single, instead of a surgeon's knot, and to his not preventing the patient from speaking or swallowing until union had taken place. Mr. A. states that the reason patients do not receive the perfect use of speech immediately after the union of the parts is that they require to be taught to place the tongue against the roots of the front teeth, in making such sounds as *c*, soft *s*, and *th*, and by diligent attention to attain the pronunciation of the different words.

I regret that my patient left me before I could test the value of these directions. I apprehend, however, that it is necessary for the *velum pendulum palati* to hang somewhat loosely across the fauces in order to close the opening of the posterior nares, in speaking. I therefore infer that Mr. Pearsall will ultimately acquire a perfect power of enunciation.

Alexander H. Stevens, M.D.
Professor of Surgery
College of Physicians and Surgeons
New York, N.Y.

COMMENTARY BY THE EDITOR

These are the first two descriptions of cleft palate closure published in America; they appeared 7 and 8 years after Roux's paper in Paris.

Considering that sailing vessels commonly required 6 to 8 weeks to cross the Atlantic in those days, and that they came infrequently and had many things to carry of more urgent necessity than medical journals published in foreign languages, this delay is not surprising. It is obvious, of course, that these authors would have had no knowledge of the lateral incisions and attempts at uranoplasty published in Germany the year before by Dieffenbach.

Nathan Smith was born in Massachusetts in 1762 and obtained his M.D. degree from Harvard College in 1790. He prompted the establishment of a professorship in medicine at Dartmouth in 1798 and taught there from 1798 to 1813. From 1813 to 1829 he was a professor at Yale College. Besides this article, he is known for a treatise on typhus, for performing one of the early ovariotomies, and for doing one of the first amputations in this country through the knee joint. He was editor of the *American Medical Review,* in which this brief note on cleft palate closure appeared.

Alexander Hodgon Stevens (Fig. 1) was born in 1789, graduated from Yale College, and then attended the University of Pennsylvania where he got his M.D. in 1811. He served then as a house surgeon in the New York Hospital for 7 months. During the War of 1812, he sailed to Europe bearing dispatches and the ship he was on was captured by a British cruiser. Stevens was put in prison at Plymouth, England. After his release, he went to London and studied under Astley Cooper, then to Paris where he served as an intern. While attempting to return to the United States he was again taken prisoner, but was not detained for long.

A few years after his return, he became Professor of Surgery in the College of Physicians and Surgeons of New York. Later he was one of the founders and then President of the New York Academy of Medicine; he served also as President of the New York State Medical Society and of the American Medical Association. Stevens translated Boyer's *Surgery* from French into English, and edited an American edition of Astley Cooper's *Surgery.* By any standard, he was one of the most prominent American surgeons of his day. Following the great scandal at Bellevue Hospital in 1847, a blue-ribbon committee was appointed to reorganize the medical staff; the two surgeons on that committee were Valentine Mott and Alexander Stevens.

It is not clear whether this early staphylorrhaphy was done in Bellevue Hospital, The New York Hospital, Dr. Stevens' office, or elsewhere. Except for this omission, his description of the work and the postoperative course is a model for clarity.

CLOSURE OF CLEFT PALATE

ROBERT LISTON, M.D.

London, England

(Reprinted from pp. 471–473 of Practical Surgery, *by Robert Liston, M.D., John Churchill, London (Soho), 1837)*

The *velum palati* sometimes is found entire, though the bones are so far deficient, and *vice versa*. In general the fissure extends through both, causing difficulty in receiving nourishment. Many children are imperfectly nourished, and perish in consequence. When the individual grows up, he still finds an effort necessary to prevent food from passing through the nostrils and his articulation is very indistinct and disagreeable.

In the majority of cases the patient must content himself with having a plate of metal properly fitted to occupy the space, and this may be constructed with a movable portion behind, or not, as circumstances seem to demand or permit. Occasionally cases present themselves in which the space is not very wide betwixt the two portions of the velum and uvula, and the deficiency of the hard palate is not considerable. At a proper age, when the patient, having attained the years of discretion, is willing to submit to some pain and inconvenience, to afford every facility for the accomplishment of the operation, and to throw no obstacle in the way of the union, an attempt may be made to bring that about. It is only, however, in very favourable instances that this velo-synthesis should be attempted; for if the edges do adhere in part, and are put upon the stretch, the patient is not much benefitted, if at all; he is not by any means rewarded for all his pain, anxiety, and self-denial. The muscles of the velum cannot act even so perfectly as before, and the proceedings of the dentist in fitting an artificial palate are rather interfered with than otherwise.

When everything is favourable and the operation is determined upon, the plan of procedure must be well considered beforehand, and the apparatus calculated to effect the different objects got in readiness. This consists of narrow, sharp-pointed knives for the incisions, long, sharp-pointed forceps and needles to carry through the ligatures, and instruments to assist in seizing and drawing them tight: the incisions may first be made or the ligatures introduced previously, according to the fancy of the operator. I have generally pared the edges, given the patient plenty of time to clear the throat of blood, and recover his composure, allowed the bleeding to stop, and the irritability of the parts to abate before interfering farther.

The first part of the operation is not attended with much difficulty. The knife, held by the further end of the handle, is introduced through the edge of the fissure at its anterior margin and run back to the apex of the half of the uvula. This may be laid hold of and made tense by means of the forceps already described. The same proceeding is repeated on the other side, the knife being used by the right and left hand, respectively, if the operator can so manage it.

The introduction of the ligature is more easily accomplished in the simple manner here represented than by the use of any of the contrivances, forceps, or port-aiguille's that have been invented. The needles of different sizes and curves, fixed in handles, somewhat resembling those shown at p. 282, are passed through the velum from about a quarter of an inch, or more, from its free edge and towards it. They should penetrate two-thirds of its thickness. This needle carries a double ligature, the noose of which is caught by a blunt hook and pulled out into the mouth, whilst the instrument is withdrawn.

A second and smaller ligature is carried through opposite to this, and by means of this second thread, the first and double one is brought through. By a repetition of this proceeding, two, three, or more points of interrupted suture are made.

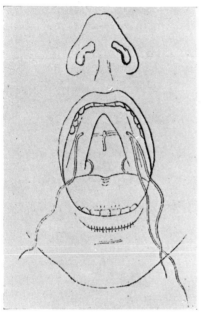

FIG. 1.

After the edges are put together by one or two points, no difficulty will be experienced in carrying others through both edges by means of a more curved instrument in a handle, or by the use of a small needle, carried in the points of a pair of strong and well-fitted forceps.

Before the ligatures are finally secured, the parts being put upon the stretch, an incision should be made on each side towards the alveolar ridge (Fig. 1) through the anterior surface of the velum. The dotted lines in the above sketch indicate the position and extent of these. By this method the edges come together more easily, and the strain is taken off the threads, so that there is less risk of these making their way out by ulceration.

All motion of the parts should be guarded against as much as possible. The patient should make no attempt whatever at articulation for many days, and his efforts at deglutition should be as slight and rare as possible. The risk of failure is considerable; the parts are not favourably circumstanced for union; their involuntary movements, the moisture by which they are bathed on all sides, are greatly opposed to the process; yet by careful adaptation of the parts, and by the precautionary means calculated to relax and keep them quiet, a favourable result may often be anticipated.

Robert Liston, M.D.
University College Hospital
London, England

COMMENTARY BY THE EDITOR

We have here, in my opinion, the first well-planned and lucidly described operation for closure of the cleft palate. In it is illustrated, for the first time, lateral relaxing incisions.

Curiously, this was a part of the Chapter on Harelip Operation in the 1837 edition of Liston's book, where it was attached as a seeming afterthought. Liston's books on operative surgery were not casual afterthoughts, however; they were carefully written and the most popular works extant in this field during the early and middle part of the 19th century. This book went through 4

editions within 9 years, and was a jewel. We tend, I think, to concentrate too exclusively on journal articles and to forget that many landmarks in surgery were first described in books.

What about the man?

Robert Liston was born in 1794 in Linlithgow, Scotland. He studied surgery in Edinburgh under John Barclay, but spent most of his working life in London. In 1834, he was appointed professor of surgery in University College, London, and soon became noted as one of the most resourceful and skillful surgeons in that metropolis.

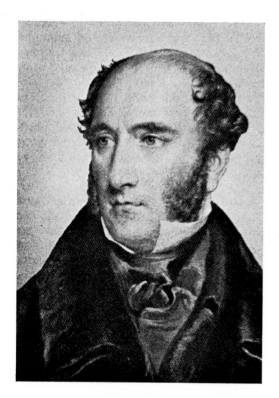

ROBERT LISTON
1794–1847

A man of great physical prowess, he had arms and hands which were often likened to those of Hercules. Bettany writes, "He would amputate the thigh single-handed, compress the artery with his left hand, using no tourniquet, and do all the cutting and sawing with his right." He was said to be very skillful, also, in the delicate operations of plastic surgery which required great dexterity.

Liston was the first in England to remove a scapula, the designer of the Liston splint for use in thigh dislocations, and he proposed a special mirror with which to examine the larynx. He is most remembered for two things, however. *1.* As the first distinguished surgeon in England to use ether as an anesthetic—on December 21, 1846 in University Hospital, London, for a thigh amputation. (John C. Warren and Morton's use of ether was first described in the *Boston Medical and Surgical Journal* of November 18, 1846.) *2.* For his astounding books on operative surgery.

This remarkable Scottish surgeon and author died in London on December 7, 1847.

—*Frank McDowell*

OPERATIONS FOR FISSURE OF SOFT AND HARD PALATE

J. MASON WARREN, M.D., *Boston, Mass.*

(*Excerpts reprinted from New England Quart. J. Med. & Surg., 1: 538, 1843*)

(*Excerpt 1*)

The form of operation which I have practised will be best illustrated by the relation of the first case in which it was put into execution.

The patient was a young man, 25 years old, with a congenital fissure of the soft and hard palate, the bones being separated quite up to the alveolar processes, with a deviation to the left side. On looking into the mouth, the whole posterior fauces were exposed, with the openings of the eustachian tubes and the bottom of the nasal cavity of the left side distinctly visible. The speech of the patient was rendered so indistinct, by this misfortune, that it was with the greatest difficulty that he could make himself understood. Deglutition had always been imperfectly performed, liquids, particularly, being swallowed with much difficulty, and often regurgitated through the nose. At the first glance the soft parts were scarcely perceptible, being almost concealed in the sides of the throat from the action of the muscles. On being seized by a forceps they could be partially drawn out, though with great resistance. So far as any of the old methods were applicable to the relief of this extensive fissure, the patient was beyond surgical aid. I determined, however, to put in practice the operation which had before appeared to me practicable.

The patient was placed in a strong light, his mouth widely opened, and the head well supported by an assistant; with a long, double-edged knife, curved on its flat side, I now carefully dissected up the membrane covering the hard palate, pursuing the dissection quite back to the root of the alveolar processes. By this process, which was not effected without considerable difficulty, the membrane seemed gradually to unfold itself, and could be easily drawn across the very wide fissure. A narrow slip was now removed from the edges of the soft palate, and with it the two halves of the uvula. By this means a continuous flap was obtained, beginning at the roots of the teeth and extending backwards to the edges of the *velum palati*. Finally, six sutures were introduced, on tying of which the whole fissure was obliterated. The patient was directed to maintain the most perfect quiet, and to abstain from making the slightest efforts to swallow even the mucous which collected in the throat, which was to be carefully sponged out as occasion required.

The following day he was doing well. He complained of some pain, or rather a sensation of excessive emptiness of the bowels, which was relieved by the use of a hot spirituous fomentation. On the third day, a slight hacking cough commenced, owing to the collection of thick ropy mucous in the throat and air passages. The cough was temporarily relieved by an injection of a pint of oatmeal gruel into the rectum; during the night, however, it again increased so much as to tear away the upper and lower ligatures. I now allowed him to take liquid nourishment, which at once quieted the irritation in the throat. The other four ligatures were removed on the following

From the Harvard University School of Medicine.

days, the last being left until the sixth day after the operation. This patient returned home into the country at the end of 3 weeks, a firm fleshy palate being formed behind, and half the fissure in the bony palate obliterated.

In the following spring I again operated on the remaining fissure in the hard palate, and succeeded in closing about half the extent of it, the tissues yielding with some difficulty, owing to the inflammation caused by the former operation. The small aperture which remained I directed to be closed by a gold plate. His speech was very much improved at once as well as the powers of deglutition, and he will, no doubt, ultimately, as the soft parts become more flexible, to a great degree recover the natural intonations of the voice.

Since performing this operation, I have had occasion to repeat it in 13 different cases, which with one exception have terminated successfully, either in the closure of the whole fissure, or of both hard and soft palate, or so far that the aperture which remained in the bones could be easily closed by an obturator fitted to the adjoining teeth.

(Excerpt 2)

The last case to which we shall allude, was operated on in the month of December, 1842. The patient was a young man, 20 years old, from Cambridge, whose prospects in life were materially affected by the malformation under which he labored, a division of the hard and soft palates, the bony separation being about three quarters of an inch. His speech was very imperfect; the deglutition not much affected. I was assisted in the operation by Dr. Hayward, Jr., Dr. Wellington, of Cambridge, and Mr. Townsend. The cutting part was done as in the preceding case, followed by the introduction of sutures. The threads were all removed in 48 hours, the adhesion being perfect. A small aperture after-

wards appeared at the upper angle of the fissure, from a slough where the threads had been too tightly drawn; by touching this with the nitrate of silver, it was obliterated in a fortnight, and his speech almost completely restored. He was seen by a number of medical gentlemen before leaving town. In this case the improvement of speech was at once more marked than in any previous case; as a reasonable amount of time must necessarily be supposed to elapse even in the most simple fissures, before the soft parts, stretched almost to the tightness of a drum-head, can be expected to regain their natural and healthy movements.

I shall now proceed to make some remarks on various interesting circumstances which have been presented, both in the forms of this affection, and in the method of operation.

(Excerpt 3)

As the dissection approaches to the connection of the soft parts with the edges of the *ossa palati,* where the muscles are attached and the union most intimate, great care must be taken or the mucous membrane will be perforated, and from these causes I have found this part of the operation to be the most embarrassing. As soon as this dissection is terminated, it will generally be found that by seizing the soft palate with a forceps it can be easily brought to the median line. If the fissure is wide, and this cannot be effected, I have found the following course to be invariably followed by success. The soft parts being forcibly stretched, a pair of long, powerful French scissors, curved on the flat side, are carried behind the anterior pillars of the palate; its attachments to the tonsil and to the posterior pillar are now to be carefully cut away, on which the anterior soft parts will at once be found to expand, and an ample flap be provided for all desirable purposes.

The edges of the palate may now be

made into a raw surface by seizing them on either side with a hooked forceps and removing a slip with the scissors or a sharp-pointed bistoury. Our next object is to insert the ligatures, and for this purpose an immense armory of instruments have been invented. After the trial of nearly all of them I have found the most simple to be the most effectual. A small curved needle being armed with a strong silk thread, confined in a forceps with a movable slide, is introduced to the upper edge of the fissure, the needle being carried from before backwards on the left side, and from behind forwards on the right, or *vice versa*. In this manner, three, four, or more ligatures may be successively introduced. The patient is now requested to clear his throat of mucous and blood, the ligatures are wiped dry and waxed, and tied with deliberation, beginning at the upper and proceeding gradually downwards, waiting a little between each ligature, in order to allow the throat to accommodate itself to this sudden and almost insupportable tension of the soft parts. No forceps are required for holding the first knot while the second is tied; the object is better effected by using the surgeon's knot, that is, by making two turns of the thread instead of one, and by enjoining perfect quiet on the patient for the moment, until the second knot is tied.

J. Mason Warren, M.D.
Massachusetts General Hospital
Boston, Mass.

COMMENTARY BY THE EDITOR

For the best biography of Mason Warren, read the fascinating one by Robert Goldwyn in this book.

Warren carried the primitive uranoplasty of Dieffenbach far forward. He became, probably, the most skilled in the world at closing the complete cleft palate, in the period of 1840 to 1860. Patients with this problem were referred to him from far and near.

Although he referred briefly to a single case in an earlier communication on rhinoplasty (*Boston M. & S. J., 22: 361, 1840*), this is his first complete description of the well-developed and successful uranoplasty. His discovery that it was easier and better to peel the soft tissues bluntly up off the oral surface of the palatine bones than to attempt to dissect the mucosa, was a real milestone. Though Liston had developed Dieffenbach's casual suggestion of a lateral incision into a definitive and routine little cut to relieve some of the tension, it was Mason Warren who extended it on back across the anterior pillar (and even the posterior pillar, when necessary) to really free the entire lateral mass.

Warren was the first to develop each side of the palate into a loose and relaxed flap which could easily be shifted to meet its fellow from the other side. It requires but little imagination for the reader to see here the mind and hands of a master surgeon at work. There are good reasons why many have called today's usual type of complete cleft palate closure the "Dieffenbach-Warren operation."

Though his success was said to have been more than 90 per cent in the closure of 100 complete cleft palates, Mason Warren fully recognized a thorny problem which remained—the difficulty in mobilizing the area near the connection of the soft palate with the palatine bones. "I have found this part of the operation to be the most embarrassing."

Others were plagued by this problem, too. In the following pages we shall learn of the measures they took to circumvent it.

—*Frank McDowell*

ON STAPHYLORAPHY

JOHN P. METTAUER, M.D. *Prince Edward, Virginia*

(Excerpt reprinted from *Am. J. Med. Sci., 21:* 309–332, 1837)

When the operation is to be executed, the subject of it should always be seated in a chair of convenient height, with a moveable back, regulated by a screw, similar to a barber's chair, upon the upper extremity of which a head piece must be fitted for the reception and support of the head, and padded or cushioned. The most favourable exposure for this operation is a southern one; the operation may nevertheless be executed and with much ease subjected to the mild light of northern exposure, in which situation we once operated without the least deficiency of light. The patient must be so placed that the light shall enter the mouth obliquely, or the surgeon so place himself as to contemplate the parts in a line passing near the commissures or angles of the mouth, so as not to intercept the light in its passage to the fauces with his head or hands. The period between the hours of 11 A.M. and 2 P.M. is the most favourable, as affording the best light.

After the patient is properly seated, and the head inclined upon the cushion of the sliding back of the chair, so as to give the light its direct passage to the fauces, the jaws are then to be separated and kept asunder by interposing between the teeth a soft bit of wood of convenient width, and thick enough at the edges where in contact with the teeth to prevent a rocking motion. . . .

When the cleft is confined to the uvula, or to this as well as the velum at the same time, any of the modes which have been adopted and practiced from the date of Graefe's first operation down to the present time, may be pursued. But the operation, as contrived and executed by Dieffenbach, unites more advantages than any other of which we have seen an account. . . . In our hands it has been successful more than once. . . .

(*Editorial note.* Dr. Mettauer followed with a 10-page description, in great detail, of his operative technique, which was based on that of Dieffenbach. After this, he described some of the "problem cases.")

The operations described in the preceding pages, as already remarked, are designed for the correction of the more simple forms of cleft palate, situated either in the uvula, or the uvula and the velum at the same time. They may also be rendered efficient in some of the examples in which the fissure involves the bony palate, or even the palatine processes of the superior maxillaries, when it exists as a fissure only, and without any material deficiency of substance. But when there is a separation of the margins to an extent which will not allow them to be approximated, besides the fissure, these methods alone will not be found sufficient, and for the correction of the deformity other expedients must be resorted to. . . .

The first operation contrived by us in a case of this description consisted of a series of incisions more or less extensive, formed exterior to the margins of the cleft, and parallel with them, extending from the faucial to the nasal surface on both sides. These incisions, being designed as granulating surfaces, were not allowed to reunite by the first intention, but kept apart by interposing between them small portions of buckskin or soft sponge, there to remain until suppuration should be well established, and then to be removed. . . .

(*Editorial note.* With the above, Mettauer introduced the use of lateral incisions in America. With the following, he just missed his chance to introduce the cutting of the tensor tendon.)

Should the parts be deficient in length, the method which we have been describing may be employed in a transverse direction, guided by the views just submitted, but not to divide the *tensor palati* muscle. . . .

The operation, which we have been describing is far less painful than *a priori* might be imagined; and with properly constructed instruments, for executing the sections, can be performed with comparative ease to the surgeon and entire safety to the patient. . . .

OBSERVATIONS ON CLEFT PALATE AND ON STAPHYLORAPHY

WILLIAM FERGUSSON, ESQ., *London, England*

(Excerpt reprinted from Medico-Chirurgical Transactions [London], *28:* 273–301, 1845)

. . . . Dr. Mettauer, of Virginia, recommends methods somewhat similar to both the plans above described (by me). He proposes to increase the breadth of the two flaps, by making a series of lunated incisions through the flaps, each about half an inch in length, along the margins of the fissure, which he causes to heal by granulation, and thereafter proceeds with the ordinary operation; or by another method, he relaxes the parts at the time of the operation, by making a longer incision on the lower surface of the palate on each side, but a little nearer the mesial line than that proposed by Mr. Liston. . . .

I have already in an early part of this paper referred to the method followed by Dr. J. M. Warren* in instances of fissure of the hard palate. . . . After describing his method of dissection of the soft tissues from the bones forming the roof of the mouth, he states that "it will generally be found that by seizing the soft palate with a forceps, it can be easily

* New England Quarterly Journal of Medicine and Surgery, April 1843.

brought to the mesial line. If the fissure is wide and this cannot be effected, I have found the following course to be invariably followed by success:—The soft parts being forcibly stretched, a pair of long powerful French scissors, curved on the flat side, are carried behind the anterior pillars of the palates; its attachment to the tonsil and to the posterior pillar are now to be carefully cut away, on which the anterior soft parts will at once be found to expand, and an ample flap be provided for all desirable purposes.". . .

If the free margin on one side of the fissure be seized with the forceps, drawn towards the mesial line, and the flap be then irritated, it will be drawn upwards and outwards with remarkable force; this movement, it is evident, can only be effected by two muscles, the *levator palati* and *palato-pharyngeus.* These muscles, then, I consider the chief mechanical obstacles to the junction of the margins in the mesial line. Hitherto I have taken no notice of the action of the circumflexus, or *tensor palati.* I am inclined to think that its action is very limited, and probably, as the dissection in my possession would indicate, is greater upon the parts outside the posterior pillar, than on those contiguous to the fissure. . . .

The incision recommended by Mr. Liston has evidently no reference to division of muscular fibres. . . . Dr. J. M. Warren, so far as I can understand his description, only separates the anterior pillar from the tonsil and posterior pillar, and makes no allusion to the division of muscular fibres. Possibly, however, by the clipping process which he describes, some of the fibres of the *palato-pharyngeus* may be divided.

Dr. Pancoast, in the language already quoted, certainly proposes "to divide the insertion of the palate muscles," but, as my demonstration proves, he cannot touch the insertion of one muscle, and can only reach the other, or a part of it, by hazard. . . .

I imagine that few who have listened to this paper throughout, will have any difficulty in anticipating what my proposals will be. I therefore, without further preamble, propose, as an important accessory to the operation of staphyloraphy, that the surgeon should . . . . so conduct his incisions as to destroy all motory power in the soft palate for the time being and thus permit that repose of the stretched velum which is so essential to a happy result; in other words, I advise the division of the *levator palati,* the *palato-pharygeus,* and the *palato-glossus* muscles. . . .

CLEFT PALATE—VELOSYNTHESIS

ROBERT LISTON, M.D. *London, England*

(Excerpt reprinted from pages 571–572 of Mr. Liston's book *Practical Surgery* [Fourth Edition], John Churchill, London, 1846)

. . . . All motion of the parts should be guarded against as much as possible. The patient should make no attempt whatever at articulation for many days, and his efforts at deglutition should be as slight and rare as possible. The risk of failure is considerable; the parts are not favourably circumstanced for union; their involuntary movements, and the moisture by which they are bathed on all sides, are greatly opposed to the process; yet by careful adaptation of the parts, and, by the adoption of the precautionary means calculated to relax and keep them quiet, a favourable result may often be anticipated.

Professor Fergusson, having had an opportunity of dissecting a case of split palate, and having observed the great developement of the *levator palati* and *pal-ato-pharyngeus* muscle, and thinking that they act forcibly in drawing the edges of the fissure apart, has recommended the division of these muscles as a preliminary step, and has invented a set of small crooked knives for the purpose. If the fleshy belly of the *circumflexus (tensor) palati* could safely be reached and cut, this would, as far as I can understand, put the parts in a still more favourable condition to come together. Its tendon is certainly divided by the incision above directed, properly and effectually carried out. The union is apt to fail under any circumstances, and I think that this was found to take place in the hands of the above named professor, even after the division of the muscles as he has recommended. . . .

COMMENTARY BY THE EDITOR

Operations sometimes develop slowly, inch by inch, and this seemed to be the situation with cleft palate closure in the 1830s and 1840s. Several surgeons in Europe and in America were able to close partial clefts successfully most of the time, but closure of complete clefts was a different story. Separation was frequent in the early postoperative period; it usually started at the junction of the hard and soft palate.

Liston's first timid lateral incisions, expanded greatly by Mason Warren, were a great advance—but there were still too many failures, even in the hands of these masters. It finally became apparent that in wide closures the contraction of the palatine muscles in swallowing and gagging tended to pull this area apart.

As so often happens, the first man to see the problem denied, almost in the same breath, the measure that would prevent it. The great John Mettauer of Virginia (and we shall hear much more of him later) was apparently the first to use lateral incisions in America and he had a phenomenal amount of success in cleft palate closure at this early date. His long paper, from which you have just read a small excerpt, was by far the most extensive treatise on the subject that had been published to this date. Naturally, it attracted much attention in America and in Europe. Apparently, his remark about not dividing the tensor tendon was enough to start Fergusson in London thinking about myotomies to temporarily still the palate in these cases.

Fergusson's 1845 paper, a brief excerpt of which is reproduced here, was a monumental work by one of the most distinguished surgical academicians of that time. It was the intensely practical Robert Liston, however, who brought attention back to cutting the tensor tendon.

—FRANK McDOWELL

OPERATION DER ANGEBORENEN TOTALEN SPALTUNG DES HARTEN GAUMENS NACH EINER NEUEN METHODE

(Operation on Congenital Total Cleft of the Hard Palate by a New Method)

PROF. DR. BERNHARD LANGENBECK

Berlin, Germany

(Reprinted from *Deutsche Klinik, 8:* 231, June 15, 1861. The following English translation is a free one which appeared in the "Foreign Correspondence" columns of the *Medical Times & Gazette,* of London, *2:* 69, July 29, 1861.)

At a recent meeting of the Medical Society of Berlin, Professor Langenbeck introduced a boy in whom he had effected a cure of congenital total cleft of the hard and soft palate by a new operative proceeding. A complete closing of this malformation has probably never yet been attained before. The trials made until now for this purpose may be classed under three different heads:

1. The separation of the mucous membrane of the hard palate at both sides of the cleft, and union by means of sutures of the parts of the mucous membrane, having been made moveable by lateral incisions. The fragility of the mucous membrane of the palate and its firm adhesion to the bone, especially at the anterior extremity of the hard palate, render this proceeding exceedingly difficult and insecure, while the circumstance of those parts containing very few blood-vessels, generally leads to more or less extensive gangrene of the mucous membrane. In two cases of total cleft of the hard palate in which M. Langenbeck made this operation in 1843 and 1844, the soft palate having been previously cured by staphylorraphy, the separated parts of the mucous membrane perished by gangrene, and he was by this result deterred from all further trials of the kind. The late Professor Dieffenbach has not been more fortunate in his efforts. In 1847, a short time before his death, he wrote to M. Langenbeck saying that the union of the soft palate was all that could be obtained by operation in cases of this kind. Mr. Fergusson, of London, has recently operated in this way with better results, as he succeeded, in small clefts of the palate, especially of the horizontal part of the *os palatinum,* in closing the defect by separation of the mucous membrane.

2. Implantation of flaps of mucous membrane into the defect. This method, which has been proposed by Krimer and Dieffenbach, is not at all to be recommended. In two cases in which M. Langenbeck tried it, the separated flaps of mucous membrane at once became necrotic.

3. Union of the broken-off edges of the bones of the deficient palate. Dieffenbach was the first to originate the idea of this operation, but he has never performed it himself. In a very large majority of cases, the cleft of the hard palate is unilateral, and there this operation could not be done; because the vomer is grown to one edge of the cleft, and would have to be broken off in order to bring the edges of

Editorial note. This is the first description of the use of mucoperiosteal flaps in cleft palate closures.

the defect near each other. The operation may, however, be performed in small bilateral clefts of the hard palate, and M. Langenbeck has done it twice in such instances, but without success. M. Bühring has resorted to this method in the operation of defects of the hard palate, caused by syphilitic necrosis, and has brought about an almost perfect cure; but, in such cases, the circumstances are very different from those of congenital defect of the palate. In total cleft of the hard palate this operation could not possibly be performed, as the osseous substance which is necessary for it is wanting.

The method recently employed by M. Langenbeck consists of separation of the mucous membrane of the palate, together with the periosteum, from the edges of the defect. The osteoplastic operations made before by this surgeon had given the result, that the mucous membrane of the palate may, together with the periosteum, be extensively separated without the bone or the separated membranes being in danger of necrosis. This fact justified the hope that a separation of these parts from the bone might be employed as a means for closing congenital clefts of the palate; and he expressed this hope on introducing a successful case of subperiosteal resection to the Society of Physicians. Since that time only clefts of the soft palate had come under his notice, and it was not until a few weeks ago that he had the opportunity of performing uranoplastics on a patient.

This patient, a boy aged 14, has been born with a cleft of the left lip and total cleft of the hard and soft palate together with the left alveolar process. The operation of hare-lip had been done soon after birth, but had failed; and a second operation made about a year afterwards, had been successful. On February 6 M. Lan-

genbeck united first the cleft of the soft palate by means of a needle-instrument especially invented by him for this purpose. On May 11 he closed the hard palate in the following manner. Close to the edges of the cleft, the mucous membrane and the periosteum of the hard palate were cut through to the bone by means of a strong knife, and the edges of the cleft freshed up. By means of a raspatorium placed into these incisions, the mucous membrane and the periosteum were then drawn off and separated by blunt levers from the two halves of the hard palate. Thus two flaps were formed which were only connected anteriorly with the gums at the alveolar process, and proceeded backwards into the soft palate which had been separated from the posterior margin of the *os palatinum*. The edges of these flaps were then united by five silken sutures in the median line, and thus the whole cleft, up to the front teeth, completely covered up. This separation of the mucous membrane of the palate and of the periosteum is troublesome, but can be done without in any way injuring other parts. The haemorrhage from the vessels of the periosteum necessitated repeated interruptions of the operation, which was, however, concluded in half an hour. After the sutures had been removed, which was done in the course of the second week, the cure by first intention was quite complete in the whole extent of the wound. The healed palate is only distinguished from a normal one by a fine cicatrix visible along its whole extent and a slight indentation at the top of the uvula. In another case of total cleft, in a woman aged 24, who came under M. Langenbeck's care a fortnight afterwards, he performed staphylorraphy and uranoplastics in the same sitting, and with the best result.

INTERMEZZO BY THE EDITOR

In a not uncommon custom of that time, von Langenbeck's original squib in the June 15 (1861) *Deutsche Klinik* was written in the third person, in a diffident manner, with a non-informative title. The Berlin correspondent of the *Medical Times & Gazette* (of London) was quick to see its importance, however, as his translation appeared in the July 29 issue of that journal.

The above evoked a quick reaction. In the "Original Communications" columns of the August 31 *Medical Times & Gazette* (*2:* 213, 1861), J. W. Hulke (of King's College Hospital and the Royal London Ophthalmic Hospital) disparaged Langenbeck's work—stating "this 'new proceeding' has long been very successfully practised by English Surgeons" and citing a partially successful case of his own, performed in 1859. (He cut the posterior palatine arteries, however, which Langebeck advised one to save. Hulke made no lateral incisions and decried the use, by Langenbeck, of blunt elevators instead of sharp knives.) In a later communication, Mr. Hulke stated that he was satisfied that the periosteum had been elevated by English surgeons, "though this may not have been done intentionally."

In the November 23 *Medical Times & Gazette* (*2:* 537, 1861), the foreign correspondent refutes Mr. Hulke, stating "Independently of the circumstance that no English Surgeon has ever mentioned the separation of the periosteum for the purpose of uranoplastics, it is very improbable that this operation should ever have been done because, hitherto, it was generally believed that detaching the periosteum was followed by necrosis of the bone . . . Mr. Hulke also states that gangrene of the flaps . . . was favoured by the use of blunt levers and raspatories. . . . This is a strange assertion, as levers and raspatories have never been used for uranoplastics until Professor Langenbeck did so, and this Surgeon has not only accomplished a perfect cure of total cleft just by means of blunt instruments, but also maintains that the periosteum can only be fully detached from the bone by levers and raspatories!"

In the *Medical Times* of January 11, 1862 (*1:* 44, 1862) Langenbeck's personal rejoinder appears. He wrote, about Hulke's statement, "Such a remark could never have been made by a person who had even once endeavoured to separate the periosteum from the palate, either in the dissecting room or in the living body. This proceeding is so laborious that it is not likely to occur accidentally . . . this can, in fact, only be accomplished by means of blunt levers by which the periosteum must be, as it were, lifted and torn off." Langenbeck mentions herein, also, the extensive treatise that he has published meanwhile in the second volume of his new journal *Archiv für Klinische Chirurgie*. Perhaps he had decided that the earlier short and diffident communique with the non-informative title would succeed only in losing the most important discovery of his life. Perhaps he over-reacted when he made this second (following) paper 82 pages in length, florid and turgid with repetitive and elaborate German prose.

In this *opus magnum*, Langenbeck starts by pointing out the differences between staphylorrhaphy and uranoplasty, and tracing the history of cleft palate surgery. He relates then the efforts of various European and American surgeons to close clefts in the hard palate by shifting either mucosal flaps, or full-thickness flaps containing bone. He notes the high incidence of failure, often due to gangrene, and then describes the anatomy of the palate in great detail—especially the blood supply. He differentiates the various types of clefts, and puts forth his reasons for believing mucoperiosteal flaps to be better—as well as the blunt instruments he has devised for raising them (Fig. 1). Finally, he describes the technique of the operation, and then repeats much of this information in 5 lengthy case reports.

This great work is far too long for reproduction here, but a few short excerpts will be presented. May the curtain please rise now, on these excerpts?

—*Frank McDowell*

DIE URANOPLASTIK MITTELST ABLÖSUNG DES MUCÖS-PERIOSTALEN GAUMENÜBERZUGES

(Uranoplasty by Means of Raising Mucoperiosteal Flaps)

BERNHARD LANGENBECK, M.D.

Berlin, Germany

(Excerpts, reprinted from *Arch. f. klin. chir.*, 2: 205–287, 1861)

No. 1. Total Cleft of the Hard and Soft Palate. Staphylorrhaphy and Uranoplasty. Healing.

Ernst Strehlow, 13½ years old, from Pollnow near Koslin, was a very intelligent and strongly developed boy who had been born with a left-sided lip cleft and a total cleft of the palate. The cleft lip had been operated on soon after birth, however without success, but in another operation in his second year this was healed. For healing of the palate cleft he was received in our clinic.

The cleft of the hard and soft palate was of precisely the same extent and generally in the same proportions as in Case 2, shown in Figure 3 (*left*). . . .

On February 6, 1861, I did a staphylorrhaphy, after which he received the usual postoperative care for this operation. The raw surfaces created on the borders of the cleft velum were held together with 5 silk sutures; the muscles through two side incisions were severed.

February 7. Unimportant reaction. Neck ache and swallowing complaints. Hydropathic envelopment of the neck. Senna infusion.

February 10. The patient finds himself well. One suture came out.

February 15. The last suture came out. The closure is complete. The side incisions are cicatrized.

May 11. The boy has recovered completely from the last operation. His speech is much more understandable; the cleft remaining in the hard palate is about 1 to 1½ lines wide.

Uranoplasty

From the upper rim of the healed soft palate to the anterior rim of the cleft in the hard palate, I cut out a thin edge throughout the entire length, at the junction of the palate covering and nasal mucosa, until I was compelled to cut on bone. Through this cut, I worked outward with the hooked elevator from the right side of the cleft, separating the periosteum together with the mucosa of the hard palate; then with the help of the bent elevators, the entire expanse of the palatine covering was separated from the *pars horizontalis* of the palatine bone, in combination with the soft palate.

A second incision was made on the hard palate near the row of upper teeth, extending back to the soft palate; this served as an attacking point, from which the periosteum and mucosa was in the same way loosened. The envelope of the palate was, from the adjacent mucosa of the nasal septum on out to the gum on the right side of the hard palate, loosened and settled downward in the form of a thick, rigid, skin flap—after loosening it from the posterior edge of the palatine bone.

The mucoperiosteal covering of the left half of the palate was, somewhat differently, separated from the gum on one side to the free rim of the cleft on the other, and from the entire tissue of the palatine process and the *pars horizontalis* of the palatine bone. It was hanging anteriorly in the region of the left canine and incisor teeth, and posteriorly from the left half of the soft palate, with which it was in continuity.

Through these loosenings, the covering of the palate was completely shifted from both sides so that a complete union with 5 silk sutures was possible; the entire length of the cleft was completely closed. The operation required ½ hour, was done with little difficulty, and was accompanied by insignificant bleeding.

May 13. Slept well, pain and swallowing difficulties minor. The wound edges are lying together.

May 14. Since yesterday, onset of light fever and somewhat more pain in the neck. The covering of the hard palate, by swelling of the periosteum, has become very massive, arching itself over the oral cavity. It is of normal pale-red color, closed precisely in the region of the sutures, and the lateral incision on the left is completely effaced.

May 19. Patient is fever-free. The first suture came out. After that, on May 23, two more followed; on May 24, the last two came out and healing by primary intention became apparent throughout the entire length.

May 27. Today, on the 16th day after operation, the patient left his bed for the first time and the drawing in Figure 2 was made. On this, the scar in the midline represents the closure; the scarred incision on the inner side of the left alveolus is still visible. However, 4 weeks after the operation these lateral scars became finally covered and the color, as well as the form and arching of the hard palate became completely normal.

On the 29th of May, the healed child was shown to the Berlin Medical Association (*Deutsche Klinik, 24:* 232, 1861), and on June 24 he was discharged to his home. On careful palpation of the newly built hard palate, in the region of the

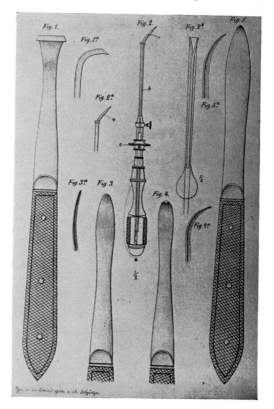

FIG. 1. Instruments designed and used by Langenbeck for uranoplasty. Fig. 1. = hooklike bent elevator. Fig. 2 = sewing tool to place the sutures (*a* = handgrip; *b* = stem; *c* = dial to release the spring, which is crowded within the tool). Fig. 2a = needle point, with the spring pulled back. Fig. 2b = thread carrier. Figs. 3, 4, 5 = raspatories (elevators) of various strengths and curves. (*Courtesy of National Library of Medicine, Bethesda, Md.*)

earlier cleft, over the greater part there was already bony consistency—but at one point the new bone formation had not

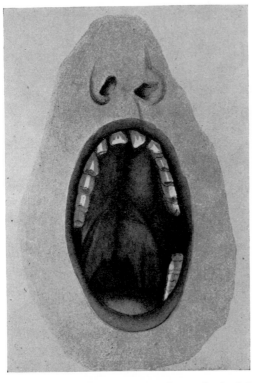

FIG. 2. *Case 1.* Shows the cicatrix on the healed palate 16 days after operation. Near the inside of the left row of upper teeth, the lateral incision appears as a scarred groove. (*Courtesy of National Library of Medicine, Bethesda, Md.*)

come to this. At the beginning of winter, the boy will enter the Institute to improve the form of his upper lip; through the opportunity thus afforded, the extent of the new bone formation will be checked.

No. 2. Total Cleft of the Hard and Soft Palate. Staphylorrhaphy and Uranoplasty in One Sitting. Healing of Hard Palate with Complete New Bone Formation. Not in Conjunction with Soft Palate (Figure 3).

Marie Müller, 24 years old, from Lubochow near Kalau, was born to a healthy family in which cleft palate had not occurred before.... She had a left-sided lip cleft, and a total palate cleft (Fig. 3, *left*).... The lip cleft was operated upon at 14 days after birth and luckily became united; how it came about, however, is a repetitive story.... Since December 1860 she had suffered from a profuse suppuration out of the right nostril; examination showed a necrosis in the region of the inferior turbinate and the nasal process of the maxilla.... On May 13, the necrotic material under the nasal muscle on the right side was extracted, and this resulted in her becoming ready for the palate operation in the following days.

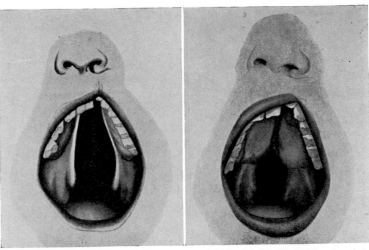

FIG. 3. *Case 2. (left)* Total palate cleft on the left side. (*right*) Healed hard palate, 3 weeks after the first operation. (*Courtesy of National Library of Medicine, Bethesda, Md.*)

On May 29, therefore, I made a uranoplasty and staphylorrhaphy. After I
freshened the rims of the cleft in the soft
palate, I used a strong scalpel similarly
along the left rim of the maxillary cleft,
cutting to the bone. Then I cut through
in the same way the covering of the right
side of the cleft rim in its entire length,
along the border of the nasal septum. A
right-angled raspatory was introduced
into the wound, with its blade placed
firmly against the bone, and the periosteum together with the palatine mucosa
was loosened up.

... Then I made an incision in the
hard palate near the row of teeth down
to the bone and loosened the palatine
mucosa together with the periosteum in
the same manner; similarly, I did the
same on the right side.... The two
lateral incisions were extended downward into the soft palate and through
them the muscles were severed. With the
help of the bent elevators, the palatine
mucosa together with the periosteum of
both sides of the cleft palate became completely loosened, and by cutting through
the mucosal upper attachments of the
soft palate to the posterior rims of the
bones, the palate flaps could be moved—
so that the connections to the bones remained only at 4 points (namely, at the
front end on either side behind the incision and canine teeth, and posteriorly in
the region of the pterygopalatine foram-
ina). However, the continuity between
the hard palate cover and the soft palate
was not interrupted. The two halves of
the palatine covering and the soft palate
were now completely displaceable, and
laid themselves firmly one against the
other.

The operation was, because of rest-
lessness of the patient and strong hemorrhage (which lasted until the tissues were
off the bones) difficult in the highest degree and was repeatedly interrupted. The
placing of the sutures was done very

quickly, so that the entire operation was
finished in 1½ hours. The first suture
was placed through the loosened covering right behind the incisor teeth, the
last through the uvula. In all, 12 sutures
were placed and afterward, as they were
tied in their sequence of anterior to posterior, the entire cleft was completely
concealed. The wound margins came
into exact contact, without overlap.

The patient then, somewhat exhausted
by the operation, took some wine by
spoon and went to bed. There was no
after-bleeding. . . .

(Editorial insert. On the 8th day, 3 sutures came
out of the soft palate and it opened. On the 11th
day, the sutures came out of the hard palate, but it
remained closed. Later, some drainage came out of
the old sequestrectomy site; a second sequestrectomy
was done there, through the nose and under chloroform anesthesia, one month after the palate closure.)

On July 29, 8 weeks after operation,
the hard palate was well healed and the
drawing in Figure 3 *(right)* was made.

(Editorial insert. Case 3 was a complete cleft of
the hard and soft palate, up to an intact alveolar
process anteriorly. Von Langenbeck closed it in the
same manner, in one sitting, but a violent infection
ensued and the closure broke down.)

*No. 4. Congenital Cleft of the Soft
and Hard Palate up to the Palatine
Process. Staphylorrhaphy and Uranoplasty. Healing to a Small Opening in the Soft Palate.*

Cecilie Lewin, 24 years old, from
Schubine, with a vigorous body but
poorly developed as a girl, was received
in the clinic on May 28, 1859. Three of
her sisters had cleft palates. She had a
wide cleft of the soft palate, extending
forward through the hard palate to the
palatine process. The alveolar process
was normally constructed, though the incisor teeth were irregular and slanted.

(Editorial insert. On June 20, 1859, Langenbeck
did a staphylorrhaphy in which he also undermined
only the mucosa of the adjoining hard palate; this
undermined mucosa was lost several days later, from
gangrene. After a long period, the soft palate healed
and the residual opening in the hard palate was 6

lines long and 4 lines wide. By a secondary repair, in which he raised mucoperiosteal flaps, this healed to a hole about half this size.)

(Case 5 concerned a congenital defect of the left maxilla, which was successfully closed by uranoplasty.)

COMMENTARY BY THE EDITOR

The designing of an operation (or operations) that would be routinely successful for closure of the complete cleft palate has been one of the most difficult feats in the entire realm of surgery. Always, it seemed, elusive success was just around the corner. For every step taken forward, another was taken backward; fortunately, some of the latter were shorter than the former.

The development of all this was incredibly tedious, spanning 150 years in time and a lifetime of disappointing efforts by countless surgeons—but progress was slowly made and some degree of success was finally attained.

As can be seen here, the "so-called" Langenbeck operation did not spring forth fully developed from his scalpel and pen. George Dorrance, in his incomparable book *The Operative Story of Cleft Palate* (W. B. Saunders Co., Philadelphia, 1933), recounts the many contributions to this operation made by various surgeons before and after von Langenbeck. What von Langenbeck did contribute was a most major step—raising the periosteum with the mucosa, by the use of blunt elevators, from just behind the incisors to the posterior edge of the palatine bones. This proved to be the long-awaited key to success.

Robert Goldwyn's article (in the back part of this book) is, I think, the most interesting biographical sketch of von Langenbeck. It contains, also, a fine portrait of this distinguished surgeon and editor.

—Frank McDowell

ON A NEW METHOD OF STAPHYLORRHAPHY

KARL SCHOENBORN, M.D., *Königsberg, Germany*

(*Arch. für klinische Chirurgie, 19: 527–531, 1876*)

Translated from the German by
DR. RUDOLF K. STELLMACH

I believe it is a known fact among most surgeons that healing of the congenital cleft palate can be achieved, with a high degree of certainty, by the uranoplasty introduced by von Langenbeck and by a staphylorrhaphy. However, after even the most successful operation the speech of these patients leaves much to be desired; there is severe nasality.

Intensive speech therapy and the use of electricity may improve this handicap to some extent, but the speech in many cases remains so poor that some people have attempted to modify the surgical method to obtain better speech. Others, however, have encouraged the patients to wear a Süersen obturator, rather than undergo surgery.

Passavant pointed out that the patient retains a nasal tone, despite the good healing achieved, because the newly formed soft palate is too short to accomplish velopharyngeal closure. He was not only the first to suggest, but also the first to try, surgical methods designed to correct this disadvantage. Joining together the palatopharyngeal muscles to partially close the pharynx, as well as to elongate the soft palate, gave him no satisfactory results. On the other hand, he achieved almost normal speech in a female patient by joining the posterior border of the soft palate to the posterior pharyngeal wall (the velopharyngeal suture of Passavant). As it proved difficult to carry out this operation, Passavant later attempted another method—a pushback of the entire soft palate.

I do not know if other cases have been successful after using one of these two methods; however, neither operation has found general acceptance.

Please allow me to bring a new surgical method to your critical attention, in which joining of the soft palate to the middle part of the pharyngeal wall can be achieved safely and simply. This consists of incorporating a flap, taken from the posterior pharyngeal wall, between the two halves of the soft palate.

About 4 years ago, as I was discussing with my friend and colleague Trendelenburg the possibility of closing an abnormally wide cleft palate (which we had the opportunity to see at the Surgical Clinic of the University of Berlin), he advanced the idea that it might be possible to join a flap from the posterior pharyngeal wall to the soft palate. If I remember correctly, he also made some important attempts on human bodies and animals; however, the operations appeared to be very difficult and, as far as I know, there were no further attempts.

Two years ago, I had the opportunity of carrying out a uranoplasty and staphylorrhaphy on a 4-year-old child under general anesthesia, after a tracheostomy was done. I was able to convince myself that under the same conditions it would be possible to detach a large, long flap from the posterior wall of the pharynx

Paper read on April 9, 1875 at the IV Congress of the German Society for Surgery, in Berlin.
Editorial note. This is the first description of the pharyngeal flap operation.

and to suture it safely, and without much difficulty, between the two halves of a dissected and mobilized soft palate.

I performed this operation on a female patient on July 2, 1874. This patient, Emma Kollecker, aged 17, had a congenital (unoperated) cleft of the hard and soft palate, extending to the incisive foramen. Both sides of the velum were underdeveloped. The patient spoke so badly that unless one was used to the strong nasal tone, she could not be understood.

After induction of general anesthesia and tamponade of the trachea (by the method of Trendelenburg), I made rim incisions along the cleft borders. With a long scalpel (similar to that which von Langenbeck used in making the first incision of the mucoperiosteum) I outlined a flap about two cm long and 4 to 5 cm wide, with its long axis vertically and its base *caudally*, from the posterior wall of the pharynx. (The flap should begin as high, cranially, on the posterior wall as possible, so that after detachment it can be brought easily and without tension at least up to the back edge of the hard palate.)

The incision was carried through the mucosa and underlying muscles. The detachment of the flap was not easy; I used a long scalpel with a two cm blade, bent at a right angle. (Since then, I have used two types of scalpels with double cutting blades, one pointed and the other blunt at the tip.) The upper edge of the flap was held with a small hook and, with the scalpel described, the flap was carefully detached (proceeding from the cranial end, caudally). (Particular attention must be paid to keeping the scalpel within the loose areolar tissue beneath the muscle, so that no part of the flap is thinner than the other.) Next, I detached the mucoperiosteal layer of the hard palate enough so that it and the soft palate were sufficiently mobile. Then I trimmed the edges of the flap so that it was in a triangular form, with the tip at the upper end. This was sutured then between the dissected two halves of the velum. I used the von Langenbeck needle-instrument, and 5 sutures were necessary on each side. The cleft in the hard palate was closed with 3 additional sutures.

As soon as the patient had regained consciousness from the chloroform anesthesia, her speech was tested and it immediately appeared to be better than it had been before the operation. The Trendelenburg cannula was replaced with a normal silver type after 24 hours. Swallowing was difficult during the first few days; otherwise, there was nothing unusual. Secretion of mucous and pus was rather heavy. All sutures were removed on the fifth day.

The take of the pharyngeal flap (between the halves of the velum) was complete on the right side; on the left side, between the tip of the uvula and the flap, there was non-union of about one cm. Non-union appeared also, remarkably enough, between the two parts of the detached mucoperiosteal layers of the hard palate—though there were neither signs of tension nor any form of difficulty in suturing them together. Consequently, there remained a cleft 3 cm long and 1½ cm wide in the hard palate. This was closed later, using the von Langenbeck procedure.

The result of the operation, as far as improvement of speech was concerned, was very important. Immediately after healing had taken place, the patient's speech was absolutely clear and easily understandable to everyone. The nasality had not disappeared completely, but it diminished from week to week as the patient learned, by speaking, to close both side openings through the activity of the pharyngeal muscles. These muscles, being on the sides of the pharyngeal flap, facilitate closing the communication between the nasal and oral cavity.

The patient had no difficulties in swallowing, nor in breathing through her nose. It is well known that such complaints are not typical of patients who have spontaneous union between the soft palate and pharyngeal wall, caused by several diseases, provided openings of not too small diameters still exist on both sides.

Until this patient, I had not seen such a remarkable improvement in speech immediately after healing took place, in a cleft of the hard and soft palate which had been closed by the usual surgical methods. For this reason, I would like to recommend this method for further testing.

The operations should be done in the following steps. The first step should be limited to achieving union between the pharyngeal flap and the velum. After healing, the second operation should be performed to close the cleft of the hard palate (uranoplasty). In this way, healing will probably be much safer than if one performs the operation in one stage, as I did on that patient.

I believe, further, that to carry out the first operation quite safely and without any risk of detachment of the flap, tracheostomy and blocking of the trachea should be preliminary precautions. In the future, I intend to operate in this way on all cases of clefts which involve the hard and the soft palate.

Karl Schoenborn, M.D.
Department of Surgery
University of Königsberg
Königsberg, Germany

PRESENTATION OF A PATIENT AFTER STAPHYLOPLASTY*

KARL SCHOENBORN, M.D., *Königsberg, Germany*

(Excerpts from Verhandl. d. deutsch. Gesellsch. f. Chirurgie, 15: 57–62, 1886)

Translated from the German by
DR. RUDOLF K. STELLMACH

Last year Dr. Julius Wolff presented a case of a cured cleft palate in which he used an obturator prosthesis to achieve a good end result. At the time, I stated that I still preferred surgical treatment and that, even in very difficult cases, a satisfactory functional result could be achieved. I am taking the opportunity to present a patient on whom I have performed a staphyloplasty.

I have now done the staphyloplasty on 20 patients. Of these, one died of septic pneumonia; in 3 other cases, the transplanted flaps became necrotic. Healing was achieved in 16 cases; in two of them it was limited to one side of the flap, but after a second operation the other side also healed. In the remaining 14 cases, healing was uneventful.

With time, the method of operation has become simple. After induction of general anesthesia, a tracheostomy is performed and Trendelenburg's tampon-cannula is inserted. The mouth is opened with Whitehead's gag, and the tongue is pressed down with the same instrument. . . .

A rather wide flap of the posterior pharyngeal wall is developed. Now, I regularly place its base cranially, high up around the pharyngeal tonsil. (Formerly I made the bases of these flaps caudally, but this is not ideal because the mucosa from the region of the adenoids is not suitable for suturing, being extremely fragile.) This flap is detached with the help of a long hooked forceps, and with Cooper's scissors. It is sutured to the raw edges of the two halves of the soft palate. . . .

As a rule, 3 sutures on both sides are needed. I never separate the muscles of

* Patient presented at the Third Session of the 15th Congress of the German Society for Surgery, on April 9, 1886, in Berlin.

the palate—so the operation is finished. It lasts about 45 minutes.

After 6 to 8 weeks, the wound in the wall of the pharynx is healed, and uranoplasty can be undertaken. However, it is better to wait for about 6 months, during which time the width of the cleft in the hard palate diminishes. . . .

The patient whom I introduce here had the staphyloplasty, as described, at the age of 8 years. It was followed by uranoplasty after 6 months, and repair of a fistula later.

The relatively small openings between the nasopharynx and the mouth do not interfere with breathing. The patient sleeps well and snores only a little. There have been no unusual instances of rhinitis. . . .

I am convinced that the operation should aim at later dividing the connection between the velum and pharynx again, if the patient maintains acceptable speech for some years. . . .

Using an obturator has the disadvantage of requiring several revisions over the years, if it is inserted in growing children. I have performed the staphyloplasty on patients from 5 to 22 years of age. It seems desirable to operate on patients so successfully that an obturator will not be needed.

Karl Schoenborn, M.D.
Department of Surgery
University of Königsberg
Königsberg, Germany

BIOGRAPHICAL SKETCH AND COMMENTARY BY
DR. RUDOLPH STELLMACH

Karl Wilhelm Ernst Joachim Schoenborn was born in Breslau, Silesia, on May 8, 1840. Later he became a medical student at the universities of Breslau, Heidelberg, Göttingen, and Berlin, getting his M.D. degree in 1863. His thesis was on "De Monstris Acardiacis," submitted to the Medical Faculty of the University of Berlin.

In 1864 he entered the surgical department of Bernhard von Langenbeck at the University of Berlin. Soon he became the favorite student and assistant of this great surgeon. Schoenborn worked there for 7 years in the field of general surgery. During the Franco-Prussian war (1870–1871) Schoenborn, being the oldest assistant of von Langenbeck, was appointed Chief of the Department of Surgery at the University of Berlin during Langenbeck's absence in battle. At the same time he took the chair of the famous surgeon von Bardeleben at the renowned Charité hospital.

After the war, being well acquainted with the Queen, he was appointed Professor of Surgery and Chief of the Surgical Depart-

ment at the University of Königsberg, in 1871. He remained there until 1886, when he accepted the opportunity to become Chief at the University of Würzburg, in Bavaria. There he lived until his death on December 11, 1906.

Schoenborn was an outstanding teacher and a splendid surgeon, but he did not write much and has left only a few articles. He helped found the German Surgical Association and was one of the founder members present at the first convention in Berlin, in 1872. Schoenborn was interested in various areas in the field of surgery, but his training with von Langenbeck, and his cooperation with von Bardeleben—both pioneers in cleft lip and palate surgery—inspired him to do much work in this field too. He followed the surgical lines drawn by his teacher, von Langenbeck.

Reading his original articles on staphyloplasty makes it clear that Schoenborn was a plastic surgeon. His clinical observations, his thinking in terms of handling tissues and tissue reaction, and his critical view of

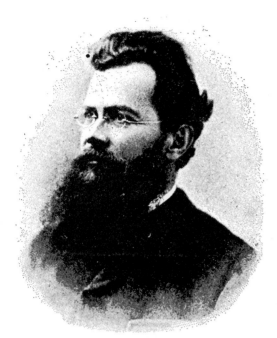

KARL SCHOENBORN
1840–1906

his own method of staphyloplasty make him a surgeon of a high level. The way he fought for his ideas at meetings of the German Surgical Society is impressive.

Reviewing all that he has said about the problem of pharyngoplasty, we find that he omitted almost nothing.

He was honest and modest enough to give credit to his friend Trendelenburg for the idea of building a flap from the posterior pharyngeal wall, aimed at bridging the distance to the velum. But Schoenborn is to be credited for his surgical innovations resulting from these discussions and other observations. He worked out the pharyngeal flap first with the base down, then up, and he gave exact explanations for the advantages of a superiorly-based pharyngeal flap. He even mentioned that the union between the velum and pharynx can and should be cut after a few years of normal speech, to re-establish the normal anatomical relationships in the upper pharynx.

Today, it seems curious that the work of Schoenborn was forgotten for almost 3 decades. The idea of pharyngoplasty was rediscovered in 1924 by Rosenthal, who did not know of the earlier work of either Passavant or Schoenborn. Rosenthal used a caudally-based flap. In the year of his death (1924) Trendelenburg (the man with the first idea of building the pharyngeal flap) wrote Rosenthal a fine letter of appreciation and congratulation, after his first publication of this type of pharyngoplasty. Trendelenburg apprised Rosenthal of the fundamental work of Schoenborn. From that time on, we speak of the Schoenborn-Rosenthal operation—meaning the velopharyngoplasty with the base downward.

Another 10 years were necessary before the rediscovery of the superiorly-based pharyngeal flap, brought forth again by Šercer in 1935. Sanvenero-Rosselli promoted the use of this type of pharyngeal flap, and he gets most of the credit for its use nowadays.

In the last years, my work in this field of plastic surgery has been to evaluate the temporary pharyngofixation of the velum (formerly used by Burian *et al*) with a cranially-based mini-pharyngeal flap. This velopharyngeal adhesion is done at the time of the soft palate repair, and we cut it through again after the establishment of normal speech.

All these ideas can be found in the papers of Karl Schoenborn. The time has come to give this great and modest surgeon his rightful place among the pioneers in the plastic surgery of cleft lip and palate.

Rudolph K. Stellmach, M.D.
Professor of Maxillofacial Plastic
Surgery
Free University of Berlin
Hindenburgdamm 30
1 Berlin 45, Germany

ON URANOPLASTY

PROF. THEODOR BILLROTH, *Vienna, Austria*

(*Wiener Klinische Wochenschrift, 2: 241, 1889.*)

Translated from the German by
DR. LEO CLODIUS, *Zurich, Switzerland*

In many cases, the results of staphylorrhaphy and uranoplasty, introduced by B. v. Langenbeck, did not fulfill the expectations for speech improvement. Good results were obtained for small acquired lesions (lues), but not for congenital defects. A complete surgical success in one operation was not always possible.

To achieve this goal, a number of trials were made. Each of these 4 patients we are presenting healed by first intention after one operation. The wound closure was done carefully, not merely by suturing the freshened wound edges, but by carefully adapting the nasal raw surfaces and by uniting them exactly by superficially placed sutures. The hitherto inconvenient purulent discharge from the open lateral wounds was successfully circumvented by packing with iodoform gauze.

In congenital defects, the muscles moving the soft palate are not just cleft, but powerless. This is the reason for the minimal postoperative speech improvement. In clefts of the soft palate alone, this muscle deficiency is minimal and, therefore, the postoperative functional result is best.

In clefts of the hard palate, the entire musculature of the soft palate, corresponding to the width of the cleft, is missing. In addition, these rudimentary muscles are transected by the lateral incisions.

During healing, the soft palate is pulled with the united soft tissues of the hard palate toward the vault of the hard palate, which, in these patients, is usually quite high. These factors explain the functional insufficiency of the muscles and the slight speech improvement postoperatively.

To avoid this bilateral sectioning of the muscles by the lateral incisions, I did not divide the entire thickness of the soft palate in my last operations. After the mucosa was incised, the medial plate of the wing of the pterygoid, above the hamulus, was cut with a narrow chisel. In this way, the hamulus was rendered somewhat mobile and could be moved (from either side) toward the midline, with its uninjured musculature.

Despite all this, the ability to completely separate the nasal from the oral cavity during speech was not achieved, in most cases, by the operation alone. Therefore, an attempt was made to close the remaining communication by a well-fitting obturator. Dr. v. Mettnitz was kind to make such an obturator, according to the commonly used models, for one of my patients.

Finally, to achieve a decent result the patients have to be reasonably intelligent. They have to learn to use muscles for speech which they did not voluntarily before. Dr. R. Coën undertook to instruct the patients in this respect. Cer-

---

Patient-presentation before the Imperial and Royal Medical Society of Vienna, March 15, 1889.

Editorial note. Herein the great Billroth describes, for the first time, the now common practice of fracturing the hamulus and moving it medially to relieve the tension created by the tensor muscle. *F. McD.*

tainly it will take months before a real success is established.

In one of the 4 patients presented, only a staphylorrhapy was performed. This patient speaks best. The 3 other patients had both uranoplasty and staphylorrhaphy. Of these, one patient wears an obturator.

I should like to add that in all 4 patients the cleft lip was closed before the end of the first year of life. You see, the cosmetic result is not quite excellent. The best cosmetic results in lip closure are obtained in adult patients.

Dr. R. Coën lets the patients read. He reports upon the status of speech, as regards which sounds were pronounced normal and which defective, before he starts instructions. Speech therapy consisted of making the patients read loudly and especially to accent the vowels, thus training the muscles. The sounds formed in the anterior oral cavity were pronounced more easily than the ones originating from the posterior oral cavity. The voiceless sounds were more difficult to pronounce than the voiced; the plosives were less distinct than the hissing sounds. $/L/$ is uttered most easily, $/G/$ with most difficulty.

Professor Exner mentions the physiological interest of these cases, because the adults, like children, must learn to speak. As opposed to the children, however, their disadvantage consists of the fact that the adults have to forget their previous language and innervation feelings and acquire new ones.

Theodor Billroth, M.D.
Chief, I Surgical Service
University of Vienna
Vienna, Austria

THE LIFE OF THEODOR BILLROTH

Billroth lived in a time of great surgical advances, when diseases thought to be purely medical came into the realm of surgery (*e.g.* diseases of the stomach). Surgeons ceased to be craftsmen and became physicians with a special therapeutic method.[1, 2]

Christian Albert Theodor Billroth was born on the Island of Rügen in the North Sea in 1829, the son of a pastor. His father died when he was only 5 years old. During gymnasium (high school), he was a mediocre student, without much concern for mathematics and ancient languages.

His main interest was music and he wanted to become a musician. Throughout life he loved and played the piano and violin, he composed music himself, and he became a close friend of Brahms.* His mother and his uncle (professor of pharmaceutics) decided, however, that medicine was a safer choice.

* *Editorial note.* If there are any who love surgery and love music, and who have not read the legendary and warm letters between Billroth and Brahms, please seek out the treat which awaits you.

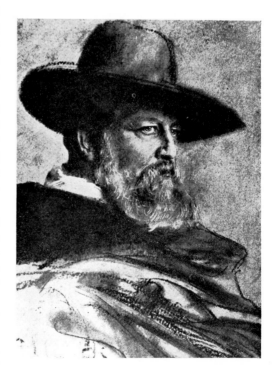

FIG. 1. Portrait of Billroth by Lenbach. (Vienna)

Thereupon, Billroth studied medicine in Greifswald, Göttingen, and in Berlin—where he became a disciple of Bernhard von Langenbeck. Frequently he visited the clinic of Albrecht von Graefe. In 1853 he began private practice in Berlin but during two months he saw not one patient. So he was happy to accept a position as assistant to von Langenbeck.

At first, his principal interest was pathologic histology. In 1856 he became "Privatdozent" and in 1858 he was offered the chair of pathologic anatomy at the University of Greifswald. However, he wanted to continue his career as a surgeon, especially since his courses in operative surgery had been most successful. Another reason was that he was allowed to continue his stay with von Langenbeck, even though married; he was allowed to live outside the hospital!

In 1860 Billroth was elected Professor of Surgery there in Zurich, where he stayed for 7 years; during this time he treated more than 8,000 surgical patients. In 1867 he was finally offered the famed chair of surgery in Vienna, which he occupied until his death in 1894. In 1870 he served as a volunteer in the ambulance corps of the German army. Later, he became one of the great pioneers in abdominal surgery and in 1881 he performed the first gastric resection for cancer. In 1873 he did the first laryngectomy.

Billroth was, as his teacher von Langenbeck was, the founder of a surgical school. He was much interested in establishing safe methods of doing typical operations, and these were spread by his disciples all over the world. He published a book on university reform and, during his time in Zurich, he prevented the medical school from falling under a rigidly controlled system.[3]

He pioneered the study of wound healing and was the first to systematically control these studies by temperature measurements;[4] he became convinced that the wound itself was not the cause of illness, but that something from outside entering the wound produced inflammation.

His most fascinating book was on general surgical pathology,[5] published during his stay in Zurich. (It was even translated into Japanese.) In it, Billroth stressed the utmost necessity of a good basic general knowledge in anatomy and physiology for one to be a good surgeon.

Billroth (Fig. 1) was reported to be a good plastic surgeon, especially in facial reconstruction, because of his artistic imagination.[6] During his time in Zurich, he operated upon 32 children, up to the age of two years, with clefts of the lip and palate—using the methods of Malgaigne and von Langenbeck. His mortality was 11.5 per cent and he concluded, from this figure, that early operation in children was justified. Concerning the speech results of his adult patients (19 cases), he noticed that they were discouraging—and that the foremost problem in palatal closure was, indeed, to obtain good speech.[7]

Billroth was known for his sincerity in openly discussing his successes and failures. "One unhappy case is better than 10 good ones, if one does not hide the mistake but (rather) analyzes it." Although his ideas on wound infection differed from Lister's, after a visit of the latter to Vienna Billroth sent one of his residents to Edinburgh; later, he adopted Lister's antisepsis. "In general, I always try to calculate my statistical and therapeutic results as bad as possible; I consider good results as self evident, even without me."

This important contribution on fracturing the hamulus was one of Billroth's later papers. Five years afterward, in 1894, he died while on a visit to the small town of Abbazia (in what is now Yugoslavia).

Leo Clodius, M.D.
Dept. of Plastic Surgery
Raemistreet 100
CH 8006 Zurich, Switzerland

REFERENCES

1. Siegrist, H. E.: *Grosse Aerzte*. Lehmann, Munich, 1954.
2. Rogers, B. O.: Carl Ferdinand von Graefe. Plast. & Reconstr. Surg., *46:* 554, 1970.
3. Huber, A.: *Theodor Billroth in Zürich*. Seldwyla, Zürich, 1924.
4. Billroth, T.: Beobachtungs-Studien über Wund-fieber und accidentelle Wundkrankheiten. Arch. klin. Chir., *2:* 325, 1862.
5. Billroth, T.: *Allgemeine und Chirurgische Pathologie und Therapie*. Hirschwald, Berlin, 1866.
6. Gersuny, R.: *Theodor Billroth*. Rikola, Wien, 1922.
6. Billroth, T.: *Chirurgische Klinik, 1860–1867*. Hirschwald, Berlin, 1869.

LENGTHENING THE SOFT PALATE IN CLEFT PALATE OPERATIONS

GEORGE M. DORRANCE, M.D., *Philadelphia, Pa.*

Reprinted from Annals of Surgery, 82: 208, 1925

There is a distinct percentage of cleft palate cases in which, even though the operation succeeds in closing the cleft, fail from a physiological standpoint in correcting the speech of the individual. The reason for this failure to aid in phonation is the fact that the soft palate is unable to come in contact with the posterior pharyngeal wall.

An ideal cleft palate operation is one that will permit the patient to speak normally and at the same time close the defect in the palate. While both may be accomplished in a certain percentage of cases, we are all aware that there is a distinct type of case with a short palate in which the speaking voice has not been helped.

I have attempted in this proposed operation of mine to first obtain a sufficient length of palate to insure good phonation and later on attempt to close the hard palate.

I advise this type of operation on all cases where a short soft palate will result from any operations hitherto described, for example, the Langenbeck. Despite the fact that most operators prefer doing their operations before the second year, in my opinion the best time to operate where we wish to lengthen the soft palate is from the fourth year on. I find that from the fourth year on the structures of the hard and soft palate contain more fat and lymphoid tissue and will stand manipulation much better than in the younger child.

My anatomical studies, both on the normal and the cleft palate, have made it quite clear to me that if the increased length is to be accomplished, it must be obtained by releasing the anterior attachment of both the hard and the soft palate. To release the structures of the hard palate, I make an incision as shown in Figure 1, at the same time freshening the edges of the cleft. I then raise the flaps as shown in Figure 2, *left.* These flaps contain all the structures down to and including the periosteum over the hard palate. The elevation of this flap is continued until the border of the hard palate is reached as shown in Figure 2, *center,* and the attachment of the palatine aponeurosis of the hard palate is divided. On reaching the tuberosity of the maxillary bone, it will be found that there is still some structure which prevents the palate from falling backwards. This structure is the tendon of the *tensor palati* muscle. If the hamular process around which this muscle turns at a right angle is broken off, the divided portions will be drawn downward by the *pterygo-pharyngeus* muscle—this muscle being a much stronger and larger structure than is usually described. After this hamular process has been fractured you dislocate the tendon of the *tensor palati* muscle, thus changing its direction so that instead of forming two sides of a right angle triangle it will form the hypotenuse, as shown in Figure 3, and will allow the lengthening of this

From the Department of Surgery of the Thomas Evans Institute of the University of Pennsylvania.
Presented at the meeting of the Philadelphia Academy of Surgery on April 6, 1925.

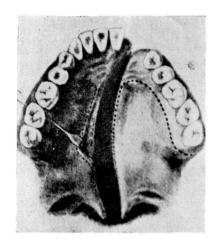

FIG. 1. Modified from Brophy's book. Incision to release the hard palate.

them to either the remains of the septum or the horizontal plate of the palate bone. While this operation gives you the desired lengthening as shown in Figure 2, *right*, it leaves a defect in the anterior portion of the hard palate. This is later closed by means of a flap.

In one case the palate was so short that my colleague, Dr. LeRoy Johnson,

muscle and transpose it from a *tensor* into a *levator* muscle. This can be demonstrated on any cadaver. After the above procedure has been performed on both sides, you will gain one-half to three-quarters of an inch lengthening and there will be found to be less tension than under the Langenbeck operation. The two flaps will be sutured together, as shown in Figure 2, *right,* using whatever suture you especially desire. The anterior edge of these flaps will have a tendency to fall downward. To hold them in place, suture

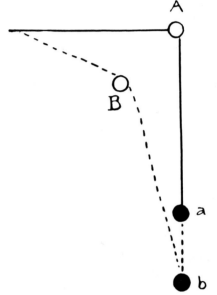

FIG. 3. Alteration in direction of *tensor palati* muscle.

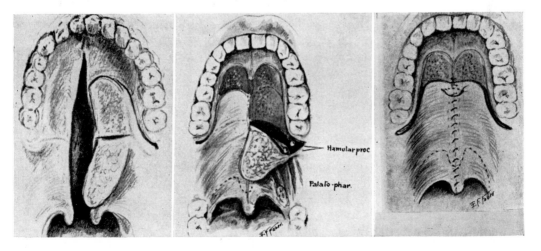

FIG. 2. (*left*) Palatal flap raised. (*center*) Hard palate completely exposed. (*right*) Alteration in direction of *tensor palati* muscle. Note increased length of palate below dotted line.

Professor of Orthodontia at the University of Pennsylvania, felt that no operation was justifiable. As he expressed it, "You will only have a stiff palate which will not close off the opening." Nevertheless, after the operation in this case one will see that the palate comes in contact with the posterior pharyngeal wall, shutting off the mouth from the nose. There is a point I have been asked about a number of times. Does not this method predispose to sloughing of the flaps? In the cases I have observed so far, I have noted less blanching of the flaps than in my usual cleft palate operations. There has been no sloughing. The blood supply comes in through the tonsillar plexus. It has always been my contention that in a correctly performed Langenbeck operation the posterior arteries are divided.

I thank Dr. Addinell Hewson for the many courtesies he has extended and the help he has given me in the Anatomical Laboratories of the Postgraduate Department of the University of Pennsylvania.

George M. Dorrance, M.D.
Department of Surgery
The Thomas Evans Institute
University of Pennsylvania
Philadelphia, Pa.

COMMENTARY BY THE EDITOR

We have here, of course, Dorrance's first description of his "pushback" operation (though he hadn't named it yet). He presented it before the Philadelphia Academy of Surgery, of which he had been a member since 1905, in April of 1925. Almost simultaneously, and independently, Alexander Limberg of Leningrad developed a similar operation which was published one year later (Nov. chir. Mosk., 2: 67, 1926). The two men met first in 1926, while attending the Oral Surgery Section of the Fifth International Dental Congress in Philadelphia. There they discussed their recent publications.

Also in the spring of 1925, at about the time he presented this paper, George Morris Dorrance was elected to membership in the American Association of Plastic Surgeons.

As you see by this first description, the operation is a modification of the von Langenbeck procedure; it is depicted variously, in the drawings, as being used for a complete unilateral cleft, a partial cleft extending forward to the alveolus, and a partial cleft involving only the velum. Its later popularity was achieved in the latter type, and in submucous clefts; closure of the hole (that remained up front in the longer clefts) by "a flap," as Dorrance suggests here, was neither easy nor acceptable.

Dorrance advocated cutting the major palatine arteries, as "it has always been my contention that in a correctly performed Langenbeck operation the posterior arteries are divided." In later papers he advocated a preliminary operation to cut and tie the arteries while raising the flap, conceiving it to be safer to thus have a delayed flap.

It was Barrett Brown who subsequently devised a method of stretching the major palatine arteries for one to two cm out of their canals, then dissecting them forward and loose from the mucoperiosteal flap for another centimeter or two—so that the palate could be set back as an island flap with intact arteries. He also left a small tag of the aponeurosis attached to the bones near the midline, on which to suture the anterior edge of the setback flap. In 1941 Dorrance watched me do this island flap type of elongation in St. Louis and exclaimed, "if I were your age and had your hands, that is

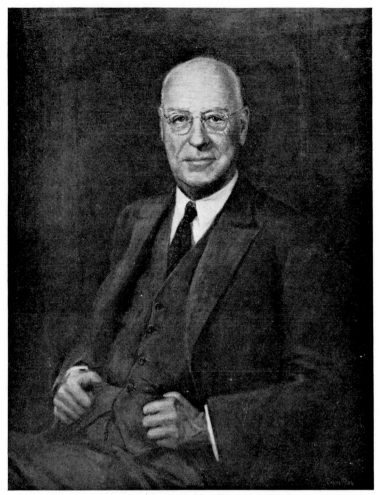

GEORGE MORRIS DORRANCE
1877–1949

the way I would do this operation!" He was a very large man—tall, with broad shoulders, a large head, and large hands.

Biographical sketches of Dorrance have been published in the *Journal* (*5:* 264, 1950 and *32:* 209, 1963). Only a little can be added, information that has come to our attention recently.

Dorrance was a general surgeon, by training and instinct, who became interested in the head and neck area while serving as a Demonstrator of Anatomy at the University of Pennsylvania, in a dissecting room that was shared by the dental and medical stu-

dents. When he came back from World War I, he could not break into the general surgical hierarchy controlling surgery in the University of Pennsylvania Medical School and Hospital at that time. However, he did obtain an appointment as Professor of Maxillofacial Surgery in the School of Dentistry, which permitted him to take patients seen in the outpatient clinic (but no others) into the University Hospital. This must have been a great disappointment in his life, and was (no doubt) due to distrust of him on the part of some of the leading general surgeons, as he was a vigorous competitor in some of their areas of interest. It did, however, act as a spur to increase his activities and abilities in head and neck surgery. In this he had the firm backing and friendship of Blair. Dorrance became one of the men who helped to organize and found the American Board of Plastic Surgery.

George Dorrance married Miss Emily Fox on October 12, 1921, when he was 44 years of age. He has one son, George Morris Dorrance, Jr., now President of the Philadelphia National Bank. His son is also Chairman of the Board of Trustees of the American Oncologic Hospital, where his father was chief surgeon and provided personally the greater part of all the latest proven methods for the treatment of malignant disease.

It may be of interest that Dr. Dorrance was also the Vice-President and Medical Director of the Campbell Soup Co., a firm founded and owned (until it "went public") by him and his brothers. His great interest, however, was in his surgery. Possibly his two greatest works were (1) the origination and further development of his "pushback" operation and the elongation concept, and (2) his scholarly *The Operative Story of Cleft Palate* (W. B. Saunders Co., Philadelphia, 1933), which has been a model for 40 years.

With this we conclude the series of Classic Reprints on cleft palate surgery. There have been other important developments, but the patience of our readers is finite. Let us leave them in peace, and the papers for possible review in the future.

—*Frank McDowell*

For much of the information on the background of Dr. Dorrance's interest in surgery of the head and neck, including cleft palate and fractures of the jaws, and some facts on his family and relationship with the Campbell Soup Company, we are indebted to Dr. Robert H. Ivy. As many will remember, Dr. Ivy was associated with Dr. Dorrance for many years in the teaching of maxillofacial surgery in the School of Dentistry of the University of Pennsylvania.

SECTION V

Cross-Lip Flaps

LIP REPAIR (CHEILOPLASTY) PERFORMED BY A NEW METHOD

(Laebedannelse [Cheiloplastik] udført paa en ny Methode)

PROFESSOR S. A. V. STEIN, *Copenhagen, Denmark*

(*Hospitals-Meddelelser, 1: 212–216, 1848*)

Translated from the Danish by
DR. NIELS C. PETERSEN

When a plastic operation is planned to replace the loss of some part of the human body, then one should judiciously choose the material which is to take the place of the lost substance. On this choice will depend not only the maintenance and luxuriant life of the transplant under the changed conditions, but also the role it will play in the future when it has formed an organic union in its new place —both with regard to the function of the repaired part and to its more or less normal appearance. If this indispensable consideration is not given to the substance— but instead an attempt is made only to cover a hole with a flap taken from the surrounding tissue—then the new-formed part may, after the lapse of some time, assume an appearance which does not at all conform to one's sense of beauty. It may even give a worse impression than the tissue loss which one has attempted to cover by a painful operative intervention.

If these considerations are now applied to cheiloplasty, it is evident that the material of choice for the replacement of the loss of a lip must be sought in the labial substance formed by Nature herself.

The fullness, the color, and the position and manifold changes in the form of the lips under the influence of muscular action are due to the musculature with which they are provided, and of which their mass mainly consists. But as such musculature is found only in the labial substance itself, this cannot be replaced in a satisfactory way by any other organic material; for all other substances, although they may physically cover the loss, will never in a life-like fashion enter into the new place—as they cannot participate in the normal muscular action of the area.

Would it be possible to transplant labial substance from one lip to the other, so that the mass is equally distributed in both, and the loss of substances in one lip is thereby covered by the relative abundance in the other?

This question was solved in a satisfactory way by cheiloplasty of the lower lip done in a patient admitted to the Royal Frederiks Hospital last year. A report on the method and the result of the operation was read before the Meeting of Scandinavian Scientists in Copenhagen in 1847.

CASE REPORT

A seaman, Peter H . . . , aged 48, of healthy appearance and robust body build, was admitted to the Hospital on March 12, 1847, with a cancerous lesion on the lower lip. There was considerable induration and hypertrophy both of the labial substance itself and of the upper median part of the chin. Only minor parts of the vermilion, close to both angles of the mouth, were as yet uninvolved. The mouth was large. The broad, full, upper lip was absolutely healthy (Fig. 1, *left*).

Cheiloplasty, with transplantation from the upper

lip, was performed on this patient on March 19—according to the principles mentioned above.

The Operative Procedure

Two incisions were made, which began a little medial to the angles of the mouth and from there continued convergently downward until they met a little below the chin. All of the affected and suspicious mass was severed from the unaffected tissue. The large, triangular interspace thus produced by the loss of substance was at once reduced by the insertion of three twisted sutures from the lower wound angles upward (Fig. 1, *center*).

After the triangular space had been thus reduced, the remaining loss of substance was to be replaced by a graft from the upper lip. To accomplish this the posterior surface of the upper lip was detached from the gum by cutting the frenulum. A pointed bistoury was then thrust through the labial substance between the angle of the mouth and the midline, at the junction of the vermilion, so that the *arteria coronaria* remained intact. The knife was then carried in an oblique direction upward and inward to the nasal septum. A similar incision was then made on the other side, meeting the first at an acute angle just below the nose. In this way a large triangular flap was formed of the midportion of the lip—representing about one-third of its mass.

By a third incision in the midline, which also cut the vermilion, this flap was divided into two smaller ones. These flaps were thus completely separated—whereas each one, while rotated downward and outward, remained in connection with its lateral mass of the upper lip through the vermilion which was left untouched by the lateral incisions (the incisions are indicated in Figure 1, *center*).

Now the two separate flaps, for which sufficient nutrition had been secured through the intact *arteria coronaria*, were turned down and drawn into the open space in the lower lip. Their tips were attached to the lower angle of this space by a needle inserted into both structures. The attachment was continued by the insertion of several twisted sutures which united the outer edges of the flaps with the lateral edges of the space. The uppermost of these sutures united the vermilion of the grafted flap with the tiny remainder of the vermilion of the former lower lip (which had been spared at the angle of the mouth). Finally, two twisted sutures were inserted just below the nose—to reduce the gaping wound in the upper lip. This concluded the first part of the operation.

The gap of the remaining part of the wound in the upper lip, and that between the edges of the grafted flaps, could not be closed until later when the organic union of these parts in their new sites had been established. The patient remained in this condition (Fig. 1, *right*) for the next 20 days—although as early as the third postoperative day the flaps were so intimately united that the needles could be removed. During this period, the patient was fed with the greatest ease, partly through the open mid-cleft, and partly by a tube through the two elongated openings. (These openings, which constituted the future gap between the upper and lower lips, were bounded on the outside by the angles of the mouth and on the inside by the turned-down vermilion.)

At the end of the aforementioned period, the two arches of the vermilion (by which the flaps were still in organic connection with the upper lip) were cut. The operation was completed by uniting the mid-clefts in both the upper and lower lips by several twisted sutures, after making the edges bleed. Union was accomplished with the greatest ease and healing occurred by first intention—except for a small portion below; however, this portion soon closed after a good suppuration.

DISCUSSION

Thus, the transplantation from the upper to the lower lip was successfully accomplished. The patient, whose appearance is shown in the portrait sketch (Fig. 2), left the hospital on May 7 with a well-

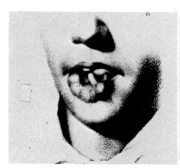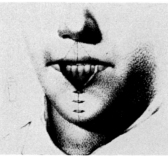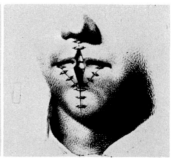

Figure 1

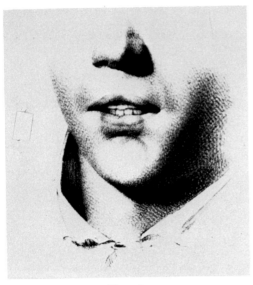

Figure 2

shaped lower lip, one provided with a natural and full vermilion. The size of the mouth had obviously been somewhat reduced; but the movements of both lips were fairly unimpeded.

Under other circumstances, transplantation may just as easily be done from the lower lip as *vice versa*. The method can be modified in various ways, according to the size and site of the loss of tissue.

Although, admittedly, this technique of cheiloplasty does not at all make other methods superfluous, it offers many advantages when it can be used. Perhaps it may be hoped that this method will be given a modest place in plastic surgery.

Professor S. A. V. Stein
Copenhagen, Denmark

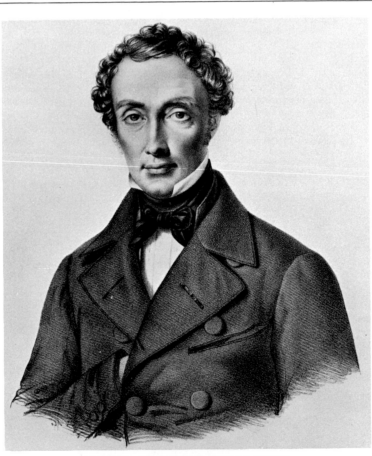

SOPHUS AUGUST VILHELM STEIN
1797–1868

COMMENTARY BY DR. NIELS C. PETERSEN

Stein's cheiloplasty, with two flaps from the unaffected upper lip, was performed in 1847—10 years after Sabattini had used a similar method, but before the cross-lip flaps reported by Estlander (1872) and Abbe (1898). All 4 surgeons seem to have devised their procedures independently of each other.

Stein occupied a central position in the development of surgery in Denmark in the nineteenth century. He was the son of a barber-surgeon and, after a scanty schooling, he received his training at the Copenhagen Academy of Surgery.

At that time, a sharp distinction obtained between training in surgery and training in medicine. Medical education proper was given at the University of Copenhagen and it required a better educational background for admission. But in the course of time it became common practice for medical students to also seek some supplementary surgical training at the Academy. Stein had to do it the other way.

At the age of 34, he entered the University—while he had to earn his living as a surgeon and family doctor.

However, it was mainly anatomy on which Stein's interest centered during these years. He began to publish a large *Anatomical Atlas*. Unfortunately, his publisher left him in the lurch; the ambitious work remained merely a torso. In 1835, he was appointed Professor of Anatomy at the Royal Danish Academy of Arts. This provided scope for his talents in drawing and modeling. A few years later he became Assistant Professor of Anatomy at the University of Copenhagen.

As an anatomist, Stein won international recognition. But in the long run his interest in surgery got the upper hand, and when the position as Head of the Surgical Department at the Royal Frederiks Hospital (the highest surgical post in the country) became vacant in 1844, he applied for it. He was appointed Chief Surgeon. The following year he became Professor of Surgery, though a group of younger surgeons protested vigorously because they found Stein's qualifications "insufficient." (The younger generation had studied surgery in Paris and in other European capitals. Unlike Stein, they regarded pathological anatomy, histology, and physiology—not gross anatomy—as the basis of surgery.)

In principle, the critics were right, but they forgot that they had to do with a man of incredible diligence and exceptional skills. During the next few years, Stein won a reputation as the leading Danish surgeon. He became an eminent teacher for the medical students and for would-be surgeons—and he took a special interest in plastic surgery. This latter field benefitted greatly from his artistic talents and his technical skill. He worked in fruitful competition with the surgeon of the nearby General Hospital, Eskildsen Larsen—another pioneer in Danish plastic surgery. Larsen was particularly interested in rhinoplasties with Indian forehead flaps. Both men seem to have been inspired by Dieffenbach who, during one of his many journeys, visited Copenhagen in 1846 and performed an operation at the General Hospital.

In Stein's time, surgery made rapid progress and it won a reputation of being equal to medicine. However, the contempt with which the surgical discipline had been regarded in the past was still near enough to make its practitioners touchy. They were anxious to emphasize that surgery should not be regarded as a purely technical specialty. Stein, the highly admired technician, was particularly susceptible to this risk. He discussed it in an introductory lecture on operative surgery.

Gentlemen: The time is long past when the surgeon was a despised person and regarded merely as a mechanically acting tool, as a simple lever for the surgical ideas of physicians. In the

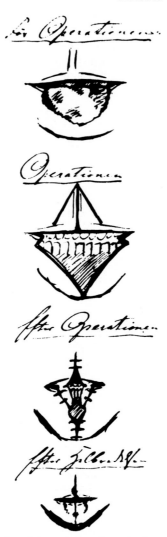

Fig. 3. Stein's sketches of the operation, drawn in the record of his patient.

past, operative surgery was placed among the bottles and jars in the *materia medica* of the physician. The saying ran: "The apothecary is the right hand of the physician, the surgeon his left."

However, Gentlemen, although this attitude is a thing of the past, the same ideas occasionally emerge in our time. Now and then we see highly esteemed physicians who are so narrow-minded in their views of the value and importance of surgery, and of the stage of development which this science has attained, that they seriously believe that one needs only a certain amount of dexterity to become a competent surgeon and operator.

No, Gentlemen, dexterity is not enough! It is not merely mechanical skills that have raised surgery to its present standard. It is, rather, the spirit which has guided—and which always must guide—the finger. It was certainly a bold and grand idea which directed the hand of the surgeon who first excised the lens from the human eye. Not less grand was the idea which made another ligate the main trunks of circulation in order to force Nature to form new routes for the blood stream—or that made another transplant parts of the body to a new site where they could find nutrition and maintain life, thus allowing living tissue to replace lost substance.

It is the implementation—and the imitation—of the great ideas of such ingenious men which have gradually developed operative surgery into a respected and independent branch of practical medicine.

Stein's cheiloplasty was performed without anesthesia. He had used ether anesthesia more than a year previously, but apparently he thought this case was not suitable.

The drawings which illustrate the operation in his report are undoubtedly trustworthy. We may compare them with the sketches made in his case record (Fig. 3). They are almost identical although the sketches show the stage with apical necrosis (this is also mentioned in the report).

Stein's two-flap cheiloplasty suffered a strange fate. Apparently, it was not repeated by him or by any other Danish surgeon until 62 years later when, in 1908, two cases were reported from Sundby Hospital in Copenhagen.

It is interesting that in 1852 he did perform the single-flap procedure, now known as the Abbe flap, but he never published it.

Niels C. Petersen, M.D.
Consultant in Plastic Surgery
University Hospital of Arhus
8000 Arhus C, Denmark

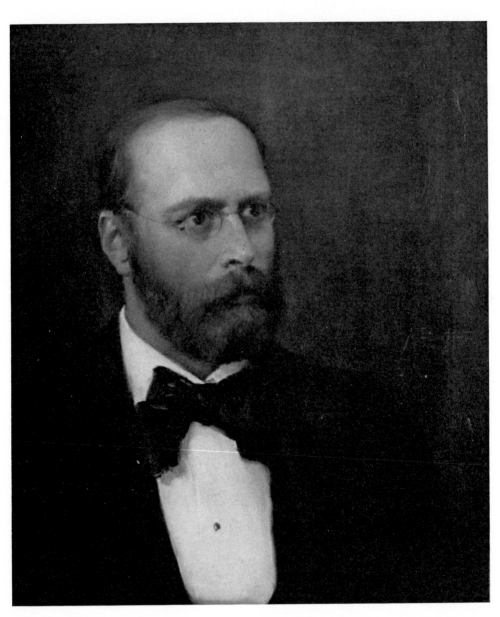

JAKOB AUGUST ESTLANDER, M.D.
1831–1881

EINE METHODE AUS DER EINEN LIPPE SUBSTANZVERLUSTE DER ANDEREN ZU ERSETZEN

(A method of reconstructing loss of substance in one lip from the other lip)

DR. J. A. ESTLANDER, *Helsinki, Finland*

(*Archiv für Klinische Chirurgie, 14:622, 1872.*)

Translated from the German by
DR. BÖRJE SUNDELL

Few operations have presented as many different methods as cheilo- and meloplastics. Bruns, in his large *Handbook of Practical Surgery* has dealt with this question more extensively than anybody else and presents no less than 44 methods, not mentioning the lesser modifications of several of them. A closer survey of these methods reveals that, in order to provide reconstructive material for one lip, surgeons have utilized all possible parts of the face—extending their incisions even to such far-away regions as the thyroid, while the closest neighbor, the other lip, has been almost totally overlooked. Yet, the substitute material presenting itself here is in all respects so superior to that provided by other locations that a method described in the heading of this report should render the majority of the other methods unnecessary. True, Bruns describes 3 methods related to this principle, but all suffer from essential shortages; one is only suitable for minor losses of substance, another requires a healthy cheek, and the third can be used on the upper lip only. I, therefore, hope that a general method used by me for several years, but which has not been described by any of the authors available to me (such as Bruns, Szymanowski, Weber, etc.) would not be without practical interest.

The loss of substance necessitating such an operation occurs most frequently in the lower lip and is more rare in the upper lip and cheek; I shall thus describe first the operation in the form I have usually performed it; as an example, I have selected a case of local recurrence of an epithelioma.

FIRST CASE

Matts Suntia, a 63-year-old farmer from Anjala, had in his lower lip for more than 10 years a small tumor which grew slowly until the beginning of 1871, when it started to enlarge very rapidly, forcing him to seek admission into the clinic. Thereby, he had an epithelioma involving the entire lower lip to the corners of the mouth and the sulcus labiomentalis. This neoplasm was removed by the assistant surgeon, Dr. Krohn, by means of a quadrangular incision; he reconstructed the lower lip with a method which is frequently used in my clinic. (The incision, constituting the lower border of the quadrangle, is extended to both sides along the edge of the lower jaw; two incisions parallel to this incision are drawn from the corners of the mouth across the cheeks towards the edges of the masseter muscles, whereafter the flaps are separated from the underlying bone and joined together in the middle line. When such a flap is completely separated from the bone it can without difficulties be brought over ¾ inch closer to the middle line.) In this case, the tension after joining the two flaps together was not very significant. The wound healed well, and after 12 days in the hospital the patient was discharged with a lower lip which entirely covered the teeth.

From the Department of Surgery Emperor Alexander University.

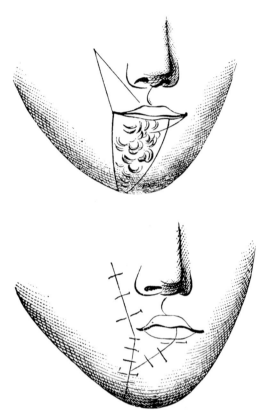

FIG. 1. (*above*) Excision of carcinoma of lower lip and repair by rotation flap from upper lip. (*below*) Completion of procedure shown above.

January 11, 1872 the patient again appeared at the clinic, with a local recurrence. The epithelioma now involved the right side of the lip and the cheek from the corner of the mouth to the edge of the lower jaw, extending even to the left side. No more than one-third of the reconstructed lip (at its border) was healthy. The tumor extended to the bone but no enlarged glands were palpable. Since the stretch of the skin and mucous membrane of the cheek had already been (to a very great extent) utilized in the first operation, and the scars following the earlier incisions rendered several other methods unusable, I decided to replace the missing substance with tissue from the upper lip. The epithelioma was removed by means of an angular incision, the apex of which extended a few lines below the edge of the lower jaw; this left behind no more than approximately one-fourth of the lip margin. The wound margins regressed more than usual; after I had separated them to some extent from the bone, the defect appeared unexpectedly large.

Thereafter I cut from the right side of the upper lip a triangular flap, whose one side (situated in the vermilion) was somewhat over 2 cm long when the lip was not stretched. As shown in Fig. 1, that part of the angular incision which extended from the edge of the lower jaw up to the corner of the mouth was continued through the skin and the mucous membrane upwards to the area of the infraorbital foramen, and from there downwards almost to the vermilion—the skin incision being about 4 mm and the mucosal incision some 8 mm distance from this margin. This latter point was then fixed with a suture to that point where the old corner of the mouth had been situated and where also the new one would find its place; the rest of the upper part of the incision was closed with sutures. In this way the substitute flap fell naturally into its place. No matter how impossible it had appeared to fill the large tissue defect with such an apparently small piece of the upper lip, it turned out that the substitute flap had so retained its usual elasticity that the wound edges could be joined without undue tension. As shown in Fig. 1 (lower drawing), the apex of the substitute flap came to fill the end point of the first incision at the edge of the lower jaw; the previous corner of the mouth was joined to the remnants of the lower lip; the previous margin of the upper lip now constituted the margin of the lower lip. The wound healed almost completely by first intention.

Fourteen days following the operation, the lip margin belonging to the substitute flap was 2¾ cm long; although it still was thick and swollen it could be stretched over ½ cm. The philtrum ran straight without being drawn to the right or left, but the mouth orifice was some 7 mm shorter on the right, a difference which became more striking when the patient opened his mouth. This, however, he was able to do so well that the distance between the front teeth was almost 2½ cm.

The patient explained that he was far more content with *this* lip than with the previous one, because with this new lip he was now able to hold a piece of bread, which had been impossible for him after the first operation. To observe the changes in the new lip, I kept him for some time at the hospital. On February 19th the swelling had rather disappeared and the motility in the newly built parts of the lip was almost normal. The patient was quite able to pronounce the labial consonants. As he was completely satisfied with his mouth and did not want to undergo another operation, he was discharged as cured.

In comparison with the lower lip, as was already pointed out, defects of the upper lip occur only rarely. In my experience, with 7 cheiloplasties, only one concerned the upper lip. The basis for this, as is well known, is that (peculiarly enough) epithelioma occurs only rarely in the upper lip. Out of 28 men and 1 woman who were admitted to our clinic over the last 12 years for labial carcinoma, the upper lip was not affected in any case, or was only affected secondarily and at the corner of the mouth to some small extent. Also the 6 papillomas over this period were all situated in the lower lip. Only for scars after traumatic lesions and lupus, or such cases where an original bone process has secondarily affected the upper lip (e.g. the large destructions after noma) is a cheiloplasty in the upper lip necessary. To describe the operation in this region, I shall report a case of the latter type.

SECOND CASE

Oskar Hanström, 17-year-old farmer's son from Hausjärvi, was admitted to the clinic on February 7, 1868 because of destruction of the face which had developed during typhus in the preceding autumn. A great part of his cheek and the entire right side of his nose had been lost; also the upper lip (with the exception of one-fourth of it, close to the left corner of the mouth). The scar extended over a part of the right side of the nose to the inner corner of the eye, continued from there in a curve over the cheek to near the edge of the masseter muscle, and terminated at the right corner of the mouth. A part of the facial plane of the upper jaw, a part of its nasal process, and the entire alveolar process with the teeth belonging to it, were bare. Also on the left side the incisor teeth and adjacent bone lay bare.

This large loss of tissue was reconstructed as follows. After the scar had been removed and the wound margins (i.e. over the zygomatic bone) had been freed, a triangular substitute flap was cut from the right side of the lower lip. The flap extended not quite to the middle of the lower lip, and from the chin to quite a bit below the lower edge of the lower jaw; its outer angle extended a few lines further to the right than the former corner of the mouth. This flap,

which was connected at the vermilion to the remaining parts of the lower lip and was kept alive by the intact coronary artery, was turned upwards in such a way that the part of it which had been taken from the lower chin came to fill the wound at the inner corner of the eye; the part close to the corner of the mouth was, however, rotated to join the remaining part of the upper lip; the latter was freed and its contracted mucous membrane was used to border that part of the flap margin which had been taken from outside the corner of the mouth.

To build the side of the nose, an incision was made into this flap; as a consequence that part of it which was supposed to build the upper lip also fitted well into its place. The wound margin in the cheek was joined without difficulties to the other side of the flap; similarly, the remaining defect of the lower lip was closed after it had been separated to some extent from the bone of the chin.

After the flap (which did not show any tendency towards gangrene) had firmly healed all over, the bridge containing the coronary artery and the scar close to it were cut through—whereby the mouth regained its ordinary form and the patient was able to open it almost to its regular size. When the patient was discharged from the hospital after two months, his face was disfigured only by a large scar, which ran from the corner of the eye in a curve through the corner of the mouth and to somewhere a bit below the chin.

A case of loss of tissue limited to the cheek alone probably occurs only very rarely; as a rule, at least one lip is at the same time largely destroyed. Consequently, meloplasty is almost always performed in association with cheiloplastics. I have only once had the opportunity of observing a case where the entire cheek and only a relatively insignificant part of the lip were destroyed. To demonstrate that the same method can also be applied here, I shall report on this case.

THIRD CASE

Olof Hiltunen, 17-year-old farmer's son from Kerimäki, was admitted on the 22nd of February, 1868, with a large tissue defect in the face which had developed a few months earlier during typhus, as a consequence of gangrene. A part of the lower lip and the entire mucosa-covered part of the right cheek were destroyed, to the anterior edge of the masseter muscle and down close to the lower border of the lower jaw. Both the upper and lower teeth lay bare.

The firm scar tissue which connected the coronary process, and partly also the inferior condylar process of the maxilla, to the zygomatic bone and superior maxilla, had compressed the teeth against each other so firmly that they protruded in an angle. The patient was very pale; he had lost much weight as he could only eat liquid foods and very small pieces of bread, which he forced through the interspaces between his teeth.

Since I was convinced that it was impossible to separate by knife the firm scar connection between the named bones, about one inch of the horizontal part of the lower jaw was resected. In the upper borders of both sawed surfaces of the bone, we burred two small holes which came to hold the sharp ends of a small metal rod;* this was constructed so that while *in situ* it could be shortened and lengthened at will. By this instrument, we succeeded during a great part of the healing process in keeping the bone ends separated, although the scar adhesion subsequently drew the lower jaw to an oblique position.

Two months later, the lower lip was separated from the jaw bone and brought about ¾ inch over to the right, using an auxiliary triangle which was cut downwards.

On June 2nd, after the first operation had completely healed, the cheek was reconstructed by forming a flap of the right side of the upper lip and of the upper part of the cheek; its bridge in the red margin of the lip contained the coronary artery and its upper roundish part extended over close to the infraorbital margin. This flap was rotated downwards, so that the part of it which had been taken from below the eye came to cover the false joint and the lower part of the defect at the edge of the masseter muscle; the new corner of the mouth came to lie somewhat below the place where the bridge was. The tissue loss was thus completely replaced. The new cheek became so elastic that it interfered in no way with the false joint; this was functioning (at the time of discharge of the patient on July 6th) so well that he was able to open his mouth until the distance between his front teeth was ¾ inch.

* *Editor's note:* This seems to have preceded another paper on a similar subject (Byars, L. T. and McDowell, F.: Preservation of Jaw Function, Surg., Gyn. & Obst., *84,* 870, 1947).

The reported 3 case histories will, I hope, be enough to present a general view on the use of this operative technique in different cases. Still, it seems necessary to emphasize certain especially important circumstances.

The most difficult point in the operation is to determine how large must be the bridge which connects the flap to the remaining part of the donor lip. The narrower this is, the easier it is to rotate the flap into place which is usually diametrically opposite to its original position—and the less will the appearance of the mouth be changed. But the closer one comes with a scalpel to the red margin of the lip, the greater becomes the danger, also, that one may cut the only thread on which survival of this substitute flap depends. Determining a certain point to which one could always proceed without danger would require that the coronary artery have a constant place in the lip. However, the measurements which I have performed (on corpses and during operations) demonstrate that this is not the case. Of the 3 distances which determine the location of the artery—namely, the distance from the artery to the mucosa, to the skin, and to the highest point of the red lip margin—only the first-mentioned is (to some extent) constant (2 mm). The second varies according to the thickness of the lip; the third, which is of greatest significance for the size of the nutritive bridge, shows extensive variations so that one can only say that in the middle of the lip, the artery usually (but not always) runs closer to the red margin than it does near the corner of the mouth. It is, therefore, safest during the operation to let oneself be guided by the pulsation which can always be felt; one avoids injury to the artery best by keeping it, as soon as the incision comes to its propinquity, constantly under one's finger. . . .

To reconstruct a completely lost lip, one might (instead of a single large substitute flap) take two smaller ones from both sides and join them in the middle line. I have no doubt about its complete success, even if the coronary artery is severed on both sides. This artery is, in the middle of the upper lip, connected to the nasopalatine artery through a constantly present and significant branch; in the lower lip, the anastomoses with the mental and submental arteries are even stronger so that there can be no danger to the survival of the substitute flap. . . .

> *Jakob A. Estlander, M.D.*
> *Professor of Surgery*
> *Emperor Alexander University*
> *Helsinki, Finland*

COMMENTARY BY DR. BÖRJE SUNDELL

When Jakob August Estlander became professor of surgery in 1860 at the Emperor Alexander University in Helsinki, he was only 28 years old. Estlander was born in the western part of Finland (in Lapväärti) in 1831. After graduating from high school in 1848, he received his medical education at various places, including Sweden and France, and graduated in 1858 as Doctor of Medicine. Next year, Dr. Estlander presented his doctoral thesis "Nécrose des os" to the medical faculty.

From 1858 to 1860, Dr. Estlander paid visits to leading medical centers in France, England and Germany. He received medical training under Nélaton, Civilian and Broca. Later, he studied surgical technique with Bastien and ophthalmic surgery with Desmarres. Subsequently, he wrote a paper for his professor's nomination in surgery: "Valeur relative des méthodes de traitement des rétrécissements organiques de l'urèthre".

During the years Estlander served as professor of surgery (which position he held until his death) the medical profession made rapid progress in Finland. This was partly due to the personal qualities of Estlander, but also due to the times. Anesthetics in surgery became routinely used and could be trusted. The meaning of antisepticism and aseptic surgery was realized, but not very well understood.

Professor Estlander took great interest in many fields of surgery, as papers written by him will show. At that time, when the professor of surgery also gave lectures in ophthalmology, ophthalmic surgery was of special interest to Estlander. Perhaps most interesting of all, however, are the papers that he published on problems in plastic and thoracic surgery.

In 1872, Estlander reported this method for reconstruction of lip and cheek defects. His clear definitions of his surgical technique have been of great importance in the development of later methods of lip reconstruction. Estlander was a stimulating teacher of plastic surgery; his successor as professor of surgery, Maximus Widekind af Schultén (who was trained by Estlander) was very interested in plastic surgery.

In 1879, Professor Estlander published a paper on treatment of resistant empyema cavities by resecting ribs and moving the thoracic wall inwards to collapse the empyema cavity—that is, thoracoplasty. This operation has been used even in modern times and is still known in the French medical literature as "l'operation d'Estlander."

Professor Estlander was a very active chief with many new ideas. In the 1860's he had to face many difficult problems—such as severe hospital infections—which could not be easily solved. He was convinced that one of the causes of severe hospital infections was the small rooms of the patients. Therefore he appealed unremittingly to the hospital authorities for a new and larger hospital; this was not granted, however, during his life time. Instead, antiseptic wound care was subjected to careful investigation and carbolic acid was the new weapon against infections.

Professor Estlander was renowned professionally for his meticulous and conscientious work, and for always remembering that he was dealing with human beings. He was an extraordinary teacher, a creative surgeon, and his very winning character (represented by kindness and patience) gave sick people confidence in him.

On a trip to Italy in 1881, Professor Estlander contracted malaria and died at the age of 50 in Messina; he was buried in the "Campo santo evangelico" cemetery in that city. In 1905, a memorial was raised by the Messina Medical Faculty to the memory of this Finnish surgeon.

Börje Sundell, M.D.
Pajalahdentie 17 F 102
Helsinki 20, Finland.

Dr. Sundell is Docent in Plastic Surgery at the University Central Hospital in Helsinki.

A NEW PLASTIC OPERATION FOR THE RELIEF OF DEFORMITY DUE TO DOUBLE HARELIP

ROBERT ABBE, M.D.*

New York, N.Y.

(Reprinted from Medical Record, 53: 477, 1898)

A lad of twenty-one years recently presented himself for a conspicuous deformity of the lips, the sequel of an operation for double harelip in infancy, consisting in an extreme flatness and scantiness of the upper lip, with an enormous pouting and redundance of the lower one (Fig. 1). He also had a complete cleft of the hard and soft palates, upon which two attempts had been made in former years to close. He desired this to be closed first, which I did, and operation was afterward done upon the lips.

Their inequality was admirably corrected by transplanting the middle portion of the lower lip into the upper, as illustrated in Fig. 2.

A median vertical incision was made in the upper lip, and the central scar portion excised so as to obtain edges of an excellent quality of skin. The gap thus created was about three-fourths of an inch in width.

A flap taken from the central portion of the lower lip, a little wider than the upper gap, was then made, in such a way as to make a hinge upon one side containing the lower branch of the coronary artery on the left, which flap was turned upward so that its lower edge on the chin was placed beneath the columna nasi. The vermilion border was exactly stitched on one side, as shown (Fig. 1), and numerous very fine stitches were applied so as to secure apposition around three-fourths of the flap. The lower part of the wound upon the chin was also brought in apposition up to the red portion.

Upon the right side of the mouth the upper half and the lower half of the red lip were left free until the inverted flap should have grown in its new position. Retention sutures were made to transfix the upper lip from side to side, and also one was passed from below the left angle of the mouth, crossing obliquely to the right upper lip, below the wing of the nose, thus preventing unconscious dragging upon the flaps. These are not shown in the sketch.

On the twelfth day, the flap having grown perfectly in its new position, its base was very carefully cut from the lower lip so as to leave an ample portion of the red middle lip, which was turned upward and exactly fitted to the freshened edge of the free half of the lip, as shown in Fig. 2. The lower lip was then refreshed and sutured.

The nutrition of this transplanted flap by its new capillary nourishment was so perfect that in color and texture it seemed to have been always a part of the upper lip. The lines of suture rapidly faded and were quite insignificant. The two lips were afterward in about their normal proportion, and gave the patient perfect satisfaction (Fig. 3).

During the twelve days between the

---

* Surgeon to St. Luke's and Cancer Hospitals; Assistant Attending Surgeon, Roosevelt Hospital.

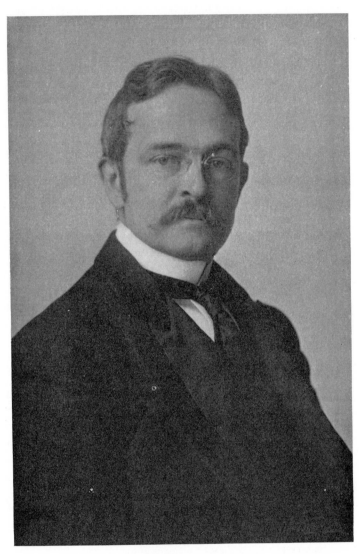

ROBERT ABBE

1851–1958

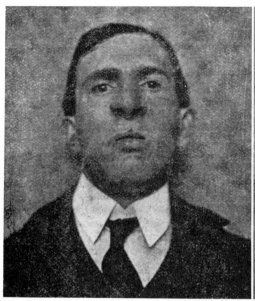
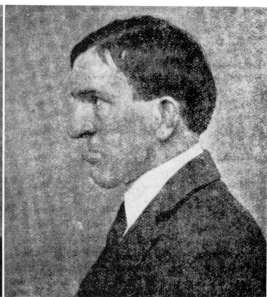

FIG. 1. Before operation

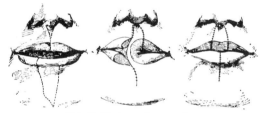

FIG. 2. Design of operation

operations, nourishment was well sustained by fluid taken through a tube inserted through the nostril.

Robert Abbe, M.D.
St. Luke's Hospital
New York, N.Y.

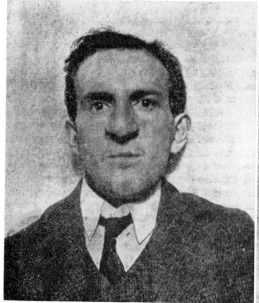
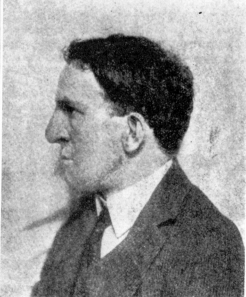

FIG. 3. After operation

COMMENTARY BY DR. RICHARD STARK

I have never met some of my best friends, simply because they were older than I, occasionally by several centuries. To know well a man like Robert Abbe is, indeed, a strong endorsement for the study of the history of medicine. Besides Abbe the quiet charismatic leader, was Abbe the innovator, Abbe the thoughtful and the inquisitive prober of unsolved problems. "Why should not you or I be the one to grasp the apparently incomprehensible idea and put it in comprehensible language?" he asked his contemporaries, and is asking those of us who read his prolific writings today.

Abbe is best known for the lip-switch flap, described in 1898. This often bears his name, although he contributed many new operations, several in the specialty we now call plastic surgery—including construction of the congenitally absent vagina and correction of the ankylosed temporomandibular joint. In addition, in 1903, he founded radiation therapy in the United States after Madame Curie presented him with a quantity of radium.

Abbe was keenly interested in the surgical correction of cleft lip and cleft palate. Nearly 75 years ago, in 1894, Abbe published a detailed description of his surgical approach to the problems of facial clefts. He advocated the use of either the Mirault or Hagedorn procedures for unilateral cleft lip. He recognized the importance in cheiloplasty of construction of the labial tubercle and of placement of the philtral dimple in the midline. In addition, although he occasionally resected the protruding premaxilla in bilateral cleft lip where retrodisplacement did not seem possible, he always retained the prolabium (no matter how minuscule) and used it for the center of the upper lip—observing that one often was "surprised at how much nature has done toward perfecting (the surgeon's) work." In bilateral cleft lip, he eschewed the Hagedorn procedure (wherein lateral lip elements are brought together in the midline beneath the prolabium) because "the resulting lip was too long."

In cleft palate, Abbe divined correctly that the highly arched palatal shelves provided more mucoperiosteum for closure than did the more lowly vaulted palate. He corrected the palatal cleft in the manner commonly referred to today as von Langenbeck's operation. Abbe used relaxing incisions about which he said, "the gaps on either side need not give you any uneasiness, because they are soon filled with granulations." To free the lateral soft tissue so that midline closure could be achieved, Abbe cut the aponeurosis between the hard and soft palates.

In his classic article upon the lip-switch flap of 1898, Abbe alluded neither to Sabattini (1838), Stein (1848), nor Estlander (1872); indeed, it is unlikely that he was aware of their work. The use to which Abbe put the flap was an advance in the surgery of facial clefts, i.e., reducing the protruding lower lip and at the same time plumping out the tight upper lip that resulted from removal (not by Abbe) of the intermaxillary segment in the repair of bilateral cleft lip. The patient, whose pre- and postoperative photographs were taken by Abbe 70 years ago, had an associated cleft palate. Abbe wisely chose the proper sequence of operations in the older patient; he performed the functional palatoplasty first, thus being virtually assured that the patient would return later for the cosmetic cheiloplasty.

—*Richard B. Stark, M.D.*

SECTION VI

Otoplasty

AN OPERATION FOR PROMINENCE OF THE AURICLES

EDWARD T. ELY, M.D.

New York, N. Y.

(Reprinted from Archives of Otology, *10:* 97, 1881)

The patient was a boy, aged 12, who came to the clinic of Dr. Roosa and myself at the Manhattan Eye and Ear Hospital, complaining that his companions ridiculed him on account of the prominence of his ears. He had this common deformity of the auricles to a somewhat unusual degree.

On March 1, 1881, I operated upon the right ear as follows: An incision was made through the skin, along the entire length of the furrow formed by the junction of the auricle with the side of the head posteriorly. This was joined at each end by a curved incision carried over the posterior surface of the auricle, and the skin and subcutaneous tissue included by these incisions were dissected off. Two incisions, nearly parallel to the former ones, were then carried directly through the cartilage, and an elliptical piece of the latter, measuring $1\frac{1}{8}$ in by $\frac{1}{3}$ in, was removed. The piece of excised skin was considerably larger than this. The edges of the wound were then united by 10 sutures, of which 7 included only the skin, while 3 passed through both skin and cartilage. Owing to the natural folds of the cartilage, it was impossible to secure perfect coaptation on the anterior surface of the auricle, and a small space was here left to heal by granulation. The dressing consisted of absorbent cotton and a bandage. Healing ensued without accident. There was no pain and very little swelling. The posterior incision united by first intention, and the anterior wound healed rapidly by granulation. The sutures were removed on the fourth day.

The operation upon the left ear was performed on April 19th. Holding the auricle so that the light from a window shone through it, I transfixed it with the scalpel, and rapidly excised a piece of cartilage of the desired size and shape, together with its overlying skin. Additional skin was then removed from the posterior surface, until the wound seemed to correspond in extent to that made at the former operation. Twelve sutures were used, of which three were passed through the cartilage on its anterior surface and one on its posterior surface, while the others were passed through the skin only. The dressing was the same as before, and, excepting the fact that complete union by first intention was not obtained behind, the healing was equally satisfactory. I did not like this plan of operating, however, as well as that first employed. Ether-anaesthesia was used on both occasions.

It was very interesting to observe how well these wounds of the cartilage healed. The position of the auricles is now (June 1st) all that could be desired. The posterior cicatrices are hidden by their position, and those on the anterior surface are hardly noticeable. No change in the hearing, which was normal, has been observed. The accompanying woodcuts are copied from photographs taken after the first operation. They will serve to show the position of the auricles before and after this treatment.

I do not know whether this is a new operation for the deformity in question or not, but, if allowed to judge from a

From the Manhattan Eye and Ear Hospital.

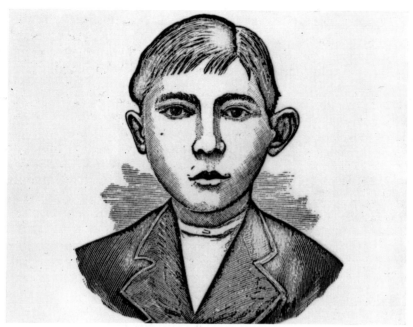

Fig. 1. Front view, after first operation to set back right ear

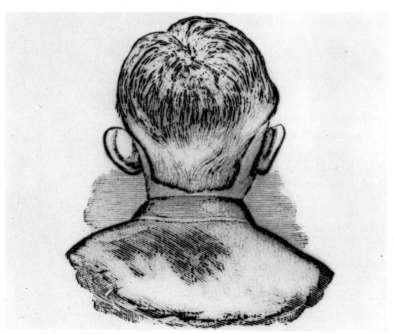

Fig. 2. Rear view, after first operation to set back right ear

single case, I can highly recommend it. Before operating, the hair should be shaved from the neighborhood of the ear, and the meatus stuffed with cotton to prevent the entrance of blood.

Edward T. Ely, M.D.
Manhattan Eye and Ear Hospital
New York, N.Y.

This article was sent to the Journal by Blair O. Rogers, M.D.

COMMENTARY BY DR. BLAIR O. ROGERS

It is, perhaps, historically noteworthy to mention in this centennial year of the Manhattan Eye, Ear and Throat Hospital,[1] that one of its early staff members, Edward Talbot Ely, probably described for the first time in the medical literature in the year 1881 *"An Operation for Prominence of the Auricles"*.[2]

Contrary to the erroneous statements of Becker[3] and others who have paraphrased him, Dieffenbach[4] was not the first to describe the correction of protruding ears. A careful translation of "Die Ohrbildung: Otoplastik", in Dieffenbach's *Die Operative Chirurgie* (1845), fails to reveal any reference whatsoever to the correction of protruding ears. Dieffenbach[4] describes only the restoration of those portions of the external ear injured by complicated wounds, lacerations, tears, amputations, and burns.

The young 31-year-old Ely, son of Dr. W. S. Ely (an upstate Rochester, N.Y. physician) was characteristically humble when he stated in his paper: "I do not know whether this is a new operation for the deformity in question or not, but if allowed to judge from a single case, I can highly recommend it." Ely was also the first to recognize the need for excising and removing a piece of the conchal cartilage, in addition to the skin excision, to obtain a more acceptable, permanent change in the position of the protruding ear.

His technique was improved upon only slightly by subsequent authors—including Keen[5] in 1890, Monks[6] in 1891, Haug[7] in 1894, Joseph[8] in 1896, Morestin[9] in 1903, and others. Joseph wrote in chapter XIX, "Die Ohrenplastik (Otoplastik)," in his classic textbook,[10] that priority for the protruding ear operation should be given to Ely. He made no mention whatsoever of his fellow German, Dieffenbach, in this chapter, although he cited Dieffenbach several times in those chapters describing reconstruction of nasal defects.[10]

Ely's life was tragically short. He was born in 1850 and died in April, 1885, at the age of 35 years, leaving a wife and an infant daughter. The cause of his death was listed in The Medical Register[11] as *phthisis pulmonalis,* or pulmonary tuberculosis. When one stops to consider the extensive medical literary output of this young surgeon, it is easy to understand that he, perhaps literally, worked himself to death in a consumptive state without realizing the seriousness of his illness.

Ely graduated from the University of Rochester in 1871 and received his medical degree from Columbia University's College of Physicians and Surgeons in 1874. Soon thereafter, he was appointed to the House Staff of Charity Hospital, where he subsequently became a Visiting Surgeon for 6 years prior to his death.

After serving his internship at Charity Hospital, he was appointed Assistant Surgeon to the Manhattan Eye and Ear Hospital in 1876. Almost immediately, he became associated with Dr. Daniel Bennett St. John Roosa, one of the founders and surgeon directors of this Hospital from its very inception in the year 1869. The two of them edited a little pocket-manual, entitled *Ophthalmic and Otic Memoranda*[12], which was intended in 1876 to give the student and practitioner of medicine a concise outline of the current knowledge available in the fields of ophthalmology and otology.

In 1879, Ely wrote about the treatment of acute suppuration of the middle ear[13]; in the following year, 1880, his plastic surgical leanings became evident when he described skin grafting in cases of chronic suppuration of the middle

From the Department of Plastic Surgery of the Manhattan Eye, Ear and Throat Hospital, and the Institute of Reconstructive Plastic Surgery, New York University Medical Center.

ear[14]. In this same year, 1880, he and Dr. Roosa co-edited another book *Ophthalmic and Otic Contributions,* a collection of papers dealing with ophthalmologic and otologic disorders (including case histories) which both of these surgeons had previously published in other medical journals[15].

Several papers written in the years 1880 to 1881 dealt with diverse subjects as the effects of tobacco on cigar makers who were, of course, cigar smokers[16] (effects which he concluded were not deleterious), a case of pyemia following a mastoid abscess which was treated without medicine and fortunately resulted in recovery[17], and finally, a rather exhaustive study on the ophthalmoscopic refraction of the eyes of newborns to try and determine whether they were born with a tendency to be near-sighted or far-sighted[18]. He concluded that there was a preponderance of far-sightedness in newborn infants. His studies of 102 cigar makers, men and women of various racial backgrounds, are historically colorful, to say the least. Of the 4 Chinese cigar makers in his investigation, 2 admitted to smoking opium at least 1 to 3 times daily—a sad comment on the living conditions of the Chinese-American in New York City during the late 1800's.

In paraphrasing Dr. Roosa's obituary tribute to Ely, "... his untimely death was a great loss to science as well as to his associates and friends," one can only conjecture that his contributions might have been even more noteworthy, had he lived several more decades. Like many other otolaryngologists, he seemed to be utilizing, more and more, the techniques in the then slowly developing field of plastic and reconstructive surgery.[19]

Blair O. Rogers, M.D.
875 Fifth Avenue
New York, N.Y. 10021

REFERENCES

1. Rogers, B. O.: The historical evolution of plastic and reconstructive surgery, in *Nursing Care of the Plastic Surgery Patient.* Edited by D. Wood-Smith and P. C. Porowski, p. 4. C. V. Mosby Co., St. Louis, 1967.

2. Ely, E. T.: An operation for prominence of the auricles. Arch. Otology, *10:* 97, 1881.

3. Becker, O. J.: Surgical correction of the abnormally protruding ear. Arch. Otolaryngol., *50:* 541, 1949.

4. Dieffenbach, J. F.: *Die Operative Chirurgie.* F. A. Brockhaus, Leipzig, I: 395, 1845.

5. Keen, W. W.: New method of operating for relief of deformity of prominent ears. Ann. Surg., *11:* 49, 1890.

6. Monks, G. H.: Operations for correcting the deformity due to prominent ears. Boston Med. & Surg. J., *124:* 84, 1891.

7. Haug, R.: Eine einfache neue plastische Methode zur Rücklagerung hochgradig abstehender Ohrmuscheln. Deutsche med. Wchnschr., *20:* 776, 1894.

8. Joseph, J.: Eselsohren. Verhandl. der Berl. med. Gesellsch., p. 206, 1896.

9. Morestin, H.: De la reposition et du plissement cosmétiques du pavillon de l'oreille. Rev. d'orthopéd., *4:* 289, 1903.

10. Joseph, J.: *Nasenplastik und sonstige Gesichtsplastik ...*, p. 698. Curt Kabitzsch, Leipzig, 1931.

11. *The Medical Register of New York, New Jersey and Connecticut ...* G. P. Putnam's Sons, New York, *23:* 236, 1885–1886.

12. Roosa, D. B. St. J. and Ely, E. T.: *Ophthalmic and Otic Memoranda.* Wm. Wood and Co., New York, 1876.

13. Ely, E. T.: Note on the treatment of acute suppuration of the middle ear. Arch. Otology, *8:* 178, 1879.

14. Ely, E. T.: Skin grafting in chronic suppuration of the middle ear. Arch. Otology, *9:* 343, 1880.

15. Roosa, D. B. St. J. and Ely, E. T.: *Ophthalmic and Otic Contributions.* G. P. Putnam's Sons, New York, 1880.

16. Ely, E. T.: Observations upon the effects of tobacco. New York Med. J., April, 1880.

17. Ely, E. T.: Pyaemia following a mastoid abscess. Treated without medicine. Recovery. Arch. Otology, *10:* 42, 1881.

18. Ely, E. T.: Ophthalmoscopic observations upon the refraction of the eyes of newly born children. Arch. Ophth., *9:* 29, 1880.

19. Rogers, B. O.: The "first one hundred years" of Manhattan Eye, Ear, and Throat Hospital in *Centennial Symposium: Manhattan Eye, Ear, and Throat Hospital.* Woodhaven Press, N. Y., pages 11–26, 1968.

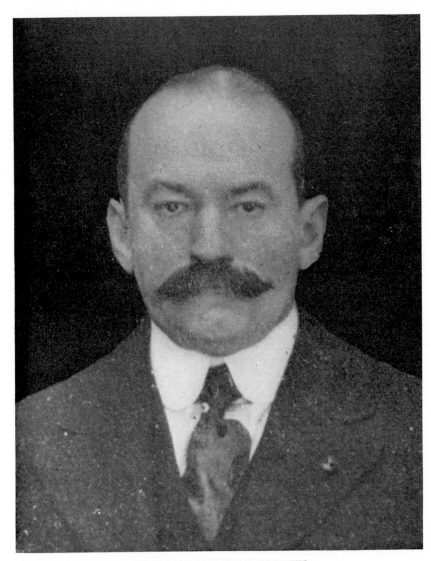

WILLIAM HENRY LUCKETT
1872–1929
(Courtesy of The New York Academy of Medicine)

A NEW OPERATION FOR PROMINENT EARS BASED ON THE ANATOMY OF THE DEFORMITY

WILLIAM H. LUCKETT, M.D.

New York, N.Y.

(Reprinted from Surg. Gynec. & Obst., *10:* 635–7, 1910.)

Prominent ears are comparatively of uncommon occurrence. It is not sufficient to tell a mother of a child that repeatedly returns home from school crying because he has been called "donkey ears" or "sail ears," to leave him alone for such advice will not be accepted, and the odium attached to these ears and the constant harassing by his class-mates frequently is the cause of so much distress as to produce a very bad mental condition in the child as well as in the parents, and to warrant our surgical interference. This deformity occurs in either one or both auricles and in either the whole of the auricle or the lower or the upper part.

Recent writers upon this subject and articles in text-books ignore entirely the anatomy of the deformity, and for that reason describe operations that may temporarily change the so-called cephalo-auricular angle, but will be followed by neither a permanent result nor by a restoration of the normal anatomy of the ear. In order to understand the operation herein described it is necessary for us to enter into the anatomy of the auricle or pinna to a certain extent.

To a careful observer "donkey ears," or prominent ears, means something more than an increase in the cephalo-auricular angle as suggested in recent text-books on surgery; it means a deformity of the ear itself, a change in its topographical anatomy. Rarely have I observed a perfect ear, anatomically, set at so great an angle from the head as to attract attention.

The external surface of the normal auricle is irregularly concave, and presents for examination several well marked depressions and elevations which depend for the most part upon the same depressions and elevations in the underlying cartilage. The concha, the largest and the deepest of the concavities, surrounds the entrance or meatus to the external canal. This funnel-like fossa is subdivided by an obliquely transverse ridge, the crus helicis, which runs forwards and upwards, curving backwards and downwards along the curved margin of the auricle, forming the helix, and terminates just above the posterior margin of the lobule in the cauda helicis. The second elevation, the antihelix, which is in front and parallel to the helix, is a curved ridge which begins at the antitragus below, forms the concave posterior boundary of the concha and divides above it into the superior and the inferior crus, between which lies the fossa triangularis or fossa antihelix. A horizontal section through the auricle just above the level of the auditory canal shows that the cartilage of the concha bends outwards at a right angle from the head until it reaches the antihelix, which it forms by being folded backwards upon itself (Fig. 1, *left*).

Now in most prominent ears which are characterized by a bending forwards of the auricle, either the antihelix is

From the Surgical Service of the Lutheran Hospital.

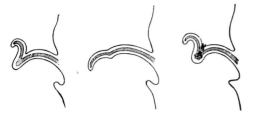

Fig. 1. (*left*) Schematic horizontal section of a normal auricle just above the level of the auditory canal. (*center*) Schematic horizontal section of a prominent ear, showing absence of the fold in the cartilage that forms the antihelix. (*right*) Schematic section of auricle after completion of the operation; sutures in cartilage and skin of reconstructed antihelix. (All are top views.)

undeveloped or entirely absent, the concavity of the concha being continuous with the concavity or fossa of the helix (Fig. 1, *center*). In those cases of prominent ears characterized by a drooping of the upper part of the auricle, we have the concavity of the concha continuous with the fossa triangularis and the fossa helicis, both intervening ridges of the crura antihelicis being absent, or in some lesser deformities of the upper part of the ear, only the upper ridge of the crura antihelicis may be absent. These ridges, the antihelix and the crura antihelicis,

are simply a fluting, bending, or folding of the cartilage, and are apparently intended as trusses for supporting the flexible ear.

The operation, as described and illustrated here, is for the purpose of reconstructing the fold or truss of the cartilage recognized as the antihelix in ears turned forwards, and the same principle is applicable for the reconstruction of the superior crus of the antihelix for the so-called drooping ears, or of both together when necessary.

Because the integument is more freely movable, and the sutures more easily passed, and the resulting cicatrix practically invisible, the inner or posterior surface of the auricle is chosen for the operation. A crescentic incision is made through the integument opposite to the line of the intended new or reconstructed antihelix. The inscribed integument is removed; the edges of the skin are now dissected free from the cartilage and retracted (Fig. 2, *left*). A similar crescentic segment is removed from the cartilage, care being exercised in incising and excising the cartilage not to buttonhole the

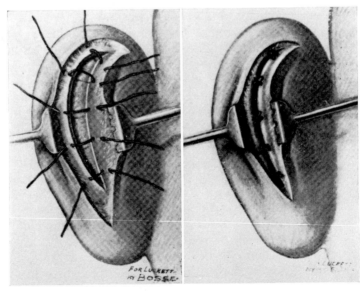

Fig. 2. (*left*) Showing removed section of cartilage, retracted skin, and method of passing sutures on the inner or posterior surface of the ear. (*right*) Showing folding of cartilage after sutures are drawn tight and tied.

skin on the external surface of the auricle. The skin and the cartilage are now sutured separately, and it is the method of suturing the cartilage that is emphasized.

The cartilage suture is passed from the cranial side from within out-and-back again (Fig. 2, *left*), care being taken not to perforate the skin on the external surface, then crossed over the excised portion and passed on the other side from within out-and-back again as a Lembert suture, in such a manner that when the suture is drawn tight and tied, not the edges but the sides or flat surfaces of the cartilage will be in apposition (Figs. 2 and 1, *right*). The edges have been turned forwards or outwards to form the antihelix and at the same time the helix is set closer to the cranium, thus diminishing the cephalo-auricular angle.

Four or five interrupted sutures are usually enough for the cartilage. A so-called fistula, one-half circle, needle is best for the cartilage. The skin is sutured with horsehair and leaves a very small cicatrix.

The greatest care must be exercised in asepsis, as the slightest infection may set up a perichondritis and an auricular perichondritis usually results in a deformed, thickened, corrugated ear. Also care must be taken in the haemostasis. There are no large vessels encountered, and usually the continuous pressure of the artery clamp during the operation is sufficient. It is well to avoid ligatures, but when they must be used only the finest and a single tie is sufficient. A haematoma auris is quite deforming.

The width of the crescentic segment of the cartilage to be removed depends upon the size of the ear, and thickness of the cartilage. In macrotia a large section is removed. In microtia a small section or no section at all is removed, only an incision is made to facilitate the turning outwards of the edges of the cartilage.

In an ear with a very thin flexible cartilage, I think it would be possible to reconstruct the antihelix and set the helix close to the head without excising a segment, or even incising the cartilage, simply by fluting or folding the cartilage at the proper site, and passing the suture in such a manner as to maintain the fold.

William H. Luckett, M.D.
Lutheran Hospital
New York, N. Y.

COMMENTARY BY DR. BLAIR O. ROGERS

William Henry Luckett, who also practiced in New York City, was probably the first surgeon following Ely to introduce a major new concept in correction of the protruding ear. He was apparently the first to emphasize that the protruding ear abnormality is essentially a failure of development of, or folding of, the antihelix. Thus, he suggested an operation which permanently altered this unpleasant contour by removing a long ellipse or crescent of skin and cartilage from almost the entire vertical length of the ear, the excision being carried up to and directly into the proposed line of the superior crus of the antihelix.

Luckett's perception of the requirements for otoplasty was remarkable, indeed. His classic paper is the basis for nearly all of the surgical procedures for this purpose which have been proposed since that time. The background of the surgeon who made such a unique contribution is of interest.

He was born in 1872 in Bastrop, Texas, and graduated successively from the Texas Agricultural and Mechanical College, the Medical School of the University of Virginia, and Columbia University's College of Physicians and Surgeons. He was a charter member of The American College of Surgeons and served as president of the Harlem Medical Association. When he died of heart disease in New York in 1929 (at the age of 57), he was Surgeon-in-Chief of the Lutheran Hospital in Manhattan; formerly he had been the chief surgeon of Harlem Hospital.

In the first World War, he served with the First Division in France and received a

Distinguished Service Citation for his duties as head of a field hospital. He had always been an expert with firearms and at one time was the champion pistol shot of the United States. It is, thus, understandable that he was widely known for his skill in treating gunshot wounds. One of his most notable cases (which was reported and illustrated in several medical journals in 1920) was the successful extraction of a bullet from the right ventricle of a woman's heart, with recovery of the patient.

As a Governor of The New York Athletic Club he was interested in many kinds of sports, including trap shooting and golf. Probably he needed all the physical energy he could muster for the extensive medical literary output which also flowed from his pen between 1907 and 1925. Twenty-one medical papers, or references, are included in the subject index of the Library of The New York Academy of Medicine; 15 were written by Luckett as the sole author. He was apparently a general surgeon in the old and complete sense of the word when, unlike today, the term implied that the surgeon knew his way in and about the human body—anywhere from the top of the frequently injured skull (at times, dented by ping-pong balls) to the tips of the post-Victorian toes.

His papers, and fields of interest, included such diverse subjects as the use of paraffin in surgery, biliary system drainage, X-ray diagnosis of fractures of the skull, pyelography in trauma of the kidney, various methods used in the treatment of tetanus (including anti-tetanic serum), rupture of the ligamentum patellae), torsion of the omentum complicated by acute appendicitis, visible acute dilatation of the stomach during laparotomy, a new instrument for scarifying in the tuberculin test, new methods of suture tying, cholelithiasis in carcinoma of the gall bladder with involvement of the abdominal wall, dislocation of the astragalus, vesico-ureteral and renal tumors, phagedenic ulcers of the abdomen, and (last, but not least) a ping-pong ball indentation of the skull without fracture. In 1910, when the ping-pong ball episode occurred, Teddy Roosevelt's influence on the concepts of "vigorous living" must have extended not only to the rough-and-tumble world of cavalry charges, devil-may-care horsemanship and big game hunting—but to the more sedate atmosphere of Edwardian table-tennis, as well.

In conclusion, we have briefly visualized the otoplasty contributions of two New York City surgeons—Ely, the brilliantly gifted but tragically short-lived opththalmologist-otolaryngologist, and Luckett, the athletic, extroverted general surgeon. Both had wide ranges of interests and contributed substantially, within the period from 1881 to 1910, to the initiation and improvement of operations to correct that very common deformity, the protruding ear.

Blair O. Rogers, M.D.

SECTION VII

Facial Fractures

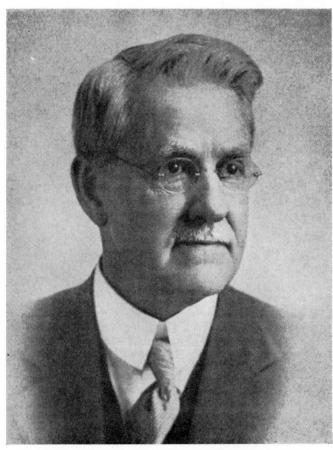

THOMAS L. GILMER, M.D., D.D.S., Sc.D., F.A.C.S.
1849–1931

A CASE OF FRACTURE OF THE LOWER JAW WITH REMARKS ON THE TREATMENT

Case Report

THOMAS L. GILMER, M.D., D.D.S., *Quincy, Illinois*

(From the Archives of Dentistry 4: 388–390, 1887.)

On June 1, 1887, Joseph H. aged 58 years, of Durham, Mo., while leading a horse through a gate, received a kick from the animal on the right side of the inferior maxilla, which drove him with great force against the open gate, causing a compound fracture of the right side of the jaw on a line with the first molar tooth, and a comminuted fracture of the angle and a part of the lower half of the ramus on the left side.

All the teeth on the right side posterior to the fractures were missing. The posterior fragment of the compound fracture was elevated by the action of the muscles. The anterior fragment, containing all the teeth of this jaw, was drawn toward the left side, and greatly depressed, giving the patient an aspect anything but agreeable.

The posterior fragment of the left side, which included the greater portion of the ramus and a part of the angle, was but slightly displaced. The treatment was as follows:

On the right side, the gum was dissected up from the bone on both buccal and lingual surface for about half an inch anteriorly and posteriorly to the fracture. In each fragment a hole was drilled of suitable size to just admit a No. 16 (standard gauge) platinum wire, which was bent in the shape of a staple; the fragments having been put in place the two arms of the staple were inserted into the holes from the lingual surface. These arms were brought together on the buccal side and tightly twisted, drawing the parts into close apposition. Next a short steel wire, No. 27, was placed around the neck of each individual tooth of the lower jaw between the second bicuspid on the right and the second molar on the left and the corresponding teeth of the upper jaw. The ends of each wire were brought together and twisted, fastening it securely to the teeth. This being done, the teeth of the lower jaw were exactly articulated with those of the upper by bringing them together and twisting, thus firmly lashing the lower to the upper jaw. To prevent lateral motion the wire of the upper left lateral was secured to the lower right lateral; this crossing being continued throughout, held the jaw immovable. The smaller fragments of the comminuted fracture were pressed in place as nearly as possible. The compress and bandage were omitted in order that the nutrition of the parts might continue uninterrupted, the before described method of treatment having enabled me safely to dispense with these otherwise necessary appliances.

The patient was advised to cleanse the teeth thoroughly each day, so far as they could be reached by a stiff tooth brush. An antiseptic wash was ordered for frequent use. The patient was fed on liquid food by means of a long-nozzled bulb syringe known to the physician as a powder blower. The bulb of this syringe was filled and its contents discharged into the mouth through the aperture made by the loss of the teeth near the compound fracture. All seemed to go well until about the third week when an abscess, probably caused by a spicula of bone unobserved when the fracture was reduced, formed just below the compound break. A free opening was made into the abscess in such a way as to establish thorough drainage. The pus cavity was syringed with peroxide of hydrogen and a drainage tube sufficiently long to reach the bone was inserted. Every day, as long as the formation of pus continued, peroxide followed by a strong solution of carbolic acid was forced through this tube. The drainage tube was held in place by three silk ligatures stitched in its lower end, the ligatures being secured to the face by adhesive strips.

The comminuted fracture being simple, united in about four weeks, without complications, while the compound fracture required two weeks longer. At this time, the sixth week, the wires were removed, the patient being advised not to use the jaw for mastication for some time longer. The contour of the face is entirely restored, the articulation is good, and there is but little left to indicate the miserable condition the patient presented when he first came under my care.

Thomas L. Gilmer, M.D., D.D.S.
Quincy College of Medicine
Quincy, Ill.

COMMENTARY BY ROBERT H. IVY, M.D.

There are two points about this case report that deserve especial comment.

1. It is the first record in the literature of fixation of a fractured mandible by holding the lower teeth in occlusion with the upper by wire ligatures twisted together. No illustrations are published with the article, but the method of application of the wires and twisting together the ends of those passed around the necks of pairs of upper and lower teeth, respectively, to hold them in occlusion is depicted in later reports by Dr. Gilmer.*

2. Another point in this 1887 report, which apparently has hitherto been overlooked, is that this same case of Gilmer's was one of the first (if not *the* first) in American literature recording the successful use of direct wiring for holding in place a long edentulous posterior bone fragment by a wire suture passed through holes drilled in the bone fragments. The abscess which occurred about three weeks after the application of this internal wire fixation could readily be accounted for by the infection from the wire foreign body, rather than

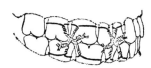

Fig. 1. Method of wiring the lower to the upper teeth.

from an overlooked bone fragment (to which it was ascribed by Dr. Gilmer).

For a full biographical sketch of Thomas L. Gilmer, one may refer to the obituary by Arthur D. Black, M.D., D.D.S. (one of his close associates in the Northwestern University Dental School, Chicago), published in Dental Cosmos *74:* 303–305, 1932. The portrait of Dr. Gilmer published herewith is from that obituary. However, I would like to record here a few important events of his life, and a brief estimate of his character derived from my personal acquaintance with him and opinions of his friends.

Thomas Lewis Gilmer was born in Lincoln County, Missouri, in February 1849. His father was a physician, as were many of his family in preceding generations (one of whom came to Williamsburg, Va., from Scotland in 1731). Gilmer had his academic education in Missouri and Illinois and received the D.D.S. degree from the Missouri Dental College (Dental Department of Washington University) in St. Louis in 1881. He then studied at the St. Louis Medical College during 1881 and 1882 and received

---

* From Gilmer's "Lectures on Fractures of the Maxillae," Chicago, 1901, p. 30—and also in his "Lectures on Oral Surgery at Northwestern University Dental School, Chicago, Session 1899–1900," page 94. In these two publications, Gilmer states that, at the suggestion of Dr. H. J. Goslee of Chicago, he now employs "German silver wire for ligating the teeth, instead of the original steel wire."

his M.D., from Quincy, Ill., College of Medicine in 1885. Afterwards he served as an Oral Surgeon at St. Mary's Hospital in Quincy and taught microscopy and histology in the Quincy College of Medicine.

Dr. Gilmer moved to Chicago in 1889. In 1891, he called a meeting which resulted in organization of the Northwestern University Dental School, in which he later became Professor of Oral Surgery and served as Dean. He specialized in oral surgery throughout his professional career and was Oral Surgeon to St. Luke's Hospital in Chicago for many years. He became a Fellow of the American College of Surgeons, one of the Founders and President of the Institute of Medicine of Chicago, and a member of the Chicago Pathological Society.

Dr. Gilmer was a Founder in 1921 (and second president, in 1924) of the American Association of Oral and Plastic Surgeons— the forerunner of the present American Association of Plastic Surgeons. In 1912, Northwestern University conferred on him the honorary degree of Doctor of Science. He died December 28, 1931, at the age of 82.

Dr. Gilmer inherited both the professional and gentlemanly traits of his ancestors, to which were added a frankness and friendliness that became outstanding features of his personality. In fighting for a principle, he managed to avoid personalities and retain the friendship and respect of those on the opposite side. He was thoroughly well-grounded in the fundamentals of medicine.

Of all the leading "oral surgeons" of the day, Dr. Gilmer stood highest in Vilray Blair's respect and esteem. When organizing courses for training Army medical and dental officers for the management of American face and jaw casualties in World War I, Blair selected Northwestern University Dental School, under direction of Dr. Gilmer, as one of the three civilian institutions to conduct these courses.

My earliest meetings with Dr. Gilmer took place about 1910. I saw him many times at meetings in Chicago and elsewhere between 1915 and 1917, during the height of his activity in the field of investigation of chronic foci of infection around the teeth and their influence upon diseases of the body in general. He was among the leaders in this important study, with Frank Billings, E. C. Rosenow, Hartzell and Henrici, Moody, and others.

Among my most valued possessions is an autographed copy of one of the two textbooks published by Dr. Gilmer, entitled "Lectures on Oral Surgery." The book is small, having only 162 pages with 59 illustrations (photographs and drawings) and covers 22 lectures on many diverse subjects.

I benefited greatly in my earlier years from occasional contacts with this great pioneer and teacher in the field which has eventually blossomed into our modern specialty of plastic surgery.

ROBERT H. IVY, M.D.

EXPERIMENTAL STUDY OF FRACTURES OF THE UPPER JAW

Parts I and II

RENÉ Le FORT, M.D., *Lille, France*

(*Rev. chir. de Paris, 23: 208–227, 360–379, 1901.*)

Translated from the French by
DR. PAUL TESSIER, *Paris, France*

Surgically speaking, we must consider as belonging to the upper jaw and face the pterygoid processes of the sphenoid bone and the lateral masses and *lamina perpendicularis* of the ethmoid—in a word, the whole bony mass hanging from the cranial base and immediately continuous with it.

In most previous works, the authors have studied the fractures of various bones of the face separately.... But the various parts that make up the upper jaw are united by sutures which do not prevent the propagation of fracture lines; consequently, they cannot be used as a basis for division of the subject. One would not dream of studying separately the fractures of the diverse bones of the skull; in the same way, it is impossible to separate the fractures of the upper jaw from those of the palatine bones, cheek bones, *etc.*

It is not the same with partial fractures, however, limited to a circumscribed area—as, for example, fractures of the true nasal bones.... All of the limited lesions are produced by a brusque blow on a small surface which alone yields to the wounding force.

I am eliminating one category of fractures from this study—gunshot wounds. Often the result of suicide attempts, these are veritable explosions in the face and are without surgical interest....

Wounds made by sharp instruments, such as those from saber cuts ... must also be excluded from this study. And finally we exclude certain fractures of the face which are only a concomitant of a fracture of the base of the skull. Often there is misunderstanding on this subject.

Frequently after marked trauma there is a simultaneous serious fracture of the skull and a fracture of the face. The fact is incontestable; the interpretation is not.... In the vast majority of cases, the facial fracture is not dependent on the skull lesion and does not necessarily accompany it; skull fractures due to force exerted exclusively on the skull do not spread to the face other than in an exceptional and always insignificant manner.... The possibility of inflicting a skull fracture from a facial fracture is most interesting; we shall return to it.

I have studied fractures of the upper jaw with their concomitant vast and notable contusions and compressions. I will use the term *indirect* fractures (if that term hasn't been used too frequently for fractures of the superior maxilla) to des-

Editorial note. The reader will recognize here the first two of the 3 long papers that Prof. Le Fort wrote on his monumental experiments on human cadavers to determine the lines of least resistance in fractures of the face. I thought it fitting to have Dr. Paul Tessier do this translation and commentary, but asked him to condense it to 10 pages. When we received his translation, the work was of such great interest that I decided to add to Tessier's condensation some of the descriptions of the actual experiments, and a few additional bits of text. These were translated by Kitty Dabney and Mary McDowell.

ignate those fractures caused by force at the level of the neighboring bones. . . . There is a regrettable confusion in terminology; a fracture is *direct* when it is produced at the point of contact with the blow—*indirect* when it is produced at a distance from the blow, even if it is on the bone itself. . . .

The laws that govern fractures are the general laws of body resistance, and the laws of action and reaction. Action is represented by the site of the application and the extent of the applied area of the force—the direction of this force, its velocity, its duration, and the mass of the wounding agent. Reaction is everything that opposes the simple displacement of the body subjected to the impact—in other words, the degree and the means of fixation of the body undergoing the strain. The effect of these two forces depends upon the architecture and the texture of the bones. For any variation in one of these causes, there may be a corresponding variation in the effects; herein lie the reasons for their infinite clinical variety, and for the torments of experimenters. . . .

The *rapidity of the wounding agent,* and the *extent of the surface which it disturbs,* influence the results; the greater the rapidity of the blow or the smaller the surface, the more the tendency to local lesions; but when a local lesion is produced, the effort is expended in this and the ulterior action simulates a slower blow if the force is sufficient to cause new damage. Here the *duration of action* intervenes.

The *mass of the wounding agent* does not play a role, except relative to the degree of the lesions produced.

There remain, then, 3 important conditions which must guide the experimenter. The first two depend on the action; they are the *point of application of the force,* and *the direction of the wounding agent.* The third stems from the re-action; it is the *degree* and the *position of the head* during the trauma. . . .

An eminently favorable condition for the experimental study of fractures of the bones of the face is the almost non-existent role of muscular contractions in the production of these fractures. . . . Of the muscles of the face, only the pterygoids have any real influence on the displacement of the fragments. These very advantageous conditions permit us to draw precise conclusions from our experiments, which can be applied clinically with certitude.

Nearly all the experiments were performed on whole cadavers, or after decapitation. In almost all cases, after having exerted a force directly on the face (or at a distance from it) I sawed the skull circularly, detached the *dura mater,* and examined the cranial bases for possible traces of a fracture. Then the head was boiled to enable me to remove the soft tissues easily.

The cleaning of a fresh head, before boiling or macerating it, is almost impossible without creating some fractures. The osseous planes are slender and yield to the least effort. . . .

Before going into detail on my experiments, I'd like to point out certain things which struck me peculiarly. First is the *intensity of the violence* necessary to produce a fracture of the face. The bony mass which constitutes the upper jaw has particular characteristics which one does not encounter at any other point in the body. It is formed by some columns of tissue, more or less spongy, between which are the very slender blades of compact tissue hung like curtains. The examination of a facial skeleton cannot give us an idea of the resistance of this mass. The bones (prepared and blanched) yield very easily to the least effort. Take a prepared skeleton and with your finger punch at the level of the canine fossa, for example, and you can go right through it without any difficulty.

On the contrary, when one takes a fresh and entire head and inflicts various traumas on it and dissects it, he will find it has resisted. Why? Because the fragile parts are not easily accessible to direct trauma, and because the projecting parts are resistant. The fragile parts are covered on all sides by soft tissues, which considerably augment the solidity by lending their elasticity to spread and dissipate the forces of trauma. . . .

The face resists these forces because of the elasticity of its bones, periosteum, and soft tissues. The extreme thinness of many of its parts does not decrease its resistance, but exaggerates its elasticity. When the limit of elasticity is finally exceeded, it breaks—but the fractures therein differ from those of the long bones. They are usually long fissures, without damage to the soft tissues; displacements of the fragments are exceptional.

And still these displacements are mentioned in almost all observations. The following will explain it.

Until 1866, when A. Guerin showed the possibility of diagnosing certain fractures of the upper jaw that were not displaced, one did not recognize the resulting hollows in the face, and gross lesions passed unnoticed. Experimental study demonstrated that almost always, following trauma to the face of sufficient strength to produce widespread bony lesions, the bones remained in their normal positions and nothing would lead one to suppose, at first glance, that there was a fracture. . . . The *fracture without displacement is the rule.* One can say of this phenomenon the same thing the surgeons say of a double transverse fracture; "If it is easy to produce on a cadaver, it is impossible that it does not appear frequently in the living patient."

This absence of displacement together with the extremely rapid healing, proved by clinical observations, indicates that *fractures of the upper jaw are the most frequently unrecognized* and, for that reason, are considered to be rare. . . .

This absence of displacement and of lesions of the soft parts often makes it very difficult to diagnose these fractures. One can say that on a cadaver it is never possible to do it completely. Serious and widespread lesions generally do not manifest themselves by any exterior sign. Often, educated doctors who helped me with my experiments advised me, after the first blow, to hit again—convinced that there was no lesion when actually the damage was most extensive. . . .

It would appear that the diagnosis could be singularly facilitated if the surgeon, when confronted by a facial contusion, knew which were the weak points, the lines of least resistance—where, at last, he must look to awaken the pain which often will be the only revealing symptom. This was the practical goal of the present work. . . .

ANTEROPOSTERIOR BLOWS ON THE UPPER LIP

A. Guerin, whose name remains attached to this variety of fracture, wrote: "When a violent blow is struck backward on the face, as if one wanted to push in the part of the upper jaw lying below the nostrils, a transverse fracture is produced which passes about one cm below the malar bone and extends through the pterygoid processes; the latter processes are always fractured at the level of the lower end of the pterygomaxillary fissure—*i.e.* where they have the least resistance". . . .

On the initiative of Guerin, Cocteau undertook at Glamart 7 experiments; these supported the convictions of the master. The experiments were repeated later on many occasions. M. Lejeune reproduced them on 5 cadavers, and 5 times he obtained the transverse fracture; M. Fillion did them 3 times and M. Papin many times, always with the same results. . . .

The authors who first described these fractures did not place any importance on concomitant lesions, such as the palatine split. Lejeune, who noted the lesion in his first two experiments, did not report it in the next 3 experiments. . . .

I did some experiments on this fracture. A considerable force was necessary to produce it. Three times (Experiments I, II, and III) I obtained only insignificant crushing of the front wall of some tooth sockets. In two other experiments (IV and V) the first blow produced a partial transverse fracture simultaneously with a complete palatine fissure running from front to back. The second blow completed the transverse fracture in Experiment IV, but in Experiment V it completed it only on one side. . . .

Experiment I

Female, approximately 50 years old. Entire cadaver, supine, face turned up. Three blows with a club were applied directly to the front of the upper maxilla, with moderate force. At examination, only insignificant lesions of the alveolar border were found.

Experiment II

Male, approximately 65 years old. Entire cadaver, lying on the ground supine, with face up.

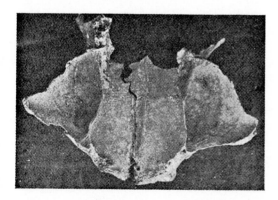

FIG. 1. Guerin's fracture, the inferior fragment resulting from Experiment IV. (Photograph made from above downward.) (*Courtesy, National Library of Medicine, Bethesda, Md.*)

One blow with the heel applied forcefully on the upper lip was accompanied by a bony cracking. Dissection revealed only a minimal crushing of the front wall of the alveolus (recently deprived of teeth).

Experiment III

Male, about 45 years old. Decapitated specimen. The head was hurled against the rounded edge of a table, so as to apply force to the upper lip. The result was negative.

Experiment IV

Male, about 65 years old. After decapitation, the head was thrown violently against the rounded edge of a marble table. The first blow did not seem to produce a fracture. After a second blow, one noted a fissure between the nasal orifice and the canine fossa . . . the palatine vault was fractured between the two incisors and the fissure extended backward to the right and near the midline to the apophysis of the palate. The pterygoid processes were broken, the left at the level of the lower portion of the pterygomaxillary fissure. . . . A third blow, administered like the first two, was necessary to achieve a horizontal fracture. It was very high, near the cheek bones, but did not cut them open (Fig. 1).

Experiment V

Macerated head, covered only with some soft parts. Supported in a hollow, on the occiput, face looking up. The first blow was directed at the upper edge of the alveolus, from the front backward. The force, administered with a club, hit below the left incisors. A fissure was produced from the front to back of the entire palatine vault. Another fissure divided the lower portion of the nose on the right side and traversed the lower part of the cheek bone, but the fracture in the cheek bone was incomplete.

A second blow lengthened the fissure, and the right pterygoid process was broken. On the left side, the malar was dislocated at the level of the frontal and the zygomatic process; the whole left maxilla, including its processes, formed a great fragment with the malar on the same side and the palate. . . .

LATERAL BLOWS ON THE LOWER PART OF THE UPPER JAW

M. Fillion, in 4 experiments, obtained in the first two a fracture of only the maxilla which was hit. . . . M. Papin repeated these experiments and he distinguished the results of blows over the canine from those delivered over the molars. . . . With horizontal blows delivered at the level of the canine tooth, he once obtained a large horizontal fracture. . . .

I did two experiments on this subject. It was difficult to wound the superior maxilla laterally without wounding the malar bone or the mandible at the same time—and it is probably rare that one encounters lesions produced by this mechanism.

Experiment VI

Male, about 45 years old. Cut off head, partly depilated of its soft parts. It was placed, right side down, on a table. Several blows with a wooden club were directed at the left side of the face, at the left part of the alveolar arch, and below it. The angle of the mandible gave way on the right side, which rested on the table.

At dissection, there was a transverse fracture of the upper jaw, separating the nasal cavity and running back toward the pterygoid processes, where it stopped. . . . The right zygomatic arch was broken, disjointed in front from the malar. . . .

A new blow, directed like the preceding ones, fractured the pterygoid processes at their bases and parted the ethmoid and vomer. Guerin's fracture was thus complete.

Experiment VII

Man, about 50 years old. Entire cadaver supine with the head hanging backward over the edge of the table. A violent blow was struck with the club on the right upper jaw, beneath the malar. The force was directed obliquely from bottom to top, as though the subject were standing. . . . When the specimen was dissected there was a transverse fracture of the maxilla on the right, cutting all of the bones as in Guerin's fracture. On the left, a fissure divided the nasal cavity fairly low, then ascended to reach the suture at the lower edge of the orbit, and then traveled obliquely to the sphenomaxillary fissure.

(From these) one obtains, usually, a large transverse fracture in which one or both pterygoid processes sometimes remain intact; at times, there is an associated fissure of the palate.

After oblique lateral blows downward, one may see a fracture of the alveolus (if the force is exerted at a short distance from the teeth), or a separation of the whole lower part of the upper jaw (if the force is exerted higher).

After a lateral blow going obliquely upward, the fracture may be an ascending one. The horizontal fracture on the side receiving the blow may be continuous with an ascending fracture passing above the opposite malar bone. In a word, the fracture follows the direction of the force.

BLOWS DIRECTED UPWARD ON THE UPPER ALVEOLUS

I did 3 experiments on this, and the results obtained were very comparable to each other. . . .

Experiment VIII

Old person, almost edentulous. The cadaver was supine, with the head protruding over the table and hanging back. The mouth was wide open. A moderate blow with a wooden club fell level on the upper dental arch—that is to say, from bottom to top and from front to back (as though the subject were standing). The force was minimal; the assistants were sure that there was no lesion.

Dissection after boiling. A large fissure skirted the malar bone; from the sphenomaxillary fossa, it traversed the orbital floor, skirted the pyramidal process while passing the canine fossa, then below the edge of the alveolus to ascend again in the back toward the posterior edge of the maxilla. About 12 mm from the edge of the orbit, a branch ran from the main fissure to reach the inferior part of the nasal cavity. . . .

Experiment IX

Man, about 45 years old. The cadaver was positioned in the same manner as in the preceding experiment, and the blow was delivered in the same way, but violently. There was a clear feeling of bony cracking. All of the palatine arch was movable and was forced back.

At dissection, two fracture lines ascended vertically to the middle of each nasal bone, then inclined outward symmetrically to traverse the ascending processes of the maxillae, reached the nasolacrimal duct on each side, passed along the floor of the orbit to exit at the suture between the malar and maxilla. From this point, the symmetry was no longer absolute. . . .

After ablation of the fractured part, there remained adherent to the base of the skull the central and superior parts of the nasal bones, and the malar bones with the tops of their pyramidal processes—allowing a view of the most external part of the maxillary sinuses. All of the middle part of the face had disappeared (Fig. 2).

In summary, there was a falling back of a large fragment which consisted of almost the entire two superior maxillae. This fragment was itself divided into secondary fragments.

Experiment X

Man, about 45 years old. The cadaver was positioned as in the two preceding experiments, and the blows were administered in the same fashion. The first blow (minimal) deviated to the left and did not produce a lesion; the second blow was more violent.

At dissection, on the right a fissure divided the orifices of the nasal fossae below the nasal bones, traversed the superior process and then went along a small part of the orbital floor, descending to the canine fossa and falling into a large transverse fracture. On the left, almost symmetrical lesions were present....As in the other experiments, the condition of the palatine mucosa did not cause one to suspect the lesion....

In Experiments IX and X, the lesions were more extensive. The fissure that goes around the malar bone was still to be found, but the lesion was double and the whole middle part of the face had yielded.

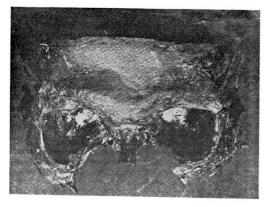

FIG. 2. The cranium of Experiment IX and the part of the face that remained after removal of the fractured parts. (*Courtesy National Library of Medicine, Bethesda, Md.*)

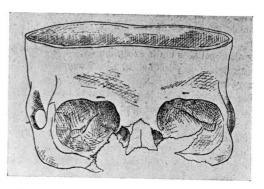

FIG. 3. Drawing (made from a photograph of the specimen) of the cranium of Experiment XI and the part of the face that remained after removal of the fractured parts. (*Courtesy, National Library of Medicine, Bethesda, Md.*)

This particular lesion (which will be met again, produced by a different mechanism) displayed clear-cut characteristics. A large fissure started upward from the nasal notch, reached the orbit, and left it to pass symmetrically around the malar bones and cut the pterygoid processes adjacent to their bases. The nasal bones, more or less intact, remained partly adherent to the skull—as did the malar bones and a part of the malar processes of the maxillae. The remainder of the face, including the pterygoid processes, formed part of a large, circumscribed fragment. Furthermore, this fragment was divided by a fissure that crossed the whole hard palate from front to back. In addition, there was a large transverse fracture* on one side in Experiment IX; it was complete and double in Experiment X.

BLOWS BACKWARD ON THE MIDFACE

It appears that forces exerted on the midface produced results comparable to those following direct blows from below upward on the upper alveolus. It is helpful to compare Experiments IX and XI, and Figures 2 and 3, which report this. In the two cases, all the midface gave way—almost following the same lines. The fa-

*Editorial note. Guerin, or Le Fort I, fracture.

cial fragment circumscribed by the large fissure had, in the two cases, suffered the same divisions—anteroposterior fracture of the palatine arch, and transverse fracture of the upper jaw. . . .

I have tried, without success, to produce fractures of the upper jaw by precipitating a whole cadaver, face down, against a padded and resistant substance. Always, the cadaver has turned aside while falling, or the shock has been insufficient to produce the lesions. . . .

Experiment XI

A woman, about 65 years old, the head, taken off, was placed firmly in a hollow on the occiput, the face looking up. A violent blow with a club was administered to the anterior part of the face, avoiding force on the cheek bones.

The lower end of the nasal bone was fractured on the left side. From there, the fracture line went up between the nasal bone and the ascending process of the maxilla, where it completely disjoined the suture. Then the line traversed the floor of the orbit at the level of the articulation with the malar, following the suture to the cheek tubercle. On this side (left) the separation of the malar and maxilla was complete and exactly at the level of the suture. All of the maxillary portion of the floor of the orbit remained adherent to the maxilla on this side.

On the right, the fracture line commenced at the external and superior part of the nasal incisure, traversed the ascending process, and followed the internal inferior angle of the orbit. Another line, coming out of the preceding one, cut the inferior wall of the orbit, then its anterior edge, and separated the malar from this side of the maxilla. A fragment of the zygomatic process adhered to the malar. The two pterygoid processes were broken at their bases. The nasal septum was fractured below and above. The two maxillae remained completely separated from the face (Fig. 3).

The large fragment which comprised the midface was itself divided by a fracture of the hard palate. There was a disjunction in the midline from the alveolar border to the level of the palatine bone; at this level, the fissure traversed the palatine process on the right obliquely, in such a way that it abutted midway between the midline and the pterygoid process.

Finally, a horizontal fracture, situated high, divided the fragment of the right side into two portions—one comprising the palatine arch and

alveolar border, the other the ascending process of the maxilla.

Experiment XII

Woman, about 50 years old. Supine, head placed on the occiput, face looking up. A blow with a club was applied directly to the top of the nose.

At dissection, the lesions were limited to the bones of the nose. The lower half of the nasal bone on the right, and the inner part of the left nasal bone, formed a small, free fragment, broken clean without splinters.

Experiment XIII

Very old woman, completely edentulous. The cadaver being supine on the ground with the face looking up, it was kicked violently on the lower part of the face, avoiding the cheekbones.

After dissection, only a broken right canine fossa was found. . . .

BLOWS DOWNWARD ON THE BASE OF THE NOSE

(*Editorial note.* The author did no experiments on this, but cites previous work by others.)

UPWARD BLOWS ON THE MANDIBLE

. . . I have tried to evaluate the question and at first I tried to crush the maxilla between the skull and mandible. One case failed completely (Experiment XIV); the skull and the mandible gave way, while the upper jaw alone resisted. In another (Experiment XV) the cervical vertebrae gave way, the force having been misdirected. . . . Attempts to precipitate the head on to the mandible (Experiment XVI) yielded only insignificant shock to the teeth. . . .

The results of applying force to the chin were more successful. In Experiment XVII, in addition to a fracture of the mandible, there was a fissure which completely outlined the pyramidal process, so that the malar was held only by its superior and posterior angles. In Experiment XVIII, the canine fossa gave way while the alveolar arch resisted, in spite of its thinness. The mandible was dislocated. . . .

(Editorial note. These experiments are then described in detail. Only part of Experiment XVII will be reprinted here.)

Experiment XVII

Old woman, about 60. The cadaver was in the dorsal decubitus position, the head lying beyond the edge of the table and hanging free. The mouth was open. A very violent blow was administered with a club to the chin. External examination revealed only a fracture of the lower jaw.

At dissection, the mandible was found to be broken a little to the right of the midline, and there was also a fracture at the junction of the ramus and the body. On the right, there was also a fracture of the condyle.

In the upper jaw, a fissure separated the maxilla from the left cheekbone at the level of the orbital border. From there the fissure descended to outline the pyramidal process, then backward and finally upward toward the base of the pterygoid process and up again to the pterygomaxillary fossa. In the orbit, the fracture followed the infraorbital canal for 1½ cm, then stopped a short distance from the pterygomaxillary fissure in such a way that the cheekbone was hardly held, except by its superior and posterior angles (Fig. 4)....

It seems logical to consider together the lesions obtained by compression of the upper jaw between the mandible and skull—whether the upper jaw is immobilized against a resistant plane (supplied by the sternum or an external agent) or the force is exerted on the mandible (as in a fall on the chin or a blow up under the mandible)....

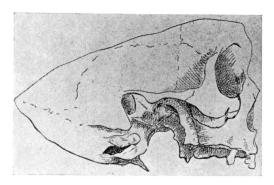

Fig. 4. Drawing of the cranium from Experiment XVII. *(Courtesy, National Library of Medicine, Bethesda, Md.)*

It matters little whether the mandible yields or not, but in all cases it is essential to distinguish between closed-mouth and open-mouth injuries. When the mouth is closed, the upper and lower teeth imbricate—adapting and corresponding to one another so that the face forms a whole, and the mechanism of fracture is that of bipolar compression (even when inertia fixes the skull). When the mouth is open, the lower jaw becomes the wounding agent by suddenly bringing together the dental arches.... The lesions are comparable to those obtained by exerting direct force on the alveolar arch, with the mouth open.

This was actually demonstrated in our experiments. In Experiment XVII (blow on the chin) as well as in Experiment VIII (direct blow on the upper alveolus) identical lesions were produced, passing around the malar bone, despite the apparently different mechanisms....

GENERAL CONSIDERATIONS OF BLOWS
ON THE MALAR BONE

Blows to the malar bone must indubitably constitute the majority of facial injuries, due to the fact that the zygoma is the most exposed part. This has been confirmed by our observations, and by the studies of previous authors....

LATERAL BLOWS TO THE MALAR, THE
HEAD BEING UNSUPPORTED

Following a force exerted laterally against the cheekbone, while the head is hanging free and not supported by a resistant plane, the dominant lesion is a breaking in of the cheekbone into the maxillary sinus by collapse of the pyramid. The breaking in is moderate, and most often the internal wall of the sinus remains intact....

Experiment XIX

Old woman. Cadaver supine. The head was off the table, hanging freely behind. A violent blow was applied laterally on the right malar by an aide, using a club.

At dissection, the inferior part of the cheekbone was found to be partially into the sinus. There was a collapse of the pyramidal process which had been reduced to splinters (these were detached in preparing the skull and are absent in Figure 5).... A small line, quite visible on the drawing, departed from the splintered region of the pyramid and fell horizontally into the nasal cavity. On the specimen, this line was difficult to see, but it was the photograph which revealed it.

Experiment XX

Man, about 50. The cadaver was supine with the head off the table, hanging backward freely. A violent blow was applied laterally to the right cheekbone by an aide, using a club at a very acute angle.

At dissection, there was a comminuted fracture of the center of the malar bone. The zygomatic arch had given way in the middle part, following a vertical line.... At the pyramidal process, the maxilla had a comminuted fracture and the cheekbone was pushed into the sinus.... Above, there was a disjunction of the malar and frontal bone at the level of the external angular process.

After removing the fragments circumscribed by the fissures, one saw (Fig. 6) that the line crossed the floor of the orbit, of which the anterior half had been fractured. The fissure passed near the nasolacrimal duct, without reaching it, and outlined the base of the pyramidal process, passing one cm from the alveolar border....

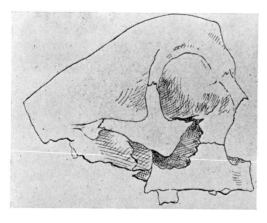

Fig. 5. Drawing of the specimen from Experiment XIX. (*Courtesy, National Library of Medicine, Bethesda, Md.*)

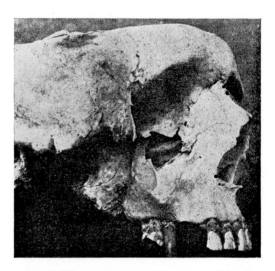

Fig. 6. The specimen from Experiment XX after removal of the loose bony fragments through the fissures. (*Courtesy, National Library of Medicine, Bethesda, Md.*)

Experiment XXI

Man, about 45. Cadaver in same position as previous one. An extremely violent blow was applied to the left cheekbone with a club. The soft parts resisted.

At dissection, all of the left side of the face was the site of an extremely comminuted fracture. The left malar was reduced to 3 or 4 fragments; a small splinter of the superior angle adhered to the external angular process.

All the splinters of the fractured region were circumscribed by a huge fissure ... (which also) traversed the alveolar arch between the canine and the left incisor, crossing the palatine arch obliquely toward the right pterygoid process.... The vomer was fractured vertically behind, and the perpendicular plate of the ethmoid, cut at the level of the skull in back, was cut obliquely from back to front and from front to bottom. The zygomatic process was broken a little behind its middle.

All the bony mass limited by the large fracture line was composed of small splinters, and there were no other lesions beyond this line. When the splinters were removed, there remained a hole capable of holding a mandarin orange.

Experiment XXII

Aged woman, edentulous. The cadaver was placed in the same position as in the 3 preceding experiments, and the aide directed the force in the same way, laterally, with a club against the cheekbone—but the blow was not so abrupt.

At dissection, we found only an insignificant bony fraying of the lower part of the malar bone.

BLOWS ON THE CHEEKBONE, PRODUCED BY MOVING THE HEAD RAPIDLY TO HIT A RESISTANT OBJECT

When the rapidly moving head hit a resistant body (the mechanism of fractures from a fall), the effects were intermediate to those obtained by blows on the swinging head and those which resulted from crushing the face between two opposing forces. . .

Experiment XXIII

Man, about 60. The head, taken off and held solidly in the hands, was violently projected toward the padded edge of the autopsy table in such a manner that the forehead did not suffer; the force was applied to the anterior part of the left cheekbone, and to the left side of the nose. After the first blow, external examination revealed nothing. After the second, we saw a fracture of the inferior orbital rim. After the third, a fracture of the nasal bones and perhaps of the ascending process of the maxilla was present.

At dissection, on opening the skull we noted

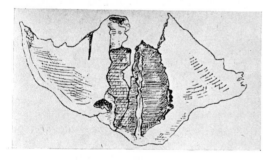

FIG. 7. Experiment XXIV. The two principal fragments are seen from above downward. On the sides, the fractured parts of the floor of the orbit appear clearly; in the center, in the longer plane, the floor of the nasal fossae is shown in a darker tint. (*Courtesy, National Library of Medicine, Bethesda, Md.*)

the presence of a fissure of the cranial vault . . . it was accompanied by a subdural effusion of blood. . . . On the side of the face, the left cheekbone was pushed into the sinus. It was a little lower and inclined, in such a way that the inferior angle was lowered, drawing near the maxilla. The orbital rim was also lowered. Above, there was a disjunction of the external angular process; behind, there was a clean-cut vertical fracture of the middle part of the arch and a fracture of the posterior angle of the malar. . . . The pyramidal process was outlined by a large fissure and adhered to the cheekbone, with which it formed a large fragment. When the fragment was removed, the sinus was wide open. . . .

Experiment XXIV

Aged woman, edentulous. The head, stripped almost completely of its soft parts, was violently projected against the round edge of a table. The blow hit transversely on the left cheekbone; the edge of the table met the bone on an oblique line from top to bottom and from front to back. Almost all of the face exploded into 3 fragments, completely detached. . . .

The fracture line commenced at the left malar . . . at the line of encounter between the bone and the table edge. From there it passed to the floor of the orbit and across the inner aspect to reach the suture between the ascending process and the frontal. It descended between the process and the left side of the nasal bone, cutting its inferior half and commencing to cut that of the right bone, then went straight down to the nasal incisure. The line started again from this orifice, cut the ascending process on the other side, reached the other orbit and traversed its medial wall from front to back, crossing its floor transversely to the sphenomaxillary fissure. From there, it went upward toward the external wall of the orbit, staying $2\frac{1}{2}$ cm posterior, toward the external angular process of the frontal bone—which it had separated from the superior angle of the malar (Fig. 7).

(*Editorial note.* Le Fort continues with another page of description of the various fractures in Experiment XXIV.)

(*To Be Continued*)

COMMENTARY BY THE EDITOR

Let us pause for a moment, divert our thoughts from this rather macabre scene, and ask ourselves what this young investigator—so busily clubbing cadaver faces in some Parisian cellar—is accomplishing. Up to now, using various kinds of forces in differing intensities, applied from diverse directions to point after point in the face, he has uncovered a large number of isolated weak points in the bony structure. As yet, there is no pattern.

In Part III, as Le Fort continues his systematic investigation some definite patterns do begin to emerge and he is able to connect the weak points into 3 "great weak lines" (or planes). These, of course, are the bases for the LeFort I, II, and III fractures.

So, let us return to the basement.

—*F. McDowell*

Part III

(Rev. chir. de Paris, 23: 479–507, 1901.)

BLOWS ON THE ANTEROLATERAL PART OF THE MALAR, WITH THE HEAD RESTING ON THE OCCIPUT

Lesions produced by this mechanism differ a bit from those which we have considered. We have observed only the breaking in of the cheekbone into the sinus, as force was exerted on the free head.... The considerable forces necessary to cause damage when the head can freely avoid the wounding agent are not necessary to produce grave disorders on the fixed head....

Blows directed against the malar have the first effect of breaking the pyramidal process of the maxilla and of separating from the rest of the face a primary fragment composed of the entire malar and a large part of the pyramidal process... then the two footings on which the zygomatic complex rests are also broken; the ascending process of the maxilla with part of the nasal bone forms a second fragment, and the base of the upper jaw, pushed back, forms a third fragment, separated horizontally and comprising all of the palatine arch, the alveolar arch and the two pterygoid processes, torn out with this fragment at the weakest point....

Experiment XXV

Woman, about 65. Cadaver ... (with) ... head lying on the table, the face turned up. A moderate blow with a club was applied to the anterolateral part of the right malar. Examination of the cadaver showed no trace of fracture ... (but) ... at dissection the right malar and the pyramidal process of the maxilla together formed a large primary fragment which was not displaced.... In summary, there were 3 fragments: (1) the right malar with the pyramidal process; (2) the ascending process with part of the nasal bone; (3) the inferior part of the two maxillae were separated, as in a Guerin''s fracture.

Experiment XXVI

Adult cadaver laid out as in the previous experiment. A blow of a wooden club was applied to the cheekbone as before. There was no bony displacement and the lesions were not recognized until after removal of the soft parts.

At dissection, the main fragment was comprised of the malar with part of the pyramidal process.... A second fragment, not mobile, was completely separated from all the rest of the face; it comprised the palatine arch, the alveolar arch, and the two pterygoid processes (separated at their bases).... A third fragment included the lateral and inferior part of the right nasal bone, part of the ascending process, and the internal and anterior portions of the nasolacrimal duct.... A fourth fragment was composed of the zygomatic arch, separated in front as we have described, and in back at 2 or 3 mm from the transverse base.

Experiment XXVII

Woman 45 to 50. Cadaver in dorsal decubitus position, the face looking up. We applied blows to the middle of the face with a metal shaft. The first blow hit the mandible and produced a comminuted fracture of the main part of this bone.... A second blow, applied with the same force, was directed anteroposteriorly along a vertical line on the lateral face of the malar.

At dissection, there was a comminuted fracture of the cheekbone. A large vertical fracture, passing behind the orbit, separated it into two unequal parts ... the pyramidal process of the maxilla was outlined by a large fissure coming from the orbital border and descending toward the first molar to within one cm of the alveolus ... when these fragments were removed, the sinus was largely open....

Finally, an important fragment comprised the posterior part of the alveolus, emanating from the second bicuspid area and going up to the pterygoid process which, separated at its base, was part of the fragment....

BLOWS ON THE LATERAL PART OF THE MALAR, THE HEAD LYING ON THE OPPOSITE SIDE

When force is exerted on the cheekbone with the head being supported on the opposite side, there is bilateral compression and the lesions present a marked symmetry on the two sides. The action is almost the same on the side which receives the blow as on the side which is supported.... I have tried to produce fractures by bilateral compression of the face between the jaws of a large vise placed at the level of the two cheekbones. It is very difficult to keep the head in position, when the jaws come together, while working with a head denuded of soft parts. When the head is stripped of the soft parts, one obtains only a local crushing of the cheekbones (Experiment XXVII)....

Experiment XXVIII

Old woman. The head was placed between the jaws of a large vise and held, as much as possible, while applying compression on both sides at the level of the cheekbones. The soft parts were crushed and, as one worked, the head turned and escaped.

Experiment XXIX

The same experiment was repeated on the head of an adult man, first removing the soft parts at the level of the cheekbones to avoid displacement. As successive crackings occurred, the cheekbones were crushed and broken in. As the compression was continued the skull, which the jaws of the vise had reached, gave way in turn at the level of the temporal bones and of the sphenoid. At dissection, there were no other lesions of the side of the face, except the broken cheekbones.

Experiment XXX

Adult cadaver, in dorsal decubitus position, the head completely inclined to the right side. The aide struck a violent blow with a wooden club on the left cheekbone.

Examination of the cadaver revealed a fracture of the zygomatic arch, but it was impossible to discover any other lesions. As usual, the soft parts remained intact.

At dissection, the zygomatic arch was found to be fractured at its two extremities and in the middle.... The malar had suffered a genuine luxation without displacement. Its superior angle was separated from the frontal; the line of separation of the angular process of the frontal from the sphenoid and maxilla did not exactly follow the suture....

FORCES EXERTED ANTEROPOSTERIORLY ON ALL OF THE ANTERIOR PART OF THE FACE

A force exerted backward on a large area, after fracturing the ends of the nasal bones (or even without this, if the surface of the wounding agent is concave or depressible), may be applied to the whole anterior part of both malar bones and maxillae. The lesions observed in such cases consist of a separation of the face from the skull, the face itself being fractured.

Thus, in Experiment XXXI, the face is entirely separated from the skull and divided into two main fragments by an anteroposterior fissure of the hard palate. The right side underwent further division into the 3 fragments which are seen in fractures resulting from forces exerted directly on the malar. There was a large fragment composed of a part of the zygomatic process, a second fragment composed of a part of the frontal process and the nasal bones, and a third fragment comprising the hard palate and the alveolar arch on the right side. This latter fragment was in itself divided into two parts. The opposite side displayed only a transverse fissure that a more violent trauma would certainly have made complete.

Experiment XXXI

Man about 60, cadaver in decubitus dorsal position. The head was supported by the table, the face looking up. A violent blow with a wooden club was applied to all of the face in an anteroposterior direction. It was directed at the center of the extremity of the nose. There was no gross displacement of the bones of the face, and mobility was doubtful.

At dissection, all of the face was separated from the skull by a vast fissure, and the facial bone mass was divided into several fragments....

One fissure passes between the two median incisors and on the left side of the nasal spine. It goes along the palatine arch, skirting the midline to approach the dental arch on the left; its posterior part bifurcates to circumscribe some small splinters at the posterior border of the arch. This gives us two principal fragments, one left and one right (Fig. 8).

The right fragment is itself divided. The cheekbone and the pyramidal process form a mass of which the V-point is directed toward the first molar. Its posterior edge, invisible on

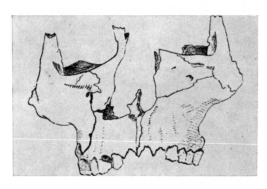

Fig. 8. Experiment XXXI. The principal fragments were glued together, photographed, and this drawing was made from the photograph. *(Courtesy, National Library of Medicine, Bethesda, Md.)*

Figure 8, is almost vertical. The ascending branch, with a large part of the lacrimal bone, is equally isolated. The inferior portion which supports the teeth is again divided into two by a fissure which goes between the second bicuspid and the first molar and is directed toward the posterior face of the palatine arch, separating the floor of the nasal fossa from the floor of the sinus.

The left fragment has also a tendency to horizontal division. A little below the most external part of the nasal fossa one sees a line which goes up toward the cheekbone. Inside, along the nasal wall, this same line stretches out backward, falling toward the posterior edge of the maxilla. That is the outline of the large horizontal fracture.

On both sides, the zygomatic arches are disjointed from the posterior angle of the malar; moreover, that of the left side is fractured in back, as has been described....

FORCE EXERTED ON THE FACE AND SKULL AT THE SAME TIME

It is not rare to see force applied to the face and skull at the same time, and often the lesions don't appear to influence each other much.

(Le Fort goes on to cite several cases of his own and others from the literature, including some exceptions to the above.)

Experiment XXXII

Head of an adult, lying on the right side. The aide, with a wooden club, applied a first blow simultaneously on the external prominence of the cheekbone and on the zygomatic arch. There seemed to be no lesions. A second very violent blow was applied in the same fashion, and one could feel a fracture of the zygomatic arch....

At dissection, the zygomatic process with its bases and a small part of the temporal and even of the sphenoid bone were mobile.

(Le Fort had here several pages of description of the extensive comminuted fractures.)

Experiments XXXIII, XXXIV, and XXXV

In each of these 3 experiments, the entire head was slowly squeezed between the very large jaws of a vise to produce fractures of the skull.... The cranial fractures, very extensive in XXXV, were always limited to the skull.

GENERAL CONCLUSIONS

If we review all the clinical facts and, above all, the experimental results (infinitely more accurate), some general conclusions may be drawn from this work.

The upper jaw, despite its multiple connections to the base of the skull, enjoys a considerable independence from it. It is disposed, essentially, to transmit to the cranial base the physiological stresses steadily exerted on it by the lower jaw.

The bony columns above the upper alveolar arch transmit to the cranial base the vertical forces resulting from collisions with the alveolar arch of the lower jaw, and distribute them on a very broad cranial area. Laterally the malar bones, disposed like keystones and nearly alone exposed to the lateral stresses, also distribute these forces into large areas of the maxillae and the base of the skull. But a great number of weak points (or better said, *lineae minoris resistentiae*) cause the facial bones to break up into fragments so that the stress is exhausted by the effect produced, preserving the integrity of the bony envelope of the brain.

There is between the two bony masses a well-defined cleavage plane at the level of which fracture lines nearly always stop, whether they come from above or below.

Trauma involving the malar bones can cause the separation of the face from the skull.* Whether the stress is anteroposterior or lateral, the effect is the same; the line of separation between the cranium and the face is identical.

This line passes through the nasal bones. The lower part of the nasal bones may be said to be facial and their upper part cranial. This upper part is very resistant. When it yields, the cribriform plate of the ethmoid bone yields also; on the other hand, there is no risk for the cribriform plate when only the lower part of the nasal bones is involved.

From the nasal bones, the fracture line runs toward the orbit—passing either

* *Editorial note.* The author is beginning to describe, here, what we now know as the Le Fort III fracture.

across the upper part of the frontal process of the maxilla or, more rarely, between the latter and the frontal bone (following the suture). Then it crosses the upper part of the lacrimal bone, then the medial wall of the orbit to widely open the ethmoid cells (the upper ones remain adherent to the cranium and the lower ones to the facial mass). At this level, the fissure always widens and circumscribes multiple splinters of the medial wall of the orbit.

The fissure runs toward the optic canal without reaching it; instead, it descends and falls into the remotest part of the infraorbital fissure. There, it forks to complete the separation of the face. Above, it runs on the lateral wall of the orbit, often cutting somewhat into the sphenoid and even the frontal bones; it ends at the level of the zygomatic process which it separates from the malar bone, sometimes leaving a very small fragment of this bone adherent to the cranium. Downward and backward, the line leaves the pterygomaxillary fissure to cut pterygoid processes, more or less close to their bases.

The face would still hold through the zygomatic arches and the nasal septum, except for the following.

The zygomatic arch often yields at several points. This arch may be said to be neither facial nor cranial; it is merely a link between the face and the cranium. Often damaged in fractures of the skull alone, still more often in fractures of the upper jaw alone, it yields usually at the malar suture (but frequently, also, at its convex midportion). The line then is more or less vertical. In the midline, the nasal septum is broken high at a short distance from the cribriform plate, closer to it anteriorly than posteriorly. There, a large triangular fragment of vomer usually remains adherent to the sphenoid bone. (Experiments by Prof. Lannelongue demonstrated its feeble resistance.)

That is the *first great weak line*—the protection barrier of the cranial cavity (Figs. 9, 10).

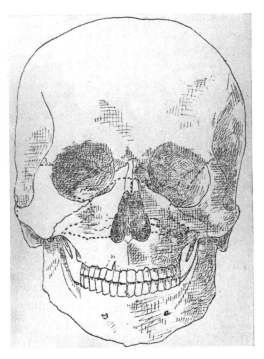

Fig. 9. The great lines of weakness in the face, and the fragments which they circumscribe. Front view. ((*Courtesy, National Library of Medicine, Bethesda, Md.*)

A *second great weak line** circumscribes the whole middle part of the face. In such cases the malar bones are not involved (Figs. 9, 10).

This second line is not entirely independent of the previous one, merging with it in its middle part. Like the first line, it crosses the lower part of the nasal bones. Sometimes, also, it begins a little below them, but in all cases it crosses the frontal process of the maxilla to reach the lacrimal bone, usually at the upper part of the nasolacrimal canal. From this point, the fracture line is wide; the orbital floor has a very weak resistance, and the line deviates easily; but, in all cases, it reaches the infraorbital rim at the junction of the malar bone and the maxilla. Then it passes around the malar bone, re-

* Editorial note. Here the author begins to describe the plane of separation in what we now term the Le Fort II fracture.

specting it, often passing through the infraorbital foramen. From there, it goes through the whole frontal process and on backward into the pterygomaxillary fissure. There, it meets the pterygoid processes and cuts through them as the first line did.

The nasal septum also yields at its upper part, as in the *first great weak line.*

A *third weak line* also cuts across the face.* It starts from the lower part of the pyriform aperture, crosses the canine fossa somewhat below the malar bone and meets the second line (which means that it rises posteriorly to cross the pterygomaxillary fissure and cut the pterygoid process).

This third line is the one involved in Guerin's fracture, one of the most frequent forms of upper jaw fracture. Guerin's fracture can be produced by various mechanisms, and is frequently incomplete. (For instance, it may be complete on one side and only outlined on the other, or even only indicated on one

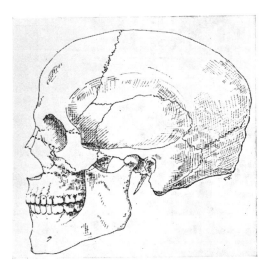

Fig. 10. The great lines of weakness in the face, and the fragments which they circumscribe. Profile view. (*Courtesy, National Library of Medicine, Bethesda, Md.*)

* Editorial note. Fractures through this plane are now usually called Le Fort I fractures, although Le Fort referred to them as Guerin's fractures.

side. In such cases, the pterygoid process yields last.

The interrelationships of these 3 fracture lines are easily understandable if one considers that the first two great weak lines circumscribe a fragment—the malar bone with the top of the nasal pyramid. The last two great weak lines also circumscribe a second fragment—the frontal processes of the maxilla. Below the third great weak line there is a third fragment—the hard palate with the alveolar arch and the pterygoid processes.

The fragment that presents the most constant characteristics is the lower one, but the level at which the pterygoid processes are fractured is rather variable.

The point at which Guerin's fracture draws closest to the teeth lies rather regularly at the level of the first molar, where the protrusion of the malar begins. The minor fissure lines that run across the hard palate anteroposteriorly rarely follow the median suture, and never from beginning to end. They usually run toward the middle of the area between the midline and the pterygoid hamulus. . . .

SUMMARY

Severe fractures of the face, far from presenting a fantasy which defies description, follow simple laws. They have common characteristics, and can be divided into a small number of well-defined types.

An understanding of the possible lesions will facilitate research and aid in the precise diagnosis of fractures which have too often passed unperceived, to the detriment of patients and sometimes even of the surgeon.

René Le Fort, M.D.
Faculté de Médecine
Université de Lille
Lille, France

COMMENTARY BY DR. TESSIER ON LE FORT'S PAPERS

There is nothing to add to the original work of Le Fort (1900), which came after that of Guerin (1866).

Everything was observed and pointed out—the anatomical descriptions, the general views about the middle third of the face, the confrontation between the experimental results and clinical observations in this area, the precision of the cadaver experiments, the interpretations of the mechanisms involved. The ideas in Le Fort's experiments followed the principles laid down some 50 years before by the great Claude Bernard—of what constitutes the scientific method.

One of the most wonderful observations and explanations made by Le Fort in 1900 is the mechanism by which fractures of the middle third of the face are produced when the mandible is jammed against the sternum. Now, with so many Le Fort II and Le Fort III fractures occurring from traffic accidents, we see everyday proof of this clever interpretation by Le Fort.

Part of Le Fort's experimental findings about fractures of the ethmoid, maxilla, and zygoma served as a basis for the later outstanding clinical work of Paul Bonnet (Lyon)—who described everything about orbital fractures in 1931 and 1932.

From this masterpiece of Le Fort, it has been easy to derive some surgical procedures. It helped us to undertake the Le Fort II and the Le Fort III types of osteotomies, for instance, for correction of faciostenosis due to Crouzon's or Apert's disease—or for correction of old deformities resulting from facial fractures. His data also suggested to us how we could simplify the Le Fort I type of osteotomy by making it between the maxilla and the pterygoid processes, instead of through the pterygoids.

Finally, we must point out that the papers being reprinted here show clearly that Le Fort II fractures, as well as the Le Fort II type of osteotomies, do not run vertically through the alveolus (as someone recently described) but traverse the maxilla.

Paul Tessier, M.D.
26 Avenue Kleber
Paris 16, France

BIOGRAPHICAL SKETCH OF RENÉ LE FORT

René Le Fort was born in 1869 in Lille, the son of a physician and the nephew of a well-known surgeon (Leon Le Fort). As a military student in Lille he won, at the age of 19, first place in the entrance examinations of the "Internat des Hôpitaux de Lille." At the age of 21 he was awarded his Doctor of Medicine degree, being then the youngest one in France to possess it. His thesis was "Topographie cranio-cérébrale, applications chirurgicales." Following this he served, first as an apprentice and then as military surgeon, at the famous military hospital "Val-de-Grace" in Paris until 1899.

It was said, "Although he loved the army passionately, he was more and more attracted by a university career and he resigned some time later to be able to devote more time to teaching." During this period he returned to Lille to teach at the medical school. Concurrently, the 3 famed papers on upper jaw fractures appeared in the February, March, and April issues (1901) of the *Revue de Chirurgie*. He was about 31 years of age when he conducted these experiments and it is not clear where they were done—but possibly in Paris before he left.

At Lille, he became more and more interested in orthopedic surgery and decided to make this his specialty (Fig. 11). He published a series of remarkable works but in 1912, with the onset of the unexpected Balkan war, he could not resist the temptation of doing surgery on the field of battle.

Two years later came World War I, in which he served in many positions. He was cited for operating under primitive and dangerous conditions at the front lines in the battle of Dinant. In the last two years of this war, he became interested in thoracic surgery and was one of the first to operate on the great vessels, the pericardium, and the heart. In 1918 he published a book, *Projectiles Enclosed in the Mediastinum*. It was also in 1918 that Clemenceau asked Le Fort to reorganize the Hôpital des Invalides, which he directed until 1919.

In 1920, Le Fort returned to Lille as Professor of Operative Medicine, later becoming Professor of Children's Surgery and Orthopedics. For many years, he was sur-

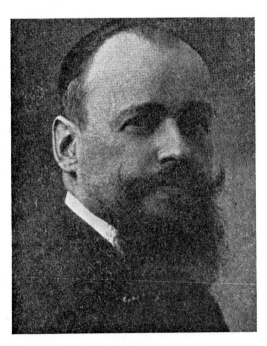

Fig. 11. René Le Fort. 1869–1951. (*Courtesy, National Library of Medicine, Bethesda, Md.*)

geon, also, to the great Sanatorium of Zuydcoote where he gave voluntary services to operate upon a large number of patients with bone tuberculosis. During this period he published many papers and was awarded the Laborie prize, the highest honor of the Academy of Surgery. In 1934 he published "Bases du traitement chirurgical de la tuberculose osseuse fermee."

In 1936, at the age of 67, he was elected President of the French Society of Orthopedics, and a bronze plaque of his likeness was cast in his honor (Fig. 12). Apparently he was not very active during the remaining 15 years of his life and he died, at the age of 82, in 1951 in Lille.

Le Fort was an indefatigable traveler, before and after World War I—in the Balkans, Indochina, Madagascar, Russia, Patagonia, and other parts of the world. He visited the Mayo Clinic and many other medical centers in the United States. At one time, he was Vice-President of the Societé de Géographie.

—*Paul Tessier, M.D.*

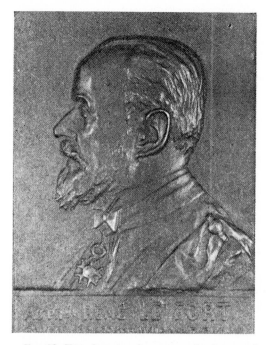

FIG. 12. The bronze plaque cast in honor of René Le Fort when he became President of the French Society of Orthopedics, in 1936. The plaque was created by A. Blaise, a sculptor who had won the Grand Prix de Rome. (*Courtesy, National Library of Medicine, Bethesda, Md.*)

SECTION VIII

Papers on
Various Subjects

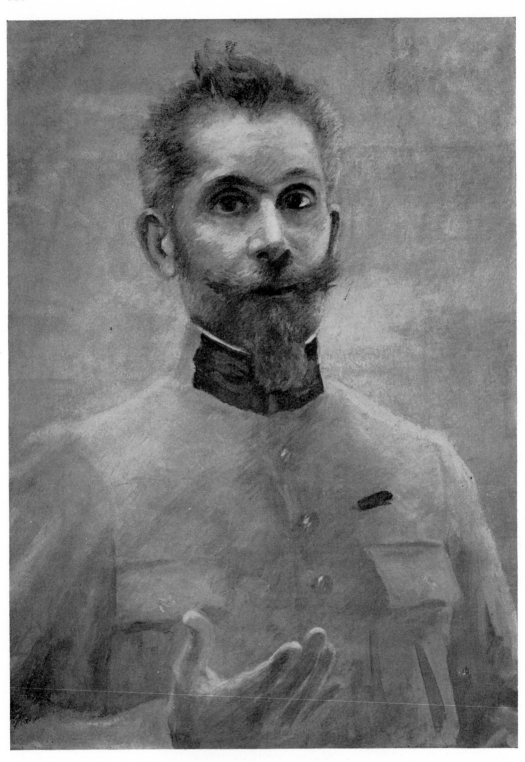

HYPPOLYTE MORESTIN (1869–1919)
Portrait painted by Roll.
(*Courtesy Hôpital Val-de-Grâce, Paris*)

LA RÉDUCTION GRADUELLE DES DIFFORMITÉS TÉGUMENTAIRES

H. MORESTIN, M.D., *Paris*

(*Bull. et mém. Soc. chir. Paris, 41: 1233, 1915*)

Translated from the French by
JOHN MARQUIS CONVERSE, M.D.

Deformities of the integuments, even when their extent is moderate, are difficult to treat. In the region of the face, in particular, a surgeon finds himself embarrassed in the choice of procedures, as the classical methods of autoplasty do not offer, in many cases, the possibility of obtaining satisfactory results.

I feel, however, that a large number of patients whom the surgeon hesitates to treat could benefit from a method which I have called the *gradual reduction method.* This consists in the progressive elimination of deformed parts by successive excisions patiently repeated at variable time intervals.

I have described earlier* the method of spontaneous autoplasty by progressive stretching of the integument in cases of loss of tissue in diverse areas where the approximation of the edges of the wound can be facilitated by certain positions assumed by the patient. A number of patients were presented to the Surgical Society and you have been able to appreciate the enormous simplification which is brought about by this method in the repair of tissue defects in the region of the elbow or of the groin. My present method is based on the same principle; it utilizes the nearly indefinite possibility of extension of the skin; it leads to spontaneous autoplasty but by quite different procedures.

* Journal de Chirurgie *8:* 509, 1911.

Let us suppose that we are faced by a large nevus, the resection of which would be possible only at the expense of an extensive and mutilating operation, or would at least require an extensive autoplasty which is difficult to achieve. Instead of this complete immediate resection that it is not essential to perform in one stage (as we are dealing with a benign lesion), could one not do the excision in successive stages? I think it is possible and this manner of proceeding has the great advantage of avoiding having to suddenly face the problem of the repair of the entire defect.

If one resects a portion of the black lesion, and if the edges of the wound are immediately approximated, one will have eliminated a tenth or a twentieth part of the lesion. After a few days the lesion can be submitted to a renewed reduction at the price of a simple small operation. The suppleness and the elasticity of the integuments allow them to accommodate and soon another resection will be possible.

In summary, one can theoretically conceive the entire destruction of a lesion by a more or less long series of small partial operations, each of which would be of an extreme simplicity and would not require an autoplasty in the ordinary sense of the word. . . .

Facts only can demonstrate the value of "gradual reduction" and I will report, first of all, two cases of extensive pigmented nevi of the face that appear to me to be excellent demonstrations of the method.

CASE 1

Iréné X., 21-years-old, a hairdresser, was sent to me by Dr. Planson, for an extensive nevus of the face that had been previously treated without success by various methods. In reality it was a case which offered considerable difficulty—a thick black plaque . . . covered with hair occupied, on the right side of the face, the entire infraorbital region, a portion of the cheek and of the upper lip, and even impinged over the malar region (Fig. 1). The plaque was uneven in surface, rough and protruding: in brief, its presence on the face constituted an abominable deformity. . . . He had been treated for a long time by high frequency electrocoagulation without any result. In addition he had submitted to a prolonged treatment by radium. But the results of these treatments were negative. In last resort, the patient consulted various surgeons, who had misgivings because of the extent of the lesion; certainly the enormous surface occupied by the nevus would explain and fully justify their reserve.

It was clear that only the destruction of the entire lesion, thickened, modified and invaded by pigment as it was, could result in the disappearance of the malformation. Destruction, however, is simple but the problem of the reparative surgery was immediately posed and was sufficiently complex to make one reflect at great length before tackling this project.

After having thought about the problem for some time, I came to the conclusion that the solution could be found by a cure in successive stages, in the progressive reduction by a series of partial excisions of the territory occupied by the malformation. . . .

The first operation took place on the 3rd of November 1913. An incision was made on the edge of the black plaque, on the lateral aspect toward the cheek, in the shape of a curved line, the concavity of which was placed antero-superiorly. I dissected the plaque from above downward and from backward forward. From time to time I assured myself that this dissection was not carried too far in order that approximation of the edges could still be effected after the resection of the dissected portion.

After having removed a portion of the plaque extending over a surface of two or three centimeters, I made a second incision which extended as far as the upper and the lower ends of the first incision. After excision of the lesion comprised between the two incisions, a surface representing approximately a third of the nevus, I proceeded to approximate the edges of the wound, this approximation requiring careful attention because the edges of the wound were not of the same length and it was necessary to adapt them to each other.

The approximation having been obtained and to avoid traction on the sutures, I carefully exerted

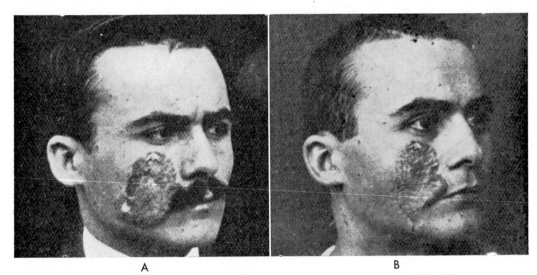

A   B

FIG. 1. *A*. Preoperative view, extensive nevus of face. *B*. After first partial excision.

upward and forward traction on the skin of the cheek and neck by means of adhesive tape which I strapped forward on to the forehead and the opposite cheek. The result is indicated in Figure 1.

On the 14th of November, another small operation consisted in the extirpation of a portion of the nevus. On the 24th of November, the 8th of December and the 20th of December, I did other resections. Every time the operation was very simple. . .

Already the appearance of the patient had been considerably modified; Iréné X. realized this himself, he followed with extreme attention the diminution of his deformity; the results obtained reaffirmed his hope and encouraged him to continue a treatment which he had accepted

without too much confidence. On the 3rd of January a sixth operation was performed. Up to now vertical sections had been removed from the nevus; this time the incisions were placed in an antero-posterior direction. The same procedure was performed again on the 19th of January, on the 27th of January, and on the 9th of February. The skin was beginning to be tight and the sections removed were smaller than at the beginning of the treatment, but under the influence of traction the remaining portions of the pigmented plaque appeared lighter in color and the deformity was, therefore, attenuated. As it was impossible to remove large fragments, I excised two or three fragments from various areas of the lesion.

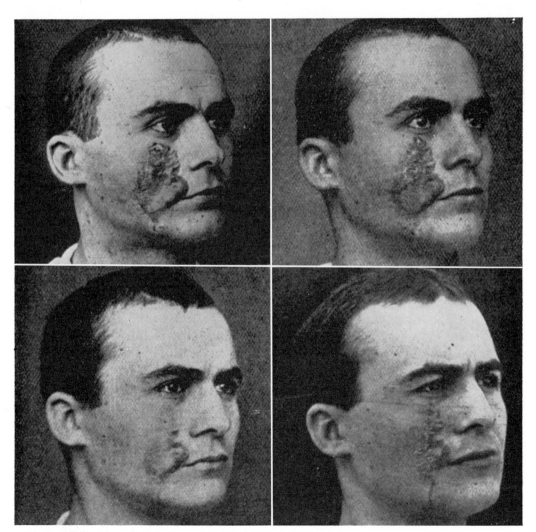

FIG. 2. Various stages of multiple partial excisions of same patient as shown in Figure 1.

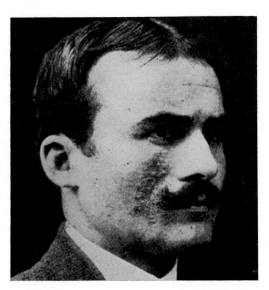

FIG. 3. Final result obtained on patient shown in Figure 1.

One must especially avoid pulling on the lower eyelid or upon the angle of the mouth; to avoid this, it is necessary to calculate each time with care the extent of the excision and the direction of the incisions.

Each new operation produced an appreciable gain and the patient gradually underwent a radical transformation in appearance (Fig. 2).

Other operations took place on the 20th of February, the 2nd of March and the 14th of March.

The patient declares that he is satisfied. What remains of the pigmented lesion has become considerably paler under the influence of the traction of the skin. The scars are relatively inconspicuous and the remaining pigmentation contributes to dissimulate them.

I would have liked to have resected a few more fragments of the lesion and finish the job but I finally agreed to leave the patient with the attained result (Fig. 3).

CASE 2

Here is another case that also offers considerable interest: Alfreda L., was brought to the Hôpital Bichat at the beginning of the year 1913, approximately three months after she was born. The baby was full term, born of robust and healthy parents; she was physically well developed but unfortunately this poor little girl was born with an enormous pigmented nevus that covered a considerable extent of the face. In fact, the cutaneous malformation occupied a large portion of the right cheek, malar region, upper lip, the entire infra-orbital region, the entire lower eyelid, the greater portion of the right half of the nose, the root of this structure, and the medial angle of the eye (Fig. 4).

In its entire extent, the plaque was elevated, thick, rough, covered with soft hair, and had a coloration which varied from dark brown to deep black. The child did not show any other malformation; no trace of deformity was found in her parents who were young and healthy. Nothing peculiar occurred during pregnancy.

The parents strongly pressed me to make every attempt to improve the appearance of the face; their impatience was understandable, because this black irregular and hairy plaque gave the child an appearance which was monstrous, bestial and frankly repulsive. I did not want, however, to undertake a cure which obviously would be rather laborious in such a young child.

It was agreed that the baby would re-

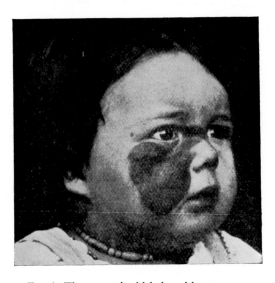

FIG. 4. Three-month old baby with an enormous pigmented nevus of the face.

main under observation until a period of one year had revolved. . . .

During the month of November 1913, the child being one year of age, I began the treatment.

The extirpation of this large plaque would have been a serious operation in this baby. It would have created a defect, the immediate repair of which probably would have been impossible. It would have required, in any case, long and certainly complicated surgical maneuvers. I had outlined a different plan, my intention being to practice successive operations to gradually reduce the plaque, hoping finally to practice only rather limited autoplasties and thus reduce to the minimum the operative risks and the consequent scars.

On the 5th of November 1913 the work of reduction by successive resections began.

A torpor was induced in the child by a whiff of chloroform and I attacked the central portion of the plaque, situated in the infraorbital region and the anterior part of the cheek. By means of two incisions delimiting an ellipse, I outlined a fragment wider than a one franc coin. This fragment having been removed by a rapid dissection, I approximated the edges of the vertical wound by a few sutures. The operation did not last five minutes; it had been extremely simple. The result of the operation was nevertheless very important; the black plaque was considerably reduced in size.

There had been, however, no traction exerted upon the lower eyelid, the ala of the nose, or the upper lip.

The results of such a surgical intervention could only be favorable. In fact, there was no local nor general reaction; the small dressing applied on the first day was eliminated on the following day; on the seventh day the sutures were removed, primary healing was obtained.

On the 14th of November, a second operation was done, soon followed by another operation on the 24th of November, a fourth operation on the 8th of December and other operations again on the 5th of January, 1914, the 2nd of February, the 18th of February and the 9th of March.

Each time the operation was very short. The child was given a few whiffs of chloroform or ether and a more or less important fragment of nevus of varying size was extirpated, after calculating the length and the direction of the incisions to avoid any malposition of the eyelid, of the corner of the mouth or of the ala of the nose. Each of these operations was simple and the postoperative recovery uneventful. To give an idea of the simplicity of the procedure, let us note this detail: each time the child was to be operated upon, she was brought from Landrecies,

near the Northern frontier, and taken home on the same day.

I took great care to make all incisions within the territory of the nevus, without ever impinging upon the healthy tissues —to avoid causing unnecessary scars. Progressively, the face of the child underwent a metamorphosis and the pigmented plaque gradually diminished in size (Fig. 5). The child grew and developed; the multiple operations that she submitted to did not influence her general health.

Repeated operations took place on the 13th of May, the 3rd of June, the 17th of June, the 8th of July. We prudently excised a small portion of the upper and lower eyelids. The pigmented surface was now reduced to a triangle, which occupied the infraorbital region, a portion of the lower eyelid and the right lateral portion of the nose.

We had now arrived at the limits of what could be obtained by gradual reduction, but what remained of the nevus could not be removed without leaving a defect, the repair of which would offer insurmountable difficulties.

War started* just as I was ready to do this operation. I remained without news of the child for a long time and it was only in April of 1915 that the child could be brought back to Paris.

I operated on her on the 12th of April, excising the last remains of the nevus and the scars left by some of the previous operations. The raw surface was immediately covered by a triangular flap taken from the forehead. The donor site of the flap was closed immediately in its entire extent, thanks to the looseness of the integuments of the forehead of the child. This flap adapted itself perfectly by its size and shape to that of the defect.

All that was left to do was to unite the edges of the flap to the edges of the defect. The postoperative recovery was satisfactory and healing occurred within a few days. On the 15th day, I did a small secondary operation which consisted in excising the twisted base of the flap.

* The onset of World War I, August 1, 1914.

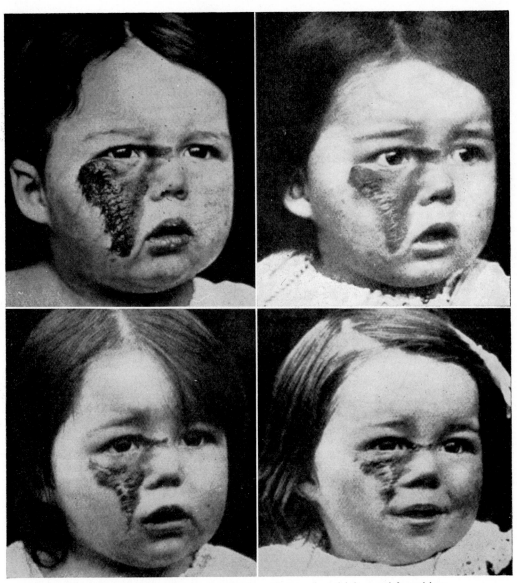

Fig. 5. Appearance shown after various stages of multiple partial excisions

At present, the flap is still quite thick but I am convinced that within a few months it will flatten out and will harmonize in a very satisfactory way with the surrounding parts. It would also be possible to adjust the flap if excessive thickening persisted. For the moment the only thing to do is to leave everything alone, particularly as the parents cannot prolong their sojourn in Paris.

The final result can be considered as obtained (Fig. 6). There is no longer any vestige of the primary deformity and the cure is obtained without any deformity of the eyelids, nostrils or corner of the mouth.

In conclusion, here were two cases that can be considered among the most difficult and the most unsatisfactory to treat and in which the gradual reduction sufficed. . . .

I have not had occasion to apply this

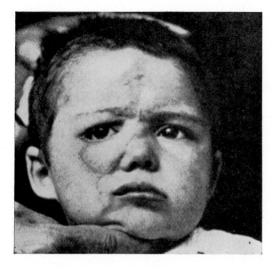

FIG. 6. Final result on patient shown in Figure 4

method to vascular tumors of the skin but I believe that it would be equally useful in such cases. . . .

Conditions are less favorable when one is dealing with scars; one can, however, obtain appreciable results, progressively reduce the scarred surfaces, remove them completely sometimes, even reduce them to linear proportions. This method can offer a considerable advantage, notably in operative scars produced by the removal of a flap in cases of reconstructive rhinoplasty for example; one can frequently reduce to a vertical or slightly oblique line the forehead scar resulting from the removal of the flap. I have often had the occasion to improve scars resulting from tuberculous ulcerations, trauma or burns by the procedure of gradual reduction.

In burns it is unusual that one can, by gradual reduction, produce a disappearance of the entire deformity; but in a number of cases, one can simplify in a large measure future plastic surgical operations. In some cases one can avoid any autoplastic procedure as a result of the considerable improvement produced by the reduction of the cicatricial area after successive excisions. This is what happened, notably in a young girl whose history I will give briefly.

CASE 3

This young girl, 20-years of age, had been horribly burned around the neck and the upper portion of the thorax, the shoulders and the anterior aspect of the left arm (Fig. 7A).

The photograph gives a poor impression of the appearance of the scar which covered these regions. The scar was hard and irregular, and covered by

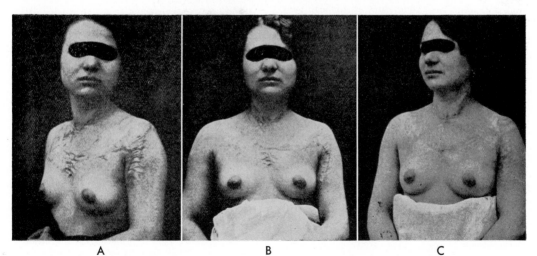

A   B   C

FIG. 7. *A.* Initial appearance of patient with burn scars. *B.* Appearance of patient after 12 operations. *C.* Final appearance after about 9 more operations.

keloidal protuberances; its appearance was truly horrible. Fortunately, despite the severity of the deformity the scars had caused no faulty positioning of the head or the neck, no limitation of movement of the upper extremities; in fact, despite its extent the scar remained mobile over the underlying tissues. Because of this characteristic it appeared to me that it would be possible, in this case, to utilize the elasticity of the tissues and gradually to appreciably reduce the scarred area.

I began by making a few injections of formaldehyde in the larger keloidal protuberances. (I would like to mention, in passing, that formaldehyde injections constitute one method of treatment of keloids.) On the 30th of January 1914, I began the operative treatment. I excised a transverse area over the anterior portion of the thorax, measuring 7 or 8 cm in the transverse dimension and 3 in the vertical dimension. I chose for this resection a portion of skin which was particularly thick and hard. This was the beginning of a series of operations which were done successively in every part of the scarred area. The patient was operated upon the 24th of February, the 4th of March, the 16th of March, the 18th of May, the 25th of May, the 3rd of June, the 17th of June, the 30th of June, the 3rd of July, the 10th and the 15th of July, the 19th of August, the 26th of August, the 3rd, the 9th, the 16th of September, the 18th of November. A few small operations were again done at the beginning of 1915.

All of these operations were done by means of local cocaine anesthesia. Each time one, two or three fragments were removed, depending upon the patience of the subject and the amount of time that was available; these operations do not require any detailed report. . . .

The result has been extremely satisfactory and we observed that healthy tissues were advanced toward the base of the neck and the anterior part of the chest; the scar on the arm and over the shoulder was reduced to a line. All of the irregularities and the keloidal scars have disappeared, the scar tissue has been reduced and simplified. In summary a happy change has occurred in

the appearance of the areas affected by the burn. Figure 7B shows the condition of the patient in July 1914; figure 7C shows the appearance of the patient at the beginning of this year (1915).

These examples suffice to indicate the idea that has guided us, the very simple technique which permits its achievement and also what one can hope in the area of reparative surgery.

One can see that the technique of gradual reduction is without danger, without risk and it is also very simple to achieve.

Local anesthesia is always satisfactory in adults; in children a light and short general anesthesia is required. The patient need not be hospitalized. . . .

There remains only to consider briefly the indications of the method.

It is applicable, first of all, to all extensive congenital malformations of the integuments, large pigmented nevi in particular, against which the surgeon was up to now completely ill-equipped, and also for vascular nevi. One can apply the method to plexiform neuromas or any other important alterations of the soft tissues. The same method could be applied to certain circumscribed sclerodermas.

It can also be used as a routine method in the treatment of scars, either as a method of eliminating the scar completely or as a preparatory and complementary method of treatment prior to autoplasties. At the present time* I am in charge of a special service for the military wounded who are facially mutilated and I have constant opportunities to apply the method in the treatment of scars resulting from war wounds.

Hyppolyte Morestin, M.D.
Hôpital du Val-de-Grâce
Paris, France

* The paper was read on June 16, 1915. Morestin was in charge of the plastic surgery service for the wounded of World War I at the Military Hospital of the Val-de-Grâce in Paris.

COMMENTARY BY DR. CONVERSE

Hyppolyte Morestin was a precursor, in the true sense of the word, of the modern plastic surgeon. He published numerous papers on surgical anatomy, surgical pathology, on techniques of abdominal surgery and surgery of the head and neck tumors during the first 10 years of his surgical career.

During the remainder of his short surgical career (Morestin died at the age of 49) he wrote numerous articles on plastic surgery. Among his many contributions were papers concerned with the application of the "Z-plasty" for the treatment of contracture of the fingers and the use of costal cartilage, both in the repair of cranial defects and as a transplant for the restoration of skeletal support of the nose.

There are, in the Museum of the Military Hospital of the Val-de-Grâce in Paris, numerous plaster casts of patient's faces in various stages of reconstruction. One of these shows the preliminary implantation of a costal cartilage graft under a forehead flap to serve as the skeletal support for a reconstructed nose. Morestin showed that extensive undermining could be done over a distance of 15 to 20 cm in every direction around a defect without impairing the vascularization of the skin.

Successively Intern, Anatomical Aide, Prosector, Chief of a Surgical Service in the Paris hospitals, Associate Professor and member of the French Surgical Society, Morestin would have been appointed full Professor had he not died prematurely at the age of 49 years.

Morestin was born on the Island of Martinique and, from information recently gathered in Paris, he was afflicted with tuberculosis. His death was attributed to pulmonary complications during the epidemic of influenza which followed World War I. He is described by his contemporaries as having a "moody" personality, as being totally dedicated to his work, and having no particular interests outside of his work.

His premature death left a void in French plastic surgery but he left behind him a lasting influence, particularly upon Harold D. Gillies. To quote Gillies: "At about this time my American dental friend 'Bobs' Roberts, who had just returned from six months' jaw surgery in the American Hospital in Paris, brought back a book by Lindemann which he had received from Germany. It being a rather informal war, the enemy did not seem to mind our learning of the good work they were doing on jaw fractures and wounds about the mouth. Bobs presented this book to me with, 'Giles, why don't you take up this work?' I became intrigued, and when an opportunity for leave came in June of 1915, I took it in Paris, where the famous Morestin from Martinique was rumoured to be performing unbelievable feats of surgical reconstruction.

"I found him at the huge, rambling Val-de-Grâce Hospital. He was a strange and moody octoroon, whose dagger-like sharpness was accentuated by his pointed moustache and tapering beard as well as the agility of his long, thin hands. In the space of a single moment he could reveal the gentleness of a kitten and the savagery of a tiger. He received me kindly, and I stood spellbound as he removed half of a face distorted with a horrible cancer and then deftly turned a neck flap to restore not only the cheek but the side of the nose and lip, in one shot. Although in the light of present-day knowledge it seems unlikely this repair could have been wholly successful, at that time it was the most thrilling thing I had ever seen. I fell in love with the work on the spot."

John Marquis Converse, M.D.

THE INFLUENCE OF MECHANICAL PRESSURE ON WOUND HEALING

V. P. BLAIR, M.D.

St. Louis, Mo.

(Reprinted from Illinois Med. Jour. *46:* 229, 1924)

In much of reparative surgery the operator will be tremendously handicapped until he realizes that the satisfactory result is more dependent upon intelligent application of the older surgical principles than upon an aseptic technic as ordinarily interpreted, though the latter is never to be disregarded. A consideration of the bearing of one of these older principles to this type of surgery will be a much more fitting and profitable subject to present for your consideration than any technical tricks or possibly out of the ordinary cases that might be at my disposal.

The maintenance of a definite external surface pressure is essential not only to the life of the body but also to the proper functioning of the various organs. The movement of the contents of the alimentary canal, the circulation of the blood and the respiration of air are all dependent upon differentials of pressures. Special provision has been made for maintaining the tension of the muscle sheaths and of the abdominal and thoracic parietes; greater or less disability will follow a disturbance of these mechanisms. In dealing with the pathological results of such disturbances, artificial pressure has long been recognized as one of our most important resources; therefore, we use the truss or the abdominal binder to compensate for a hernia or bandage the leg for varicose veins or for lymph stasis. In the healing of wounds, it is one of the great helps which we may add to the natural reparative forces. Where a disturbance of the pressure balance within the tissues is complicated by an infection, there is no chemical or emollient that has the antiseptic value of properly applied mechanical pressure, as illustrated by the efficiency of complete circular strapping of the leg for a varicose ulcer or the application of a firm pressure dressing to any granulating surface.

The application of most any dressing produces pressure, but he who employs this pressure in a selective, purposeful manner will get bigger returns than he who applies it incidentally or even as a matter of routine.

There are chiefly four basic things to be gained by the use of properly applied mechanical pressure to wounds:

1. The elimination of dead spaces.
2. The control of oozing.
3. The limitation of venous and lymph stasis.
4. Limitation of the amount of plastic material that pours into the wound.

In wounds about the face and mouth the above factors combine to form a much more efficient preventive of sepsis than the most painstaking attempts at an aseptic technic.

The amount written in the previous two decades on the technic of the "Thiersch" graft* would fill volumes, no

From the Department of Surgery, Washington University Medical School.

Oration of Surgery delivered at the annual meeting of the Illinois State Medical Society, May 8, 1924, at Springfield, Ill.

* *Ed. Note:* This paper was written before the development of the larger and thicker "split-skin graft" by Blair and Brown.

small part of this being related to the aftercare and dressings. Our observation leads us to believe that properly applied and maintained pressure is the one essential and that it will usually neutralize the possible effects of accidental wound contamination; that size, thickness and the location of the graft are matters of little relative importance. Without stopping to trace the development of this plan of grafting, it is sufficient to mention that if one or several pieces of "Thiersch" graft containing one or ten square inches of epidermis are wrapped, raw surface outermost, on a wax form and buried in the floor of the mouth, as high a percentage of perfect "takes" may be expected as with any graft applied to a surface with the most elaborate technic. The wax form must be of the proper size and shape and must be sutured in under proper tension but, on the other hand, salivary contamination apparently may be disregarded. In applying "Thiersch" grafts to a recently made clean raw surface, to a granulating surface, or one from which the granulations have just been cut, the use of well controlled pressure is our main reliance to insure the best chances of a good result. An explanation of the freedom of sepsis under this treatment may be that the close contact maintained between the raw surfaces of the bed and of the graft permits the efficient tissue action upon the bacteria and their products. This is in no way meant to belittle the value of the standard aseptic technic but rather to emphasize the fact that, in the healing of wounds, the latter is not the only adjuvant at our disposal.

An attempted aseptic technic combined with pressure dressing has not always saved our grafts, but in the comparatively few instances where failure of the graft has been due to sepsis there has been a strong suggestion of an auto-inoculation. The patient in almost every instance has been the subject of active septic lesions in some more or less remote parts of the body at or shortly before the application of the graft. On the other hand, the number of cases in which success has followed the implantation of free grafts in non-sterile fields is now fairly large and I believe that in this success properly applied mechanical pressure was an essential factor.

Our technic for using the full thickness skin graft was at first based on two premises; first, that if the transplanted skin were sutured at its normal tension or at slightly plus tension the cut ends of the cutaneous vessels would remain open and would more quickly take up a blood supply; the second, that as each particular part takes its blood supply from the immediately subjacent tissue, the only logical limit to the size of a graft would be the amount of operating and hemorrhage the patient could stand. Subsequent experience justified both of these conclusions, but very soon after these two hypotheses were put into practice it became evident that there were additional factors of almost equal importance that still remained to be catalogued. The first of these stumbling blocks was a fact long ago recognized in dealing with large, thin flaps; that it is one thing to have blood supply and quite another to have an adequate venous return. In the first several of our cases the full thickness grafts were applied to the bridge of the nose or to the forehead. In the former the tension of the sutures drawing the graft over a curved firm surface, and in the latter pressure of the bandage that held the dressing, both helped to limit the amount of blood that could stagnate in the skin while the new venous return was being established. It was not until the attempt was made to place a large graft on the cheek that we were forced to conclude that in the previous cases good luck had outrun calculation. In this particular case the retaining dressings were removed at the end of two days for fear mouth secretions might seep under them and the newly adherent graft was left exposed. Within a few hours the pale pink skin became deeply blue and repeated scarifications, carried on night and day, and citrate of soda packs failed to save us from the painful necessity of explaining to the patient the loss of $\frac{7}{10}$ of a 3×4 inch graft. That part of the graft survived which lay over a wax form in the hollow of the cheek which furnished counter-pressure to the bandage that held the pack in place.

Based on this experience, a marine sponge pressure dressing was evolved which, if carefully applied and made of sponges of proper quality, will maintain an even pressure over an irregular surface or one without underlying bony counter-support. Further use of this pressure dressing demonstrated an unforeseen virtue and an inherent danger. It permits of the application of the graft over a freshly made raw surface, such as results from the removal of a scar, without tying any but large vessels, but if the pressure is too great, especially over a bony prominence such as the outer part of the supra-orbital ridge or dorsal surface of the middle metacarpal bone, it can kill the compressed area by ischemia. Maintenance of the proper pressure for four or five days will prevent the graft dying from engorgement, but its early discontinuance favors the formation of blebs which later may lead to another catastrophe. The blebs are apt to become infected; continuance of the sponge pressure for several days longer helps to control the formation of blebs.

The common plan of transplanting rib cartilage into the bridge of the nose is through an incision made within the nostril. Compared with the frequency with which apparent breaks in "technic" occur, a high percentage of "takes" follow this procedure. This suggests that here too pressure from the elasticity of the skin or of superimposed padding may have some influence on the average outcome.

In the preparation and transplantation of pedicle flaps, one of the most disastrous incidents is the failure of union of the flap to its original or its new bed and one of the most efficient preventives, even in the presence of a moderate amount of contamination, is evenly applied pressure. The safest and most efficient plan of applying this is the incorporation in the dressing of one or several large, soft marine sponges that have been wet, wrung out in a twisted towel, and immediately bandaged in place. It is particularly useful where the graft is bedded on a surface of irregular topography and consistency. To a less certain extent this sponge pressure can help to control venous stasis which threatens the vitality of the flap.

These observations are backed up not only by our experience but also by that of the general surgical service where the marine sponge pressure dressing has been adapted for holding the skin flap up in the axilla after a radical breast amputation. We have found it equally efficacious in maintaining contact after extensive neck dissections.

In applying this sponge pressure, one must use his surgical sense to gauge the desired tension but he can use it with the assurance that he has more leeway in making this pressure than with any other padding substance with which we are familiar.

Vilray P. Blair, M.D.
Metropolitan Bldg.
St. Louis, Mo.

COMMENT BY THE EDITOR

The origin of pressure dressings must be very old, but they did not achieve wide popularity until well into the 20th century. After the important contributions of Pasteur and Lister, surgeons rightly became busy with developing antiseptic and aseptic techniques, to the great benefit of their patients. Only after some decades did it become apparent that absolute sterility is seldom possible in many surgical situations, or that the presence of micro-organisms (even pathogenic ones) and the development of clinical infections are not synonymous. (I remember one surgeon who used to cry "You've infected me!" whenever his "sterile" gown was inadvertently touched by a circulating nurse or orderly.)

Still longer was required for a significant number of surgeons to learn the chain of events that leads to many clinical infections—that "nature abhors a vacuum,"—that "dead spaces" will become filled by lymphatic or venous oozing with seromas or hematomas—that these, in turn, almost inevitably become abscesses, or foci of spreading cellulitis.

In attempts to prevent hematomas, many surgeons then resorted to "meticulous technique." One dictionary definition of *meticulous* is "extreme or excessive care in the treatment of details." In practice, the "meticulous technique" of that era (and of today?) often consisted of excessive rubbing of tissues with sponges to promote excessive oozing which, in turn, was controlled by excessive clamping and tying. This technique was self-defeating. Wounds containing large amounts of necrotic (ligated) tissue and foreign material were fertile culture media for the growth of any itinerant organisms. If the remaining tissues were devitalized by 5 or 6 hours of exposure and wiping, an infection could be well established by the time the final skin suture was in place. Even if this did not occur, when dead spaces or loose flaps were left, the chances of supervening seromas or hematomas were great—especially if the wounds were "dry" or "dried out" at the time of closure.

Now, all of this remained pretty much of a mystery (and still does) to some surgeons who operated mostly in deep areas, to some surgeons who were concerned more with teaching than doing, and to some who were primarily "record room surgeons." It could not remain long a mystery, however, to those curious and observant surgeons who did a great deal of operating at or near the surface, and who followed their visible operative sites closely and personally. Blair was one of these. He soon found that wounds healed nicely and infections were practically nil when operations were expeditious and seromas or hematomas did not occur. The latter, he found, were better prevented by limiting clamping and tying to vessels of visible caliber, relying on a few minutes of pressure and blood coagulation to stanch the others, and applying a pressure dressing to seal the tissues together and discourage further lymphatic or capillary oozing. Searching for a medium which would transmit an elastic pressure from a rigid external bandage, which would distribute it evenly up over the hills and down into the valleys, and which would retain resiliency whether wet or dry, he made the happy initial choice of marine sponges. All of this popularized the procedure.

Apparently, Blair thought when he gave this paper that the subject material was too well known for presentation before a national group, or publication in a national journal. Nevertheless, though many had adopted this technique from word-of-mouth communication, or possibly from their own discoveries, little had been written about it. This paper has been more widely quoted on the subject than any other, by far. For this reason, it is included in *The Source Book*.

The editor would hesitate to suggest that it be required reading for any Infection Committee that is having trouble deciding why one surgeon has a much higher incidence of infections than others, even while working in the same operating room and under the same conditions. However, any reader is free to do so.

—*Frank McDowell*

DE LA RÉTRACTION DES DOIGTS PAR SUITE D'UNE AFFECTION DE L'APONEUROSE PALMAIRE

BARON GUILLAUME DUPUYTREN, *Paris*

(*Jour. Univ. et Hebdomadaire de Méd. et Chir.*, 5: 348, 1832)

Translated from the French by
DRS. ALEXANDRE PAILLARD AND MARX

We present here in detail the lecture given at the Surgical Clinic of M. Dupuytren, December 5, 1831. This is a true report upon an entirely new subject, and presents a new theory, and a new method of treatment for a disease generally regarded as incurable.

We are going to endeavour to report the Professor's words exactly, in order to give an idea of his approach.

"I am going to speak to you today about a single patient and a single disease. The patient presented for your observation is named Jean Joseph Demarteau; he is about forty years of age; his profession a coachman; he lives at No. 63, Ste-Marie. His illness is a permanent contraction of the ring finger and adjacent fingers of both hands, which appeared spontaneously without any injury or previous illness. For some years he has seen these fingers contracting imperceptibly toward the palm, and the skin of this area form several folds similar to the arc of a circle. These folds merge the one into the other, and the concavity of the fold is turned toward the base of the fingers.

"Upon extending the fingers one sees a cord-like structure which passes from the fingers to the palm of the hand; its tension increases in proportion to the efforts one makes to extend the affected fingers.

"In this man the contraction has progressed to such a point that the digits make a right angle with the palm of the hand. It is impossible for the patient to extend them himself; and any force applied to the fingers would succeed only by producing a rupture of the tissues.

"This form of contraction, completely different from that which one observes so often following inflammation, wounds, fracture, etc., is a very common malady, for I have been able to observe thirty or forty examples during a period of twenty years.

"In spite of its frequency, the causes, the nature and the treatment of this disease have remained unknown until this day; at least I have searched in vain among the works of authors who have written upon diseases of the hand. It is true that my life, almost completely employed in active work, has not perhaps permitted me to make investigations sufficiently extensive."

. . . . . .

"This disease develops without having been preceded by any rheumatic or gouty affection, or any inflammation of the tendon sheaths, of the synovial joint capsules, without sprain, without distention of the ligaments, without ankylosis, without fracture or any external injury whatever.

"One sees it especially in individuals who often grasp hard objects with the

---

From a Surgical Clinic presented at the Hôtel Dieu; transcribed by Drs. Brierre de Boismont and Buet. Published later in German, English, Italian and Danish.

This article was located, obtained, translated, and furnished to the Journal through the kind and scholarly efforts of Dr. Sumner Koch.

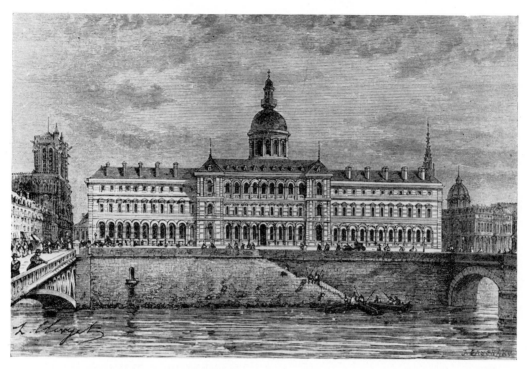

FIG. 1. The great Hôtel Dieu in Paris, in 1830 when Dupuytren was chief surgeon. The first hospital at this site on the Ile de la Cité was constructed about 650 A.D. Ambroise Paré was chief surgeon in the 16th Century Hôtel Dieu. (Photograph shown here is reproduced by the courtesy of Madame Dubois, Chief of Centre d'Optique et d'Electronique de l'Assistance Publique de Paris).

hand, and work with them applied to the palm for long periods. Thus, our patient is a coachman, obliged, as a result, to hold almost constantly in the hands a whip with a large and hard handle to spur the activity of two bad horses. The palm of the hand and the palmar surface of the fingers are thus constantly exposed to pressure and a form of persistent contusion.

"I have observed this contraction in a wine merchant, obliged to sip often of wine, who is in the habit of giving often in the course of the day blows with an awl to a large number of casks. The handle of the awl is large and hard, and strongly contuses the palm of the hand."

. . . . . .

"I have seen it also in masons and other individuals obliged to lift heavy weights with the tips of the fingers. In other cases I have been unable to discover any cause for this disease.

"The disease begins ordinarily in the ring finger; it extends to the adjacent fingers, and particularly to the little finger; it increases by imperceptible degrees. The patients notice first a little stiffening in the palm of the hand, and difficulty in extending the finger, soon the fingers remain flexed to a fourth, to a third or a half. Flexion is sometimes carried even farther; and the finger tips then come to rest on the palm of the hand. From the beginning a cord is felt upon the palmar surface of the fingers, and of the hand; this cord is more tense when one attempts to extend the fingers; and it disappears almost completely when they are entirely flexed.

"What is the seat, and what is the cause of this unusual affection? This is important to determine in order to establish the treatment on a solid base.

"Some individuals have thought it should be attributed to a thickening of the palmar skin, but this envelope, compelled as it is to comply with the movements of the fingers, does not draw back upon itself in following their contraction, and has nothing to do with the disease. Others have attributed it to a spastic condition, to a contracture of the muscles of the volar surface of the forearm, but this is no better based, for the muscles enjoy complete freedom to contract and obey the will. Others, and there are many, have thought it is a disease of the flexor tendons, a thickening, a chronic inflammation of organized structures. I myself long had this opinion but I have abandoned it since the dissection of these tissues has shown that the tendons show no form of alteration. . . .

"The number of these causes, for the most part insignificant, improbable or contradictory would alone be sufficient to reject them. There remained only one method to dispel the obscurity which prevailed concerning the diagnosis, and afterward the treatment, of the contraction of the fingers; it was the careful dissection of the tissues which are affected in this disease."

. . . . . .

He then goes on to describe the findings when he obtained the opportunity to dissect the hand of a man who died after having had a contraction of the fingers for many years. . . .

Ed. Note—In a later and longer version of this lecture, Dupuytren made the following statement. "Such was the general view of our knowledge upon this point, when a man, who had been for a long time affected with this disease, happened to die. I had kept my eye on him for some years, and was determined not to lose this opportunity of investigation. Accordingly, I possessed myself of the arm of this man, had the state of the parts ac-

curately drawn by an artist, and then proceeded to dissect them. . . . When the skin was removed from the palmar surface of the hand and fingers, the folds which I had before noticed, disappeared altogether. . . . The dissection was continued by exposing the palmar fascia, and I was astonished to perceive that this fascia was tense, retracted, and shortened. . . . I cut through the prolongations extending from the fascia to the fingers; the state of contraction immediately ceased, and the slightest effort was sufficient to bring them to complete extension."

"The flexor tendons within normal sheaths were shining, smooth and of normal size and thickness. On dividing one, and then both flexor tendons, no change in the contraction took place. The joint capsules were normal. . . ."

These findings gave the clue to the corrective treatment.

"The cause of the contraction once recognized and established, it remained then to find the appropriate remedy for its correction and restore the mobility of the fingers. The failure, often demonstrated, of all the methods employed against this disease has proved the uselessness of trying them again. These remedies could not have acquired any greater value after it was discovered that the contraction of the fingers was due to the puckering up and contraction of the palmar fascia.

"It seemed to me that section of the bridles formed by this aponeurosis would be the most prompt and effective remedy for this disease."

He then describes the operative treatment.

"With the hand of the patient held firmly we began to make a transverse incision of ten lines opposite the metacarpophalangeal joint of the ring finger. The bistoury divided first the skin, then the aponeurosis, with an audible cracking sound. The painful incision completed, the ring finger straightened, and one could extend it almost as easily as a normal finger." Hoping to avoid for the patient the pain of a second incision, M. Dupuytren attempted to extend the division of the aponeurosis by sliding the bistoury transversely and deep under the skin toward the ulnar side of the hand so as to free the little finger also. This was in vain."

In spite of transverse incision opposite the metacarpophalangeal and proximal interphalangeal joints, it was only when an incision was made opposite the middle of the proximal phalanx that the little finger could be easily extended, probably because this was at the point of insertion of the aponeurosis. Considerable bleeding followed the incisions, and was controlled by compression.

The postoperative course was slow and painful—acute inflammation, swelling of the entire hand, suppuration, were finally controlled and healing of the open wounds gradually took place.

The operation was performed June 10. Cicatrization of all the wounds was complete July 2. The swelling of the hand gradually receded; on August 2 the patient was beginning to use his hand. On December 5 "the patient is in a state of complete recovery."

M. Guillaume Dupuytren
Hôtel Dieu
Paris, France

COMMENTARY BY THE EDITOR

There has long been some question of priority of Cooper vs. Cline vs. Dupuytren in describing this affection of the palmar fascia. In a longer version of this same lecture, Dupuytren makes the following statement. "Astley Cooper, in his work 'On Dislocations and Fractures of the Joints' says, that a finger or toe may be drawn by degrees from its normal position by the contraction of the flexor tendon and its sheath; and that, in consequence of this distortion, the

first and second phalanges of the toes project upwards against the shoe." For a succinct discussion of this priority question, the reader is referred to Hueston's book (Hueston, J. L.: *Dupuytren's Contracture.* The Williams & Wilkins Co., Baltimore, 1964).

More interesting is the man, so well portrayed by Goldwyn in this book, and the milieu in which he worked, described partially in the following excerpts. They were written when Dupuytren was "visiting professor" at Guy's Hospital in London (reprinted from Lancet, *10*: 861, 1826). (The first patient is a man with ileus.)

. . . . Ordered twenty-five leeches to the abdomen; he continues to take the calomel and opium pills, and sulphate of magnesia in mint water. . . . . At one o'clock, the patient was visited by Sir A. Cooper, in company with Baron Dupuytren. Having ascertained the previous history of the case, Sir Astley proceeded to examine the abdomen, pressing his hand firmly on the umbilical region, and then carefully feeling each inguinal canal, and the scrotum. Having done this, Sir Astley remarked, that he could not discover any swelling, and under these circumstances, he fully concurred in the plan of treatment which had been adopted. When the bed-clothes were drawn down, Sir Astley proceeded to make some observations on the case to Dupuytren, who seeing the abdomen distended, inquired if the bladder was not full. On inquiry, it was found that the patient had not passed any urine since the preceding morning; Mr. Callaway introduced a catheter, and drew off about a pint and a half of clear urine. (This had no connexion with the symptoms or with the swelling of the abdomen; the inquiry of Dupuytren, we suppose, therefore, was accidental.). . . . .

VISIT OF BARON DUPUYTREN AT GUY'S HOSPITAL—OPERATION OF LITHOTOMY BY MR. KEY

On Tuesday last, that illustrious French surgeon, Baron Dupuytren, visited Guy's Hospital, and went round the wards with Sir Astley Cooper. The circumstance of his being about to visit the Hospital being generally known on the preceding day, a large concourse of pupils assembled to meet him, by whom he was received with marked attention and politeness.

He immediately proceeded round the wards with Sir A. Cooper; amongst the cases which were pointed out as particularly worthy of notice, were the case of strangulated hernia related in this week's reports, a case of empyema, and compound fracture of the cranium.

A long discussion ensued between Dupuytren and Sir Astley Cooper in Accident Ward, on the subject of fracture of the neck of the thigh bone. We understood the former to assert the possibility of ossific union taking place; he said that he had a preparation illustrative of this fact, which he would take care to forward for Sir Astley's inspection. The treatment usually adopted by him in fractures of the neck of the thigh bone, he said was, to place the limb on a double inclined plane, and he usually found that the parts had united at the termination of eighty days, that is, about double the length of time usually assigned for the union of fractures in other parts of the thigh bone. When Dupuytren was about to enter the Accident Ward, Sir Astley Cooper turned round, and addressing Mr. Key and Mr. Callaway in his usual jocose manner said "Now if you have got a *good* fracture of the thigh, and one *properly* done up, let the Baron see it, but for God's sake do not shew him one of the *ram's horn* cases which every now and then happens."

Dupuytren objected generally to the beds used in this Hospital; he recommended first a straw mat, then a flock mattress, and lastly on this a flock bed. After seeing several other cases, he proceeded to the operating theatre, in order to witness the operation of lithotomy by Mr. Key.

The patient, a boy about five years of age, was placed on the table; the straight staff was passed without difficulty, and Mr. Key effected his incision into the bladder with his accustomed dexterity. The forceps were now introduced and speedily afterwards, Mr. Key withdrew them, and passing his finger through the wound into the bladder, turned round, and looking aghast, exclaimed, *"the stone is not in the bladder, it is in an abscess at the neck of the bladder."* It was somewhat unfortunate that

Mr. Key should have made this remark, for on raising the forceps, he found that the calculus had been withdrawn, and was then actually between the blades of the instrument, but it was so small that it had previously escaped observation. The satisfaction depicted in the operator's countenance on making this discovery may readily be conceived. Sir Astley Cooper afterwards remarked to a pupil, (apparently with great feeling) "it is fortunate for the honour of Guy's Hospital, that the operation terminated in this satisfactory manner."

"The best thing you could have done," said Sir Astley to Mr. Key, "if you had not found a stone, would have been to hang yourself up by the neck." (What says Ben Travers to this?)

Dupuytren expressed his approbation of Mr. Key's operation in the highest possible terms of praise; he said that he had frequently seen the operation performed with much dexterity, but never "more promptly, more decisively, or more happily (*bonheur*) than on the present occasion."

Baron Dupuytren, after the operation, visited the museum, the lecture room, and other parts of the new buildings. When he took his leave of Sir Astley Cooper, he saluted the worthy Baronet on each cheek; the manner in which Sir Astley submitted to this ceremony, afforded no small share of amusement to the pupils standing round, which was heightened by his observing, "Well, I am even with the Baron, for I saluted his daughter yesterday, when he was out of the way."

A scene worthy of the pencil of Hogarth occurred in the presentation of the Pharmacopoeia Guyensis to Dupuytren by the venerable Stocker—the standard-pestle of Guy's Hospital.

Reading all this, one is reminded that amidst all the hustle and small talk of daily chores, surrounded by the boundless good humor and cheeriness of well-rounded people, *how lonely are the great!*

—FRANK MCDOWELL

BRIGAND OR GENIUS?

Newton's Third Law, "to every action there is an equal and opposite reaction," may have application in the field of human relations, as well as in the physical universe. Success begets envy; genius, by its mere presence, may beget scallions.

Dupuytren is remembered first for the palmar contracture which bears his name, but secondly as "an arrogant man." The latter reputation stems more from the barbed eponyms bestowed by Lisfranc and Percy, than from anything that Dupuytren himself wrote.

Lisfranc called him "the Brigand of Hôtel Dieu;" Percy's acid phrase was "the greatest of surgeons and the least of men." These two may not have been entirely objective in their appraisal.

Lisfranc was chief surgeon at La Pitié, a well-known Parisian hospital, but scarcely another Hôtel Dieu. Of Lisfranc, John Billings writes (in his *History and Literature of Surgery*) "he sought to reduce operative surgery to mathematical rules . . . he was . . . envious of the greater success of some of his contemporaries, particularly Dupuytren and Velpeau, and died dissatisfied with himself and with everyone around him."

Percy was an ambitious military surgeon, made a baron by Napoleon, and was surgeon-in-chief to Napoleon's armies at Waterloo in 1814. In 1815, Dupuytren was awarded the most coveted post in France, Surgeon-in-Chief at the Hôtel Dieu. He was a friend of, and personal physician to, Louis XVIII, who created a baronetcy for him; later he was physician to Charles X. It is likely that Percy was *persona non grata* in the circles in which Dupuytren moved; conversely, Dupuytren was no egalitarian.

But what do we expect of a great surgeon? At 17, this one was studying with an intensity and singleness of purpose rarely seen in any century. Destitute, he studied by the light of candles which he made from the fat of cadavers, under bedcovers in winter to keep from freezing in his unheated quarters, fed for weeks by the leavings of a neighborhood water carrier. At age 18, he was put in charge of all autopsies at the medical school, an unrivaled opportunity of which he made the most. At 24, he became chief of anatomy and wrote a treatise on pathological anatomy, based on findings in 1,000 autopsies. The following year he became second surgeon at the Hôtel Dieu. The schedule there began with his arrival at 6:30 a.m. (it is said

that he would not tolerate tardiness), rounds with students and a large number of visitors until 9 a.m. (he prided himself on seeing every surgical patient in the house every day), a lecture from 9 to 10 a.m. attended by 300 to 400, operations for some hours, office patients in the late afternoon, emergencies at night. By what lack of understanding could we expect that anyone with this history would be a genial soul?—"the well-rounded man?" —or even a pleasant person?

But who has ever said that great surgeons, as a species, are amiable folk? On what basis did such giants as Cushing, Halsted, Evarts Graham and Will Mayo achieve their fame? Can we still applaud, or even tolerate, their successors?—and successors to Chopin, Van Gogh, Poe, Einstein, Winston Churchill or George Patton? Or must our leaders of the future all be shaped in the molds of "well-rounded men," as conceived by psychologists, educators, and their computers?

Of Dupuytren, Billings says "he was a cold, reserved, unscrupulous and ambitious man, with contemptuous and offensive manners who can hardly be said to have had any personal friends; but he was an incessant worker, thoroughly self-reliant, a bold operator, and unsurpassed as a clinical teacher. . . . He was the most distinguished surgeon in France—and, for that matter, in the world." Can we see in this, both the greatness of his surgical genius and the Chaplinesque tragedy of his personal life which, in a way, was the price of that genius?

—*Frank McDowell*

UNDERDEVELOPED LOWER JAW, WITH LIMITED EXCURSION

Report of Two Cases With Operation

VILRAY PAPIN BLAIR,* M.D., *St. Louis, Mo.*

(Reprinted from J.A.M.A., 53: 178, 1909)

My reasons for reporting the two following cases are, first, that one of them is, as far as I know, unique in its pathology, and the other presented a degree of deformity that is extremely rare; and, second, that the procedures resorted to for their relief have, as far as I know, never before been employed or suggested except by myself.

Case 1.—*Patient.*—A young woman, referred to me by Dr. C. Dewitt Lukens, who gave the following history: When five years of age she was crushed under a falling bale of hay, was generally injured, remained unconscious for forty-eight hours, but made a good immediate recovery. Between the ages of 11 and 12 years it was noticed that she could not open her mouth freely, and on examination it was found that the excursion of the lower jaw was limited. From that time on it was noticed that the chin became relatively more receding (Fig. 1, *left*) and the downward excursion of the lower jaw lessened.

When she consulted me the patient was 21 years old, delicate, and very thin. The mandible was undeveloped and the downward excursion was limited to the extent that the greatest possible vertical opening between the upper and the lower incisor teeth was one-eighth of an inch. Owing to the receding jaw, the lower incisors were one-fourth inch behind the upper, which with the one-eighth opening gave a possible feeding space. I thought that probably the lack of development was related to the early injury, but this did not explain the limited movement, which presented the following peculiarities: The movement was free until the opening between the incisor teeth was one-

eighth of an inch and then stopped suddenly. During this movement the right condyle traveled forward as much as it would do in normal full opening of the mouth. The left remained apparently stationary and the chin moved to the left more than it did downward. A poor X-ray taken at the time failed to throw light on this point, but I figured out that some obstruction impinging on the dorsal part of the right ramus of the jaw near the angle could cause just that movement by transferring the center of motion on that side from the center of the ramus to the angle. The indications here were to give a free opening of the mouth, to establish a normal occlusion of the teeth and to improve the profile by carrying the chin forward and holding it there. Granting that my idea of the obstruction was correct, all of these things would be accomplished by the operation for receding jaw which I have described elsewhere.[1]

Operation.—At St. Luke's Hospital, on Nov. 8, 1905, under ether an incision of five-eighths of an inch was made in front of the lobe of each ear, the parotid gland turned back, a curved needle passed under the ramus and out through the cheek and a Gigli saw introduced, the soft structures protected and the ramus cut through on both sides. Owing to an abnormality of the ramus on the left side the mucous membrane of the mouth was pierced by the needle and we had an infected wound on that side which later caused a temporary paralysis of the upper branches of the seventh nerve, but this cleared up in about four weeks. The wounds were packed, the muscles of mastication stretched, the body of jaw brought forward

1. Surg. Gynec. and Obst., January, 1907; Dental Era, April, 1907.

*Clinical Professor of Surgery in the Medical Department, and Professor of Oral Surgery in the Dental Department, of Washington University.

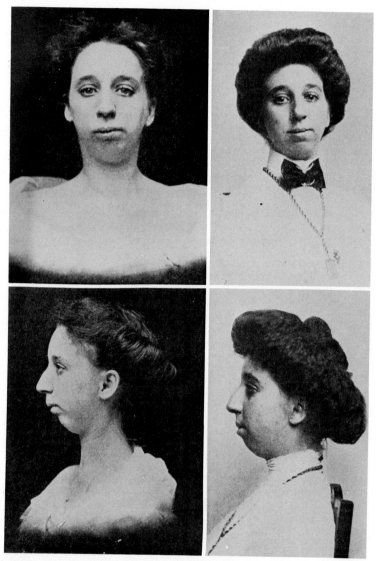

FIG. 1. *Patient 1.* (*left*) Before operation. In the full face view, notice the lateral position of the chin. (*above right*) The lateral position of the chin has been corrected. (*below right*) Notice the change in the relative position of the lips resulting from the new position of the body of the lower jaw.

until the lower incisors were a little in front of the uppers and the chin symmetrically placed. It was wired in this position.

Postoperative History.—The packing was removed from the face wounds on the third day. The right one was closed with a suture that had been previously placed and the left dressed open. The paralysis on the left side appeared on the second day, but cleared up as previously stated. The patient left the hospital November 18, ten days after operation. In four weeks the union was examined and found not to be strong, so the teeth were rewired for eight weeks more. Later Dr. Lukens, by orthodontic operations, brought the teeth into more perfect occlusion. In removing the wires from the teeth, it was found as expected, but, nevertheless to my relief, that the mouth opened freely one-half inch and that the limit of movement was in the soft structures. When examined a year later, it was found that lateral movement was normal and the possible opening between the incisors was seven-eighths of an inch, which is more than is necessary for good function. As mentioned in the articles already referred to, bringing forward the body of an underdeveloped mandible does not entirely correct the obliquity of the chin. I proposed, by further operative procedure, to construct a menton eminence, but the patient expressed herself as well satisfied with her results (Fig. 1, *right*).

The peculiarity of this case was the limit of excursion of the mandible, which was due, as demonstrated later by a good X-ray taken after the operation by Dr. H. P. Wells (Fig. 2, *above*), to the

fact that the styloid process on the right side was the size of my little finger and abutted against the inner side of the angle of the jaw, which corresponds with my original deduction. By moving the body forward a space was obtained between the angle and the styloid process which gave room for the angle to travel backward during normal movement. The other results are a symmetrical chin, an improved profile, good health and mental relief. The patient's own brother did not recognize her when she returned home and within a few months she gained twenty-eight pounds over her pre-

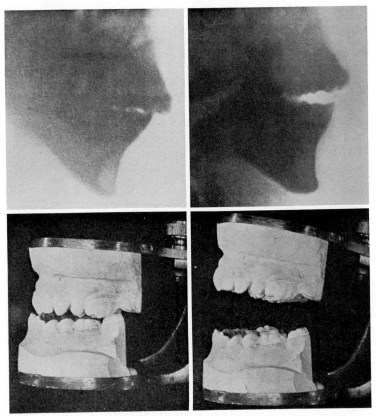

Fig. 2. *Case 1.* (*above*) X-rays before and after operation, showing how much the lower jaw has been brought forward, and the amount of opening possible before and after operation. (*below*) Comparing left with right, the increase in the possible opening can be measured. Before operation the possible opening was one-eighth of an inch; a year after operation it was, as stated, seven-eighths of an inch. Since then there has been a contraction of the bone scars which has reduced the opening to five-eighths of an inch, but it will contract no more. The cast showing the present condition was taken this year by Dr. J. L. Newborn of Memphis, Tenn.

vious weight which she has retained. She has been in good health ever since, which was not the case before, and she seems very happy. Removal or fracture of the abnormal styloid would give her freer opening, but the patient does not feel the need. She had been seeking relief for some years before I saw her, and, including the members present at medical and dental associations before which, at the request of her dentist, she had appeared seeking advice, she had been seen by a large number of men of both professions.

The photographs of this patient and the next (Figs. 1 and 3) are unretouched and show the exact condition of features, but exaggerate the color of recent scars.

Case 2.—*Patient.*—A girl, aged 23, who came to my clinic at the dental department of the Washington University. She had had scarlet fever at the age of 2, with a suppuration behind each ear, probably mastoid. At 6 the opening of the mouth was noticed to be limited and some attempt at stretching with wedges was made. At 9 the opening was very limited and at 15 some lower incisors were removed to allow her to take solid food.

Examination.—In January, 1908, the patient presented herself at the clinic with this condition: She was rather thin, with suppuration of both middle ears, scars from old cervical abscesses, a fair percentage of sugar in the urine. The facial contour was shown in Figure 3, *left.* There was absolutely no visible excursion of the lower jaw, which was in an extreme degree of underdevelopment. The canines and remaining incisors of the lower jaw protruded straight forward and held the lower lip in the position shown in Figure 3, *above left.*

The indications here were to improve the general health, including the ear condition, establish a joint on each side, draw the body of the jaw forward and hold it there. On strict diet, under the care of Dr. Walter Baumgarten, the sugar disappeared from the urine. The same operation on the jaw was indicated as in the previous case, but as here we had also to establish a joint on each side, I proposed to the patient to allow me to transplant the interphalangeal joints of one toe to the spaces I would leave between the cut ends of the bone.

Permission to do this was refused and I was afterward glad, as every wound but one that I ever made on her suppurated. The operation was done before the class at the Washington University Hospital on Feb. 11, 1908.

Operation.—After sawing the ramus transversely in this case, and bringing the body forward as far as I could hope to retain it, I found that there was such a great separation between the ends that bony union would not be probable. The jaw was held in its new position by wiring the lower to the upper teeth.

Postoperative Treatment.—In this case, with the large space between the cut bone ends, it seemed to me that the greatest difficulty was going to be in retaining the jaw permanently forward. To meet this I determined to keep the bone wired in its new position for a considerable time and later, if necessary, establish the joints. On April 26, on account of evident illness, the mouth was unwired. I found a considerable degree of opening, sufficient to make out a diphtheria of the pharynx. On recovery the patient returned to the clinic and I found the jaw forward in its new position with an excursion that allowed of an opening of the mouth that was three-sixteenths between the bicuspids and limited by soft structures. Attempts at instrumental dilatation with and without anesthetics were unsuccessful and I hit on the plan of inserting pieces of laminaria uterine tent between the teeth and allowing them to remain over night, which was so successful both in the lack of pain and in the result that I consider it a distinct advance over the methods ordinarily used for this purpose.

Result.—We now had the patient's jaw forward and she could open her mouth sufficiently for function, but, owing to the obliquity of the mental portion, the facial outline was still far from what was desired. The correction of this was a problem about which I had been thinking for some years. Three possible methods presented themselves to me: First, paraffin injection into the soft structures, which I dismissed early in the consideration; second, an osteoplastic resection to tilt forward a piece of the chin bone and fill in the space behind with a paraffin iodoform mixture, or silver frame and blood clot; and, third, the transplantation of cartilage. I finally settled on the latter procedure.

Second Operation.—On September 1, at the Washington University Hospital, under ether given through tubes introduced through the nose into the pharynx after the method of

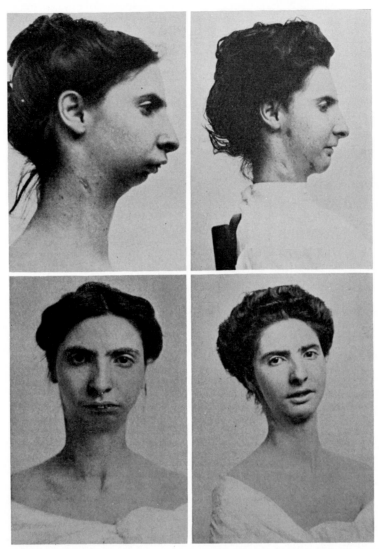

FIG. 3. *Patient 2.* (*left*) Before operation. (*above right*) Owing to their red color at the time of being photographed, the prominence of the scars on the cheek and under the chin is exaggerated by the camera. Later, when the red color fades, the scars will be practically invisible. The change in coiffure in both cases is in conformity with the mode. (*below right*) After operation the happier expression about the eyes is one of the results.

Crile, the mouth was packed and a cloth was sewed across the face below the mouth to prevent contamination from the mouth. The curved part of the eighth costal cartilage with its perichondrium was dissected loose and for temporary protection was left in its original position. Then a transverse cut to the bone was made in the crease under the chin and all the structures covering the front of the mental part of the mandible, including the periosteum, were dissected upward in one flap. The curved piece of cartilage one and a half inches long was laid on the bare bone and, after wiring it there, the flap of soft tissue, including periosteum, was replaced, and a very respectable chin resulted.

Postoperative History.—The whole wound suppurated, but I did not remove the sutures, and for days pus in large quantities poured out between them. Later the suppuration became less, and from local symptoms and appearance I came to the conclusion that the infection had occurred between the perichondrium and bone, which was a dead space, but not between perichondrium and the periosteum. Some sinuses persisted which healed nicely after the wires were removed and the sinuses had been injected with a paste of subiodide and subnitrate of bismuth and petrolatum, which is a slight modification of the plan introduced by Beck of Chicago for chronic sinuses. Later the X-ray demonstrated the bismuth in the space between the cartilage and bone. I preserved the perichondrium because it is in normal relation on the one hand with the cartilage and on the other with the soft structures; I thought that the leucocytes would be less likely to regard the covered cartilage as a foreign body, and that the nourishment of the cartilage would be preserved. I turned up the periosteum and buried the cartilage under it, because I thought that if I did loose (*sic*) the cartilage it might stay long enough to hold the periosteum in its new position until it had formed a shell of bone. Here I seem to have calculated badly, for the subsequent X-rays show no effort at bone formation on the part of the reflected periosteum.

To my mind, the most remarkable thing in the whole procedure is that the cartilage did stay in place after suppuration occurred. The scar is linear and hidden well under the chin. The anatomic operative results in this case are the facial outline shown in Figure 3, *right*, a very fair occlusion of the natural teeth that have been preserved, and false joints that permit an up-and-down excursion of the lower jaw, which is limited by soft structures and which is increasing while a lateral movement is developing. A slight amount of the movement on the right side is in the temporomandibular joint, which seems to have been restored by the dilation with tents.

Dental Operation.—Dr. LeGrand Cox, who is associated with me in that clinic and who assisted me all through with this case, removed the upper incisors to

allow the lip to retract and the remaining lower incisors and cuspids on account of their extreme malposition. He also crowned the lower bicuspids to bring them up to occlusion. The prosthetic work which shows in Figure 4 was done by Dr. F. A. Niehoff, who has charge of that laboratory, and it and the casts do great credit to his skill and patience. The treatment extended over a year and the patient's circumstances were such that much of the time she was, by the courtesy of the dean, in the hospital at the expense of the dental department. Since the movement of the jaw has been re-

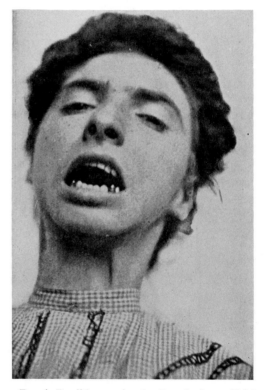

FIG. 4. Possible opening in *Case 2*, the artificial dentures, and the crowned bicuspids. The strain of the platysma was the result of the desire to have the mouth open as fully as possible, but it was unnecessary and did not contribute to the result as the mouth opens with perfect freedom till the limit is reached. The artificial incisors are so placed that they do not quite occlude.

stored and the teeth have been replaced, on ordinary general diet the sugar in the urine has disappeared. When the patient first presented herself, and all through the first months of treatment whenever she got out of the hospital and on general diet, it ran very high. The disappearance of sugar is possibly one result of the improved digestion, metabolism and spirits which have followed the operation.

Vilray Papin Blair, M.D.
Washington University
St. Louis, Mo.

Metropolitan Building.

COMMENTARY BY THE EDITOR

This paper was "the shot heard around the world," the one which lifted Blair's reputation from a not-too-well-known St. Louis anatomist and general surgeon to that of a foremost plastic surgeon. Moreover, it did much to refurbish the reputation of plastic surgery as a decent and acceptable branch of surgery, so it is a milestone in our heritage.

After the brilliant pioneering work done in this field by inspired surgical geniuses for two centuries, in the twilight of the 19th and the dawn of the 20th century an assortment of "featural surgeons" and "cosmetic surgeons" appeared—distinguished more by their brazen advertising and unwarranted claims than by their ability or their results. They were busily injecting or implanting paraffin, gutta percha, petrolatum, ivory, or what have you—often with tragic results. This dragged the name of *plastic surgery* down so far that few surgeons of high repute were then willing to admit they were doing "plastic surgery." Note that Blair did not use the term in this article, nor did he adopt it until World War I when he insisted his title be "Chief of Plastic and Oral Surgery" of the U.S. Army (rather than Chief of Maxillofacial Surgery).

In the early years of the 20th century, Blair, a "late bloomer," returned from his odyssey as a ship's surgeon between London and West Africa (or the Amazon), married, and settled down to practicing surgery in St. Louis and teaching anatomy in both the medical and dental schools of Washington University. During "spare time" he conceived and worked out the details of a new closed ramisection of the mandible for micrognathia or prognathism, using cadavers in the anatomical laboratory.

Though he had published one small book on anatomy and some 12 articles between 1897 and 1906, the articles were on malaria, the care of premature infants, and all sorts of subjects except those we would regard as plastic surgery. In the fall of 1906 he published a short case report of his ramisection operation (this time for prognathism) in a dental journal, and also in a mediocre medical journal. Apparently these aroused little interest. In 1907 he published a long, rambling paper in the then new journal *Surgery, Gynecology, and Obstetrics* entitled "Operations on the Jaw-Bone and Face." The paper contained pictures of famous statues and paintings of beautiful persons, from art museums—discourses on the ideas of beauty held by ancient Greeks, Romans, Russians, and Assyrians—pictures of prognathism in primitive races and in sub-human species, *etc.* It had no focus, was greeted with yawns, and Blair never made that mistake again. (Perhaps his greatest asset was his keen ability to learn from mistakes, especially when they were his own.)

Blair was 38 years old when the paper you see here appeared. He was still stammering in his writing ("the fact that," *etc.*), and the editor arranged the illustrations miserably (not as they are reprinted here). However, it was in one of the leading medical journals of the world, and it had an arresting focus. While the text modestly included all the difficulties and complications, the striking photographs of astounding results quickly captured the interest and imagination of readers the world over. They had never seen anything before as dramatic as the positively documented change in *Case 2;* it seemed little short of a miracle. Within a short time, physicians from all over the United States started sending patients to Blair for jaw surgery and other facial surgery. A little later patients began arriving from Europe (several weeks' travel by ship and train). With this paper, he had "hit the jackpot."

Why did the article attract such worldwide attention? Among the reasons are *(1)* it was in a major journal with worldwide circulation, *(2)* the text was in plain words and with a modest tone which evoked the immense power of understatement, and *(3)* the astounding results were irrefutably documented in the photographs. The obtaining of the latter required herculean efforts in those days—as patients had to sit still for 3-minute time exposures made under "good daylight" with big box cameras containing wet, glass plates. The surgeon had to learn to do his own, from start to finish; there was no such thing as a flash bulb, an electric flash, or an enlarger. The wonder is that the "sizing" of the befores and afters is as good as it is. Blair believed that clear, convincing photographic documentation of results was worth whatever amount of personal effort it took.

Beginning with this article, Blair's work attracted the attention of many leading surgeons—including Will and Charles Mayo; at first he visited them, then they visited him. Meanwhile he worked nights writing his first major book (the first major one by anyone on this subject), *Surgery and Dis-*

eases of the Mouth and Jaws. Again, these difficult photographs were necessary, in profusion; also he had to hire an artist to do the drawings. When the large book appeared in 1912, it was an immediate and huge success, one which had a wide sale both in America and in Europe (where war clouds were gathering). It went through 3 editions within 4 years.

In England, Sir Arbuthnot Lane (Chief of Surgery at Guy's Hospital and at the Hospital for Sick Children in Great Ormond Street) was particularly interested. He was doing cleft lip and cleft palate surgery (*cf.* "Lane cleft palate needles"), and some mandibular surgery, along with a lot of abdominal surgery and work on skeletal fractures. In time they visited each other, and Lane sent some patients to Blair. Quite naturally, when Blair arrived in England in 1918 as Chief of Plastic Surgery for the American Expeditionary Forces, he went to see Lane—who, by·this time, was Chief of Surgery for the Aldershot Command.

Lane commented that plastic surgery was not really established as a specialty in Britain yet, that because of the large number of facial injuries and their residuals arriving from the battlefront he had caused to be established a center for their care, Queen Mary's Hospital at Sidcup (within his command), and he had hoped to do much of the work there personally. However, his time had been preempted by administrative duties so he had delegated the face and jaw work at Sidcup to a young ENT man from New Zealand, one Harold Gillies, who had recently assisted Lane on face and jaw cases at Cambridge Hospital, Aldershot. Lane thought Gillies had great promise, but he asked Blair to appraise the work being done at Sidcup and to report confidentially back to him. Blair was impressed with the man and the work, noted that the British had had much actual experience with war wounds while the Americans had not, and he encouraged surgeons from his own command to visit Sidcup for a few days whenever they could get time off.

The high quality of the work done on facial injuries and burns, and their late restoration, in World War I did much to restore the reputation of plastic surgery and to demonstrate that it *could* be an honorable and worthwhile specialty, and *should* be a separate specialty. Thus, on his return from the war to St. Louis, Blair was able to establish the first separate Plastic Surgery Service in the United States (perhaps in the world) at Barnes Hospital and Washington University. He was careful to keep it closely allied to general surgery; he demanded that the work done on it, and the actions of the staff, be (like Caesar's wife) beyond reproach.

Soon afterward, in 1921, came the formation of the first plastic surgical society in the world, the American Association of Oral and Plastic Surgeons—composed, principally, of men who had served in Blair's plastic surgery section in World War I. These men were dedicated to high quality performance in a broad spectrum of surgery, to the finest educational standards, and to a conservative demeanor characterized by understatement. Through their efforts the specialty became firmly established.

—*Frank McDowell*

PLASTIC PROCEDURE USING A ROUND PEDICLE

PROFESSOR V. P. FILATOV, *Odessa, Russia*

(Published in Russian in Vestnik Oftalmologii 34 (4–5): 149–158
(April–May) 1917.)

(Translation Reprinted from Surgical Clinics of North America, *39:* 277, 1959.)

Translated from the Russian by
Miroslav Labunka, Martha Teach Gnudi, and Dr. Jerome P. Webster

I am here bringing to the attention of my colleagues a method of plastic surgery which has as its basis the preparation of a round, nutrient stalk pedicle for a skin flap to be used to cover a defect.

Thus far, I have applied this method only to one case, a plastic operation on an eyelid. The following description of this case will present the manner in which it was done.

CASE REPORT

The patient, Ivan Vasil'ev, 62 years old, was admitted to the Eye Clinic of the Novorossiisk University in September 1916 with the lower lid of his right eye covered by an edematous cancerous tumor, which had destroyed about half the length of the eyelid. From the border of the conjunctiva it had almost reached the transverse fold. Scars around the tumor, and the medical history, indicated that this was a recurrence of a neoplasm that had previously undergone a plastic procedure (sliding flap).

In planning an operation, I found that it would be necessary to remove, along with this neoplasm, two-thirds of the eyelid in its whole thickness — nearly to the orbital margin, including a part of the skin over the malar bone — and that the defect would have to be covered by means of a plastic procedure. To accomplish this, I turned to a tubed pedicle flap which I took from the patient's neck, one which I had previously devised by experimenting on a rabbit.

First Operation

With tincture of iodine, I outlined a wide strip of skin (5 cm) on the right side of the neck — from the mastoid process to the sternal end of the clavicle, along the sternocleidomastoid muscle. A 1 percent solution of Novocain with Adrenalin was injected at its edges; the outlined strip of skin was pinched into a fold, which an assistant held with his hands while I made large [mattress] sutures with two needles in a transverse direction, and tied them at the base of the fold (Fig. 1).

As the assistant consecutively replaced his hands along the fold, I sutured it in its entire length with 8 stitches, after which it remained intact [in a fold] when support was discontinued. Starting at the upper end, I incised the skin *above the sutures* along the lateral side of the fold from one end to the other; then again from the upper end of the fold I incised the skin along its medial side, and with sawlike movements of the scalpel I separated the fold from the neck, moving along it above the sutures to its sternal end.

In this way I obtained a strip of skin (with the layer of subcutaneous adipose tissue) which remained connected to the upper part of the neck at the mastoid process and to the lower end at the sternum.

The long wound on the neck, thanks to the preliminary sutures, scarcely gaped. Careful approximation of the neck wound was carried out with sutures. *The skin strip along its entire length was converted into a band strand, a "stalk," by suturing its edges to each other.*

A large bandage on the neck was carried over the axillary region and around the head, with a warm compress placed over the operative site. The pedicle was allowed to lie directly on the skin of the neck, without the interposition of gauze, to insure better warming. Wads of cotton were placed lengthwise to avoid pressure on the pedicle.

Thus the first stage of the formation of the future layer [carrier?], the basic part of the method, was completed.

Presented before the Odessa Ophthalmological Society on November 16, 1916.

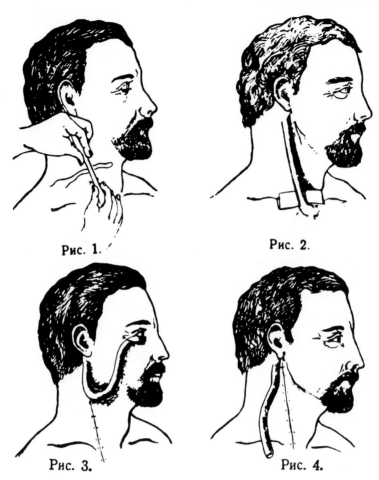

Рис. 1.   Рис. 2.

Рис. 3.   Рис. 4.

FIGS. 1–4. (*1*) The first operative stage, the preparation of a tubed flap on the right side of the patient's neck. (*2*) The second operative stage, when the flap at the lower end was lined with a mucous-membrane graft taken from the lip. (The letters at the lower end of the flap, indicating its parts, are scarcely legible.) (*3*) The third stage, when the tubed flap was migrated to the lower eyelid, after the lesion on the lower lid had been excised. (*4*) The fifth operation, severance of the pedicle. (The fourth was transplantation of additional mucous membrane from the lip to the flap.)

According to the data gained from my experiments with rabbits, the skin pedicle should adjust itself to the new conditions of blood circulation, the necessary anastomoses should develop along the cut vessels of the subcutaneous layer and, after this, the pedicle should become a solid nutritional base for the flap.

The Postoperative Course

Two days later (September 11), during the first dressing, it appeared that the pedicle was progressing well—its upper half was not edematous, there was no obstruction, and while its lower half was slightly swollen it was but slightly reddish. With a light touch of the finger it paled, but on removing the finger it again became rank.

On September 13, four days after [the first procedure], it was noticed that the lower third of the pedicle had become pinker, and therefore about ten scarifications were made with a scalpel, causing it to bleed lightly.

On September 15, six days after [the first procedure], some complications of a purely accidental nature occurred, having no connection with the method itself. The edges of the neck wound became reddish towards the center, a few sutures suppurated, and following this the middle part of the pedicle suture line became infected, as indicated by inflammation and swelling. The infected sutures were immediately removed from the neck and the pedicle, and the dressing was arranged to prevent the pedicle from touching the neck wound, which was separately covered by waxed paper over the gauze. In spite of this accidental complication, the pedicle was not damaged, which indicated its great viability.

Eleven days after the operation the neck wound had completely healed, leaving a narrow scar. The pedicle had an excellent healthy appearance; no edema was present; when touched it was very soft at the upper part and slightly thickened, and it was soft in the lower half. The lower part was a little thicker than the upper, but this was accounted for by the fact that during the incision to form the flap its breadth had been accidentally widened towards its base — and the flap, as a consequence, was made slightly wider.

Second Operation

On September 29, preparation of the future eyelid was carried out (Fig. 2).

Under local anesthesia an incision about 3.5 cm long (*a*) was made at the lower part of the pedicle. A second curved incision was made at a right angle to the first (*b*). The angle of skin outlined by these incisions was undermined, and mucous membrane from the lip was sutured onto the inside surface of this flap. Sutures were fixed at the flap edges and at its base, with two needles. The flap, lined with mucous membrane, was returned to its place and secured by one suture [at the corner] to prevent unfolding. Dressing.

Third Operation

On October third (*i.e.* four days later) a plastic procedure of the eyelid was performed under local anesthesia. Two-thirds of the lower eyelid was excised in its full thickness; the lower border of the defect reached almost to the orbital margin, where part of the orbicularis muscle was saved. The defect also partially included a section of the ascending zygomatic process, in the region of the malar bone. On the chest the cut was prolonged in a curve to the base of the pedicle foot, the flap was separated up to the base, and the latter was freed. The transverse section of the base [of the pedicle] looked like a heel of the flap.

Some bleeding was noticed on the surface of the flap and on its heel.

The pedicle was slung over the cheek, and the flap was placed on the defect (Fig. 3). It was well sutured, but for the smooth placement of

the heel it was necessary to excise a little more of the skin of the malar region, after which the edges of the flap and heel were sutured to the edges of the defect. The margin of the upper eyelid was freshened and was sutured to the upper free edge of the flap.

Finger pressure on the flap caused it to pale, but again it became reddish when the finger was removed (thus indicating some blood circulation within it). Dressing: dry gauze, cotton on the orbital region, and over this a metallic wire splint to prevent pressure on the flap and the end of the pedicle. The splint was supported only at its ends, so that blood circulation in the adjacent areas would not be impaired (Fig. 5). The middle section of the pedicle was wrapped in a strip of gauze as a suspensory; this was stuck with collodion to the skin of the temple, and the whole was covered with cotton, waxed paper, and a bandage. At subsequent dressings, the suspended strip of gauze proved to be satisfactory: the gauze strip supported the pedicle, both its ends being brought together and tightened by means of an American pin [safety pin?]; the lower free end [of the gauze] passed under the jaw to meet the upper end, which passed over the temple and crown of the head. These ends were tied, and the gauze was stuck to the temple with collodion.

During the first dressing, on the next day, the flap and the pedicle had a perfect appearance, neither pale nor purple.

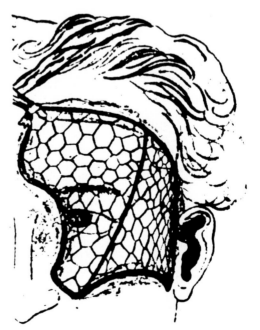

FIG. 5. The cage type of dressing used, shown here on the left side (though the operation was on the right side).

On October 6, three days later, a complication occurred which I consider accidental – an infection of the flap from the conjunctival sac. The flap was swollen, pus was exuding from its outer half, and the end of the pedicle was edematous and slightly purpled. During the next few days the sutures suppurated at the upper edge of the flap, which was necrosed in a small area. Despite this infection, which arose in part from the fact that the inner surface of the flap was insufficiently protected by the mucous membrane against conjunctival secretion, the flap at its lower edge and at the internal end healed entirely satisfactorily (*per primam*), and the edges of the heel also healed well. Naturally such a happy termination of this infection of the flap was possible only because the pedicle performed excellently its function of supplying blood to the flap.

During the infection of the flap, the pedicle was swollen in its upper third, it became slightly hyperemic, and it bled when scarified. During the dressing it also happened that, because of the improperly made suspensory, an overbalance [of fluid pressure?] occurred, causing it to become swollen. After the suspensory strip was removed and a hot water bottle was placed on the flap, it quickly regained its normal appearance. The infection of the flap lasted for nine days.

Fourth Operation

Three weeks after the plastic procedure, an additional transplantation was performed of the mucous membrane from the lip to the edge of the flap, where the surface was granulating.

Fifth Operation

One week after the additional plastic surgery procedure, the pedicle was severed at the base of the flap by an oblique cut. Since the transplanted piece was a little too thick at the distal end, the excess tissue was removed from its under surface and it was sutured back into place. Healing occurred *per primam*.

Immediately after the pedicle had been severed (Fig. 4), it was observed that it appeared pale, but a few seconds later it started to bleed; evidently the anemia at its end was of a spasmodic character. Microscopic examination of a section revealed that its cneter contained fat tissue. I recommended that the flap be returned [to its original site] in the following way. (Make an incision on the neck along the line of the scar and on the pedicle along its scar line, thin down its skin [*i.e.* excise scar tissue] and, unrolling it in the form of a strip, return it to its

previous place on the neck.) The patient, however, was not willing to agree to this.

In view of this, after cutting off a piece of the pedicle for microscopic examination, I sutured the edges of the amputated part of the pedicle with three stitches and, having protected it with a dressing, let it hang free down the neck. The lower end of the pedicle became slightly swollen and purple, but this lasted only two days. Its color then returned to its previous condition (*e.g.* normal), and the suture line healed *per primam*, thus indicating the important fact that the pedicle was excellently nourished by the blood supplied by its single [attached] end.

Six days later I amputated the pedicle at its upper end also – but I deliberately made a few preliminary oblique incisions on various parts of it. Thus I observed that for its entire length there was not only capillary bleeding present, but also there were three vessels of more significant size that were seen at each incision. When the base [upper attachment] of the pedicle was severed, blood immediately flowed from the three vessels, and they had to be clamped. I observed an interesting occurrence. At each oblique cut the pedicle instantly became pale for 2 cm along its length from the point of incision; after one to two minutes, it again reddened (reflex spasms of vessels?). (Incidentally, I might remark that the hair, which had been shaven from the patient's neck before the first operation, had grown in again.*)

Postoperative Course

The condition of the patient on the day of his discharge, November 20, was as follows.

On his neck there was a narrow scar from the mastoid process to the *manubrium sterni;* movement of his arms and neck was not impaired; the lower eyelid was of satisfactory size, the orbital aperture being slightly larger than that of the healthy side and closed well. The profile contour of the newly formed part of the eyelid was thicker than that of its unremoved part, but there was no need (because of the thickness) to thin down the transplanted flap with another operation (which would have been easy enough to do). The color of the skin was the same as that of the surrounding skin. The skin was smooth; the lid margin and a part of its inner surface were covered by mucous membrane;

* The rabbit, which had a tubed flap taken from the shaven side of its back (from the shoulder to the tail), has its hair grown back and now has a normal appearance. The incomplete preliminary microscopic examination of the "pedicle" of my patient revealed that the pedicle contained, in addition to skin and subcutaneous fat tissue, fibers and platysmal muscle in some of its parts; and a considerable number of arteries and veins, and *capillaries,* were disclosed.

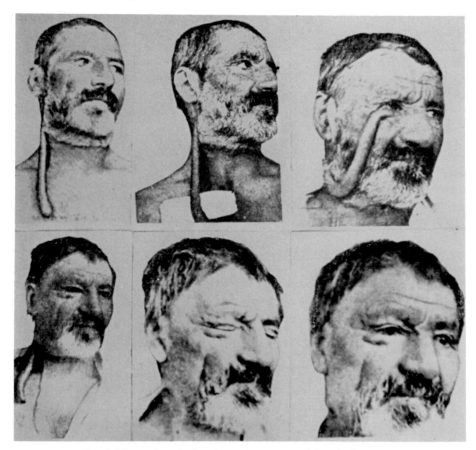

FIG. 6. The patient during the various stages of the plastic surgery.

the other parts of the inner surface were epithelized. There was no entropion of the eyelid towards the orbit; the vault of the conjunctiva was entirely sufficient; there was no friction of the lid against the orbit. The stages of the plastic surgery procedure of the tubed flap on our patient are shown in Figure 6.

DISCUSSION

On the basis of the above described case I assume: (1) that the formation of a stalklike round nutrient pedicle for the flap performed prior to the operation guarantees almost perfect nourishment for the flap; (2) that the danger of over-all infection is reduced with such a round pedicle-like root. This attribute is especially valuable when the flap has to be taken from a distant part of the body, and when the pedicle has to be carried over a region of the body which is not easily kept aseptic (as, for example, the hairy part of the cheek which, along with the hairy part of the head, was in our case infected by eczema. The possibility of infection is greatly reduced, one can say, because it is limited to the region of the flap itself (which, in no plastic procedure, is wholly protected).

These two circumstances, then, allow more freedom (through the use of a pedicle base) in the use of flaps taken from areas of the body distant from the site of the plastic procedure itself. This is especially important in operations on the face, where one wishes to avoid unnecessary incisions. Anyone who has experienced the suppuration of a flap and its necrosis in a complicated facial plastic procedure (*e.g.* in the blepharoplastic procedures of Fricke) will doubtless appreciate the merits of such a possibility.

The time spent on my patient was quite considerable, but it was somewhat longer than necessary. Each postoperative period might be reduced by a few days.

As far as I know, the use of a round stalklike nutrient pedicle in plastic operations to the eyelids has not been proposed previously. And in surgical literature I have not found a procedure proposed for transforming a skin strip into a "stalk" by prior suturing.

In a consideration of the proposed method in this form, as it was applied to my patient, the reader's thoughts might turn to Snydacker's method and its variation according to Morax's modification, which at first glance bear a similarity to the method proposed by myself. I will therefore allow myself to draw a parallel between them.

Snydacker's method[1] consists in the formation of a skin flap on the neck, from the maxillary angle to the clavicle along the sternocleidomastoid muscle (12 cm long and 2 cm wide). The lower free end is split longitudinally, and the flaps thus obtained are used in the formation of the upper and lower lids. The striplike foot, lying over the cheek, is severed on the sixth day and can be returned to its original place when necessary.

Morax[2,3,4] brought the following changes to Snydacker's method for more extensive plastic procedures. The flap from the skin of the neck can be made longer (even below the sternal end of the clavicle) and broader (up to 5 to 7 cm). The distal end of the strip is laid, without splitting, on the defect formed when part of the scar or neoplasm is removed from the forehead or eyelid. When the flap is well healed, 12 to 15 days after the first operation, a second step is performed which consists in cutting the skin that passes from the neck over the cheek (at a distance from the actual site of the plastic procedure), removing the remaining scars, and curving and placing the free end of the strip over the new defect. The granulations on the inner surface of the strip are removed with a curette, and the nourishment of this end of the pedicle now comes from its previously transplanted end. Morax used this method for the formation of two eyelids (Fig. 7D, after Wood) in covering defects after the removal of an extensive nevus on the forehead (Fig, 7, A, B, C, after Morax).

The basic principle of the Snydacker and Snydacker-Morax methods is the formation of the skin strip; they differ from the usual plastic procedure with a pedicle only in the length of the pedicle and the site of its excision. *In the method described by me, the pedicle is round, stalklike.* While not denying the many excellent features of Snydacker's method, I nevertheless maintain that of all plastic procedures (using a pedicle flap), his method, more than any other, inspires fear as to the fate of the flap and pedicle because of the distance that the blood has to flow and because of the large area exposed to infection. In expressing these hypothetical apprehensions, I would like to underline the difference in the principle of the construction of the nutrient pedicle, which gives better protection against infection and better [vascular] protection to the flap.

The excision of the skin from the neck in the plastic procedure of the eyelid described here was, of course, made on the basis of Snydacker's method, and the quilting of the fold, before its excision is, it is true, only a technical detail, but one which diminishes considerably the dramatic nature of the operation and the fear of infection in the neck wound, which in the Snydacker-Morax method is very great because of the gaping of the wound's edges.

The formation of a *round stalklike nutrient pedicle* in plastic operations, as it was applied in my case, is not to be regarded as merely a variation of Snydacker's method. There is a matter of a *new principle* which guarantees nour-

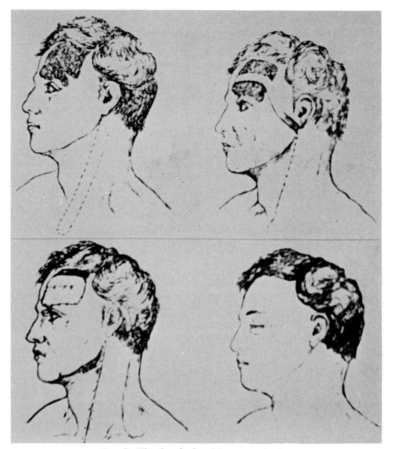

FIG. 7. The Snydacker-Morax method.

ishment of the transplanted flap. In describing my case, it is not so much the plastic procedure of the eyelid that I am proposing, as it is a method for the formation of a nutrient pedicle. This is irrespective of the type of plastic procedure and its location, provided there is an evident need for a long pedicle flap. It can be used in various plastic procedures of the eyelid, lips, nose, *etc*.

If future observations confirm my hopes as to the stalklike round pedicle (and every reason supports this), then plastic operations (not only ophthalmological, but also some surgical ones) will be considerably simplified. Although I do not wish to predetermine the type of condition to which the round stalklike pedicle can be applied,

I can already foresee some additional usages and modifications in its application.

1. In the case of a plastic procedure on both eyelids, it is possible either to resect the flap at the end of the pedicle wide enough so that (after splitting it according to Snydacker) it can be placed on both defects [at the same time]. Or the plastic procedure can be limited to one eyelid first, while the second is formed according to Morax (*e.g.* the pedicle could be severed far enough away from the eyelid, and the free end unfolded and placed on the new defect). I feel that preference should be given to the latter method.

In regard to Morax's method of plastic surgery on the eyelid, I would like to remark, however, that it is not merely a supplement to Snydacker's method — because it is applicable generally to every complicated plastic procedure with a long pedicle. But it is particularly applicable, for example, in Fricke's* operation, as previously demonstrated by Professor Golovin (independently of Morax's work) in a case of a plastic procedure on both eyelids a according to Fricke's operation (the case was not published).

I would like to add that the Morax method is a partial application of the so-called jump flap procedure, which has been widely used in general surgery (Hacker, Steinthal).

2. The second modification that can be made in the preparation of the stalklike pedicle is the following. If a very long pedicle has to be prepared (as for example in a case similar to that described), it may be useful not to resect it in its entire length at one time, but (it seems to me) rather to leave a part of the skin fold attached to the neck in the middle. This will facilitate nourishment of its detached parts, and after a few days it is easy to sever the isthmus from the neck. This somewhat prolongs the postoperative time, but it would simplify the operation and postoperative care.

3. Using the principle of the jump flap, it will perhaps be possible to modify the operation in the following way. The pedicle is not made so long (for the eyelid, for example, up to the middle of the neck). After its delay, its lower end is severed and is sutured for a time to the incised skin somewhere halfway between the ear and eyelid. At a later time (10 to 15 days), the upper end of the pedicle flap is severed at the ear and is brought to the defect on one eyelid. And, if it is necessary to do the same for the second eyelid, then the second end (that from the cheek) might be used.

[* Fricke, J. C. G.: Die Bildung neuer Augenlieder (Blepharoplastik) nach Zerstoerungen und dadurch hervorgebrachten Auswaertswendungen derselben. Hamburg, Perthes und Besser, 1829.]

This consideration is entirely based on the fact that in our case the end of the freely hanging pedicle healed *per primam;* it will naturally adhere onto the cheek incision.

The flap, one can say, will have made several jumps.

4. It is possible that, in plastic procedures that are not too extensive, it will not be necessary to form an [additional] flap to the nutrient stalklike pedicle, and that it will be more suitable merely to unfold its end over the defect.

5. One can suture cartilage, bone, *etc.* onto the end of the pedicle or flap; or they can be taken [excised] together with it.

6. The maximum length of the pedicle, of course, is not predetermined by my case. The width of the excised skin strip can also be modified, according to the case.

Vladimir P. Filatov, M.D.
Department of Ophthalmology
Novorossiisk Univ. School of Medicine
Odessa, Russia

Dr. Filatov is Professor of Ophthalmology and Director of the Eye Clinic at Novorossiisk University.

BIBLIOGRAPHY

1. Snydacker: Klin. Monatsbl. f. Augenheilk. *44:* 71, 1906.
2. Snydacker (quoted from Wood): *A System of Ophthalmic Operations, Vol. II.* Chicago, Cleveland Press, 1911. (Modification of Morax is described here.)
3. Morax: L'Autoplastie palpebrale ou faciale à l'aide de lambeaux pédiculés empruntés à la région cervicale (procedé de Snydacker) et autoplastie en deux temps avec utilisation du pédicule. Ann. D' Oculistique *89:* 18, 1908.
4. Morax et Béal: Naevus pigmentaire du front, *etc.* Autoplastie en deux temps. Ann. d'Oculistique *89:* [should be 189]: 31, 1908.
5. Hacker: Arch.f.Klin. Chir. *37:* 91, 1888 (also in Bier, Braun, Kümmel: *Chirurgische Operationslehre.* Leipzig, 1914).
6. Steinthal (in Bier, Braun, Kümmel: *Chirurgische Operationslehre,* p. 158).

BIOGRAPHICAL SKETCH BY DR. ARTHUR BARSKY*

Vladimir Petrovich Filatov was born on February 28, 1875, in the village of Michailovke, near Saransk, in the Penza province of east-central European Russia. He was

* *Editorial note.* From "Filatov and the Tubed Pedicle" by Arthur J. Barsky, M.D., Plast. & Reconstr. Surg., *24:* 456, 1959.

the son of Piotr Federovich Filatov, who practiced ophthalmology in the district. The elder Filatov's brothers were also doctors and one of them, Nil Fedorovich Filatov, was a pediatrician of great distinction who described what are known in the United States as "Koplik spots" and in Rus-

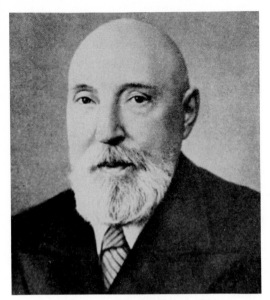

VLADIMIR P. FILATOV
(1875–1956)

sia as "Filatov's spots," an early physical sign of measles.

In his early childhood, Vladimir Petrovich's family moved to the city of Simbirsk, on the Volga River some 485 miles from Moscow. (Simbirsk is now called Ulianovsk, after the family name of Lenin, whose birthplace it was.) There young Filatov attended the gymnasium (or secondary school), and upon his graduation in 1892 he entered the medical school of the University of Moscow. His early devotion to his specialty was shown during his vacations, when he assisted his father in his ophthalmological work, both medical and surgical.

After graduation from medical school, Filatov became (in 1897) ordinator to Professor A. A. Kriukov, Chief of the Ophthalmological Division at the medical school. In 1899 he was appointed to the Moscow Eye Hospital staff. In 1903 he became ordinator to Professor Golovin, Chief of the Eye Clinic at the Novorossiisk University of Odessa. (This is now the Odessa Medical Institute in that important Ukrainian center on the Black Sea, which was to be Filatov's home to the end of his life.) In 1904 he took his medical examina-

tions and in the autumn became house surgeon at the Eye Clinic; in 1906 he was elevated to the rank of assistant. In 1908 Filatov defended his dissertation, "A Study of Cellular Toxins in Ophthalmology," which was dedicated to his father. And in August 1911, when Professor Golovin moved to Moscow, Filatov succeeded him as Director of the Eye Clinic and Professor of Ophthalmology in the Medical School of the Novorossiisk University.

During these years, Filatov made a number of trips abroad to visit and observe at the clinics in Paris, Berlin, Vienna, Munich, and Prague. These were fruitful years for him. He had, in his student days, expressed eagerness to work along the lines of corneal transplant; it was early in 1912 that he performed his first corneal transplants and presented a case. And on September 9, 1916 (Julian calendar), Filatov performed the first tubed-pedicle flap operation—although he had been contemplating the technique since 1914 and had tested the operation on rabbits.

On November 22, Filatov reported his operation and presented his patient at the Odessa Ophthalmological Society meeting; he published his account in the *Vestnik Oftalmologii* of April-May, 1917.[1] The quality of the paper is poor and the illustrations are somewhat crude, but this is not surprising when one considers what was happening in Russia at the time. So troubled were the times that it is indeed amazing that anything could have been published in Odessa.

In 1916, Russia was on the Allied side in World War I. At the close of the year, she had suffered from repeated military reverses and acute food shortages, and was ripe for revolution. In February and March of 1917 there was a general food strike, the Revolution flared, and the Kerensky government came into power. But then in October 1917 the Bolshevik Revolution broke out, and the Lenin-Trotsky group seized control. Meanwhile, Filatov's city of Odessa was in turmoil. In 1917 Odessa organized a local government and mobilized troops of Ukrainians, who adhered to the Ukrainian Central Council in Kiev. These troops continued to fight the Bolsheviks until March of 1918, when Austro-Hungarian troops entered Odessa.

It seems incredible that any investigative or clinical work could take place in such horrendous times. That the Western world then heard nothing of Filatov's work is not surprising. Yet during this time Filatov continued to work steadily in surgery, research, teaching, and writing.[2–6] In 1923, he became Director of the Odessa Institute of Clinical-Experimental Medicine. In 1931 he established a glaucoma clinic. In 1936 he was appointed Director of the Ukrainian Research-Experimental Institute of Eye Diseases and Tissue Therapy.

The trite expression, "Necessity is the mother of invention," is supported here by the fact that in 3 different places, the tubed flap was discovered almost simultaneously, hastened perhaps by the pressure of wartime surgery. First came Filatov's operation in 1916. Then, quite independently, Dr. Hugo Ganzer of Berlin recommended to the Laryngological Society of Berlin, at its meeting of March 30, 1917, the use of a tubed flap for repairs about the mouth and jaws—citing as donor areas the chest, shoulder, upper arm, or back.[7] On November 5, 1917, Ganzer reported to the same Society his use of a tubed flap from the upper arm to close a palatal defect.[8]

In England, the third area of the invention, Major Harold Gillies performed his first tubed flap operation on October 3, 1917, transferring from the neck to the face of a seaman who was suffering from severe facial burns. Gillies reported his operation verbally in late October of 1919, and published his work in various places during 1920.[10–14]

Interestingly enough, apparently quite independently of Gillies—although working at the same surgical center (the Queen's Hospital at Sidcup)—Captain J. L. Aymard, working with Leutenant G. Seccombe Hett, performed a tubed flap

transfer on November 12, 1917, using a chest flap as the second stage of repair of a nasal defect, begun on October 15. Captain Aymard published an account of his operation in the *Lancet* of December 15, 1917.[9]

Filatov was a prophet with honor in his own country; he achieved for his contributions, of which the tubed flap was only one, the highest honors and distinctions that his country could bestow upon him.[15] The list is too long to detail, but included the Stalin Prize of 100,000 rubles which he received in 1941, and the Metchnikow Medal of 1951. He was a Fellow of the Ukrainian Academy of Sciences and of the U.S.S.R. Academy of Medical Sciences, and President of both the Ophthalmological Society and the Surgical Society of Odessa. He even held political posts, as a member of the Odessa City Council and as Deputy to the Supreme Soviet of the Ukrainian Republic.

When Vladimir Petrovich Filatov died in Odessa on October 30, 1956, at the age of 81, he brought to an end a long and distinguished professional, pedagogical, and administrative career. Also he left behind him a notable reputation as a poet and a painter.

—*Arthur J. Barsky, M.D.*

REFERENCES

1. Filatov, V. P.: Plastika na kruglom stebl. Vestnik oftal., *4–5:* 149, 1917.
2. Filatov, V. P.: Plastik mit rundem stiel. Klin.Monatsbl. Augenh., *68:* 124, 1922.
3. Filatov, V. P.: Zur frage der plastik mit einem wandernden stiel. Klin. Monatsbl. Augenh., *68:* 557, 1922.
4. Filatov, V. P.: Operations plastiques a tige ronde ambulante. Presse med., *101:* 1061, 1923.
5. Filatov, V. P.: Runder wanderstiel bei komplizierten plastiken der lider und des gesichts. Aach. klin. Chir., *146:* 609, 1927.
6. Filatov, V. P.: O plastike na kruglom stebl v oftalmologii. Lijecnicki vjesnik, *2:* 1928.
7. Ganzer, H.: Weichteilplastik des gesichts be kieferschuss-verletzungen. Deutsche Monatschr. f. Zahnh., *35:* 348, 1917.
8. Ganzer, H.: Die bildung von langgestielten stranglappen bei gesichtsplastik. Klin, Wchnschr., *54:* 1096, 1917.
9. Aymard, J. L.: Nasal reconstruction. Lancet, *2:* 888, 1917.

10: Gillies, H. D.: The tubed pedicle in plastic surgery. N.Y.J. Med., Jan. 3, 1920.

11. Gillies, H. D.: *Plastic Surgery of the Face*. Oxford
Medical Publications, Oxford, 1920.

12. Gillies, H. D.: Present day plastic operations of
the face. J. Nat. Dent. A., *7:* 3, 1920.

13. Gillies, H. D.: Plastic surgery of facial burns.
Surg., Gynec., & Obst., *30:* 121, 1920.

14. Gillies, H. D.: The tubed pedicle (letter to the
editor). Lancet, *199:* 320, 1920.

15. *Vestnik Oftalmologii* (dedication issues in honor of
Filatov), *11:* no. 6, 1937; *29:* no. 2, 1950.

SECTION IX

Some of
the Great Builders

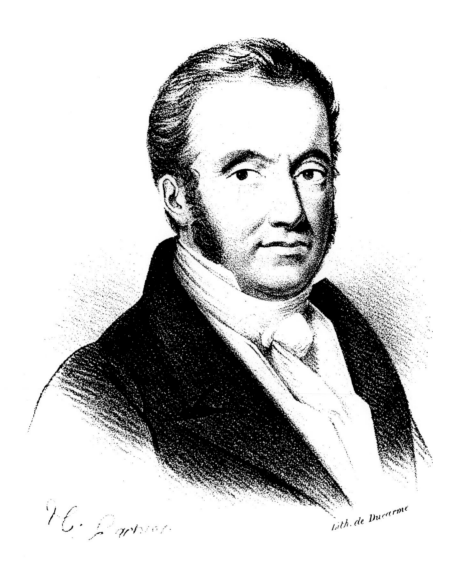

G. DUPUYTREN

(Le Baron)

Membre de l'Institut

Chirurgien en chef de l'Hôtel-Dieu,

Né à Pierre-Buffière (Haute-Vienne) le 3 Octobre 1778.

Galerie Universelle   Publiée par Blaisot

(Plate furnished by courtesy of Mme. Dubois, Chef du Centre d'Optique et
d'Electronique de l'Assistance Publique de Paris).

GUILLAUME DUPUYTREN

ROBERT M. GOLDWYN, M.D.

Brookline, Massachusetts

"Nothing should be feared so much for a man as mediocrity."

Guillaume Dupuytren

Guillaume Dupuytren is remembered principally for the hand condition which bears his name. That posterity has ignored his other numerous and more important contributions would have piqued this arrogant master surgeon.

He was born in 1777 in the small village of Pierre-Buffière, near Limoges in south central France. His father, a poor solicitor, almost lost his son at age 4 when a wealthy lady from Toulouse attempted unsuccessfully to abduct him.[1] Dupuytren's "considerable charm and intelligence" caught the attention also of a cavalry officer stationed at Pierre-Buffière. He requested Pére Dupuytren to allow Guillaume, then 12, to go to Paris to attend the College de La Marche, a Jesuit school in which the brother of this officer was an administrator. The elder Dupuytren consented, probably happy to have one less responsibility; Guillaume finished his studies in Paris a few years later.

Stimulated by the spirit of the French Revolution, Dupuytren seriously contemplated a military career. His father protested and reminded him of the many surgeons that had been in the Dupuytren family. "Tu seras chirurgien" ("You will be a surgeon"), he commanded.

Dutifully, Guillaume began his medical curriculum in a hospital in Limoges but, realizing the deficiencies of that training, he returned to Paris and entered the École de Santé. This period of his life was arduous and bitter because of extreme poverty. He had, for example, to use the fat of cadavers to make oil for his study lamp. Through enormous industry and stamina, always his attributes, he persisted to become Prosector in charge of autopsies at the medical school in 1795, when he was 17 years old.

In 1801 he was appointed Chef des Travaux Anatomiques and coupled his anatomical observations with an interest in pathology and physiology. He was the first to identify fibrin in chyle.

His competence as a teacher led to his giving his own course in pathology. Gaspard-Laurent Bayle (1734–1816) and Rene T. H. Laennec (1781–1826) were his assistants, but Laennec and Dupuytren later became enemies, each accusing the other of plagiarism and ingratitude.[2, 3]

The noted Boston surgeon, John Collins Warren, father of Jonathan Mason Warren, attended Dupuytren's first lectures and "was surprised at the minuteness and extent of his knowledge; but I was not suspicious at that time that he was destined to stand at the head of French surgery . . . I recollect remarking to him, that he spoke with great facility, and that I understood him better than any other lecturer. He replied with a modesty quite peculiar, and which he certainly got wholly rid of at a later period of life."[4, 5]

In 1802, the position of "surgeon of the Second Class" was vacant at the Hotel Dieu. Dupuytren's principal opponent was Philibert-Joseph Roux, (1780–1854),

From the Departments of Surgery (Plastic) of the Harvard Medical School, Peter Bent Brigham Hospital, and Beth Israel Hospital.

who, in 1819, was to perform the first staphylorrhaphy. In Warren's words:

"... As usual in Paris, a *concours*, or comparative trial of ability, was opened and maintained with great skill. I was present at this conflict, which took place at the Oratorie, and was astonished at the facility with which the candidates, on drawing an unknown question from the urn, entered without hesitation on a response which extended to a variety of topics branching out from the original inquiry. At the end of two days, the balance of opinion inclined to the side of Roux. Dupuytren had his mind so strongly fixed on obtaining the place, that he was almost distracted at the appearance of probability in Roux's favor. In this state of mind, he visited the gentleman who gave me the information—a person of influence, and a friend of Dupuytren. Rushing into his room, he burst into tears, struck his head violently with both hands and cried out, "I am lost!" His friend tranquillized him and said, "Take courage. Go this evening to Madam B. She thinks favorably of you; will be flattered by your application, and gratified to exert her influence in the medical intrigue. She can turn the scale in your favor, if she chooses. Kneel to her. Pray to her. Say everything you can think of to excite her interest, and you will obtain the prize. Fly! There is not a moment to be lost!" [5]

At the Hôtel Dieu, Dupuytren continued his characteristic productivity and after another contest with Roux, in 1812, he gained the Chair of Operative Surgery and became Chief Surgeon in 1814. This competition with Roux was not confined to medicine; Roux married Dupuytren's fiancee, the daughter of the surgeon Alexis Boyer, (1757–1833). Boyer had taken a paternal interest in Dupuytren's career but never forgave him for having called off the wedding the night before. Roux finally succeeded in becoming Chief Surgeon at the Hôtel Dieu, following Dupuytren's death in 1835.

Although Dupuytren was called "the Brigand of the Hôtel Dieu," his jealous enemies acknowledged his competence and contributions.[6] He was first to excise the mandible (1812) and to treat torticollis by subcutaneous section of the sternomastoid muscle (1822). He was one of the first to drain a brain abscess and to remove the neck of the uterus for cancer. His skills in surgery of aneurysms were well known—successful compression and ligation of the external iliac artery (1815) and of the subclavian and carotid arteries (1819–1829). He devised original methods for creating an artificial anus, extracting cataracts, performing dacryocystorhinostomy, and for treating hydroceles and recto-vaginal and recto-vesical fistulae.

He wrote extensively about orthopedic problems and fractures, in particular those of the lower end of the fibula (1819) and congenital dislocations of the hip (1826). He described Madelung's deformity before Madelung. His formal medical writings, however, were few; he had difficulty in even composing a refusal of a dinner invitation. Yet, from his famed *Lecons Orales*[7] (a collection of his lectures at the Hôtel Dieu) we know the variety and range of his medical interests—from the treatment of cholera, vaginitis, and the ingrown toenail to the management of carcinoma of the nasal sinuses and war wounds. His experience with the injured of the Napoleonic Wars and the Revolution of 1830, led him to write:

"The treatment of these wounds, like that of other surgical diseases, is divided into general and local. The former comprises rest of body and mind, diet in its different gradations, drinks of diverse nature, pure atmosphere, loss of blood & c. The latter is directed to ... arresting hemorrhage, preventing or removing strangulation, inflammation, and gangrene: the enlargement of the wound, extraction of foreign bodies, amputation, ligature, dressing and cicatrization of wounds, position of the limb, topical applications, &c. *Rest,* especially when there is a fracture, is of the highest importance. *A tranquil mind* is no less necessary ... *A pure atmosphere* is also of the greatest moment. Therefore, the most healthy situation should be selected and the

Wards kept scrupulously clean. *Ventilation* should, however, be cautiously conducted lest dangerous consequences ensue. Currents of air, established by means of air holes or windows opposite each other, are frequently fatal, by giving rise to inflammation of the internal organs. We have already said that tetanus often follows the action of these currents and the sudden transition from the heat of the day to the freshness of the night . . . Patients should be prevented from throwing off their bed clothes . . . After diet, rest, and drinks, *venesection* is the most effectual means of subduing fever . . . Wounds of the important organs, as the lungs, brain, liver . . . require large and repeated bleedings. The old surgeons were not afraid to bleed ten, fifteen, twenty times, or even oftener in the early stages of these wounds, and were sometimes successful in apparently desperate cases . . . Experience has proved the absurdity of sucking a wound of the chest in order to extract the effused blood, and shown that the chances of cure are much greater when it is closed immediately by a suitable dressing and the introduction of the air prevented as much as possible . . . The first problem to be solved in wounds of the limbs, is to point out the cases requiring amputation; for when this operation is deemed indispensable, it should be performed without delay, unless there exists great stupor or disturbance . . ." [8]

Dupuytren's concern with wounds led to his being the first to describe the lines of skin tension.[9, 10] In 1831, a 33-year-old man unsuccessfully attempted suicide by striking himself in the chest with an awl. Dupuytren noted that the wounds were not round, as is the point of an awl, but were elliptical as if caused by a knife. With one of his interns, the made similar wounds in a cadaver and concluded that skin "fiber alignment" was responsible for the shape of the inflicted punctures. He further observed that the pattern of these wounds varied with body area. About 30 years later, Langer[11] published his studies and acknowledged the primacy and importance of Dupuytren's work.

Because Parisians at the turn of the 19th century employed primitive and dangerous means to heat their drafty quarters, Dupuytren treated many severely burned patients. He was the first to classify burns into a logical and useful scheme. He

"divided burns into six degrees . . . *First,* erythema or superficial phlogosis of the skin without formation of phlyctenae. *Second,* cutaneous inflammation, with the loss of epidermis, and the development of vesicles filled with serum. *Third,* the destruction of a portion of the papillary body. *Fourth,* the disorganization of the whole dermis to the subcutaneous cellular tissue. *Fifth,* the formation of eschars, of all the superficial parts, and of the muscles, to a greater or less distance from the bone. *Sixth,* the carbonization of the whole thickness of the burned part . . .

"However slight the burn may be . . . when it attacks broad surfaces, the pulse sometimes rises and becomes frequent, the tongue reddens, and the phenomena of gastro-intestinal irritation develop themselves.* When 'it is situated in the head, the irritation may extend to the encephalon, and cause wakefulness, delirium, convulsions, coma, and even death . . . We must here lay down as a principle, that in all burns the pain is always severe; but it is much more intense when only the surface of the skin is burned, and when it is destroyed more deeply; and this fact is important in the prognosis." [12]

He did not employ skin grafting but used debridement and "nitrate of silver" as well as "perforated compresses spread with cerate, lint, emollient cataplasms, and calming drinks." He recorded a case of a 36-year-old epileptic who sustained a burn of the "third and fourth degrees . . . from the upper third of the thigh to below the middle of the leg and . . . more than half the circumference of the limb, especially near the ham . . ." He obtained "a perfect cure after 145 days." Following release of a burn contracture, he used immobilization and traction devices to restore limb position and function.

Dupuytren's comments and contributions relative to plastic surgery came from

* Ed. note: Dupuytren described ulceration of the gastro-intestinal tract in burned patients 10 years before Curling did.

his broad directions in general surgery rather than from a specific inclination toward reconstructive surgery. Concerning the cleft lip, he had this to say:

"There are two important points as yet undecided in the operation for harelip, generally so simple; namely the proper time for its performance, and the treatment applicable to a complication hitherto but little noticed.

"Various opinions exist as regards the first question. Many have thought it most advisable to wait until the child was able to appreciate the deformity. They relied on the greater thickness of the lips and the strength of tissue necessary to support the suture. Some surgeons have preferred waiting until the end of the third year, except in cases in which the child was prevented from sucking. The tissues, say they, have become more solid, without losing any of their extensibility, can better resist the needles; and at that period, the child having more reason submits with more docility to the precautions necessary to the success of the operation.

"Others have thought it proper to operate on children immediately after birth, because the lips being furnished with blood-vessels, of which a great part soon disappear, heal, at that period of life, more promptly. Besides children then are more passive and have not as yet acquired the habit of sucking. But the operation is not certain so soon after birth, because the flesh is too soft and easily divisible by the needles, and because the general mortality, independently of any particular reason, is greater at that period of life than at any other, and it would be imprudent to increase the chances of death. Such are the objections, are they counterbalanced by the advantages? It would undoubtedly be important to operate so early, in order to give the child the faculty of sucking; but this very inclination to suck, is one of the most powerful opponents of the success of the operation. Could this be avoided, the operation at birth would have a powerful argument in its favor; but the child sucks instinctively, even before having taken the breast: the obstacle is therefore as powerful then as at a later period.

"That, however, is by no means the least favorable period for the operation: and I cannot understand why so many writers have preferred the age of four or five years, alleging that the child being reasonable enough to feel the necessity and foresee the success, will submit to the operation with more cour-age. Experience must have undeceived them. At that age, children have just sense sufficient to feel and remember the pain, without reason to support it; they, therefore, endeavor to avoid it as much as possible, and do all they can to frustrate the operation.

"At a later period, reason and courage are indeed more developed; but if the bones be implicated, their increased solidity gives less hope of success. In all cases, it is preferable to operate early; the deformity is less, and even that proceeding from the separation of the bones disappears. Therefore, I think the most suitable time is at the age of three months, life is then more firmly established, and the chances of death less than at birth; the infant feels the pain, but forgets it immediately, and does not oppose the success of the operation.

"There is another point in the operation for harelip, to which I would call your attention. When there is a middle tubercle projecting, with two well defined lateral divisions, either the bony portion supporting is removed, or we endeavor to restore it to its place.

"If the median tubercle project in front, we must observe where it is inserted into the septum nasi, as on this frequently depend the degree of projection and the treatment. When the insertion is near the point of the nose, and the lateral portions of the lip are attached to the tubercle, the latter is drawn backward; the point of the nose follows the movement; the alae are separated, and the nose becomes flattened, resembling more the snout of an animal than anything else. What is the consequence of its insertion precisely into the end of the nose? Now this occurrence overlooked by writers is not uncommon. In such a case, struck by the deformity which would ensue, I adopted the following plan: The fleshy tubercle was separated from its bony attachment, the latter removed by the forceps; the edges of the fleshy portion having been pared, it was raised horizontally backwards, and used to form the septum, or a portion of the inferior septum of the nostrils. Then whether we wait for reunion, or complete the operation, the harelip is reduced to its greatest simplicity, and the operation performed in the ordinary manner; a bandage is sufficient to keep the tubercle in place.

"It is only when the labial tubercle is inserted near the bony nasal spine, that it ought to be preserved as an integral part of the lip. In this case I remove a portion of the subjacent osseous tubercle. M. Malgaigne in an article published by him in the Medical Gazette, thinks that this plan is liable to objections. The most serious, according to him, is the removal of the germ of two, three, or even the four incisors . . ." [13]

Dupuytren outlined the use of adjacent rotation flaps in covering defects of the nose and lower lip after cancer surgery.

Describing in detail fractures of the zygomatic arch, he warned against reducing such fractures because of the danger of infection.

"... The operation of introducing an elevator beneath the zygomatic arch would involve an incision through the integuments, perhaps also through the temporal aponeurosis, or even through the masseter muscle: and it is not very easy to foretell what amount of mischief might follow such free use of the knife. I have never seen but one case in which such a mode of treatment was admissible . . ." [14]

Aside from his surgical skill, what made Dupuytren legendary was his singular life-style. Ruthlessly, he tolerated no rival—no dissent. He rarely lost an opportunity to self-aggrandize and even allowed the use of his name for a preparation to reduce "itch" and an "ointment against baldness." He was called the "Napoleon of Surgery" and reigned alone at the Hôtel Dieu. Contemporaries described his face as having "la froideur du marbre" (the coldness of marble.[15] After Louis XVIII created a baronetcy for him in 1816, he was addressed as "Monsieur Le Baron" but his intimates were allowed to call him "Le Baron."

Jean Cruveilhier (1791–1874), the anatomist, reminisced about his "Chief." "His enemies—that was the secret of his sad life; he saw them everywhere, in a coalition to do him harm . . . infiltrating among his dearest pupils and entering his lecture hall to seize his words in order to twist them." [16]

Dupuytren had few male friends but

many devoted female acquaintances, including a mistress of Honoré de Balzac, who characterized him well in a short story "La Messe de L'Athée" (The Mass of the Atheist).[17] Dupuytren's atheism, in fact, almost prevented his appointment as First Surgeon to Charles X.

Whatever his foibles, his strength was his ability to work well and hard. "Read little, see much, do much" ("Peu lire, beacoup voir, beaucoup faire"), he would tell his students. At 6 o'clock every morning he arrived at the hospital; in 25 years he missed hardly a day. Sloppily attired in an old green coat, socks over the tops of his boots, he led an entourage of students, 5 interns and residents, and many visitors. These rounds lasted until 9 o'clock and he saw every surgical patient. An hour lecture followed and as a teacher, he had few peers in Europe. His observations and thoughts were clear, presented in a stimulating fashion, using patients for illustration. From the lecture hall, he proceeded to the Operating Room where he worked until noon before going home to see more patients. Throughout each operation, he lectured.

Concerning his surgery and personality, Jonathan Mason Warren, then in Paris, wrote his father:

"His operations are always brilliant, and his diagnosis sometimes most extraordinary. He is one of the most suspicious persons I have ever encountered. He is continually seeking to convince us that he is a great man, and that we do sufficiently value his talents. He likes much to make a show, and generally talks throughout the whole operation . . . For brutality I do not think his equal can be found. If his orders are not immediately obeyed, he makes nothing of striking his patient and abusing him harshly. A favorite practice of his is to make a handle of a man's nose, seizing him by it and pulling him down onto his knees, where he remains half in sorrow, half in anger, until he is allowed to arise and describe his symptoms . . . Dupuytren is now becoming rather careless in his operations, from too great confidence in his own powers. He was brought to his senses the other day by an accident which will make him more careful in the future. While operating for strangulated hernia, at the second cut he penetrated directly into the intestine. Raising his head with great coolness, he said, 'Voila, messieurs, la matiere fecale' and without another word quietly stitched up the wound ...'' [18]

Dupuytren emphasized to his students that an operation was "an evil alternative which nothing short of positive necessity should induce the surgeon to adopt." Furthermore, he insisted that knowing when to operate and knowing how to give proper post-operative care were as important as the operation itself. Nevertheless, one should not imagine that he was a reluctant surgeon. In 1818, for example, he set 178 fractures, drained 300 abscesses, and performed 368 other operations.[19] During that year, the total number of patients admitted to the surgical ward was 2,353. In addition he saw hundreds of out-patients; his annual patient load was estimated at 10,000. He soon amassed a fortune and doubtless his early poverty was a reason for his alleged avarice. On one occasion, he duped himself:

"Once a duchess, widow of a marshall of the Empire, came to his office after recuperating from a successful operation he had performed upon her.

'My dear doctor,' she said, 'I have brought you this purse which I myself have embroidered as a slight token of my deep gratitude.'

The purse was obviously very light, and Dupuytren, instead of accepting it, said coldly, 'That is all very well, my surgery saved your life and you owe me five thousand francs.'

The duchess smiled gently, and, without any sign of embarrassment, opened the purse and both slowly and ostentatiously withdrew from it five bills of a thousand francs each, which she pocketed. Then, closing the purse, she again extended it to the surgeon, saying lightly, 'My dear doctor, you are entirely too modest. This purse is still not empty; it now contains the exact sum which you mentioned.' " [20]

When Charles X went into exile, Dupuytren was able to offer him a gift of one million francs but the king declined this *beau geste*. Another story is more complimentary to Dupuytren and provides evidence of his knowledge of people as well as of surgery.

A woman entered his clinic with a dislocated shoulder. Dupuytren told her, "Your pain comes from the fall you have had but you did not tell me you were drunk when you fell; your son told me." When she heard this statement, the woman fainted and Dupuytren reduced the dislocation in an instant. When the woman recovered, Dupuytren said, "Your shoulder is in place, and I know perfectly well that you drink only water." [21]

He once quizzed an elderly man whom he suspected of having syphilis.

"Have you been with prostitutes?"
"No, how could you even think it?" the patient replied.
"Then they have been with you," said Dupuytren. [22]

In 1832, the first volume of his *Lecon Orales* appeared and contained his experience with "division of the palmar aponeurosis" in order to relieve contracture of the ring and little fingers in a Parisian wine merchant.[23] It is important to emphasize that Dupuytren dissected a cadaver with this condition before operating clinically.*

In November of 1833, while lecturing, Dupuytren suddenly felt a slight paralysis of the right side of his face. He covered his face with his fingers and did not interrupt his discourse. However, he was forced to take a leave of absence for 6 months; with his daughter and son-in-law (a French count) he toured Italy. Unaccustomed to leisure, he sadly remarked, "Le repos—c'est la mort" ("Rest —that's death"). When he returned from Italy, he delivered an excellent lecture

* See "The Classic Reprint" in this book.

but was unable to repeat the performance.[24]

He had to remain at home where he recorded his own symptoms and signs of congestive. failure and pleural effusion. He wrote his father,

"I was prepared to give up this rat race at 60, but not before, and to have to leave my first rank won after so much pain and effort is more terrible than I can say." [25]

In a letter, Jonathan Mason Warren recorded Dupuytren's death in 1835:

"Since my last letter we have lost a great authority in surgical science, M. Dupuytren, who died the day before yesterday...It seems that (at autopsy) the heart was diseased, the remains of the epanchement which caused the attack of apoplexy in the spring were found in the brain, and some calculi in the bladder and kidneys. He did not allow any person to know what his exact state was; it is said that until the last days of his life no one knew whether he was to die or get well, as he put on a feigned appearance when visited by his physicians, thus carrying out to the end his stern independence and eccentric disposition. By his will he has left the great bulk of his property, 7 or 8 millions to his daughter and only child, married to a peer of France; 200 thousand francs for the foundation of a chair of Surgical Pathology and for a museum in the École de Médecine; and 300 thousand francs for a hospital or asylum for 12 old retired physicians. It is said that he suffered much during the latter part of his life from noise in the street and in his hotel, there being a ball in the room over his head the night preceding his death. This was, in fact, the cause of his bequest (asylum for retired physicians)...His funeral took place yesterday and was attended by the professors and nearly all the students of the School of Medicine. The students...took the horses from the hearse, dragged it themselves to the tomb. At present I can see no one who can at all aspire to his place. His lectures on surgical pathology were unique, and I have never heard any person attempt to treat the subject in the manner which he introduced into his clinique. It is said that before he died he sent for Lisfranc and Richerand, his old enemies, and made friends with them. Whether this be true or not, I am ignorant. Lisfranc,

however, in his leçons, has of late quoted Monsieur Dupuytren—a thing which he has never done before. Dupuytren's life seems to have been passed perhaps as bitterly, considering the illustrious place he has attained, as could possibly be imagined. He had few friends,—no doubt from the repulsive manners which belonged to him, produced by the battles for distinction and the domestic troubles at the commencement of his career." [26]

This last reference is to the fact that Dupuytren and his wife separated after much acrimony.[27]

Musing on his productive and tempestuous professional life, Dupuytren once said, "I have been mistaken, but I have been mistaken less than other surgeons." [21]

Robert M. Goldwyn, M.D.
1101 Beacon Street
Brookline, Mass. 02146

ACKNOWLEDGMENTS

I am grateful to Mr. Richard J. Wolfe, Rare Books Librarian, and his staff at the Countway Library of Medicine for their generous assistance.

REFERENCES

1. Mondor, H.: *Anatomistes et Chirurgiens*, pp. 259–320. Fragrance, Paris, 1949.
2. Mondor, H.: *Dupuytren*, pp. 53–57. Gallimard, Paris, 1945.
3. Kervran, R.: *Laennec: His Life and Times*, pp. 55–57. Pergamon Press, New York, 1960.
4. Warren, E.: *The Life of John Collins Warren, M.D.*, Vol. I, p. 58. Ticknor and Fields, Boston, 1860.
5. Warren, E.: *The Life of John Collins Warren, M.D.*, Vol. II, pp. 114–115. Ticknor and Fields, Boston, 1860.
6. Garrison, F. H.: *An Introduction to the History of Medicine*, Ed. 4, pp. 488–490. W. B. Saunders Co., Philadelphia, 1960.
7. Dupuytren, G.: *Lecons Orales de Clinique Chirurgicale Faites à l'Hôtel-Dieu de Paris*, 4 Vols. J. B. Baillière et Fils, Paris, 1832–1834.
8. Dupuytren, G.: *Lectures on Clinical Surgery Delivered in the Hôtel-Dieu of Paris*, pp. 534–535. Duff Green, Washington, 1835.
9. Kraissl, C. J.: The selection of appropriate lines for elective surgical incisions. Plast. & Reconstruct. Surg. *8:* 1–28, 1951.
10. Dupuytren, G.: *Traite Theorique et Pratique des Blessures par Armes de Guerre*, pp. 60–63. Vol. I, J. B. Baillière et Fils, Paris, 1834.
11. Langer, K.: *Zur Anatomie und Physiologie der*

Haut. I. Ueber Die SpaltBarkeit der Cutis, p. 1. Karl Gerold's Sohn, Vienna, 1861.

12. *Clinical Lectures in Surgery Delivered at Hôtel-Dieu in 1832.* Translated by A. Sidney Doane, pp. 234–236. Carter, Hendee & Co., Boston, 1833.

13. Dupuytren, G.: *Lectures on Clinical Surgery Delivered in the Hôtel-Dieu of Paris,* pp. 321–322. Duff Green, Washington, 1835.

14. Dupuytren, G.: *On the Injuries and Diseases of Bones.* Translated and edited by F. LeGros Clark, p. 10. The Sydenham Society, London, 1847.

15. Gaillard, F. L.: *Dupuytren,* 16 pp. J. B. Baillière et Fils, Paris, 1865.

16. Lutaud, A.: Les medecins dans Balzac. Desplein-Dupuytren. *Bull. Soc. franc. hist. méd., 14:* 373–381, 1920.

17. Maurois, A.: *Prometheus: The Life of Balzac,* pp. 293, 315, 405. Harper & Row, New York, 1965.

18. Arnold, H. P.: *Memoir of Jonathan Mason Warren, M.D.,* pp. 84, 85, 87. University Press, John Wilson and Son, Cambridge, 1886.

19. Dupuytren, G.: *On the Injuries and Diseases of Bones.* Translated and edited by F. LeGros Clark, pp. 333–336. The Sydenham Society, London, 1847.

20. *Medical Director's Notebook,* Eaton Laboratories, December, 1967.

21. Coues, W. P.: Guillaume Dupuytren (1777–1835). Boston M. & S. J., *75:* 489–494, 1916.

22. Mondor, H.: Dupuytren, p. 142. Gallimard, Paris, 1945.

23. Dupuytren, G.: *Lecons Orales de Clinique Chirurgicale Faite à l'Hôtel-Dieu de Paris,* Vol. I, p. 1. J. B. Baillière et Fils, Paris, 1832–1834.

24. Goldwyn, R. M.: Le Baron and the Doctors Warren. Harvard M. Alumni Bull., *42:* 24–27, 1968.

25. Mondor, H.: *Dupuytren,* p. 2. Gallimard, Paris, 1945.

26. Arnold, H. P.: *Memories of Jonathan Mason Waren, M.D.,* pp. 90–91. University Press, John Wilson & Son, Cambridge, 1886.

27. La Siboutie, P. de: *Recollections of a Parisian,* pp. 113–116. John Murray, London, 1911.

28. Delhoume, L.: *Dupuytren,* 494 pp. Imprimerie Societe des Journaux et Publications du Centre, Limoges, 1935.

The next two surgeons were famous competitors of Dupuytren, in this golden era. Then came other greats, on both sides of the Atlantic, of a little later period. The plastic surgeon of today can do what he does only because he is standing on the shoulders of these men and a few other giants. If he had to start on square one, it is unlikely that he would advance to the level of Imhotep.

CARL FERDINAND VON GRAEFE (1787–1840)

BLAIR O. ROGERS, M.D.

New York, N.Y.

In the year 1818, two articles were published by Carl Ferdinand von Graefe in which the titles included the words "Rhinoplastik" [1] (in German) and "De rhinoplastice" [2] (in Latin). Gibson[3] believes, therefore, that as a result of these articles von Graefe was probably the first to introduce the word "plastic" for our specialty. Some medical historians, including Garrison,[4] consider von Graefe to be the founder of *modern* plastic surgery because of the scope of his early contributions to this field—including articles on palatoplasty, rhinoplasty, blepharoplasty, *etc.*

Some two years earlier, in 1816, for the first time in medical history von Graefe devised an operation for the successful closure of a soft palatal cleft.[5, 6] In 1820 he was one of the founding co-editors of the prestigious *Journal der Chirurgie und Augen-Heilkunde.*[7] Except for a brief paragraph in Garrison[4] describing a few of his contributions, very little concerning the life of von Graefe can be uncovered in most modern standard English references. Several articles written by his English contemporaries[8, 9] and in the German literature[10, 11] give us a better insight into his early life and training.

Von Graefe was born on March 8, 1787 in Warsaw, where his father was secretary to Count Moszynsky. Sometime after his birth, the family moved to Dolsk, a small Polish town near Poznan, where the young von Graefe was taught by a tutor until the age of 14. He then attended the Gymnasium at Bautzen (in Oberlausitz near Dresden); subsequently he attended the City School in Dresden.

He apparently acquired a very good working knowledge of Latin and Greek classics, showing such great promise early that he attracted notice. According to Bullen,[9] he "... gave the promise of future celebrity."

His medical studies began in Dresden at the Collegium Medico-Chirurgicum, where he showed an early predilection for surgery—attending the lectures and the practical instructions given by Hedenus, the professor of surgery, and by Forenz, the professor of obstetrics and gynecology. In 1805 he continued his medical studies in Halle, where his masters in surgery were Froriep, Loder, and Bernstein. He so distinguished himself in a clinical course of accouchements that Reil, a celebrated teacher of pathology and therapeutics, appointed him in exclusive charge of the city hospital.[8]

When Napoleon's French armies invaded the Halle region, the University was dissolved. To complete his studies, von Graefe traveled to nearby Leipzig in neighboring Saxony. His formal education was almost completed there, under the famous Platner (professor of philosophy), Rosenmuller (professor of anatomy), and Eckhold and Reinhold (heads of the clinical institution). In 1807, at the age of 20, he graduated with the title of "Doctor of Medicine and Surgery," after defending his thesis "De notione et cura angiectaseos labiorum." The thesis dealt with the extirpation and cure of a nevus of the lip which had been poorly understood and badly treated, consequently taking on malignant characteristics.

In an 1834 medical portrait of von

From the Department of Plastic Surgery of the Manhattan Eye, Ear and Throat Hospital and from the Institute of Reconstructive Plastic Surgery of the New York University School of Medicine.

Graefe, the writer in *Lancet*[8] described von Graefe's training as

...a very fair example of a German education. The medical student first enters the burges' school, then the gymnasium (classical school), and, finally, the University, where he resides 3 or 4 years, and after an extensive range of scientific and practical pursuits, graduates, as "Doctor of Medicine and Surgery,"—devoting himself afterwards to general practice, or any particular department to which his mind is determined by inclination or circumstances. The graduates who have means, often attach themselves to eminent teachers, or to the clinical institutions, where they practice many of the operations under the eye of the professor. The majority travel in their native country. Some go as far as Paris; a few reach Italy and London. This course of proceeding which, from the time and capital of the student, and from the institutions of the country, produces the greatest sum of knowledge and practical powers, has been the means of sending forth into the large towns, and into almost every district of Germany, a body of men who exercise their profession with skill, and often continue to cultivate science with ardour and success.

Despite this accolade to German surgery, the English author of the article stated quite categorically that 40 years earlier, when medicine was taught with great care at the German universities,

...surgery was left in the lowest depths of degradation.

In the rebirth or regeneration of German surgery, von Graefe played a very conspicuous role. In the beginning of the 19th century most of the professors of surgery were instructed simply as

ordinary mechanics—nurslings of trading companies—and they were cast upon the world ignorant, not only of anatomy and medicine, but often of the ordinary operations of this art. Some persons had to travel 80 (German) miles to be operated upon for fistula lachrymalis. Hare-lips were left without cure; cataracts were couched by itinerant Frenchmen. In the hospital of a populous city, no one could operate for lithotomy.[8]

With this quotation as a colorful example of the state of German surgery in the early 1800's, let us now return to the further progress of the young von Graefe at the age of 21. In 1808, Reil (his constant friend, patron, and one of his best teachers) recommended him for appointment to the court of the then-reigning Duke Alexis of Anhalt-Bernburg at Ballenstedt. As Physician-in-Ordinary to the Duke, and as a Privy Councillor, he organized the Ballenstedt Infirmary and founded and brought into fashion the Alexisbad. This curative spa was the direct outgrowth of von Graefe's analysis of the waters of a spring in the wild Selkenthal, which gushed forth from a rock at the foot of the Unterhartz Mountains.

Von Graefe found that these waters were very rich in iron and published an account of his analysis in 1809 (entitled "Der salmische Eisenquell im Selkenthal am Hartz") which helped to make this spa of Alexis one of the most famous and flourishing watering places of Germany. It was said that in this first decade of the 1800's and thereafter, visitors flocked from many parts of the European continent every June, July, and August. "...to breathe the fresh air of the mountains and bathe in the waters—to live under the clear sky of this valley." [8] Afterwards, von Graefe published yearly reports containing descriptions of patients treated by mineral waters, as well as an analysis of the cases; these reports were extensively circulated in Germany, where they were highly esteemed.[9]

During this period, von Graefe was offered many desirable appointments and was invited to become Professor Ordinarius of Surgery at Königsburg in East Prussia, and also Professor of Medicine and Surgery at the University of Halle. Both of these invitations he declined, because he felt it improper to leave his patron (the Duke Alexis) who was then quite ill. In 1810, however,

Reil once again induced him to accept a chair at the newly established University of Berlin (founded in that same year). There, at the age of 23, he was appointed the full Professor of Surgery and Director of the Clinical-Surgical-Ophthalmologic Institute.[10, 11] The University of Berlin soon became one of the foremost medical centers of the 23 universities existing in Germany at that time.

Von Graefe's name and reputation attracted numerous pupils to the University; this proved a great advantage, of course, to the new school in its early years. His own practice was also very successful. Because he developed a rather profitable connection with the Prussian court, and had no trouble in winning the confidence of the public, it is said that he managed to become both envied and hated by most of the resident physicians and surgeons who were his contemporaries in Berlin.

In 1812 he published a book on amputations, dedicated to Friedrich Wilhelm III. Von Graefe's skill was quite apparent as, in this period of the early 1800's, not one patient, out of 13 who had amputations performed, was lost by either morbidity or mortality. All of the stumps had healed by cicatrization in 3 weeks' time—most of them in a mere 12 days.[12]

In the year 1813, von Graefe relinquished his professorship in Berlin to take part in the German wars of "liberation" (Fig. 1). He volunteered his services to the Prussian army and became Surgeon-General of an entire division. He commanded the reserve and field hospitals of the army itself, all the military infirmaries which lay between the Rhine and the Vistula in Poland, and all the Prussian hospitals in The Netherlands.[8-11] In the Vistula-Rhine complex itself, von Graefe's direction and supervision extended over every major field hospital, provincial hospital, and reserve military hospital of the 3 governments and in the 38 regions which lay between these two rivers. Despite the impoverished circumstances in the emerging German states, and because of his talents and his tremendous energy, von Graefe accomplished many major improvements in the medical department of the Prussian army. He organized it so skillfully that it was able to render effective care to more than 100,000 sick and wounded persons.

Despite the difficulties of working both as an administrator and as an operating practical surgeon, he still had time to write several works much valued by the medical directors of military hospitals—and useful as practical guides to help army surgeons dealing with typhus fever, Egyptian ophthalmia, and other specific military surgical problems among the troops. One of these publications, *Instructions for the medical directors of the hospitals,* ... (published in 1813) contained many rules to be ob-

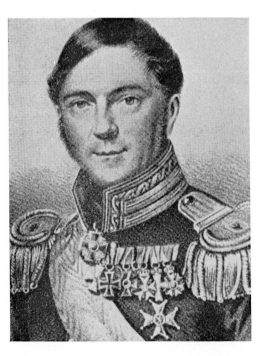

FIG. 1. Carl Ferdinand von Graefe (1787–1840). (From Garrison.[4])

served in military hospitals. These concerned the separation, selection, and proper placing of the sick, the application of various corrosive acids so necessary in the removal of necrotic tissue (techniques which subsequently became quite popular in many European centers), methods for purification of hospital air, and many other benefits which improved the military hospital services. All this brought him once again to the attention of the Prussian royalty—as well as to the members of the other contemporary European governments. He was awarded the Officers' Cross of the French Legion of Honor, and the Orders of St. Wladimir and of Gustavus Vasa from the Russian and Swedish kings, respectively.

His titles and honors became so numerous in subsequent years that Rostock,[10] reviewing the surgery performed and directed by von Graefe between 1810 and 1840 at the University of Berlin Clinic, emphasized that von Graefe's full title (with all its flourishes and *accoutrements* so beloved by German and other Central European nationals) was as follows: "Royal (Privy) Councillor and Director General of the Army Medical Services; Co-Director of the Medical Surgical Academy and of the Friedrich-Wilhelm Institute of Berlin; Full Professor of Medicine and Surgery (at the same University); Full Member of the Imperial and Royal Academies of Paris, Padua, Naples, Moscow—as well as of the Universities of Pest (Hungary), Wilna, and Cracow; Commander (1st Class) and Knight of the Prussian, Russian, French, Swedish, Bavarian, Hanoverian, and Royal Hessian Orders (decorations)— *etc.*"

Von Graefe resumed his professorship at the University of Berlin during a temporary cessation of the war, but soon after its renewal he returned and assumed his former rank and position as Director of the Military Services. He devoted himself again to his duties, with the same success and unremitting application as before.

In 1814, soon after the establishment of peace, he visited Paris where he was met with gratifying receptions by numerous scientific bodies and organizations. It was at approximately this period in his life (at the age of 27 and 28) that he received the decorations cited above. Blucher and other famous European generals wrote admiring letters of approval, expressing their esteem and their gratitude toward him for the manner in which he had performed his duties during the war. It is not surprising, therefore, that his wealth of wartime experience and the reputation that he had among the crowned heads of Europe soon made von Graefe's professional career in Berlin an unprecedented success—both from the standpoint of the volume of his practice, and of his increasing wealth.

By the year 1815, at the age of 28, he was directing all of the military hospitals in the scene of operations and in the neighboring provinces between the Weser and the Rhine. Also, he was commanding all of the reserve army hospitals in the realm. After 1815, he became a Royal Medical Councillor. In 1822 he was appointed the third Director-General of the Army Medical Services Department and Co-Director of the Military-Medical Educational Institutions. In the latter position he guided the instruction and the scientific development of the entire military medical services.[11]

The clear and practical commonsense viewpoint of von Graefe toward the tasks involved in military medicine were applied equally well to other fields of medicine (*e.g.* to the science of health-spas, as well as to other aspects of medicine— especially ophthalmology). Medical historians emphasize that his two chief contributions were primarily in the fields of ophthalmology and clinical surgery. Perhaps it is not surprising that his son, Albrecht von Graefe (born in 1828), became one of the greatest ophthalmologists of the 19th century.[4]

At the end of the war, which extended from 1813 to 1815, von Graefe was considered one of the best surgical operators in Europe.[13] Castiglioni[14] credits von Graefe with developing improvements in the technique of blood transfusion. Garrison[4] and Gnudi and Webster[13] speak of him as either the "founder" or "pioneer" of modern plastic surgery in Germany. Garrison credits him with being the first to devise an operation for closure of the congenital cleft palate (soft palate) in 1816. In reviewing his other accomplishments he continues:

> In 1818, he introduced rhinoplasty (simultaneously with Bünger) and blepharoplasty (simultaneously with Dzondi). In the same year (1818), he improved the technique of cesarean section and excised the lower jaw for the first time in Germany. He was also the first German surgeon to ligate the innominate artery (1822); his patient lived 68 days. His Rhinoplastik[1] (1818) was the first handling of the theme of artificial nose making after Tagliacozzi (1597) and Carpue (1816).

Just as Carpue[16] revived interest in rhinoplastic procedures in England in 1816, medical historians credit von Graefe with reviving interest in Germany by publication of his comprehensive survey of the 3 methods of rhinoplasty—the Italian, the Indian, and what he termed the "German" method—in his small monograph. "Rhinoplastik; oder Die Kunst den Verlust der Nase organisch zu ersetzen . . ." [1]

Thus, his early contributions to cleft palate surgery (in 1816) and to rhinoplastic surgery (in 1818) were, in themselves, enough to guarantee him a niche in the hall of fame. After the cessation of war in 1815, when he resumed private practice as well as university teaching, he was frequently consulted by many of the royal families of Europe. Among them were the King of Hanover, the Grand Duke Michael, and the Grand Duke Constantine (the latter a tyrannical oppressor and governor of the subjected Poles[9]). He operated successfully on the King of Hanover for a cataract and received the title of Commander as a token of the King's gratitude; George IV made him a Knight of the Guelphic Order. In 1826 the Senate of Warsaw proposed him for the title of Knight (Ritter), which title was then recognized by the King of Prussia.

Perhaps it would be well now to describe in more detail his cleft palate contributions, which began in the year 1816.

> In 1817, von Graefe first described his attempt to close a congenital soft palatal cleft, the operation having been performed in 1816. The closure in this case apparently failed; his technique consisted essentially of cauterizing the edges of the cleft velum with a tincture of cantharides to "freshen" them, and then suturing them with interrupted twine threads.[5] He modified this technique later and obtained a successful closure in 1820 by paring the cleft defect with a "uranotome" knife[7] (Fig. 2). The free ends of the sutures were held to the cheeks with adhesive plasters, and were left there until they sloughed out.[6, 18]

Von Graefe's report of successful closure of the palatal defect in 1820* soon raised a surgical storm, heard throughout Europe. Only one year before, in 1819, Philibert J. Roux of Paris reported his first successful closure of a similar defect in John Stephenson, a Canadian medical student.[17] German colleagues of von Graefe and French supporters of Roux then charged each other with the crime of surgical plagiarism. It was suggested in the early 1820's that Roux knowingly took credit in 1819 for first devising a truly "successful" closure of the soft palate, although a similar operation had been performed (unsuccessfully) 3 years earlier in 1816 by von Graefe.[6, 18]

Interestingly, the first successful clos-

* For illustration of this, see p. 263.

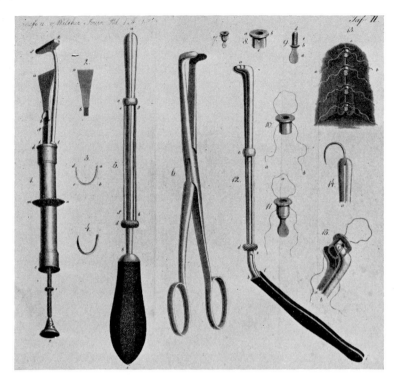

FIG. 2. Plate II. From von Graefe's first illustrated article of soft palate closure.

ure of a cleft soft palate in America was apparently performed in 1820 by John Collins Warren, on a 16-year-old girl in Boston.[18, 19] Not knowing what had been performed successfully only a year earlier by Roux, Warren invented his own instruments for the operation. Despite the injured national feelings of the French and the Germans however, the boldness of von Graefe, Roux, and Warren seemed to suddenly open up a host of new surgical approaches to the cleft palate and lip. The remaining 80 years of the 19th century saw the introduction of many new techniques and revisions of methods. (The reader is referred to Dorrance[20] for an exhaustive review of these historical events.)

In von Graefe's 1818 "Rhinoplastik ..."[1] he discussed the history and general principles of the operation and then described 3 successful cases. The first of these, performed in 1816, duplicated the "Italian," or Tagliacotian, method. The second case, similarly successful, was performed according to the "Indian" method (a flap from the forehead). The third case was once again in the "Italian" method, but advantageously modified, therefore it was called, by von Graefe, the "German" method. In brief, it can be described as follows:

A nose of fair proportions was formed in wax, and adjusted on the original site, where two longitudinal incisions were made, terminating in a point, superiorly. A piece of just dimensions was cut from the arm, and immediately grafted on the nose, with ligatures. The inferior edge of the piece, still joined to the arm, was cut as soon as adhesion had taken place. The nostrils and septum were fashioned after the model. An apparatus is fixed on the renovated organ till its form is set; the apparatus must be worn during the first winter: in summer the new nose must be exposed in the sun, to acquire color and vigor, according to the precepts of Tagliacozzi.[13]

The modifications which von Graefe

made in the Italian, or Tagliacotian, method of rhinoplasty were described by Gnudi and Webster[13] as follows.

...his rejection of the forceps used by Tagliacozzi for freeing the arm flap, which von Graefe accomplished with two free-hand incisions is an attempt to spare the larger veins. Von Graefe's determination to improve the Italian method, which derived from his unwillingness to accept the forehead scars produced by the Indian method and perhaps by an exaggerated fear of the dangers of such a "head wound," led him finally to attempt a shortening of the Italian procedure by the immediate application of the flap to the nose, without allowing a period for granulation and thickening, and by a shortening to six days, when possible, of the period during which the arm was attached to the head. However, the pretentiousness of naming this the "German" method antagonized other surgeons, particularly the French, and it was also felt (by Dieffenbach) that the norms and apparatus which he devised were unnecessarily complicated.

In 1821, von Graefe was apparently the first in Germany to successfully partially resect the lower jaw.[11] In the second volume of the Journal which he and von Walther edited,[22] he reported the successful reconstruction of a defect of the cheek, lower eyelid, and adjacent nasal region by the Indian forehead flap

method (Fig. 3)—and a partial reconstruction of a nose by the "German" method described above (Fig. 4). On March 1, 1822, he was the first in Germany to tie the innominate artery at its division into the common carotid and the subclavian artery; thus, he effectively cured the patient of an aneurysm in this region.[8, 10, 11]

In 1823, he published what many consider his principal literary production—an excellent monograph on Egyptian ophthalmia, which was the direct outgrowth of his wartime experiences from 1813 to 1815.[23] He was apparently skillful in the extraction of cataracts[8] but his eighth case, the Duke of Cumberland, recovered only the use of his right eye—due to circumstances not stated in the reports. (For those interested in von Graefe's other contributions to ophthalmology and eye surgery, a review article by Adam[24] is recommended. Similarly, a more complete summary of von Graefe's contributions to general surgery is included in the survey of Rostock.[25])

In 1830, von Graefe felt that his health was being shattered by continual work and he took a trip to a warmer climate in the hope of regaining some of his

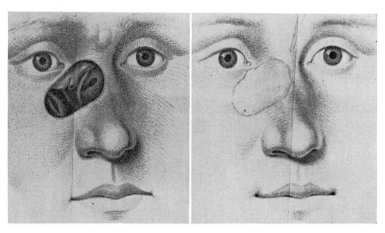

Fig. 3. The "Indian transplantation method," using a forehead flap to fill in a defect of the cheek, eyelid, and nasal region and their underlying bony parts—caused by a chronic ulcerative necrotic process. (From Graefe.[22])

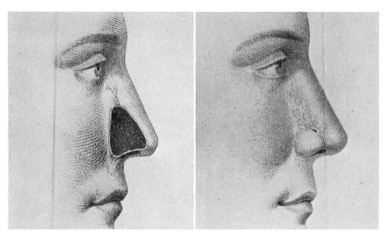

FIG. 4. Repair of defect, after excision of a nasal skin cancer in a 26-year-old woman, by the "German transplantation method." (From Graefe.[22])

energies. On this trip he apparently did not forget his scientific interest. A contemporary biography[8] narrates:

On the way he visited his favorite Alexisbad, tried the effects of the light air breathed on the high mountains of Tyrol and Italy; and after passing under Virgil's Tomb and through the dark grotto of Posilipo, examined the Grotto del Cane on the shores of the Agnano. Leaving his wife and children in Naples, and charging his nephew Andrejewskiy to investigate the nature and effects of the gasses issuing into the grotto, he sailed for Sicily. Near Mount Aetna he was shot through the shoulder by the accidental discharge of a companion's musket, and returned severely wounded to Naples, whence, without waiting till his health was perfectly restored, he hastened homewards.

In the autumn of 1832, while visiting England, a full-length sketch of him was made by an artist in St. James's Palace, where he had apartments during his residence in London (Fig. 5).

Von Graefe died in 1840 in Hanover, where he had gone to operate for cataract on George, Crown Prince of Hanover. His personal friend, Simeon Bullen, writing an obituary memoir in *Lancet,*[9] summarized his eulogy in two final sentences as follows: "He had acquired in practice immense wealth. His loss is uni-

versally deplored, and his fame immortal."

The editor of *Lancet,* in familiarizing his readers with the personality of Mr. Bullen, stated that the latter was among the first of the young medical men in England to devote his services to the unfortunate Poles several decades following the Napoleonic Wars. The editor wrote: "During his [Bullen's] subsequent stay in Berlin, he had frequent opportunities of observing the uprightness of character, the nice discrimination of disease, and dexterity in operation, for which Graefe was so justly celebrated." [9]

In summarizing his contributions to the fields of medicine and surgery, a contemporary article in *Lancet*[8] made the following salient points with which this biography will close:

As a writer, Graefe displays great acuteness and power of observation. A fact is no sooner received into his mind, than all its relations are called up, and it is referred to some general principle. His powers of invention are very great....

...Graefe is a zealous and enlightened teacher. He lectures on "surgery," in its most extended sense—on operative surgery...and on ophthalmia he bestows special attention....

...Graefe is one of the best operators in

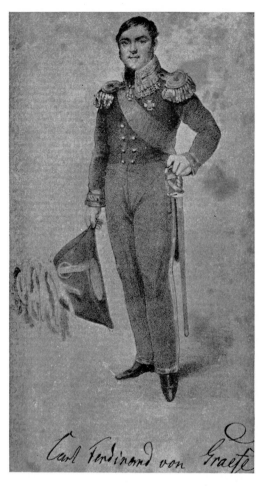

FIG. 5. Sketch of von Graefe made by an artist in St. James's Palace[8] "...where the Baron (von Graefe) had apartments during his residence in London, and where he had more convenient opportunities of treating the ophthalmic disorder of Prince George of Cumberland. The Baron was dressed on the occasion in the full uniform of the Surgeon-In-Chief of the Prussian Army. The autograph of the Baron is taken from a communication addressed by him to the Editor during the brief sojourn of the Baron in London. (From *Lancet*.[8])

Europe. In mechanical contrivance, presence of mind, and manual dexterity, he is unsurpassed. This last faculty, characteristic of the surgeon, is distributed to different men in very variable proportions, and is never more required, nor more triumphantly displayed, than in the finer operations on the living frame. Yet the knife can but cut and destroy; the mechanical part forms the rudest and least of that series of phenomena which bring healing and restora-

tion. The living organization, in which innumerable processes are constantly going on, is united by continuity of substance, by nerves and blood, so that the whole is concerned in each particular act, and the regulation of all its processes, of its relations to the external world, to light, heat, air, and food, with the administrations of specific agents, has more influence on the cure of disease than any simple manual performance. Hence, Graefe has evidently depended as much on the medical treatment of his cases, as on dexterous manipulation.[8]

No greater accolade could be paid to von Graefe, the surgeon, than that by the medical editor of *Lancet* magazine— whose final sentences perhaps reveal some of the disdain with which many English and European internists looked upon surgeons in the first half of the 19th century, and even in later years. Have these attitudes really changed?

Blair O. Rogers, M.D.
875 Fifth Avenue
New York, N.Y. 10021

REFERENCES

1. Von Graefe, C. F.: Rhinoplastik; oder, Die Kunst den Verlust der Nase organisch zu ersetzen, in ihren früheren Verhältnissen erforscht, und durch neue Verfahrungsweisen zur höheren Vollkommenheit gefördert. In der Realschulbuchhandlung, Berlin, 1818.

2. Von Graefe, C. F.: De rhinoplastice sive arte curtum nasum ad vivum restituendi commentatio, etc. Latine edidit J. F. C. Hecker. Reimer, Berolini (Berlin), 1818.

3. Gibson, T.: "Plastic" surgery. Brit. J. Plast. Surg., *9:* 249, 1957.

4. Garrison, F. H.: *An Introduction to the History of Medicine,* 4th Edition, p. 494. W. B. Saunders Co., Philadelphia, 1929.

5. Von Graefe, C. F.: Kurze Nachrichten und Auszuge. J. Pract. Arznek. u. Wundarzk., *44:* 116, 1817.

6. Rogers, B. O.: Palate surgery prior to von Graefe's pioneering staphylorrhaphy (1816): an historical review of the early causes of surgical indifference in repairing the cleft palate. Plast. & Reconstr. Surg., *39:* 1, 1967.

7. Von Graefe, C. F., and Walther, P. H.: Journal der Chirurgie und Augen-Heilkunde, p. 1. Verlage von Duncker und Humblot, Berlin, 1820.

8. Baron Graefe. Lancet Gallery of Medical Portraits. Lancet, *I:* 969, 1834.

9. Bullen, S.: Memoir of the life of the late Professor Gräfe. Lancet, *I*: 364, 1840–1841.

10. Diepgen, P., and Rostock, P.: *Das Universitätsklinikum in Berlin: Seine Ärzte und seine wissenschaftliche Leistung (1810–1933)*, pp. 55, 134. Johann Ambrosius Barth, Leipzig, 1939.

11. Hirsch, A.: *Biographisches Lexicon der hervorragenden Aerzte aller Zeiten und Völker . . .*, p. 618. Urban, Vienna, 1884–1888.

12. Von Graefe, C. F.: *Normen für die Ablösung grösserer Gliedmassen, nach Erfahrungsgrundsätzen entworfen.* Hitzig, Berlin, 1812.

13. Gnudi, M. T., and Webster, J. P.: *The Life and Times of Gaspare Tagliacozzi: Surgeon of Bologna: 1545–1599*, pp. 320–322. Herbert Reichner, New York, 1950.

14. Castiglioni, A.: *A History of Medicine*, 2nd Edition, p. 720. Alfred A. Knopf, New York, 1958.

15. Rogers, B. O.: Historical development of free skin grafting. Surg. Clin. N. Am., *39:* 289–293, 1959.

16. Carpue, J. C.: *An Account of Two Successful Operations for Restoring a Lost Nose from the Integuments of the Forehead . . .* Longman, London, 1816.

17. Roux, P. J.: Observation sur une division congénitale du voile du palais et de la luette, guérie au moyen d'une opération analogue à celle du bec-de-lièvre. J. Univ. Sc. Méd., *15:* 356, 1819.

18. Rogers, B. O.: History of cleft lip and cleft palate treatment. In *Cleft Lip and Palate.* Edited by W. C. Grabbe *et al.* Little, Brown and Co., Boston, 1971.

19. Warren, E.: *The Life of John Collins Warren, M.D.: Compiled Chiefly From His Autobiography and Journals*, Vol. 2, p. 125. Ticknor and Fields, Boston, 1860.

20. Dorrance, G. M.: *The Operative Story of Cleft Palate.* W. B. Saunders Co., Philadelphia, 1933.

21. Davis, J. S.: *Plastic Surgery: Its Principles and Practice.* P. Blakiston's Son and Co., Philadelphia, 1919.

22. Gräfe, C. F.: Neue Beiträge zur Kunst, Theile des Angesichts organisch zu ersetzen. J. der Chir. u. Augen-Heilk., *2:* 1, 1821.

23. Von Graefe, C. F.: *Die epidemisch-contagiöse Augenblenorrhöe Aegyptens in den europäischen Befreiungscheeren . . . .* Reimer, Berlin, 1823.

24. Adam, C.: Die Augenheilkunde unter Carl Ferdinand von Graefe und Johann Friedrich Dieffenbach 1810–1847. In Diepgen, P., and Rostock, P.,[10] p. 134.

25. Rostock, P.: Die Chirurgie unter Carl Ferdinand von Graefe 1810–1840. In Diepgen, P. and Rostock, P.,[10] p. 55.

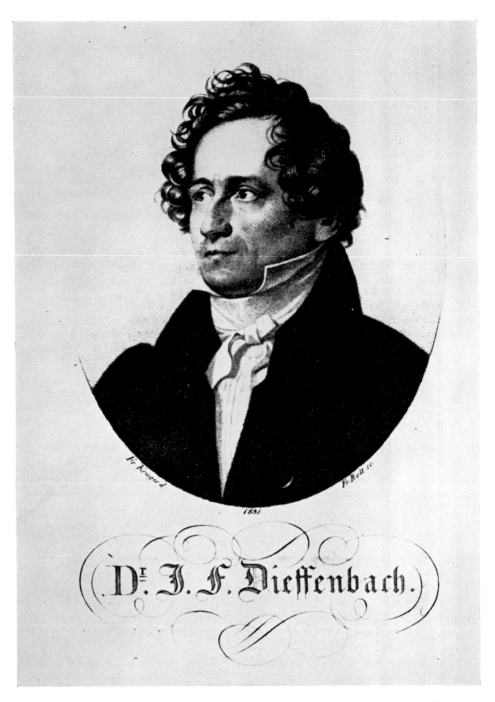

FIG. 1. Johann Friedrich Dieffenbach at 37. (From *Magazin für die Gesammte Heilkunde,* 35: edited by J. N. Rust. G. Reimer, Berlin, 1831.)

JOHANN FRIEDRICH DIEFFENBACH (1794–1847)

ROBERT M. GOLDWYN, M.D.

Boston, Mass.

Johann Friedrich Dieffenbach believed that a surgeon should be "a many-sided Odysseus, full of native inventions and resources not to be found in books.[1] His life admirably satisfied his criteria.

At Königsberg, Prussia, in 1794, Dieffenbach was born into a family which valued learning and had produced well-known scholars of history, language, and law.[2] His father taught philosophy at the *gymnasium;* his mother, a poet's daughter, nurtured in Johann an appreciation for the arts.

When Johann was very young, his father died and the family moved to his mother's home in Rostock. There he received his primary education, and in 1809 entered the *gymnasium.* An unusually talented student, he quickly obtained his baccalaureate and began the study of philosophy and the humanities at the University of Rostock.

In 1813, he joined the Mecklenberg cavalry and served in its campaigns against France. After his discharge from the army, he wrote that he was fortunate to have remained unharmed and that he pitied mothers who had to see "their children returning crippled . . . to be handicapped is worse than death. . . ."[2] His observation of battle casualties furthered his empathy with the maimed and crystallized his interest in medicine.

After returning home, he began medical studies at the University of Königsberg. One of his teachers was Carl Von Baer (1792–1876), called "the father of modern embryology" because of his discoveries of the mammalian ovum and his theory of germ layer development. Dieffenbach's leaning toward plastic surgery is reflected in the nature of his first experiments: the transplantation and regeneration of hair and feathers. The transplant investigations of John Hunter (1771) and Giusseppe Baronio (1804) were the background for these early efforts, which later became his doctoral thesis *Nonnulla de Regeneratione et Transplantione.* His laboratory work required not only scientific imagination, but manual skill. He extended this mechanical aptitude to wood carving and designed improvements for wood-lathes.

In the spring of 1820, Dieffenbach went to the University of Bonn to devote himself entirely to the study of surgery. His decision to leave Königsberg involved a financial sacrifice, as shown by his observation "a doctor could do very well in this area of 18 doctors for 70,000–80,000 people."[2] Another reason for his departure, less often mentioned, was his difficulty in an *affaire de coeur* with an older, married woman.

At Bonn, Dieffenbach closely observed the lectures and demonstrations of Philipp Von Walther (1782–1849), a physiologist and surgeon with a particular interest in the eye. A noteworthy professor, also, was Christian Nasse (1778–1851), a pathologist and anatomist largely responsible for the physiological direction of German medicine in the nineteenth century. Dieffenbach wrote, not modestly, "I worked especially hard in surgery because I am born for surgery. Technical and mechanical skill in my fingers allows me to do every operation with the experience of an older surgeon. . . . All my patients love me."[2] It should be added that his students were very

From the Department of Surgery (Plastic Surgery), Harvard Medical School.

fond of him, as well; when he left Bonn, they gave him an unprecedented send-off—they bought him a horse and accompanied it a mile outside the city gates.

A fellow student, who would always remain his friend, was Heinrich Heine, the great romantic poet.[2, 3] When Heine later became paralyzed (? tabes), he said, "I tell my illness, 'Do not molest me too much because the Healing God is my friend.'" Heine, incidentally, could not obtain permission to reenter Germany from France in order to receive treatment from Dieffenbach.[3]

In 1821, Dieffenbach had an unusual opportunity to go to Paris; he became medical advisor to a rich, blind Russian lady, the widow of the general who burned Moscow to thwart Napoleon. Dieffenbach and his patient, whom he irreverently called the "blind polar bear,"[2] got along poorly and she dismissed him after 6 months in Paris, but not before he had a chance to attend lectures by Boyer, Larrey, Magendie, and Dupuytren, for whom he especially held a life-long respect. From Paris, Dieffenbach went to Montpellier to spend a few months with Jacques Delpech (1772–1832), then well known for his ability in vascular, orthopedic, and reconstructive surgery. Delpech had devised some methods for nose and lip restoration.[4]

Always quick to side with the oppressed, Dieffenbach seriously considered participating in the rebellion of the Greeks against the Turks. His principal reason for not going was the sudden appearance of his female friend, now divorced, whom he soon married. Dieffenbach wrote that his marriage was obviously based on his bride's "unending goodness" since "she is not beautiful, young, or wealthy."[2] Unfortunately, or perhaps predictably, they separated several years later and he remarried.

Having passed his state boards in medicine, Dieffenbach settled in Berlin in 1823 and practiced general medicine as well as surgery. His clientele came from the poor and "his first rise" was

"owing to the following curious circumstance:— Rust, the celebrated surgeon and anatomist, and at that time Proto-medicus of Prussia, one night missed his way on leaving the apartment of a patient, and coming down by a backstairs in one of the great houses or hotels in Berlin, was attracted by a light which proceeded from a small chamber, not larger than a dog kennel, at the foot of the stairs. On looking in, he was not a little astonished to see the apartment occupied by two old women and a young man, who, by the glimmer of a small flickering lamp, was operating for strangulated hernia, on one of the crones, who lay upon a wretched pallet, the operator was Dieffenbach. . . ."[5]

Within the next few years, Dieffenbach began to concentrate his surgical skills on reconstructive problems. His practice grew and his achievements in dealing with facial defects, following trauma and tumor excision, won the attention of Carl Friedrich Von Graefe (1787–1840), the Professor of Surgery at the University of Berlin since 1810. Von Graefe's accomplishments in reconstructive surgery reinforced Dieffenbach's interest and provided a favorable milieu for his later efforts. Von Graefe had already described his method of palatoplasty (1816), blepharoplasty (1818), and nasal reconstruction (1818). In 1818, he had performed the first mandibular resection in Germany.

In spite of Dieffenbach's reputation and competence, however, he lacked an academic position for several years. One reason was his desire for independence; he did not wish to be, as he said, "a slave to a professor."[2]

In 1826, Dieffenbach[6, 7] published his method for repair of clefts of the hard palate, thus extending the techniques of Joseph Roux (1780–1854) and Von Graefe, who had treated defects of the soft palate.[8] Dieffenbach was obviously familiar with Von Graefe's work and also with that of Roux, whose articles he had translated into the German medical literature. Dieffenbach's palatoplasty involved dissection of the mucosa, division, and immediate or gradual approximation of the bone by twisting silver or lead sutures passed through holes in the bone by needles of his design. He advised lateral relaxing incisions in 1826, but did not employ them until 1828. In 1845, two years before his death, he summarized his experience with cleft palate repairs:

"... The principal object of the operation is to improve the speech and to eliminate the difficulty in swallowing food.... In cases of very wide cleft in the hard palate, where there is only a rudiment of the soft palate, the closing can be affected by previously lessening the cleft of the palate bone. The edge of each palate bone is pierced through with a strong, straight, 3-cornered punch and a thick, soft silver wire put through the opening, the ends of which are twisted together. The mucous membrane is divided near the place where the palate bones join the alveolar processes; a thin, smooth, concave chisel is then put to the bone, and it is cut through on both sides. The wires are then twisted again, till the edges of the bony cleft approach each other a little, or all together; the first alone can be generally done. The ends of the wire are then cut off. The effect of the closer approximation of the edges of the cleft in the bone is immediately perceptible in the soft palate. The side slits in the bone, which are at first filled up with lint, close themselves by means of copious granulation, according to the usual process. The edges can sometimes be brought still closer by twisting the wire: by the application of a hot iron, or Tincture of Cantharides, which renders them purulent, and the bony spaces are lessened. When the space in the bone is either closed or diminished so much that the cleft in the soft palate is considerably lessened, the sewing of the palate may then be undertaken, according to the directions already given, and side incisions made in the soft palate before the sutures are put in.

The rest of the operation, besides the excising of the granulations on the borders of the bony cleft, consists in the removal of the mucous membrane and pressing it into the slit; the loosened edge is then pierced with fine leaden sutures, and the place where the skin has been removed is filled up with dry lint.

The sutures, after a few days, generally break through, and the granulations that arise in the place where the skin has been taken off, prevent it from retracting altogether, and a part always remains in the cleft. This operation is to be continued from time to time, until the cleft is removed." [9]

Before the discovery of ether, he seated the patient "facing a window, his head being held by an assistant, and instructed to open his mouth and breathe in deeply, thereby pressing down on the floor of the mouth. After each incision he is allowed to recover, gasp for air, and wash his mouth with cold water but not gargle because this would irritate the velum." [10] Peer and associates[10] have described the subsequent vicissitudes of Dieffenbach's bone flap technique, and its modern use.

In 1827 and 1834, Dieffenbach reported new methods for lip reconstruction.[4, 11] Still used, although modified, is his technique of creating a triangular defect in the lip and chin and closing it by shifting two adjacent square flaps around one point of rotation.[11] Dieffenbach's cheek flaps were full thickness, including even mucous membrane for making the new lip.

Dieffenbach commonly employed the V-Y principle, applying it to reconstruction of the lower lid after tumor excision and to correction of ectropion.[4]

His talents finally won him an appointment as Surgeon at the Charité Hospital of Berlin, where he eventually succeeded Von Graefe as Professor in 1840.[12]

During the period 1829–1834, Dieffenbach published a series of brilliant articles under the general title "Surgical Experiences, Especially on the Restoration of Destroyed Parts of the Human Body Using a New Method." [13, 14] These papers dealt with reconstruction of the ears, nose, lips, palate, urethra, and eyelids as a result of burns, cancer excision, and congenital defects. He wrote even on the repair of the lacrimal duct, and the

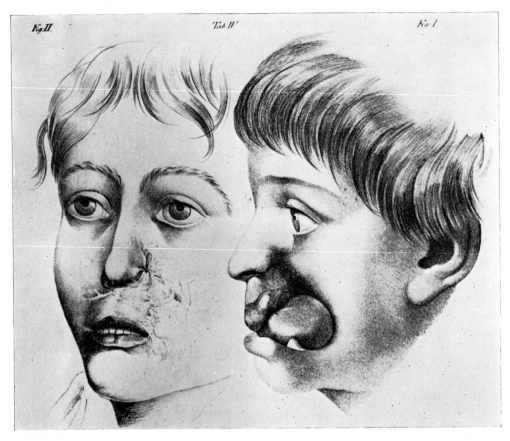

Fig. 2. Seven-year-old boy with noma: before and after closure by local flaps. (From *Chirurgische Erfahrungen besonders über die Wiederherstellung zerstörter Theile des menschlichen Körpers nachneuen Methoden.* Theodore Christian Friedrich Enslin, Berlin, 1829.)

resurfacing of exposed testes and open leg ulcers by skin grafting. In an English translation of several of these papers, he detailed his method of rebuilding the nose—chiefly by the use of a forehead flap (Fig. 3). He acknowledged the previous contributions of Von Graefe and also admitted that the reconstructed nose occasionally did not present a good appearance.

"It was on this account, that the celebrated Dr. Klein objected to the operation, asserting that a nose made of boxwood, when painted and varnished, appeared far more natural than the misshapen one of flesh. Klein has been justly censored; his opinion was too general, and liable to the same objections as his exaggeration in everything else. The failure of unskillful persons does not warrant us in banishing the Rhino-plastic operation from our code of Surgery; on the contrary . . . the difficulty of the undertaking should excite us to . . . improve the operation." [13]

Dieffenbach further advised surgeons to model in "wax or clay." His practical judgment is shown in his sage consideration of donor areas: ". . . in all operations on the face . . . , it is of equal importance with the restoration of the lost part to preserve the existing one; and that, Surgeons are not warranted in causing a considerable deformity in one place, in order to cover a defect in another. . . ." [3] Urging the necessity of "'recreating the defect," he outlined the utilization of local flaps to repair deficiencies of the nose, lip, mouth, palate, and columella

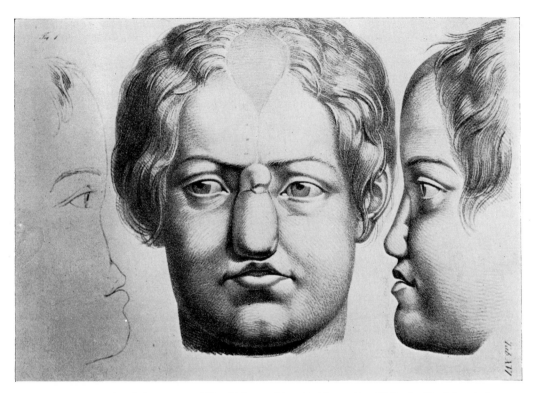

FIG. 3. Forehead flap. (*From XXI Lithographirte Tafeln zu Dr. Dieffenbach's chirurgische Erfahrungen.* Theodore Christian Friedrich Enslin, Berlin, 1830.)

following "scrofula," wounds, birth abnormalities, and cancer surgery. He concluded that section of his book by stating "... should the surgeon find my description not sufficiently circumstantial, and be unable to supply anything, from his own knowledge of general principles, that he may find wanting, he had better altogether abstain from operating. ..." [13]

In that book, Dieffenbach also offered another record of his transplantation experiments. He noted failure in transplanting pig skin to pigeons and in re-uniting severed tails in cats and dogs. Three of 50 amputated ears in dogs and rabbits, however, regained viability after reimplantation. In 5 humans, he did not succeed in putting back amputated digits. With few exceptions, "... all my attempts to re-unite portions of skin that were entirely separated from the body failed. ..." By "skin," he meant composite grafts containing cartilage, tendons, muscle, and/or bone. He observed that the application of cold to a transplanted part helped its survival. Regarding flaps, he wrote, "... the decay and death of the flap generally proceed from its being gorged with blood, which flowing in copiously and unable to find egress, or to be returned by the veins, causes great distention and mortification." [13] His follow-up of clinical cases was careful and honest. For example, he noted that the reconstructed nose fails to gain "sensation" for at least 12 months.

Dieffenbach also had his postoperative complications as the following dramatic report testifies:

"C. SCHNEIDER, a tanner, aged forty-one, a tall and robust man presented himself at La Charité to undergo an operation for the restoration of his nose, of which a severe attack of syphillis had deprived him. ... The whole nose was lost, as also the lower half of the nasal bones. The large cavity was bounded by red and indurated skin, which scantily covered the bones, except at the lower part, where the lip, in consequence of ulceration, had contracted, turned up and become united with the nasal cavity. This distortion of the mouth considerably increased the horrible appearance of this unfortunate individual, which was not lessened by the remains of old ulcerations upon the forehead and around the mouth and nasal cavity.... In consequence of the entire loss of the nose, it was necessary to procure a very large flap, which, as in the two former cases, was obtained from the scalp. I commenced the operation by making incisions round the cavity for the reception of the flap, these I formed at some distance from the margin, encroaching upon the cheek, where I could obtain a firm and healthy portion of skin to which the flap might be united; and, which was now very skilfully formed in the usual way, by Staff-Surgeon Grossheim. Being turned round, it was fixed by thirty-two pins in the furrows previously prepared to receive it. Three twisted sutures united the Columna to the lip, and four pins brought the edges of the wound on the forehead intimately into contact. The large wound on the scalp was covered with pledgets of lint. The patient, who had most heroically borne the operation, was now carried to bed; cold was applied to his head; and, as the new nose was icy cold and pale, a lotion of wine and tepid water was used for it. In a few hours the nose had swollen and become warm and red. A small branch of the temporal artery had been cut, the bleeding from which was not checked until near midnight. The patient passed a very sleepless night.

The following morning considerable re-action had taken place. The pulse was full, hard and quick, and the whole face, but especially the mouth, eyelids and lips, were greatly swollen. In most places union had taken place, and I therefore extracted the greater number of the pins. Towards evening I took a pound and a half of blood from the arm.

The second night passed as sleeplessly as the first. Notwithstanding the constant cold applications, the patient complained of an intolerable burning pain of the head, and I found him next morning suffering more than on the preceeding day, labouring—he was addicted to spirits—under delirium tremens. He was ordered brandy, administered in small quantities. Though the nose was greatly swollen, it was still approximated to the neighbouring parts, and applied twenty-four leeches around it....

During the following days, the delirium tremens having disappeared, and the fever abated, it became necessary to administer a more generous diet.

The wound of the scalp and of the brow—the edges of which had separated—were granulating freely, the swelling had decreased, and union by the First Intention taken place, except at the lower part of the new Columna, where a slight degree of gangrene had occurred. At the line of junction on the left side of the nose a very inconsiderably suppurating furrow appeared.

On the ninth day the nose, although swollen and inflamed, had much improved in appearance, its sides were more drawn together and the ridge in consequence become prominent.

On the tenth, all inflammatory symptoms had disappeared, and the whole nose seemed healthy and in a highly favourable way. The hairs were easily removed with small tweezers.

Although the operation appeared to be about to terminate successfully, the general health of the patient was greatly disturbed; a distressing cough, dyspnea and considerable diaphoresis proclaimed the lungs affected, and the wounds on the scalp and forehead, soon began to assume a sluggish, flabby aspect. It were needless to follow this case through all the stages of intermittent and continued fevers which followed; a large abcess formed in the axilla, and on the eighth of September the patient expired. The dissection exhibited considerable adhesions between the pleurae. The lungs themselves were aedematous, being actually gorged with a quantity of brownish-red fluid of a very disagreeable odour. The bronchi were ulcerated, and the heart enlarged, withered, pale, soft and empty.

The head was given to Professor Schlemm." [13]

In addition to his concern with restorative problems of the face, Dieffenbach wrote on the treatment of urethral stricture (1826), suggested better methods of bandaging (1829) and nursing (1832), and was among the first to recognize the value of intravenous infusion and blood transfusion (1828).[12] He confirmed the experimental findings of Louis Prevost (1790–1850) and Jean Dumas (1800–1888), who showed that homologous blood was more effective in reviving an exsanguinated animal than was water.[15, 16] Dieffenbach believed also that arterial blood could resuscitate more quickly than venous blood. He gave "three supfuls of blood" from a healthy man to a "hydrophobic man." Later, without benefit, he transfused an asphyxiated neonate. His article "Physiological-Surgical Observations in Choleric Patients" (1832)[17] emphasized the value of blood transfusion in this condition. He further reported experiments by himself and Van Brom in the venous infusion of various drugs, such as opiates in animals.[12]

His reputation was enormous. He received many types of reconstructive problems that others had judged incurable. As a result, Dieffenbach used his skills in the treatment of imperforate anus (1834), hypospadias (1837), urethral fistulae, and vesicovaginal fistulae. For the last problem, he tried "every known method," often without success. In his papers, he expressed his sympathy to his patients for enduring these operative failures.

Another area of surgery in which Dieffenbach excelled was in the technique of subcutaneous myotomy and tenotomy. George Stromeyer (1804–1876) performed his first subcutaneous section of the tendon of Achilles for clubfoot in 1831. Although Delpech had done the same thing 15 years before, Stromeyer developed this kind of surgery[1] and his results became known to Dieffenbach through an unusual circumstance. A young English physician, named Little, who later described congenital spastic paraplegia (Little's disease) came to Dieffenbach for treatment of his clubfoot.[12] With characteristic honesty, Dieffenbach said that he had meagre experience with this problem and referred him to Stromeyer. When Little returned very much improved. Dieffenbach was impressed; by the next year he had performed the operation 140 times with considerable success.[12, 18]

The efficacy of myotomy in lower extremity problems led him to employ it in strabismus,[19] as Stromeyer had also done. By 1841, Dieffenbach had carried out 1200 of these operations. For unilateral facial paralysis Dieffenbach divided the muscles of the healthy side.

A more curious result of his zeal in myotomy was his method of curing stuttering (1841).[20] Aware of the "painful condition of the stutterer or stammerer . . . the idea lately suggests itself to me, that an incision carried completely through the root of the tongue, might possibly be useful, by producing an alteration in the condition of its nervous influence, allaying the spasm of the Chordae vocales, etc. The brilliant success of this new operation more than realized my most sanguine expections." [20] Interestingly, his first patient was a highly educated 13-year-old boy who "stuttered in both Latin and French" ! It is significant that Dieffenbach made anatomical studies of this operation. He documented that he was cutting the genioglossus, and styloglossus, and hyoglossus muscles; he showed that his procedure had no permanent influence on taste and that it was not successful if only the frenulum was divided, or the lingual tip excised. Later, he admitted that the operation had not produced the desired permanent relief which he had initially anticipated.

Writing in the *Medical Times*, an English physician gave an interesting account of his visit to Dieffenbach's clinic.

". . . I have seen the most effectual cures by Dieffenbach's operations. Clubfeet of every description; contractions of the knee, hip, and elbow joints at obtuse or acute angles: All these I have seen restored to their normal form and use. And whence these surprising and almost invariably successful results? Simply because no one case is treated exactly like another. It is one of Dieffenbach's greatest qualities to individualize quickly and even during his operation.... Another means for accounting for Dieffenbach's happy results, is, that he is never tempted, like some surgeons, by the love of display; he never in these cases forces the limb immediately into its proper position so as to astonish his class by a kind of miraculous conjuring; on the contrary, some days always elapse before he commences any orthopedic treatment further than that of a slight enveloping bandage. . . . In the case of lagophthalmos, Dieffenbach protects the eye by a small piece of wood—in the case I witnessed, he cut it from the cover of a cigar box—passed under the lid and up to the supraorbital ridge of the frontal bone; he then pierced the eyelid at its outer angle, passed a very narrow and slightly curved knife up to the levator palpebrae superioris, which with one stroke he cut through, and then withdrew the instrument at the point of incision. The instantaneous result was truly surprising: the eyelid was immediately closed and the orbicularis had regained its power. In blepharoptosis, in like manner, the too power-ful orbicularis is divided; and both operations have been invariably attended with the most perfect success. In both, a careful orthopedic after treatment is practised. . . ." [21]

The King of Prussia, Wilhelm IV, was Dieffenbach's friend; frequently, he and members of his family attended Dieffenbach's operations. Many surgical clinics throughout Europe invited Dieffenbach to lecture and to operate. In Paris in 1832, Jonathan Mason Warren attended his demonstrations and brought back to America Dieffenbach's methods of palate repair and nasal reconstruction.[22, 23] As one of the most famous men in Berlin, Dieffenbach was the object of a popular children's song:

"Who does not know Dr. Dieffenbach?
The doctor of doctors. He cuts off arms and legs.
And makes you new noses and ears." [2]

Even a plant was named after him: *Dieffenbachia.*[24]

Although he was usually gracious, he abhorred flattery. On a day dedicated to his honor, he fled to the country side with his family. To his second wife, the daughter of a doctor, and to his son and daughter, he was an attentive husband and father. During the summers their delight was to tour Europe together. Despite the demands of his professional life,

he tried to exercise regularly: skating, swimming, and riding. So avid an eques-trian was he that it was alleged he would ask to see a wealthy patient's horses be-fore seeing his disease. He insisted that his patients exercise and "even old and fat gentlemen had to learn riding and swimming."

Like most famous men, he also had his detractors. When the first volume of his celebrated *Operative Surgery*[25] appeared in 1845, his enemies said that he had hired a ghost writer. As rebuttal, Dieffen-bach made the editors display the origi-nal manuscript. This two-volume work dealt not only with reconstructive prob-lems, but with almost every surgical event: e.g., amputations, paracentesis, laparotomy, hysterectomy, dental extrac-tions and methods for treating hydro-cephalus, fistula-in-ano, and phimosis.

One of Dieffenbach's most significant contributions was his role in the intro-duction of ether anesthesia into Ger-many.[26] Following Morton's demon-stration at the Massachusetts General Hospital in October of 1846, Dieffen-bach became very much interested in the possibilities of this technique. His first use of ether was in reconstructing a nose destroyed by "scrofula" in a 16-year-old boy. Enthusiastic, Dieffenbach wrote Stromeyer (fall of 1847) "the wonderful dream that pain has been taken away from us has become reality. Pain, the highest consciousness of our earthly exist-ence, the most distinct sensation of the imperfection of our body, must bow be-fore the power of the human mind, be-fore the power of ether vapor." [26] Al-though Dieffenbach was not the first to use ether in Germany (Heyfelder did in January of 1847), his satisfaction with the method and his stature in the medical community led others to try it.

Shortly after his letter to Stromeyer, Dieffenbach began to have premonitions of death. On the morning that he died,

"...Dieffenbach was quite well, in his usual health and spirits, and took exercise in the riding school with his wife and daughter. But for some time he had been greatly interested and excited by the affairs of Switzerland, and had frequently expressed himself very warmly in favour of a liberal party. And to this undo excitement may, perhaps, be attributed to the proximate cause of his sudden death. He repaired as usual, at two o'clock, to the Klinik, where he found two French physicians waiting him. To these gentlemen he presented a young man on whom, the day previously, he had operated for aneurism. He seated himself on his usual sofa, and explained to them the steps of the operation. Suddenly he ceased speaking, and his head fell forward, as if he was whispering to one of them. But alas! His voice had hushed forever. He had ceased to live." [21]

So great was the surprise and disbelief at his death that throughout Berlin it was rumored he was "still alive but in a continued swoon." A magnetic battery was then applied to his body, "—without success." [27] Dieffenbach was accorded a State Burial and "thousands from all classes" joined the funeral procession. Someone who knew Dieffenbach wrote that—

"...He was a bad dissembler, speaking his mind with such freedom and honesty that kept him from many high places to which men less worthy were appointed; and hence, too, like other poor children of genius, he was improvident. Although his income was considerable, he has left no fortune to his family, for his hospitality was great, and his generosity unbounded: tales of distress and necessity were never told to him in vain. Of the many who solicited his assistance, none left him unrelieved in the most effectual manner...." [21]

Dieffenbach's scientific and surgical accomplishments were numerous and varied. He discovered techniques and codified others in reconstructing the face, the mouth, the palate, and other parts of the body; with unusual skill, he employed myotomy and tenotomy to correct clubfoot, torticollis, and other disorders; he explored methods of treating vesico-vaginal and urethral fistulae, and hypospadias; early he recognized the value of infusion, transfusion, and ether anesthesia; he anticipated the benefits of transplantation and even conducted experiments in this area.

He advanced plastic surgery beyond a "decorative art" or a surgical curiosity. In his writings and lectures, he frequently used the term "constructive surgery" in contrast to "destructive" or "ablative," which characterized that period in the history of surgery. *He continually sought surgical excellence.* He had composure, courage, and self-reliance. "A surgeon should learn to do much with little; only then will he be free and independent ... Among surgical instruments, the most simple are the best since it is a surgeon who operates and not his instruments." [2] To his students, he emphasized that "there is no such thing as a minor operation." As evidence, he presented in detail the technique and the complications of piercing ears. [2]

Dieffenbach correctly predicted the direction of medical progress: "The best surgical instrument is the pencil with which the surgeon records his thoughts. Such a surgeon will base his thinking upon physiological principles and will direct his steps according to the laws of the eternal, natural healing process..." [2]

Dieffenbach's surgical and intellectual abilities were obviously impressive. No less outstanding, however, were his warmth toward patients and his pervasive desire to help them. This combination of skill and sympathy gave an unusual and happy impetus to the development of plastic surgery in the nineteenth century.

Robert M. Goldwyn, M.D.
1101 Beacon Street
Brookline, Mass. 02146

Dr. Goldwyn is Assoc. Prof. in Surgery at Harvard Medical School, Attending in Surgery at Peter Bent Brigham Hospital, and Chief of Plastic Surgery at Beth Israel Hospital.

ACKNOWLEDGMENTS

Figures 2 and 3 come from books left to Harvard Medical School by Jonathan Mason Warren.

I am grateful to Mr. Richard J. Wolfe, Rare Books Librarian, and his staff at the Countway Library of Medicine for their gracious assistance.

REFERENCES

1. Garrison, F. H.: *An Introduction to the History of Medicine*, ed. 4, pp. 495–496. W. B. Saunders Company, Philadelphia, 1960.
2. Rohlfs, H.: *Die chirurgischen Classiker Deutschlands: Johann Friedrich Dieffenbach*. Vol. 4, Part 2, pp. 1–138, C. L. Hirschfeld, Leipzig, 1885.
3. Butler, E. M.: *Heinrich Heine*, p. 195. Hogarth Press, London, 1956.
4. Kolle, F. S.: *Plastic and Cosmetic Surgery*, pp. 104, 157, 181, 183, 353. D. Appleton and Company, New York, 1911.
5. Note in Lancet 2: 586, 1847.
6. Dieffenbach, J. F.: Beitrage zur Gaumennath. Litt. Ann. D. Ges. Heilk, 4: 145, 1826.
7. Dieffenbach, J. F.: Über das Gaumensegel des Menschen und der Saeugethiere. Litt. Ann. D. Ges. Heilk, 4: 298–317, 1826.
8. Dorrance, G. M.: *The Operative Story of Cleft Palate*, pp. 5–6, 13, 134. W. B. Saunders Company, Philadelphia, 1933.
9. Dieffenbach, J. F.: Practical Observations on the Operations for Cleft Palate. Dublin J. M. Sci., 28: 227–249, 1845.
10. Peer, L. A., Walker, J. C., and Meiger, R.: The Dieffenbach bone-flap method of cleft palate repair. Plast. & Reconstr. Surg., 34: 472–482, 1964.
11. May, H.: The modified Dieffenbach operation for closure of large defects of lower lip and chin. Plast. & Reconstr. Surg., 1: 196–204, 1946.
12. Hirch, A.: *Allgemeine Deutsche Biographie*, Vol. 5, pp. 120–126. Dunder & Humblot, Leipzig, 1877.
13. Dieffenbach, J. F.: *Surgical Observations on the Restoration of the Nose and on the Removal of Polyps and other Tumors from the Nostrils* (Translated with the history and physiology of rhinoplastic operations, notes, and additional cases by J. S. Buschnan), pp. 49, 59, 129–131, 151. Samuel Highley, London, 1833.
14. Dieffenbach, J. F.: *Chirugische Erfahrungen. besonders über die Wiederherstellung zerstörter Theile des menschlichen Körpers nach neuen Methoden.* Theodore Christian Friedrich Enslin, Berlin, 1829–1834.
15. Dieffenbach, J. F.: *Die Transfusion des Blutes.* Theodore Christian Friedrich Enslin, Berlin, 1828.
16. Maluf, N. S. R.: History of blood transfusion. I: The use of blood from antiquity through the eighteenth century. J. Hist. Med., 9: 59–107, 1954.
17. Dieffenbach, J. F.: *Physiologisch-chirurgische Beobachtungen bei Cholera-Kranken.* Theodore Christian Friedrich Enslin, Berlin, 1832.
18. Dieffenbach, J. F.: *Ueber die Durchschneidung der Sehnen und Muskeln.* Albert Fostner, Berlin, 1841.
19. Dieffenbach, J. F.: *Ueber das Schielen und die Heilung desselben durch die Operation.* Albert Forstner, Berlin, 1842.
20. Dieffenbach, J. F.: *Memoir on the Radical Cure of Stuttering.* Translated by Joseph Travers, pp. 7–10. Samuel Highley, London, 1841.
21. Buschnan, J. S.: Death of Dieffenbach. M. Times, 17: 135–137, 1847.
22. Arnold, H. O.: *Memoir of Jonathan Mason Warren, M.D.* University Press, John Wilson and Son, Cambridge, 1886.
23. Goldwyn, R. M.: Jonathan Mason Warren and his contributions to plastic surgery. Plast. & Reconstr. Surg., 41: 1, 1968.
24. Barnes, B. A., and Fox, L. E.: Poisoning with Dieffenbachia, J. Hist. Med., 10: 173–181, 1955.
25. Dieffenbach, J. F.: *Die operative Chirurgie*, 2 Vols. F. A. Brockhaus, Leipzig. 1845. 1848.
26. Frankel, W. K.: The introduction of general anesthesia in Germany. J. Hist. Med. 1: 612–618, 1946.
27. Note in Lancet 2: 664, 1847.

BERNHARD VON LANGENBECK

His Life and Legacy

ROBERT M. GOLDWYN, M.D.

Boston, Mass.

Bernhard Rudolph Conrad Langenbeck was the productive nucleus of German surgery in the mid-nineteenth century. As significant as were his operative accomplishments his greatest achievements were his pupils: Bergmann, Billroth, Bose, Esmarch, Gürlt, Huter, Krönlein, Lucke, and Trendelenburg.

The founder of this surgical dynasty was born in 1810 in Padingbüttel, a small town near the North Sea. His father, a pastor and a teacher, supervised his early education in preparation for the ministry. However, the future direction of his life was undoubtedly influenced by his father's step-brother, Conrad J. M. Langenbeck, an eminent ophthalmologist and Professor of Surgery at the University of Göttingen.[1] His uncle's work and his own boyhood interest in dissecting small animals stimulated him to begin medical studies at Göttingen in 1830, where he remained 4 years. With his uncle's guidance, he prepared a dissertation on "The Inner Structure of the Retina" (Fig. 1), which earned him a two-year study fellowship, spent in Belgium, France, and England. In London, he was welcomed enthusiastically by Benjamin Brodie, Lawrence Green, and Astley Cooper. Langenbeck always acknowledged gratefully their influence on his professional life.

After returning to Germany, Langenbeck was appointed Docent in microscopy and physiology. One of his earliest contributions was to demonstrate, in thrush, a yeastlike, budding fungus which was later named *Candida albicans.*

In 1840, aged 30, he became Professor of Pathological Anatomy and also began teaching a course in surgical anatomy. Soon he attracted so many students that he tactfully left Göttingen to avoid eclipsing his uncle. Bernhard later dedicated a book to him: "I have learned from you that every minute not spent investigating the mysteries of the human body is a wasted one." [2]

Bernhard Langenbeck then accepted the chair of surgery at the University of Kiel. His competence as a clinician brought patients from all parts of Germany. Even when visiting his father, he had no respite. Once he confessed to a student that he used to escape his eager clientele by "going out of the window on a ladder." [2]

When the Holstein wars broke out, Von Langenbeck sought appointment as a staff surgeon. His singular abilities on the battlefield made the University of Berlin consider him as replacement for Johann Friedrich Dieffenbach, who had recently died (1847). That student demonstrations are not new is evidenced by the fact that the students at the University of Berlin signed petitions and held public meetings in Langenbeck's behalf. They protested against the older faculty members' distrust of Langenbeck because of "youth" and "lack of book learning." Langenbeck was appointed and gave his first lecture in 1848 to a large, enthusiastic audience (Fig. 2).

According to Billroth,[3] Langenbeck's rapport with pupils arose from his genuinely considering them colleagues. Never

From the Plastic Surgery Services of the Harvard University Medical School, the Peter Bent Brigham Hospital, and the Beth Israel Hospital.

despotic, he was always willing to point out his own mistakes. His trophic effect on youth continued, even throughout his old age. By his warmth and enthusiasm, as much as through his position, he molded German surgery to think scientifically—to draw upon biology, pathology, and physiology. He consistently urged, for example, testing an operation in animals before employing it in humans.

The agreeable associations he had while attending the meetings of the London Medico-Chirugical Society led him to organize the German Surgical Society. His capacity to discuss, as well as to discourse, made these get-togethers more than a professor's podium. With his pupils Billroth and Gürlt, he founded (in 1860) the *Archiv für Klinische Chirurgie*, which continued as a principal source of exchange among German and other European surgeons until shortly before the end of World War II.

Despite his great clinical experience and the teutonic custom of prodigious publication, Langenbeck published relatively little. He disliked doing formal writing; yet most of his 47 papers showed originality. The range was wide: "Origin of Venous Cancer and the Possibility of Transferring Cancer from Man to Animals;" "The Permanent Warm Water Bath in the Treatment of Large Wounds, Especially on the Stumps after Amputation;" "Immediate Union of Wounds by Exclusion of Air;" "On the Extirpation of Interstitial Uterine Fibroids;" "On Gummatous Tumors;" "Stammering and the Employment of Myotomy in Defects of Speech Arising from Spasm."

The enormous challenge of dealing with thousands of casualties during the Holstein Wars, the conflict with Austria in 1866, and the Franco-Prussian War of 1870 led him to perfect the technique of subperiosteal resection (Fig. 3), advocated earlier by Stromeyer and Heine. This procedure avoided amputation in

DE

RETINAE STRUCTURA PENITIORI

DISSERTATIO INAUGURALIS ANATOMICA

QUAM

CONSENSU ET AUCTORITATE

GRATIOSI MEDICORUM ORDINIS

IN

ACADEMIA GEORGIA AUGUSTA

PRO SUMMIS

IN MEDICINA, CHIRURGIA ARTEQUE OBSTETRICIA

HONORIBUS

RITE IMPETRATIS

ERUDITORUM EXAMINI SUBMITTIT

BERNH. CONR. RUD. LANGENBECK.

BREMENSIS.

GOTTINGAE,

TYPIS DIETERICHIANIS.

MDCCCXXXV.

FIG. 1. Title page of his dissertation, *Concerning the Inner Structure of the Retina,* presented upon graduating from medical school at the University of Göttingen.

certain patients; it enabled others to return sooner to active duty. Langenbeck wrote:

"... The choice of method is less important than careful performance of the procedure. The surgeon who performs a subperiosteal resection must avoid, in shoulder and elbow resection, the misuse of the periosteal elevator, and thereby prevent tears and bruises which delay healing ... The term 'subperiosteal resection' implies maintenance of the proximity of muscles and tendinous insertion at the periosteum of the diaphyses. The advantage of this method is prevention of luxation of the joint at the completion of resection; the ends of the resected bones are not pulled apart by the attachment of the muscles, but are held together by the supporting structures." [4]

Von Langenbeck urged the establishment of proper sanitation for the army, mobile treatment units, and an effective ambulance system to retrieve the wounded.[5, 6] One of his most significant achievements was to maintain the neu-

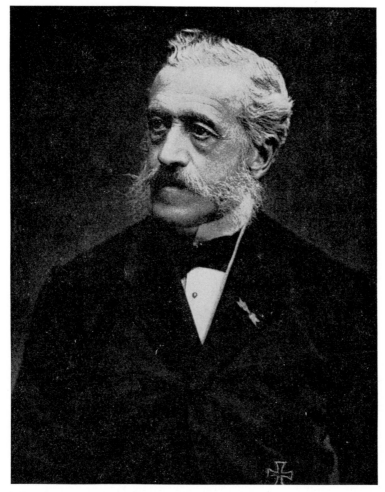

FIG. 2. Bernhard von Langenbeck (1810–1887). (From *Vorlesungen uber Chirurgie.* A. Hirschwald, Berlin, 1888.)

trality of the wounded.[2,3] He agreed with his Emperor: "A wounded enemy is no more an enemy, but a comrade needing help."[2] He attempted to elevate war surgery above the level of battle butchery. "While we may not expect the military surgeon to know everything, there are things he must know to a degree approaching perfection."[2]

An English surgeon who knew Von Langenbeck during the Franco-Prussian War reminisced:

"At this period Langenbeck arrived amongst us with a headquarters staff of the 3rd Prussian Army. We, as Englishmen, were much impressed by the marked deference everywhere shown to him by his professional brethren of all ranks and ages, whether by his countrymen or surgeons of other nationalities. From early morning until late in the evening his services were in constant request, both as consultant and operator; he was in demand everywhere, and did not spare himself even at his age. Ever careful, ever jealous of the interest of others, and more especially of juniors, he would only consent to perform operations at the special request of the particular surgeon in charge of the case. His especial skill in the performance of subperiosteal resections was so well known that he was most frequently called upon to perform them. More especially in connection with these

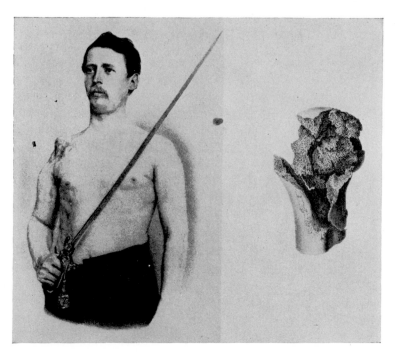

FIG. 3. Secondary resection of humeral head, after extensive soft tissue loss and comminuted fracture. (From B. v. Langenbeck. *Chirurgische Beobachtungen aus Dem Kriege,* Plate 1. A. Hirschwald, Berlin, 1874).

operations his extraordinary capacity as a clinical teacher asserted itself and soon a numerous and attentive clinique followed him . . . He was performing a subperiosteal resection of the shoulder joint, when, the knives at his disposal being considerably the worse for wear and tear and the rough usage to which they had recently been subjected, turning round to his assistant, he said, *'Dieses Messer its nicht scharf.'* Fortunately, we were able to offer him an English-made scalpel in good condition . . . Langenbeck, deeply impressed with the importance of the many debatable and moot points of military surgery, . . . urged the desirability of establishing a Surgical Society; it was mainly owing to his intense activity and great personal influence that a 'Militar-aertzliche Gesellschaft' was organized . . . Professor von Langenbeck's introductory address was on the subject of Prophylactic Tracheotomy in Cases of Gun Shot Injuries of the Larynx, even though there might be no urgent dyspnea. He was induced to select the subject from the fact that he had seen in the action near Pithivers, a few days previously, a Dragoon who had been wounded in the region of the larynx suddenly die from asphyxia, due to edema of the glottis, though apparently not dangerously injured; . . ." [7]

Von Langenbeck was not a reluctant participant in war surgery. His student, Trendelenburg,[8] observed that he liked the challenge of battle trauma and the formalities of military life. The Franco-Prussian War inflicted, however, a personal tragedy when his son, an officer, died at Gravelotte. Informed of his loss, Von Langenbeck replied, "I cannot leave; my duty keeps me here. What better could have happened to him than to have died for the King and the Fatherland?" Von Langenbeck's devotion to his Kaiser arose not only from patriotism but also from friendship as his personal surgeon.

In 1859, Von Langenbeck resected a maxilla but left the periosteum intact. His observation that bone regenerated led him to move palatal periosteum in cleft palate repairs.[9] His early predecessor, Von Graefe, described closure of the soft palate in 1816; Dieffenbach, who replaced Von Graefe and whom Langenbeck succeeded, was the first to close the hard palate.[10] Dieffenbach's method mobilized the soft tissues—mucosa, principally. Langenbeck's contribution was to realize the importance of elevating the periosteum with the mucosa, the "mucoperiosteal flaps." He divided the levator and palato-pharyngeus muscles and used lateral relaxing incisions. This technique and the patient were first presented in 1861 at a meeting of the Berlin Medical Society, of which he was then President:

"This patient, a boy aged 14, was born with a hare-lip on the left and a total cleft of the soft and hard palate and with a cleft in the left alveolar process. The operation for hare-lip was performed soon after birth, but was unsuccessful, and only a second operation performed during the second year of life healed properly. On February 6th of this year (1861) Dr. Langenbeck divided the split parts of the soft palate by suturing. On May 11 of this year, Dr. Langenbeck performed uranoplasty in the following manner: Close to the edges of the flap, the mucosa and the periosteum of the hard palate were incised in the bone with a large blade, uncovering the edges of the cleft. With a raspatory, the mucosa of the palate was elevated, together with the periosteum, and was freed from the bone on both sides. Two flaps, formed in this manner, were united anteriorly at the gumline below the alveolar process. The posterior portion of the flaps extended into the soft palate which was separated from the posterior edge of the hard palate. The free edges of these flaps were united in the midline with five silk sutures; the whole palate was closed to the incisors. The separation of the mucosa of the palate, together with the periosteum, can be carried out by tedious and careful dissection without additional injury... When the sutures were removed between the 8th and 14th postoperative day, the healing throughout the length of the suture had been achieved by first intention. The reconstructed palate differs from the normal only by a small scar through the length of the palate and by a slight deformation at the tip of the uvula." [4]

A later report mentioned that the operation lasted a half-hour.[11] Ice was the anesthetic.

"In another case of total cleft, in a woman aged 24 who came under M. Langenbeck's care a fortnight afterwards, he performed staphylorraphy and uranoplastics in the same sitting, and with the best result." [11]

An English surgeon, in a letter to the *Medical Times & Gazette,* challenged Langenbeck's claim of originating the procedure. The writer further asserted that British surgeons had separated the periosteum from the palate "though this may not have been done intentionally."

"Such a remark," Langenbeck replied, "could never have been made by a person who had even once endeavoured to separate the periosteum from the palate, either in the dissecting-room or in the living body. This proceeding is so laborious that it is not likely to occur accidentally..." [12]

Von Langenbeck performed his operation in one stage usually, but recommended it to the less experienced as a two-stage procedure. The introduction of chloroform and ether anesthesia increased the use and success of the Langenbeck technique, basic still to cleft palate repair.

In the course of his varied surgical practice, Von Langenbeck performed other kinds of head and neck surgery, especially for cancer. One observer recorded: "He never failed to neatly cover the large defect left after removing extensive malignant growths of the face, bringing up or turning in flaps of skin from apparently impossible places and sending out the patient entirely presentable." [1] Langenbeck also reported on the removal of the tongue for cancer, and "The Extirpation of the Pharynx," with the formation of a subhyoid pharyngostome.

Those who knew Von Langenbeck remembered him as a small energetic man, whose actions were precise but never harried.

"He was fluent of speech, possessed of sympathetic voice, great charm and impressiveness of manner, with a most intimate knowledge of every detail of his subject, and produced an effect upon his hearers which no pen can adequately describe..." [1] He had "an exquisitely refined face and a noble look in his eye; he was an aristocrat by nature and in feeling." [1]

He rose at five in the morning and, after coffee, went horseback riding when weather allowed. At six, he gave a course in operative surgery on the cadaver to graduates and to advanced students. At eight, he saw his office patients. From ten to two he operated upon private patients and made hospital rounds. He was due in his clinic at 2 p.m. but arrived a half-hour before to arrange the order of cases that he would see and to greet colleagues and visiting physicians. He spoke excellent English and French.

At 2 o'clock precisely, he entered the operating room. He always wore a specially made, tightly fitting coat of black-green material, scrupulously cleaned each day.

His favorite method of teaching medical students was by questioning.

"Where does the psoas major insert?"
"On the greater trochanter of the femur."
"Yes, Sir, it could but it does not." replied Langenbeck. [5]

In the operating room, on the sofa where Dieffenbach died, Von Langenbeck sat and demonstrated cases—while everyone but the patient stood. With sympathy and respect, he treated the poor as well as the rich. Billroth, his pupil of many years, was surprised not to see the same humane concern shown by other professors when he traveled.

Following his lecture, Langenbeck operated. He was fond of using small knives, which his assistants sharpened immediately before surgery. So that he could again get the knife that had served him well, he would order a notch cut into its handle.

A surgeon who saw Von Langenbeck operate characterized him "in the very first rank, original, bold without recklessness, and of great anatomical knowledge ..." [7] He stressed the delicate handling of tissues. *Invariably, he applied his own dressings.* During the procedure, his assistants truly assisted and they always found him sympathetic to their mistakes. Eagerly they would wait until autumn, when Von Langenbeck took his vacation, so that they would have free access to the operating room for their own cases. [8]

After the end of surgery, at 4:30 p.m., he spent the rest of the day either writing or relaxing with friends and family, to whom he was very devoted. His life was singularly free of affectation and eccentricity.

Of the many honors he received, the most meaningful one to him was his 70th birthday celebration—when 16 full professors of surgery who had been either his own assistants or those of his followers gathered in tribute. The students also honored him with a torch-light procession; hundreds of Berlin citizens joined. Soon after that "love fest," Von Langenbeck resigned because of failing vision due to cataracts. He retired to his beautiful villa overlooking Wiesbaden.

In 1881, he returned to London—but on this occasion he was not the unknown young doctor of 45 years before. The reception and honors that England enthusiastically accorded him befitted his international stature. Von Langenbeck nostalgically recalled his earlier trip and his previous good health. "Now I know," he said, "why Cooper complained in his old age." [2]

In 1887, after "an attack of apoplexy," he died. His nation, grateful for his contributions, mourned his death with ceremony and affection.

Von Langenbeck himself furnished his

own *leit motif:* **Nunquam Retrorsum**—
"Never Backwards."

Robert M. Goldwyn, M.D.
1101 Beacon Street
Brookline, Mass. 02146

ACKNOWLEDGMENTS

I am grateful to Mr. Richard J. Wolfe, Rare Books Librarian of the Countway Library of Medicine, and to his staff, for their cheerful and extensive help. I wish also to thank Mr. Thomas Smith, Tufts University School of Medicine, for his excellent translation of German sources.

REFERENCES

1. Platt, W. B.: Baron Von Langenbeck, surgeon-general of the German army, professor of surgery in the University of Berlin. Johns Hopkins Hosp. Bull., *40:* 62–64, 1894.
2. Bergmann, E.: Zur Erinnerung an Bernhard v. Langenbeck. Verhandlung. der Deutsche Gesellsch. f. Chir., *17:* 1–24, 1888.
3. Billroth, T. B.: Von Langenbeck. Wien. Med. Woch., *37:* 1353–1356, 1887.
4. Bernhard von Langenbeck (1810–1887), German surgeon. Editorial, J.A.M.A., *200:* 1124–1125, 1967.
5. Korting: Bernhard v. Langenbeck. Deutsche Militararzt. Zeitschr., *16:* 465–474, 1887.
6. Rehn, L.: Die Gedachtnisrede zum andenken an den 100. Geburtstag B. von Langenbeck. Arch. f. klin. Chir., *95:* 743–758, 1911.
7. Personal reminiscenses of the late Professor Von Langenbeck. Lancet, *2:* 828–830, 1887.
8. Trendelenburg, F.: Erinnerungen an Bernhard v. Langenbeck. Deutsche Med. Woch., *28:* 233–236, 1902.
9. Dorrance, G.: *The Operative Story of Cleft Palate,* p. 7. W. B. Saunders Company, Philadelphia, 1933.
10. Goldwyn, R. M.: Johann Friedrich Dieffenbach (1794–1847). Plast. & Reconstr. Surg., *42:* 18–28, 1968.
11. Professor Langenbeck on uranoplastics. Med. Times & Gaz., *2:* 69–70, 1861.
12. Langenbeck, B.: On uranoplastics (a letter). Med. Times & Gaz., *1:* 44, 1862.
13. Hirsch, A. (ed.): *Biographisches Lexikon der hervorragenden Ärzte Aller Zeiten und Volker,* ed. 2, vol. 3, pp. 669–671. Urban & Schwarzenberg, Berlin, 1931.

JONATHAN MASON WARREN AND HIS CONTRIBUTIONS
TO PLASTIC SURGERY

ROBERT M. GOLDWYN, M.D.*

Boston, Massachusetts

The year of Jonathan Mason Warren's birth, 1811, James Madison was president of the United States; Napoleon was secure in his reign; and America was about to enter another war with Great Britain. World events were undoubtedly known and discussed by the Warren family, who occupied a patrician position in Colonial America.[1, 2] Jonathan's grandfather, John Warren (1753–1815), had offered his surgical services to George Washington's army and later became the first Professor of Anatomy and Surgery at Harvard College. He was also the first surgeon in America to perform a disarticulation of the shoulder and was among the first to do a successful laparotomy.

Jonathan Warren's great uncle, General Joseph Warren (1741–1775), was also a physician. It was he who sent Paul Revere and William Dawes on their celebrated ride to Concord and Lexington. Two months later, Joseph Warren died at the Battle of Bunker Hill.

Jonathan's father, John Collins Warren (1778–1856), was an eminent surgeon who, like his father, was also a Professor of Surgery at Harvard Medical School and helped to found the Massachusetts General Hospital, the American Medical Association and the *New England Journal of Medicine*, then called the *New England Medical Journal*.[3]

The direction of Jonathan Warren's life was obviously ordained by his unique environment. His education was that of many of his own socioeconomic position: Boston Latin School, private tutorship, then Harvard College, which he entered in 1827.

Never as robust as most of the Warrens, he was forced to interrupt his studies because of his "delicate constitution."[4] After a voyage to Cuba and a quiet summer in Rhode Island with his grandfather, then governor, he began his medical career as an apprentice to his father, who instructed private students in his own home, as was the custom. Jonathan Warren (or Mason as he was called) enrolled in Harvard Medical School in 1830. Two years later he graduated. Recognizing the limitations of American medical training, Mason's father urged him to observe and study in Europe as he himself had done 30 years before. The unpublished notebooks[5] of Mason's 3 years abroad provide fascinating commentaries and unique anecdotes about some of the great European physicians of the late eighteenth and early nineteenth centuries: Bell, Brodie, Bright, Astley Cooper, Denonvilliers, Hodgkins, Lisfranc, Magendie, Marjolin, Roux, Travers and Velpeau. Larrey, formerly Napoleon's Surgeon-in-Chief, was then 67. Warren wrote:

It would not do to leave Paris without referring to that splendid surgeon—Baron Larrey with his long long, grey curling locks and his Napoleonic costume going round his wards at the Hotel des Invalides & attending his old soldiers. His courteous manners made him a friend of all students who visited there. His particular forte at that moment was the use of the actual cautery in many diseases and most especially its application to the back of the neck with the cure of incipient carbuncle. Generally attended in the wards by a small wagon carring a portable furnace—on the slightest occasion, he would withdraw a red and white hot iron according to the circumstance and apply it without hesitation..."[5]

Of Dupuytren, he had much to say:

The celebrated Dupuytren was at this time at the zenith of his fame. He was the best lecturer and

* Assoc. Prof. of Surgery, Harvard Medical School; Attending in Surgery, Peter Bent Brigham Hospital; Chief of Plastic Surgery, Beth Israel Hospital.

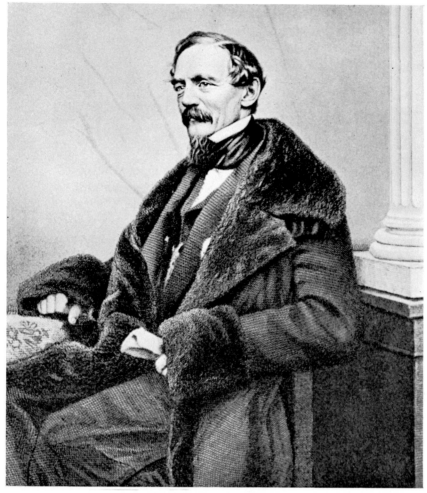

JONATHAN MASON WARREN
at age 46
(From an engraving)

though perhaps appropriating to himself the labors of others to which he gave his name, (he) brought forward many new discoveries in surgery ... Dupuytren, though a lion at heart, spoke the French language with a slow and musical diction and addressed his patients in the most endearing terms; at the same time, if irritated by his interns through any deficiency of their work ... did not fail to lash out ... like a wild horse ... For brutality, I do not think his equal can be found. If his orders are not immediately obeyed, he makes nothing of striking his patient and abusing him harshly. A favorite practice of his is to make a handle of a man's nose, seizing him by it and pulling him down on his knees, where he remains, half in sorrow, half in anger, until he is allowed to rise and describe his symptoms ... His operations

are always brilliant, and his diagnosis sometimes most extraordinary. He is one of the most suspicious persons I ever encountered. He is continually seeking to convince us that he is a great man, and that we do not sufficiently value his talents. He likes much to make a show, and generally talks during the whole operation." [5,6]

Before leaving Paris, Mason took a course in midwifery, and soon after his return to Boston in 1835, he entered his father's extensive practice. In 1839, he married Anne Crowninshield, whose father had been Madison's Secretary of the Navy.

Mason Warren's interest in reconstructive surgery was stimulated by his father's work in this area and by his contacts with Dieffen-bach and Roux while he was in Paris. Earlier, in 1828, Mason's father, John Collins Warren, had published a description of "an operation that he performed in 1819 for the cure of natural fissure of the soft palate." [7] In this paper, he wrote that he had heard of cleft palate operations being done "in Poland and Germany" and by Professor Roux but he "sought in vain for details of it." John Warren then described removing a tumor from the soft palate of a woman and subsequently closing the defect. Other early accounts of staphylorrhaphy in America were by Nathan Smith[8] of Connecticut in 1826, Alexander Stevens[9] of New York in 1827, John Mettauer[10] of Virginia in 1837 and Mason Warren[11] in 1840. This was Warren's first publication in plastic surgery and it dealt principally with methods of nasal reconstruction by the "Taliacotian operation" and the forehead flap. However, it did include a brief report about closing a cleft of *both* the soft and the hard palate.

In describing his use of Tagliacozzi's flap, he noted that the "operation was not precisely that recommended by the Italian surgeon." The lower forearm was the donor site in Warren's procedure. "The transplanted skin was separated from its connection— . . . on the 5th instead of the 14th or 15th day."—incidentally, without loss. This remarkable article contains also a description of a successful skin graft (full thickness), thus antedating the work of Wolfe[12] in 1875 and Krause[13] in 1893. Warren's concept of transplanting skin preceded the accounts of Reverdin (1869),[14] Ollier (1872)[15] and Thiersch (1886),[16] who had all utilized split-thickness skin. A patient whose nose had been restored by the Italian method presented the occasion for the skin graft.

> . . . the patient having exposed himself to the sun during a walk out of town, experienced considerable itching in the right ala of the nose where, it will be remembered there was a slight redness remaining. He came to me, very desirous to have the skin of this part at once removed because he greatly feared that he might be troubled with it

hereafter. He was also anxious that the experiment should be tried of cutting a piece of skin from the arm and immediately placing it in the wound to supply the loss of substance. Although I did not consider this part of the operation necessary, as the wound, in all probability, would have filled up by the granulating process, I yielded to his desire and made the attempt. The skin covering the ala nasi was removed so as to leave no appearance of redness remaining, and a piece of skin being immediately resected fore arm, was confined in the wound by means of lint moistened in blood, which answered a much better purpose than the common adhesive plaster. On removing the dressing, at the end of 4 days, a perfect union was found to have taken place.[11]

Later in that same account, Warren gives his opinion of autoplastic operations:

> Autoplastic operations for the restoration of parts that have been lost either by disease or from accident, are now attracting much attention both at home and abroad, and they may be had recourse to in a number of cases which previously had been given up as wholly incurable. It would be going too far beyond the limits of this paper to mention all the cases to which these operations might be applied; we therefore refer to a few only. Among the most important of these, may be instanced that the operations for restoring the lower lip and the eyelid after the ablation of cancerous tumors, frequently practised by Dieffenbach; and in cases of fistulous openings of the larynx and trachea, of the vagina and urethra, cases where the mere bringing the parts together, or making raw their surfaces, as in the hare-lip operation, almost invariably fails in performing a cure. The autoplastic method which has been most generally adopted as applicable to these cases, is that in which the flap required is taken in the immediate neighborhood of the part destroyed, slid along, and confined in the desired situation by the twisted suture. This has been called, by the French, *"autoplastie par glissement du lambeau."*[11]

He then described the use of a nasolabial flap to restore the ala nasi and advancement flaps to close a "congenital fissure of both the hard and soft palate" in a young man, 24 years of age, whose speech was "so much affected by this unfortunate conformation as to make it scarcely intelligible. . .

The operation was commenced by making raw the edges of the soft palate, after the method usually employed in cases of staphalorrhaphy, and three points of suture [silk previously soaked in tincture of benzoin] introduced. The mucous membrane covering the roof of the mouth was then carefully raised on each side of the fissure in the hard palate, brought across this opening, and confined by means of the interrupted suture. The flap formed by the mucous membrane of the mouth, it should be understood, was continuous with that of the soft palate. A firm union took place throughout the whole extent, with the exception of a small portion at its upper angle; the suture being torn away at this point on the 3rd day succeeding the operation, from violent efforts at coughing.[11]

For handling postoperative fistulae, he suggested the application of a caustic (cantharide, silver nitrate, sulfuric acid) and the insertion of an obturator or a simple prosthesis:

The small aperture remaining in the hard palate was closed in this, as in most of the cases where I had found it necessary, by a bit of India-rubber, as recommended by Dieffenbach. Two portions of Goodyear's patent India-rubber may be cut a little larger than the aperature to be closed; they are stitched together in the center: one portion is slipped into the nasal aperature, it keeps the second in the mouth in place. It can be removed and replaced at the pleasure of the wearer. Everything being accomplished, my patient departed to the West to seek his fortune, with a new palate, a new lip, and as good as a new nasal ornament.[17]

Warren's closure of complete clefts of the palate went an important step beyond what he had seen Roux do in dealing with only soft palate defects. Although postoperative fistulae were frequent, he had only one complete dehiscence in 23 or 24 operations for complete clefts.[17] Because of his competence in this area of surgery, many patients were referred to him from all parts of America. He is known to have treated surgically over 100 clefts.[18] In 1863, summarizing his experience,[18] he noted that 90 per cent of the clefts that he saw were complete. He always avoided the use of general anesthesia because of danger to the unconscious patient from "the constant flow of blood down the throat." Since he had to depend upon the cooperation of an awake patient, he deferred his palatoplasty until the child was at least 6 years old. To obtain relaxation of the tissues and to

eliminate the "violent muscular contractions which cause so much trouble in the performance of the operation in the soft palate," he transversely divided the "posterior pillar of the palate made up chiefly of the palatopharyngeus muscle." He did not employ lateral, releasing incisions. In answering the question of whether the voice will be "immediately restored by operation" Warren stated that time is required for the patient to learn "the art of using the palate in articulation." However, he wrote, "I do not remember to have seen a case in which the patient was not benefited."[18]

In 1846, at age 35, he was appointed Visiting Surgeon to the Massachusetts General Hospital. Later that year, he became involved in a major event of medical history.

In the autumn of 1846, Dr. W. T. G. Morton, a dentist in Boston, a person of great ingenuity, patience, and pertinacity of purpose, called on me several times to show some of his inventions.[19]

Having recognized the potential of Morton's discovery, Mason Warren urged his father to see him.

Dr. Morton . . . visited him, and informed him that he was in possession of, or had discovered, a means of preventing pain, which he had proved in dental operations and wished Dr. Warren to give him an opportunity of trying it in a surgical operation.[18]

With Morton administering ether and Mason Warren as his assistant, Dr. John C. Warren painlessly removed a "vascular tumor from the neck of the patient and surgical anesthesia was thereby introduced."[19] Mason Warren also wrote

There are many cases, however, especially minor operations which present themselves at the house of the surgeon, which scarcely authorize the disturbance of the system or delay which administration of ether would require. For these, local anesthesia is a great value—ice and salt.[20]

Dr. Warren participated in early activities of the American Medical Association and, in 1853, while on a train returning from a New York meeting, was in an accident which led to the death of 60 persons. He aided the injured and his son noted that "the strain of the events of this day bore heavily upon him for many years afterward." [4] He became sufficiently depressed to leave for Europe and spent several months there with his family. After his father's death in 1856, his duties became much greater. From his writings, one senses that his confidence in his own capabilities grew significantly in the absence of his stern and internationally prominent father.

During the Civil War, Mason Warren treated many of the injured at the Massachusetts General Hospital. From these cases, and the experience of 30 years in practice he published in 1867 his *Surgical Observations with Cases.* His son, John Collins Warren, who also became an eminent surgeon, wrote:

This was literally a last word on the surgery of that period and has lasting especial interest from an historical point of view for it marks the close of an era of surgery as Lister's antiseptic system was already in the making.[4]

In that book, Mason Warren presented his cases succinctly, thoroughly and honestly. Of particular relevance to the plastic surgeon are his accounts of rhinoplastic operations (four head and two arm flaps), restoration of the lower eyelids by rotation and advancement flaps following excision of tumors, release of scar contractures, procedures for excision of "epithelial cancers and rodent ulcers" of the skin and lips (over 100 cases) and removal of extensive tumors of the sinuses, tongue, the mandible and the maxilla, as well as of the parotid gland. When possible, he advised preservation of the facial nerve. Warren devoted 17 pages to repair of the "hare-lip." Concerning the cleft lip, Warren stated:

It is of much importance for the future appearance, even for the health, of the child, that this operation should be well done, and the proper time selected for it. I have performed it, with success, as early as 7 hours after birth; and its early performance was advocated by my grandfather, Dr. John Warren . . . On the whole, after

much experience, I should advise the age of 3 or 4 months, just previous to teething, and after the tissues have acquired sufficient firmness, as the best age to select. For many years, I have advocated nursing immediately after the operation, and while union is still going on . . . The muscular action of the lip, induced by nursing, rather favors the coaptation than the separation of the edges of the wound, though formerly the contrary was supposed. I am convinced that sutures are much preferable to needles, no matter how wide the separation, and consequently great the attention required to bring the parts into contact. They had these advantages: First, they are more easily introduced; second they produce less irritation; and, third, they can generally be removed at the exploration of forty-eight, or, at the most, of seventy-two hours without danger of disturbing the tender adhesions. On the other hand, if needles are used, they must be left until they are sufficiently loosened by ulceration, otherwise there is great danger of tearing open the wound . . . In regard to the method for avoiding the irregularity which so often takes place where the edges of the lip are brought together, I should say (having tried the various means that have been suggested by cutting the edges of the lip irregularly), that the only sure way is to remove a liberal portion of the margin of the fissure and beyond the red border just before it begins to curve upwards . . . [21]

In double hare-lip, complicated with a fissure in the bones, and a projecting tubucle I have preferred to operate on one side of the lip, and allow it to heal before operating on the other . . . When I have attempted both at the same time, and in fact, in almost every instance I have witnessed, a fistula has been the result, the tissue being too much stretched, and the inflammation becoming suppurative. By the preceding method one side has generally united, and, if left for a month before second operation, the protuberant intermaxillary bone will be found more or less dragged into place.[17]

Mason Warren also attempted to do something about the deformity following closure of a cleft lip.

The base of the opening of the nostrils was expanded, a flaring, and an aperature, an inch and a half long, existed between the jaw and lip, allowing a communication at that point. All these were remedied. The patient having complained that the tip of the nose was too broad, at his earnest request, I dissected the skin forming the septum from it in a pyramidal shape, elevated the tip, brought the cut surfaces in contact, re-applied the pedicle underneath, and then accomplished the object.[17]

Concerning the problem of the deviated septum, Warren wrote:

We seldom observe in books on surgery any reference to the question of the treatment of this affection; it being principally noticed in connection with the differential diagnosis of polypus and mucous thickening of the nasal cavities. It is, however, an affection of some importance, and one in consequence of which patients often apply for treatment. It would be supposed, that what is lost in freedom of respiration by the obstruction of one side would be made up on the other; but this is not the case.[22]

His method of treatment was bouginage, forcible when required, for "several days in succession," [22] and then instructing the patient to do it himself daily at home.

Mason Warren's interest in relieving congenital deformities extended to syndactyly.

. . . I was requested, in October of 1857, to see a child, who had been born a few days before with an intimate union of the middle and ring fingers of each hand . . . The conjoint finger of each hand had but a single nail, somewhat elongated on one hand, and showing a slight disposition to break-up into two. No fissure or depression could be distinguished marking the distinction between the two fingers, as may be observed in what is called webbed fingers. The finger was susceptible to flexion and extension; but no appearance of separate joints could be observed, or separate boney structure: in fact there was apparently but one finger in place of two. I therefore advised that the operation should be delayed, to afford sufficient time for the development of the different organs; . . . at the end of six months, the boney structure, joints, and other textures, were sufficiently developed to show the elements of two fingers in the mass, and warrant the attempt at an operation with a reasonable chance of separating them, without cutting into the joints, and producing stiffness or anchylosis . . . The child being etherized, the ends of the fingers, where the boney structures seemed to be united, were separated up to the first joint, by the cutting pliers. A careful dissection then separated the fingers, fortunately without entering the joints, except possibly the last joint of one finger and one hand, which might have been opened; but this was doubtful, not at all indicated by the subsequent progress of the case. The dissection was carried rather farther towards the hand than natural division, in fact

nearly down to the first knuckle joint, in order to allow for a certain amount of adhesion or contraction, which it was thought no art or labor would be able to prevent. It was then attempted, at the angle and sides of the finger, to bring the skin on the back and the palm of the hand in contact by means of sutures. This was effected, but with great strain on the integuments, on account of the thickness of the parts. A long piece of adhesive plaster was placed between the two fingers, and made to exert as great a pressure as possible on the angle of the wound. . . . The cicatrix, which extended from the angle of the fingers upwards on each side, had a tendency to contract, and curl the fingers inwards; and this, rather than the disposition of the fingers to again unite, was the principal point which required attention towards the end of the treatment. It was thought useless, at the early age of the patient, to attempt any mechanical means to obviate this contraction, which was counteracted by the constant attention of the mother, in soaking, and forcibly bending them out. The result of the operation was, in place of a very great deformity, to restore the hand to a useful condition, and to an appearance which would pass without remark.[23]

Warren also stated that he removed on several occasions supernumerary fingers and "invariably" had "good results."

The year that this book *Surgical Observations with Cases* appeared, 1867, Mason Warren died. Eight weeks before, he had written in his journal: "During the last four months have performed ninety operations at the hospital and thirty private ones." This he did despite the pain of a progressive gastrointestinal malignancy.

Oliver Wendell Holmes, a life-long friend who had been with him when they were both students abroad said,

In Paris, in London, wherever we found ourselves, he never for a moment lost sight of his great object, to qualify himself for that conspicuous place as a surgeon which was marked for him by the name that he bore and the conditions to which he was born. This was his constant aim in the hospitals which he assiduously followed, in the museums which he faithfully explored, and in the society of the distinguished practitioners to whom he had access and to whom he often introduced his less fortunate friends. We who know this laborious man, loved him, because he was good and natural in all his ways. I do not remember that any of us, even though we travelled with him, ever had a hard word with him.

One of his patients, the poet Henry Wadsworth Longfellow, told Mason Warren's father:

Truly it may be said of him that he has a high degree, 'the eagle's eye, the woman's hand'! I know he needs no commendation of mine but it is so pleasant for me to say it. I trust it will not be unpleasant to you to hear it.[4]

Jonathan Mason Warren's position in the history of medicine has generally been overlooked. Perhaps this is due to his having been the son and grandson as well as the father of illustrious surgeons. Yet by his own accomplishments, Mason Warren should stand alone. His contributions were more than isolated surgical feats.

Systematically, he explored the possibilities of reconstructive surgery. Through his techniques and writings and his prominence in American medicine, he made his profession aware of what this kind of surgery could offer the patient.

Acknowledgments. I am grateful to Dr. Richard Warren for his helpful criticisms and suggestions and to Dr. Joseph E. Murray for his careful reading of the manuscript. I wish also to thank Mr. Richard J. Wolfe, Rare Books Librarian, and his staff at the Countway Library of Medicine for their diligence and patience in locating sources, both unpublished and published.

Robert M. Goldwyn, M.D.
1101 Beacon Street
Brookline, Massachusetts 02146

REFERENCES

1. Stalker, H.: The Warrens of New England and their friends. New England J. Med., *222:* 517–529, 1940.

2. Cheever, D.: The Warren stock and some of its scions. New England J. Med., *200:* 857–863, 1929.

3. Warren, E.: *Life of John Collins Warren: Compiled Chiefly from Autobiography and Journals,* 2 vol. Ticknor and Fields, Boston, 1860.

4. Warren, J. C.: Jonathan Mason Warren. Surg. Gynec. & Obst.; *44:* 273–279, 1927.

5. Warren, J. M.: Clinical surgery in Europe 1834–35. Unpublished Warren Collection, Countway Library, Harvard Medical School, Cambridge, Mass.

6. Arnold, H. O.: *Memoir of Jonathan Mason Warren, M.D.,* p. 85–86. University Press: John Wilson and Son, Cambridge, Mass., 1886. (printed for private distribution)

7. Warren, J. C.: On an operation for the cure of natural fissure of the soft palate. Am. J. M. Sc., *3:* 1–3, 1828.

8. Smith, N. : Suture of the palate. Am. M. Rev., *3:* 396, 1826.

9. Stevens, A. H.: Staphyloraphe, or palate suture, successfully performed. North American M & S. J., *3:* 233–236, 1827.

10. Mettauer, J. P.: On staphyloraphe. Am. J. M. Sc., *21:* 309–332, 1837.

11. Warren, J. M.: Taliacotian operation. Boston M. & S. J., *22:* 261–269, 1840.

12. Wolfe, J. R.: A new method of performing plastic operations. Brit. M. J., *2:* 360–361, 1875.

13. Krause, F.: Ueber die Transplantation Grosser, Ungestielter Hautlappen. Arch. klin. Chir., *46:* 177–182, 1893.

14. Reverdin, J. L.: Greffe epidermique. Bull. Soc. chir., *10:* 493, 1869.

15. Ollier, L.: Greffes cutanes ou autoplastiques. Bull. Acad. Nat. Méd., *1:* 243–250, 1872.

16. Thiersch, C.: Ueber Hautverpflanzung. Verhandl. deutsch. Gesellsch. Chir., *15:* Part I: 17–19, 1886.

17. Warren, J. M.: Operation for fissure of the soft and hard palate, with the result of twenty-four cases. Am. J. M. Sc., *15:* 329–338, 1848.

18. Warren, J. M.: On operations for cleft palate. Am. J. M. Sc., *46:* (new series) 305–313, 1863.

19. Warren, J. M.: *Surgical Observations with Cases and Operations,* p. 614–615. Ticknor and Fields, Boston, 1867.

20. Idem. p. 621.

21. Idem. pp. 143–144.

22. Idem. pp. 62–63.

23. Idem. p. 609.

GEORGE H. MONKS, M.D.: A NEGLECTED INNOVATOR

ROBERT M. GOLDWYN, M.D.

Brookline, Mass.

George Howard Monks, who was born in 1853 and died in 1933, witnessed the rapid development of present-day surgery and contributed to its growth.

The place of his birth was South Boston, where his father, an Irish immigrant, had established a successful lumber business. George Monks was one of 5 children, born after his father, a widower, had remarried. In an unpublished autobiography, Monks wrote: "We were a very united family with few disagreements." [1] When he was 6, his father died and his mother assumed an even more important role in his upbringing. An able painter, singer, and musician, she stimulated his artistic talents.

"...she was passionately fond of beauty and art in all its forms...," he wrote. [1]

Monks attended Boston Latin School and entered Harvard College in 1871. He was active in the Hasty Pudding Club and made posters for its theatrical performances. He participated also in chess and crew. After graduation, in 1875, he went to Europe for several months. His most memorable experience was a night visit to the London slums and, in particular, to an opium den. He encountered an elderly addict who told him that Dickens had depicted her as Sallie in *The Mystery of Edwin Drood*.

After having returned to Boston, he studied architecture for a year at the Massachusetts Institute of Technology, which had been founded just a decade before. A growing interest in medicine led him to leave MIT to enter Harvard Medical School. Monks was especially fond of anatomy—doubtless due, in part, to his unique teacher, Dr. Oliver Wendell Holmes. Monks later published Holmes' medical sayings and writings:

"In the course of his demonstration of the female pelvis, he, at one stage, held it aloft, and pointing to the pubic arch, announced with dignified emphasis: 'Gentlemen! this is the arch underneath which every youthful candidate for immortality has to pass!'" [2]

In the physiology course given by Dr. Henry P. Bowditch, Monks made a model of the larynx which Bowditch then duplicated for future classes. Like most medical students, Monks was aware of the trivia he was forced to master. He recalled having to learn that a certain poison "smelled like mice's feet." However, he was grateful for the "excellent instruction" from his professors, all of whom, he noted, were Bostonians.

The next step in his medical career was becoming a surgical house officer at the Massachusetts General Hospital. At that time, there were only 4 surgical interns. Henry J. Bigelow, noted for his procedures dealing with bladder calculi and hip dislocations, was the Professor of Surgery and contributed significantly to Monks' training. [3] Following his internship, Monks went to Europe for further study in medicine and surgery and remained 4 years. He visited Vienna, Dresden, Heidelberg, Leipzig, Paris, and London. Comparing the study of anatomy in England and in America, he wrote:

"There appears no valid reason why the English student should be better prepared in anatomy than the American, but such is without the slightest doubt the case. It may be said that only a small amount of the practical and anatomical knowledge possessed by American surgeons has

From the Department of Surgery (Plastic Surgery) of the Harvard Medical School, Peter Bent Brigham Hospital, and Beth Israel Hospital.

been acquired from the regular course at a medical school. How much time would have been saved had it been otherwise."[4]

After securing his degree from the Royal College of Surgeons in 1884, Monks returned to Boston and opened an office for the practice of medicine. He later specialized in surgery following an appointment to the Boston Dispensary. As an extra activity, he lectured to the YMCA about the emergency care of the injured. In his autobiography, he recalled this incident:

"...I walked out on the stage, faced the audience, made my bow and began my lecture. After a few words about anatomy in general, I approached the skeleton with the idea of illustrating some point I was making. I pulled off the sheet, and turning again to the audience, continued to talk. It was far from reassuring to notice...that everyone was smiling—a smile which soon broadened into a loud laugh! Turning again to the skeleton, I noticed that it was spinning around very fast, with arms and legs extended. I then realized, of course, that someone as a joke had previously twisted the cord; ...removal of the sheet started the rotation of the skeleton whose feet did not touch the floor and this rotation increased in velocity...more and more...I thought that it would soon stop, and so I waited. Imagine my disgust after the skeleton finally stopped, to see it begin to spin in the opposite direction. This process of twisting and untwisting continued until finally the dizzy skeleton came to rest, and allowed the disconcerted lecturer an opportunity to proceed with his remarks..."[1]

Because of his knowledge of anatomy and his competence as a sculptor (Figs. 3, 4), he was asked to lecture in anatomy at the Boston Museum School of Fine Arts. His surgical abilities won further recognition when he was appointed to the staff of the Boston City Hospital, where he eventually became Surgeon in Chief in 1910, serving 4 years.

At the age of 44 he married Olga Gardner, the niece of Boston's Isabella Stewart Gardner, art patron and philanthropist, famous for her eccentricities and *beaux gestes*. In her biography of "Mrs. Jack," Louise Tharp mentions that Monks had been considered such "an unflinching advocate of bachelorhood that he was long given up by scheming mammas...He was a leading light at the Tavern Club, very popular with both men and women and a right good fellow."[5]

Dr. Monks and his bride went to Europe for a few months and then began housekeeping on Beacon Street. Their marriage, a long and happy one, produced two sons and a daughter. One son, John Peabody Monks, an internist at the Massachusetts General Hospital, has since died.

George Monks was appointed prosector and lecturer in operative surgery at the Harvard Medical School (Fig. 1). His cadaver demonstrations were famous for being thorough but not boring.

For 40 years, he taught surgical pathology and surgery at the Harvard Dental School; he was Professor of Oral Surgery from 1910 to 1926. Hapgood, in his *History of the Harvard Dental School,* characterized Monks as "a most valuable member of the faculty from other than educational standpoints. Owing to the fact that he held a medical rather than a dental degree, he served in a double capacity as a liaison officer on medical and dental faculties. He brought a sound medical point of view to the administration of dental school problems, and his great interest in dentistry materially furthered his interests with the ruling powers of the medical faculty."[6]

Monks' contemporaries noted that he always had "an unruffled manner." Nevertheless, he accomplished a great deal throughout his life. He published 55 papers of wide range: rupture of the biceps tendon,[7] carcinoma of the appendix,[8] fractures of the humerus,[9] abdominal trauma,[10] acute pancreatitis,[11] aseptic surgical technique,[12] hip dislocation,[13, 14] finger avulsion,[15] a method of

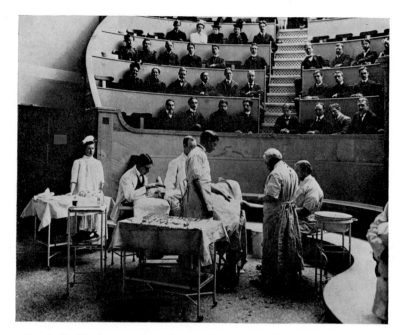

FIG. 1. Dr. Monks operating (*photograph, courtesy of Dr. V. H. Kazanjian*).

one-handed knot tying,[16] the use of the magnetic needle locator,[17] and even a way to prevent thumb-sucking in children.[18] All of these, in addition to his contributions in plastic and reconstructive surgery, will be discussed later.

The work that Monks considered to be his most important was his investigation of "intestinal localization"—". . . the determination . . . in certain abdominal operations, as to what part of the intestinal tube any given loop of it occupies (*i.e.* its 'position'); and, incidentally, as to which end of the loop is nearest to the duodenum, and which to the ileocaecal valve (*i.e.* its 'direction')." [19] When presented in 1903, his ideas created sufficient enthusiasm to result in his giving the Mutter lecture at the College of Physicians in Philadelphia the following year.

George Monks' activities in plastic and reconstructive surgery were partly the result of his interest in the head and neck from the esthetic, as well as the surgical, point of view. He made an extensive col-lection of photographs and drawings of friends and patients who illustrated various types of facial expression. In addition, he was challenged by the new field of surgical rehabilitation. His extensive knowledge and his uncommon talent for invention helped him considerably. His article "Correction, by Operation, of Some Nasal Deformities and Disfigurements," which appeared in 1898,[20] may be found on page 156 of this book. Since this paper summarized several years of work, it would be useful to trace his efforts chronologically.

His earliest article dealing with restorative surgery concerned "enormous hypertrophy of the nose." [21] In 1890, he presented a patient with this condition to a district medical meeting. His audience was pleased with what they called ". . . a very successful, and more than that—a wonderful result. . . ." [21] His methods of treatment are used today (see reprint).

In 1891, Monks published an article concerning the correction of "the deformity due to prominent ears." [22] He began by stating:

> "I do not propose . . . to discuss the question as to the desirability of doing an operation for the correction of this deformity; but shall assume that any operation, at once simple and safe, which bids fair to accomplish this result, is justifiable."

His first case, a girl, 3 years old, was referred by the prominent neuropsychiatrist, Dr. Morton Prince, his classmate at Boston Latin and at Harvard.[23] Monks first constructed a brass device which fitted the head and held the ears back. "This contrivance was tried faithfully, off and on, for several months; but at the end of this time we could not see any great improvement in the position of the ears."[22]

On the next patient, a man, he excised skin and cartilage through a postauricular incision but did not close the wound primarily. The ear was immobilized in the desired position by a heavy dressing:

> " Although the result in the case of the ear operated upon was all that could have been desired, so far as keeping the auricle back against the head was concerned, yet there were certain features about this operation, which I did not wholly like. There was formed a vertical fold of skin on the front aspect of the ear where the edges of cartilage had been brought together. Though this was not a serious objection, yet the ridge was to a certain extent a disfigurement. Another noticeable feature was that the cartilage required a long time to heal. However, on the whole, I considered the operation a very successful one, . . ."[22]

In 3 other patients, all children, he excised skin alone and reported excellent results but with a follow-up of no longer than 8 months. He concluded that both skin and cartilage should be removed in most adults and in children with stiffer cartilage. He had devised his procedures without being aware of the earlier work of W. W. Keen of Philadelphia and E. T. Ely of New York.

An article by Monks appeared in 1896 recording "A Plastic Operation on the Nose by Tagliacozzi's Method" in a 16-year-old girl whose nose was "very unsightly . . . presumably the result of inherited disease."

> "For twenty-four hours before the operation the left arm was bandaged to the head in such a position that the forearm would touch the nose. The purpose of this was to accustom the girl to the irksomeness of the position."[24]

He used plaster for immobilization and divided his flap on the 23rd day. His reasons for using "this old Italian method of rhinoplasty in place of some of the more modern methods" he stated:

> "I considered the different rhinoplastic operations, where flaps are taken from the forehead, or from the cheeks—but only to discard them . . . The appearance of the nose may be somewhat improved, but at the expense of other and new disfigurements. I was unwilling, for instance, to leave an enormous and unsightly scar upon this young girl's forehead simply for the sake of covering the bridge of the nose. All this inclined me strongly to get the necessary tissue elsewhere in the body—from a part not exposed to view."[24]

Monks also corrected nasal deformities resulting from injury. He used subcutaneous incisions and removed unsightly dorsal humps (see reprint). In addition, he tried implants of celluloid to restore contour.

In 1898, he employed "a new method" for reconstructing a lower eyelid.[25] After having acknowledged his debt to Theodore Dunham, Monks precisely described and illustrated the technique of the scalp island flap. With justifiable satisfaction, he noted that "The eyelid did not slough, but healed kindly in its new bed."[25]

Because of his interest in the larynx, he was referred a patient with a squamous cell carcinoma of the right vocal cord. Monks performed a "unilateral laryngectomy" and reported no recurrence at the end of 3 years.[26, 27] He devised a glass tracheal tube with an inflatable rubber cuff to prevent aspiration. Reporting this case in 1895, Monks wrote:

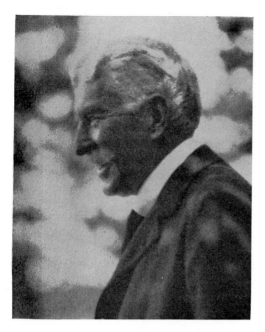

FIG. 2. George Howard Monks (1853–1933).

"The patient ordinarily wears a cork in the outer opening of the tube, so that almost all the air to and from the lungs passes through the mouth. It is extremely interesting to notice how easily the man can talk and make himself understood with only one vocal cord. A few days ago he talked with me over the telephone, and I was able to understand all that he said without the least difficulty." [27]

I have spoken to several people who knew George H. Monks. Uniformly, they recall him as a gentleman, thoroughly versed in his specialty (Fig. 2). Dr. Varaztad H. Kazanjian operated with him often and once was his patient, when Dr. Monks drained his infected finger.[28]

Monks' independent means allowed him to avoid the harried habits of the overburdened practitioner. Yet he was always mindful of his obligations to patients and colleagues. He was a diligent president of the Boston Medical Library

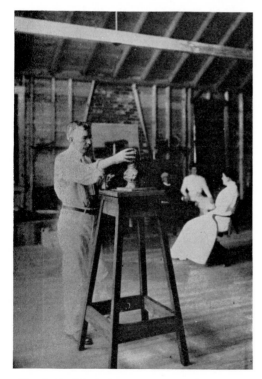

FIG. 3. Dr. Monks in his studio (*from an unpublished autobiography*).

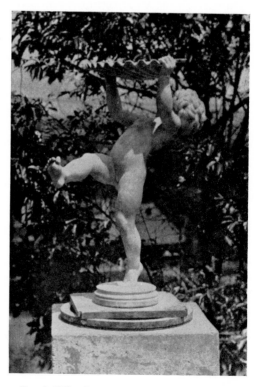

FIG. 4. "The Fountain," by Dr. Monks. This figure was one of his favorite pieces.

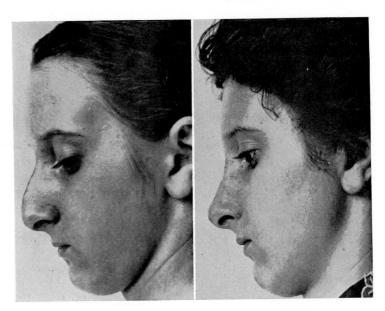

Fig. 5. Patient before and after rhinoplasty (*from Dr. Monks' files*).

and the local medical society; he was vice-president of the American Surgical Association and first president and co-founder of the Boston Surgical Society. He was medical adviser to the Red Cross during World War I, when he was over-age for military service. For many years he was in charge of the Bugle-and-Drum corps of the Boy Scouts.

Next to his profession and family, sculpturing held his allegiance (Figs. 3, 4). He was more than an amateur and several well-executed pieces attest to this proficiency. When he was in Dresden in 1881 he studied with Ernst Hahnel, and in Boston with John Wilson. He exhibited frequently in local art shows.

A surprising facet of Dr. Monks' life was his interest in games. In 1883, while visiting his brother in Normandy and preparing for the examination of the Royal College of Surgeons, he invented "Halma" (Greek "leap"). This game became extremely popular throughout the world and was the forerunner of Chinese checkers.

Monks retired from active practice

(Fig. 5) in 1914 but still lectured at the Harvard Dental School until 1926. During this time, he wrote articles, many of which dealt with prominent surgeons he knew.[29, 31]

He died in 1933 at age 79. The obituaries were noteworthy for mentioning not only his surgical accomplishments but his enviable traits.

"Of high intelligence, high ideals, high standards, curiously unself-conscious, without a trace of timidity, but always modest and self-effacing, he brought a certain fineness of finish to all he did." [32]

"He was one of the most unselfish men who have ever lived. Every instinct was that of a gentleman, and, if I may add, of an artist, and his own profit or advantage was the last thing for which he thought. In personal appearance he was strikingly handsome, nor did his appearance belie his character." [33]

The acceptance of plastic surgery in this country was aided greatly by the work of its productive proponent, George Howard Monks.

Robert M. Goldwyn, M.D.
1101 Beacon Street
Brookline, Mass. 02146

ACKNOWLEDGMENTS

I am very grateful to Dr. George Howard Monks' son, Reverend George Gardner Monks, for generously allowing me the use of his father's papers and unpublished autobiography and for checking my manuscript for inaccuracies.

I am indebted also to Mr. Richard J. Wolfe, Rare Books Librarian, and his staff at the Countway Library of Medicine for their gracious advice and assistance.

REFERENCES

1. Monks, G. H.: *Autobiography* (unpublished).
2. *Idem:* Selections from the medical writings and sayings of Dr. Oliver Wendell Holmes. Boston Med. & Surg. J., *197:* 1385–1394, 1928.
3. *Idem:* Henry Jacob Bigelow: a biographical sketch: Surg. Gynec. & Obst., *39:* 112–116, 1924.
4. *Idem:* The study of anatomy: its position in medical education in England and in America. Boston Med. & Surg. J., *113:* 104–107, 1885.
5. Tharp, L. H.: *Mrs. Jack,* pp. 198–200. Little, Brown & Company, Boston, 1965.
6. Hapgood, R. L.: *History of the Harvard Dental School,* pp. 57–59. Harvard University Dental School, Boston, 1930.
7. Monks, G. H.: Rupture of the long head of the biceps brachii muscle. Boston Med. & Surg. J., *120:* 61–62, 1889.
8. *Idem:* Carcinoma of the appendix vermiformis. Ann. Surg., *48:* 563–564, 1908.
9. *Idem:* A case of fracture of the upper end of the humerus just below the tuberosities, with dislocation of the head of the bone into the axilla. Boston Med. & Surg. J., *134:* 138–139, 1896.
10. *Idem:* A case of stab wound of the abdomen with wound of the intestines, protrusion of intestine through the wound, operation, recovery. Boston Med. & Surg. J., *133:* 87, 1895.
11. *Idem:* A case of acute pancreatitis, and necrosis of fat tissue; laparotomy; drainage; death nine days after the operation; autopsy. Boston Med. & Surg. J., *148:* 86–89, 1903.
12. *Idem:* Aseptic surgical technique. Ann. Surg., *40:* 464–474, 1904.
13. *Idem:* Dislocation of the hip complicated with fracture of the femur: report of two cases. Ann. Surg., *54:* 393–401, 1911.
14. *Idem:* Some practical points in connection with dislocation of the hip, and its reduction by the method of Bigelow. Boston Med. & Surg. J., *164:* 262–264, 1911.
15. *Idem:* Avulsion of the finger, with a case in which this accident occurred to an infant twenty months old. Boston Med. & Surg. J., *144:* 201–203, 1901.
16. *Idem:* Tying the knots of ligatures and sutures with one hand. Ann. Surg., *56:* 780–784, 1912.
17. *Idem:* The use of magnetism for localizing needles in the tissues; with the report of cases. Boston Med. & Surg. J., *173:* 37–42, 1915.
18. *Idem:* A new method for the prevention of thumb-sucking in children. Boston Med. & Surg. J., *135:* 673, 1896.
19. *Idem:* Intestinal localization: a review of certain studies (on the cadaver) in the surgical anatomy of the small intestine and its mesentery. Surg. Gynec. & Obst., *49:* 213–219, 1929.
20. *Idem:* Correction by operation, of some nasal deformities and disfigurements. Boston Med. & Surg. J., *139:* 262–269, 1898.
21. *Idem:* Enormous hypertrophy of the nose: a case presentation. Boston Med. & Surg. J., *123:* 592, 1890.
22. *Idem:* Operations for correcting the deformity due to prominent ears. Boston Med. & Surg. J., *124:* 84–86, 1891.
23. *Idem:* Morton Prince. Harvard Graduates' Mag., *38:* 185–193, 1929.
24. *Idem:* A plastic operation on the nose, by Tagliacozzi's method. Boston Med. & Surg. J., *134:* 643–644, 1896.
25. *Idem:* The restoration of a lower eyelid by a new method. Boston Med. & Surg. J., *139:* 385–387, 1898.
26. *Idem:* Unilateral laryngectomy; a case of excision of the right half of the larynx for carcinoma; recovery; no recurrence at the end of a year. Ann. Surg., *18:* 18–25, 1893.
27. *Idem:* Unilateral laryngectomy for cancer; no recurrence after three years. Ann. Surg., *22:* 785–786, 1895.
28. Kazanjian, V. H.: Personal interview.
29. Monks, G. H.: John Homans. Surg. Gynec. & Obst., *45:* 844–848, 1927.
30. *Idem:* Edward Hickling Bradford. Surg. Gynec. & Obst., *45:* 564–566, 1927.
31. *Idem:* John Collins Warren. Surg. Gynec. & Obst., *53:* 557–560, 1931.
32. Obituary: George Howard Monks, M.D., New England J. Med., *208:* 860–861, 1933.
33. Obituary: George Howard Monks 1853–1933. Tr. Am. S. A., *51:* 528–531, 1933.

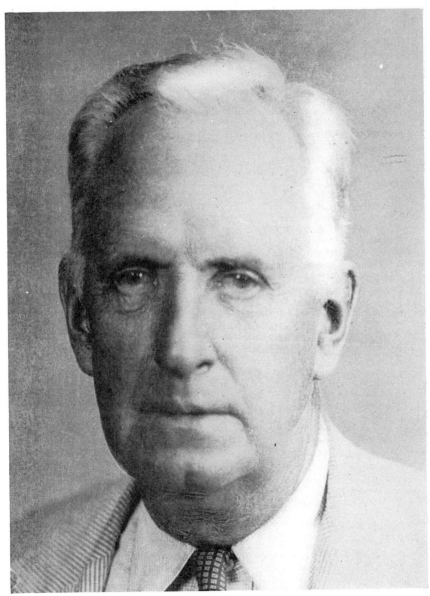

FIG. 1. Dr. Vilray Papin Blair, 1871–1955

VILRAY PAPIN BLAIR, 1871–1955*

JEROME P. WEBSTER, M.D.†

Dr. Vilray Papin Blair, at the age of 84, died on Thanksgiving Day, November 24, 1955 (Fig. 1). He was an Honorary Member of the American Association of Plastic Surgeons. The words he wrote of his teacher and friend, Dr. Elisha Hall Gregory, may well be repeated here for him: "There will be many tributes to his memory, but no matter how talented the orator or silvery the tongue, none will be given with more sincerity than this, that he was a simple man leading a simple life, seeking truth for its own sake, and doing good because it was right (1)."

Vilray Blair was one of the pioneers of plastic surgery in this country. He organized a plastic surgery unit for the U. S. Army in World War I and, almost single-handed, he was responsible for the formation of the American Board of Plastic Surgery, a most potent factor in raising and maintaining high standards in this ancient, but newly recognized, specialty.

Dr. Blair's original American ancestor, Robert Blair, who was born in Ireland in 1683, came to this country and settled in Worcester, Massachusetts in 1718. Two years later he married Miss Isabel Rankin, who lived to the age of 91, on the eve of the Revolutionary War. Dr. Blair, six generations later, was the son of Edmund Harrison Blair and Mary Clementine Papin, a descendant of an old French family which came up from New Orleans as one of the earliest settlers of St. Louis. Her father was Dr. Timothy Loisel Papin, a well known St. Louis gynecologist who had studied in Paris after graduating from the St. Louis Medical School and, in Paris, was an interpreter for the British obstetrician, Sir James Simpson, who was the first to use chloroform in obstetrics. He helped administer this anesthesia for Sir James the first time general anesthesia was given on the Continent.

In 1796 the Spanish Governor of St. Louis, a representative of His Majesty, the King of Spain, granted by royal decree to Marie Louise Papin a farm on the banks of the Rivière des Pères. When the United States purchased the Louisiana Territory, this tract of land, surveyed as Lot No. 378, comprised what is today the choicest residential district of St. Louis.

While Dr. Blair was of a highly distinguished family, his attitude towards his ancestors was not always one of unmitigated veneration. In 1944 a St. Louis art dealer wrote him that there was on exhibit in his New York gallery a portrait of a certain John Blair, painted by Chester Harding. He enclosed a photograph and offered the portrait to Dr. Blair for $3500. Dr. Blair, realizing that he had no American ancestor named John Blair, replied (2) with his typical dry humor:

* Presented at the meeting of the American Association of Plastic Surgeons, Toronto, Canada, May 18, 1956. From the Division of Plastic Surgery, Department of Surgery, Presbyterian Hospital and College of Physicians and Surgeons, Columbia University, New York.

† Consultant, Presbyterian Hospital, and Professor Emeritus of Clinical Surgery, College of Physicians and Surgeons, Columbia University.

I appreciate your writing me about the portrait of John Blair. I am returning the photograph herewith.

Approximately three hundred years ago a man named Blair came from Antrim County in Ireland and settled in New England. He had twelve sons. The particular son I came from died at the age of 92 years from a broken leg which he got while digging post holes! He left 190 descendants, and I think the other eleven did about the same. I just mention this so you will understand why I haven't the least idea who John Blair is. He may possibly come from the Virginia branch of Blairs with which we have no known connection.

Thank you just the same for writing me.

Blair attended Christian Brothers' College, from which he graduated with a B.A. degree in 1890, and from which he received an M.A. degree in 1894. Of this period he wrote in 1940 (3):

At the time I was in school it was largely surrounded by country. . . . I rode horseback out and in from Grand Avenue—to do this was one of the main reasons I was sent out there to school—and on bad snowy days John DeMoss and I would walk from the college to his home. . . . We usually were able to shoot a few birds on the way home.

Young Vilray Blair matriculated at the old St. Louis Medical College, where teaching consisted largely of formal lectures. He claimed that his Gray's Anatomy had been his only medical textbook. He was greatly stimulated by the Professor of Surgery, Dr. Elisha Hall Gregory (1824–1906), who had been Professor of Anatomy from 1852 to 1867. He wrote to Gregory's son (4):

The work in the dissecting room and the late winter afternoons I so commonly spent in your father's sitting room listening to him discourse on surgery are the nearest to formal training that I have ever had in medicine.

After one year at medical school, Dr. Blair spent a year in the Colorado Rockies stringing telephone wires for high potential hydroelectrical installations. Upon returning to St. Louis he wanted to give up medicine and go into the Westinghouse Electrical Engineering School, but was persuaded by his family to return to medical school. Despite his entire year's absence, he obtained his M.D. degree in 1893, three years after his matriculation. This tends to reflect the condition of medical education in this country at that time, and of so-called "diploma-medical schools" which Abraham Flexner corrected by his report for the Carnegie Foundation for the Advancement of Teaching in 1910.

Dr. Blair had his internship at Mullanphy Hospital, where his mentor, Dr. Gregory, was Surgeon in Chief for fifty years. His first teaching post at Washington University was as instructor in practical anatomy, and he taught anatomy as well as surgery for the first eighteen years of his graduate medical career. He introduced the method of teaching anatomy by the use of modeling clay, and this resulted in the publication in 1906 of his first book "A Textbook for the Modeling of Human Bones in Clay (5)." This experience in anatomy gave him the inestimably valuable foundation for the creative surgery that he later performed when he was called upon to do all types of "headache problems" in his surgical work. My medical artist, Mr. Ivan Summers, recalled to me that when he was a young art student working with Dr. Blair on his book "Surgery and Diseases of the Mouth and Jaws" in the spring of 1907, Dr. Blair took him one hot day to the anatomical lab and, while dissecting the trigeminal nerve on a far-gone colored cadaver, happily remarked "There's nothing prettier than dissecting."

Dr. Blair was first associated in practice with Dr. Paul Yoer Tupper (1858–1928), an assistant to Dr. Gregory at the Mullanphy Hospital who later organized and headed the staff of the Missouri Baptist Sanitarium, and in 1892 accepted the chair of anatomy in the Medical Department of Washington University. The story goes that while Blair was an intern with Tupper, he would have his horse and buggy hitched near the corner of Grand and Olive Streets, and would absent-mindedly get in the buggy and try to start off without unhitching the horse. This animal is said to have acquired a wry neck from quizzically turning his head to view the driver. Blair's first paper, "Two Practical Wrinkles in Through-and-Through Drainage (6)," was written as co-author with Tupper and published in 1897. He wrote a moving "In Memoriam" at Dr. Tupper's death in 1928 (7), and in 1948 he wrote to Dr. Gregory's son (8):

You know I started out working for Tupper. Tupper was a mild man, but I think I must have been very trying. For want of real training, I tried to make up by attention, and I "broke flat" in about five years of it, and that's when I went to sea and found out that life was really worth living.

He refers here to an illness that caused him to go to Italy to recuperate. He served for a time on tramp ships in the Mediterranean, and then went up to enter Edinburgh Medical School, where over a century earlier many American doctors received their medical training. The Boer War was in progress, and Blair applied for a place as surgeon on a British ship. As Barney Brooks says (9):

His application was refused because he did not have with him his medical credentials. He was out of money and pawned his watch chain, a family heirloom, for a pound. On his return to Edinburgh, he received a telegram offering him the position of surgeon to a ship sailing to Para. He wired acceptance and went to the Public Library to find in what part of the world Para might be (Fig. 2).

During this South American voyage he traveled 1000 miles up the Amazon and its Negro River branch. He returned to Liverpool with beri-beri, yellow-fever, small-pox and malaria aboard ship, but within three days he had signed for a second voyage, this time for a "three month's cruise to the 'white man's graveyard' ", the Gold and Ivory Coasts of West Africa. In his paper "Some Personal Observations of Malarial and Blackwater Fever on the West Coast of Africa (10)," written for the Medical Society of City Hospital Alumni, Oct. 3, 1901, he presented to his friends and close associates a fascinating description of the experiences that he had as ship surgeon and troop surgeon on this voyage during the Ashanti War. This was in part autobiographical, for he himself came down with malarial fever which he learned to treat with intravenous doses of quinine. He painted a picture of his experiences with strokes that might have come from the pen of Joseph Conrad:

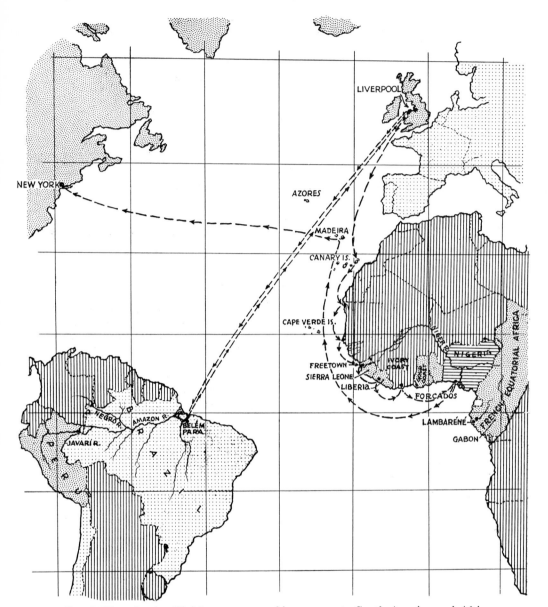

Fig. 2. Map showing Blair's voyages as ship surgeon to South America and Africa

I had not been at sea a month before my curiosity was permanently piqued by the partly fabled, partly true tales of the wealth, the dismal forests, the great rivers, the savagery, the mahogany, the gold and the curios of the surf-bound, fever-stricken west coast of Africa, which has furnished gold, ivory, and slaves to the civilized world from time immemorial; the Phoenicians traded beads for gold, and the Portuguese and Dutch swapped firelocks for human flesh. . . .

I had not only the curiosity of an ordinary traveler, but my opportunities of observation of the fevers of the Javery,* yellow-jack, and beri-beri in the Brazils and leprosy in the islands, had taught me that there were advantages in studying endemic diseases in their native habitat. . . .

The high verdure-covered mountains of the Sierra Leone give place to the low hills and flats of the Liberian and Gold coasts. The delta of the Niger, except by the creeks, is an impenetrable mangrove swamp; while to the south, is a desert as sandy and as arid as Sahara. In places, great salt marshes poison the air with a most sickening stench, while its tracts of dark forests are primeval. In spite of this variety, it presents such an unvarying picture of death and desolation as to bring it all under the one generic term. Throughout its whole extent it is tropical. . . .

On this return trip he had a shipload of soldiers suffering from quartan malaria and other tropical diseases as well as wounds from the battles of Ashanti. He signed off at Madeira and returned to St. Louis at the urging of his family. He was then about thirty years old and, for the second time, this man who was later to become a surgical giant, nearly abandoned the medical profession.

When I came back, he wrote (11), I tried to go in business with my father but he gently "shooed" me out of it, so I went back to try medicine.
I don't know if you remember Willard Bartlett who was a student of Bernays and who spent sufficient time in Germany to get their slant on surgery which was probably the best done, though I preferred the English—I spent some months in the London General Hospital in 1903 which was a seething sea of opportunity, and that kept me from throwing up medicine altogether. I had nerve enough to get married; Kathryn had some income, at the time more than mine. About the time we had four babies and I was beginning to realize that I was not making enough to go around, Bartlett. . . proposed a partnership which to me looked like things that happened in the Old Testament. . . . Kathryn went to her old friend Sluder and he told her it was fine, that it would help Willard and would teach me how to earn a living at surgery, so for five years I "hooked up" with him. We separated perfectly cheerfully and Sluder had had the right slant on it.
I also, through Bartlett, became intimately acquainted with Dr. Will Mayo and visited up there, and when there were 73 applications in the Surgeon General's Office for the job of Head in Plastic Surgery in World War I, he settled the matter by giving it to me.

From 1907 to 1912 he was preparing his classic book "Surgery and Diseases of the Mouth and Jaws," published in 1912 (12). This made an outstanding contribution to the subject and raised Blair's name to the eminence of an authority, so that eventually he was selected by Surgeon General Gorgas to head the Section of Oral and Plastic Surgery in the U. S. Army in this country and to be Chief Consultant in Maxillofacial Surgery with the American Expeditionary Forces during World War I. He wrote of this (13):

Kathryn was nearly crazy because I had been taken into the Army. I went to Ft. Oglethorpe as Captain where I spent a month and would have been there for the whole war except for orders I got to go to Washington where I spent a year trying to build up some framework of an organization; then spent nine

* Javarì (or Yacarana), a branch of the Amazon River forming a part of the border between Brazil and Peru.

months in France and England going around from place to place trying to sell the stuff to the different hospitals, backed with orders signed by Pershing which swept away any difficulties I might otherwise have had. I was taken on General Finney's staff, and Finney was one of the most lovable men I ever knew; he corrected the spelling on all the letters I sent out because the sergeants they gave us were about that kind.

In the preface to his "Plastic Surgery of the Face" (1920), Sir Harold Gillies states that "With the arrival of American surgeons in 1918 under Colonel Vilray P. Blair, M.R.C.,U.S.A., our wounded had call upon surgical skill from the whole Anglo-Saxon race. Each surgeon had the assistance of one or more colleagues from the New World, to their mutual advantage (14)." In his forthcoming work "The Art and Principles of Plastic Surgery (15)," Sir Harold recalls, in speaking of the country estate at Sidcup in Kent where he worked during World War I: "It was on these same lawns that the American plastic team played baseball during their fortnight observation visit with us. Vilray Blair, as I remember, did the major part of the pitching and it is interesting that thirty years later that great man reported his 'Hits, Strikes and Outs' in pedicle flaps (16)."

Blair felt the necessity of utilizing dental surgeons with their knowledge and skill to cooperate with general surgeons in the treatment of soldiers with jaw injuries, particularly Dr. Robert H. Ivy, who had had dental as well as surgical training and had been doing maxillofacial and plastic surgery. Blair's own knowledge of dentistry, the anatomy of the jaws, and the correction of jaw injuries, caused him to be recognized by the dental profession as an expert and to be honored subsequently with the Clinical Professorship of Oral Surgery at Washington University Dental School, in addition to his Clinical Professorship of Surgery in the Medical School.

When he returned to this country he organized several centers for the Army for the treatment of face and jaw injuries with the very valuable assistance of Dr. Ivy. These two men were very closely associated, and in fact Dr. Blair asked Dr. Ivy to work with him in St. Louis, but Dr. Ivy had already accepted a post at the University of Pennsylvania. One of the Army centers organized for the treatment of face and jaw injuries was Jefferson Barracks, outside St. Louis, where Dr. Blair worked personally for several years and was a Consultant for twenty-four years. He was called upon more and more to do operations particularly on the face and jaws for conditions which were really not adequately attacked in civilian practice in this country or elsewhere at that time. This led also to the performance of what Blair laughingly called "beauty surgery," although he was most insistent that he be called a general surgeon and not a plastic surgeon.

When Dr. Evarts Graham was selected as Bixby Professor of Surgery of the Medical Department of Washington University in 1919, four years after the completion of Barnes Hospital, numerous new men were appointed to the rejuvenated staff, but Blair was asked to remain as being a most valuable member of the staff. At this time he began to perform plastic operations almost exclusively, although he was prevailed upon occasionally to perform inguinal herniotomies, thyroidectomies, section of the sensory roots of the trigeminal nerve, radical mastectomies, bladder resections, and a variety of other such operations.

Blair had established a large suite of offices at 400 Metropolitan Building in St. Louis with Dr. Ellis Fischel, and had working with him a series of assistants who later became outstanding plastic surgeons in this country. The first of these was the late Dr. Earl C. Padgett, who subsequently headed the Plastic Surgery Department at the University of Kansas Medical School, and who is today largely known for the Padgett dermatome, which he and the engineer, Hood, devised for the removal of sheets of skin.

Prior to this, more free grafts for the rapid covering of wounds had been used by William S. Halsted and his group in Baltimore than by any other group in this country. These were chiefly small deep grafts, a thicker modification of the Reverdin graft, and the so-called Thiersch grafts, in which sheets of epithelium and upper layers of derma were removed. These grafts were cut by free hand with a long sharp knife from the skin on the outer or inner side of the thigh which was held between two flat surfaces. This was a more or less satisfactory procedure, if the thigh were well covered with muscle and fat, but only narrow strips of skin could be removed if the thigh were thin and wasted away. It was also impossible to take broad sheets of skin from the curved surfaces of the trunk. For a long time, Blair had been thinking of a method to facilitate removal of split skin grafts. At least by 1927, with the aid of a St. Louis instrument maker, he had devised the Blair suction box and the Blair knife (Fig. 3). With the suction box, when it was connected with a negative pressure pipe with an adjustable valve to regulate the pressure, the skin could be drawn up from a thin thigh, abdomen or chest to make these areas available as donor sites.

While I was observing at his clinic from the Fall of 1927 to April of 1928, Blair was undoubtedly still trying to devise a solution to a more mechanical method of cutting large skin grafts. One day, while scrubbing for an operation, dressed in his white shirt and trousers, and old white sneakers, with a gauze swathe tied about his face and head, he walked away from the sink and paced up and down, scrubbing his hands and humming to himself. Suddenly he whirled about and burst out in his high reedy voice: "Webster, did you ever see 'em split leather with a machine?" It was undoubtedly his interest in an invention of this kind that stimulated Padgett to produce the dermatome ten years later. Since that time many types of dermatomes have been devised. Often, when he was operating, he would be mulling over some problem such as this, and might sit there and make as many as ten knots in the horsehair suture he was tying in the skin (Fig. 4).

Dr. James Barrett Brown was another assistant to Blair. In World War II he was Chief Consultant in Plastic and Maxillofacial Surgery in the European Theater of Operations, and later successfully headed the Section of Plastic Surgery at Valley Forge Hospital, where as many as 1800 patients were on his rolls at one time. At present he is Chief Consultant to the U. S. Army in Plastic Surgery. He subsequently succeeded Blair as head of the Clinic.

Another surgeon who trained with Blair and remained on his staff was Dr.

Louis T. Byars, who has been a brilliant disciple and, with Brown, has carried on the tradition started by Blair. For a period of time Dr. William G. Hamm was on Blair's staff. He later moved to Atlanta. Dr. Bradford Cannon, another trainee, who practices plastic surgery in Boston, was also in the Army at Valley

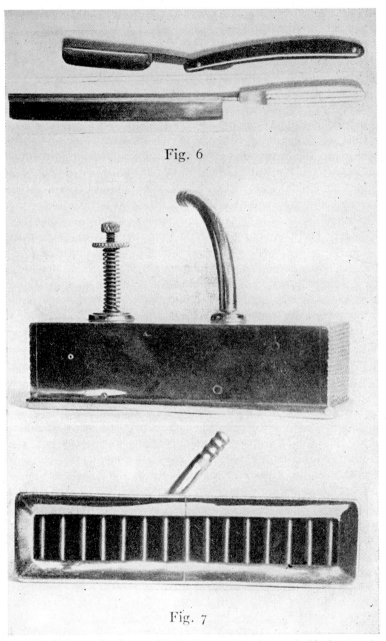

Fig. 6

Fig. 7

FIG. 3. The Blair suction box and knife for cutting sheets of skin by free hand

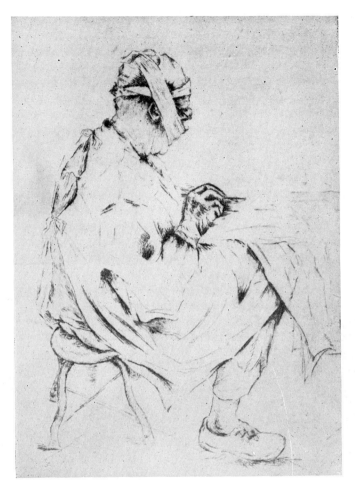

FIG. 4. Sketch of Dr. Blair while operating, by his artist Miss Gertrude Hance

Forge with Barrett Brown. Dr. Frank McDowell, another to start with the "three B's" (Blair, Brown and Byars), has remained as an associate on the staff. Among others who trained with Blair and are practicing independently are Doctors George Kenneth Lewis, Robert R. Robinson, Jr., Bernard Sarnat, Merton T. Hatch and Gordon Letterman. My own debt to Blair is incalculable for the teaching and guidance received from him and his associates while I was observing there before the opening of the Columbia-Presbyterian Medical Center. Most of Blair's trainees who went into plastic surgery have also written extensively and meaningfully in that field.

Dr. Blair was fortunate in 1910 in securing the services of Miss Della O. Cooper, who remained in his office while he was in the Army. After his return she continued the administrative functioning of his large suite of offices, a corps of secretaries, nurses and technicians. Miss Cooper took care of all his appointments and financial arrangements with the help of Miss Caroline Fahrni, who came to the office in 1922 and remained as his personal secretary until 1950. Miss Cooper left the office in 1950 to open and operate a Radium rental agency, but she continued with unstinting and selfless devotion to oversee Dr. Blair's personal affairs, including his complicated menage in the country, until his death. The artist, Miss Gertrude Hance, took photographs of his patients, made plaster casts and prostheses, and made drawings of the various steps of his operations for his numerous publications. She also used electrically driven needles for tattooing the skin, a technic which was first adapted for selected plastic cases at Blair's clinic.

Dr. Blair set up a system of having his chief operating room nurse, Miss Everil McDavitt, make available at a central sterile table in the operating room all the necessary instruments, dressings, etc., for the various types of operation scheduled for the day. From this central position she was able to keep not only one, but two, and sometimes three, operating tables supplied with sterile instruments, dressings and threaded sutures, with no time lost in waiting for special instruments to be boiled. In his operating rooms Blair had the novel idea of decorating the walls with paintings of figures from nursery rhymes for the amusement and edification of his younger patients, and also for adults who might be undergoing operation under local anesthesia (Fig. 5).

Dr. Blair was a member of the American Association of Oral and Plastic Surgeons, which, in 1941, became the American Association of Plastic Surgeons.

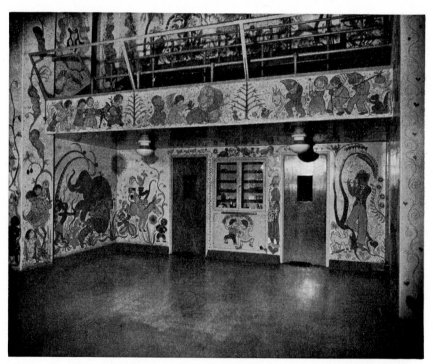

FIG. 5. Dr. Blair's operating room as he had it decorated

When this organization was small and it was possible without undue crowding to visit operating rooms where various members worked, most valuable symposia were held in the late 20's and early 30's on the problems of treatment, first, of cleft palate, and later, of cleft lip. Having had to deal with several late results of the Brophy treatment of wiring the jaws, Dr. Blair was a vociferous exponent of less rough and damaging procedures. The surgical hair, so to speak, was taken down and well shaken out in these small gatherings, and each man expressed himself frankly and without rancor. Blair thought early lip closure brought the premaxilla back. He decried Brophy's method, by which the anterior cleft was readily closed by wires, but the developing tooth buds were so injured as to become malformed or distorted. The procedure also caused such later malformations that the problem of proper occlusion was almost unmanageable. These symposia persuaded Brophy's son-in-law, Dr. William H. G. Logan, whose name is known today largely for the "Logan bow," to caution against indiscriminate wiring of the jaws (17). After the study of two infant cadavers with cleft palate, Logan concluded that there might be possible areas where wires could be applied without undue damage to the tooth buds, but came to the conclusion that closure of the jaws by this procedure was not feasible.

After this problem had been thrashed out at two or three meetings of the Association, the problem of lip closure was taken up in similar symposia over a period of years. It was at this time that Blair "sold" his modification of the Mirault operation to the outstanding plastic surgeons of this country by demonstrating at these meetings and in his own clinic the most beautiful results which he and his associates obtained by this procedure. I was fortunate enough to see Dr. Blair at work during the preparation of his paper on this subject (18). He had Miss Hance collect all the cases of harelip upon which he had operated, and he checked these over with the pre- and post-operative photographs and his operative notes, and with Miss Hance's drawings made at the operating table. In this way he could compare each step of every procedure. This operation, which should have borne his name, he modestly declined to have called the Blair operation, although it was almost entirely a new procedure devised and perfected by him. For years this operation was conceded in this country to be ideal, although subsequently Le Mesurier with his beautiful operation has had many enthusiastic followers. Barrett Brown in 1930 and 1931 was co-author with Blair in two papers on this subject (19), and later he added modifications which he published in a paper with McDowell (20).

At one of the early meetings of the American Association of Plastic Surgeons, in a city where there was only one member, this surgeon had arranged that, while he was operating in one room, a general surgeon was operating in another on an eight or ten year old boy who had a scar contraction about one inch wide in the right axilla as the result of a burn. The general surgeon proceeded to raise a flap four inches long and one inch wide posterior to the scar and parallel to the trunk. We were astounded to see this narrow flap raised for, when the arm was brought up after excision of the scar, the defect was about six inches wide, far greater than the pedicle flap could possibly cover. The gallery of assembled experts gasped, while the operator perspired profusely and became exceedingly flustered. Without a word, Dr. Blair went to the operating room floor, was gowned and masked, and suggested in a quiet kindly voice that, if the case were his, he would clean up the thigh and take a split thickness skin graft to fill the defect. He remained to give the operator explicit directions how to proceed with the removal, fixation and dressing of the graft. He thus performed a triple service: to the surgeon, to the patient, and to surgery itself. It was a heart warming experience for everyone present, and it demonstrated the fine spirit and gentle thoughtfulness that was innate in Blair.

The American Board of Ophthalmology was the first specialty board to function, and the American Board of Surgery completed its organization in January of 1937. From August of 1935 Dr. Blair had been considering ways and means of developing plastic surgery as a recognized specialty. By February 24, 1937 this thought had crystallized into a tentative invitation to a small group of representative men from all over the country to meet in St. Louis to "consider the advisability and some of the details incident to launching a Plastic Surgery Board (21)." He stated that he had recently made an address before the American Board of Surgery and would send copies of the talk he was making "to groups of plastic surgeons throughout the country (22)." These talks by Blair were published recently in Dr. Robert H. Ivy's article (23) on the formation of the American Board of Plastic Surgery.

The first meeting of the organization was held in St. Louis, June 14, 1937. After a clinic at the Barnes Hospital, the group of men selected by Blair drove out to his country home surmounting the bluffs over the Missouri River, just above its junction with the Mississippi (Figs. 6, 7, and 8). Dr. Blair refused the honor of being elected Chairman and Dr. John Staige Davis of Baltimore was chosen for this office, with Dr. Dorrance of Philadelphia as Vice-Chairman. Dr.

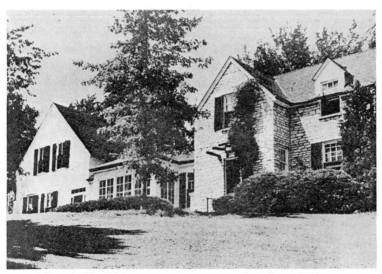

FIG. 6. The Blair country home above the Missouri River

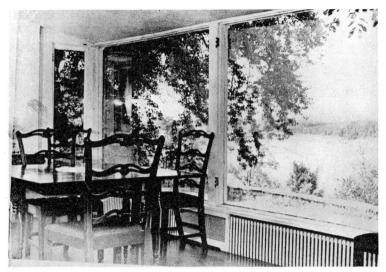

FIG. 7. The outdoor dining porch

Blair was willing to accept the responsibilities, the problems, and also, incidentally, the ability to guide the policies of the Board as its Secretary.

At that time the public generally considered plastic surgeons as "face lifters" and "nose whittlers." To be sure, a few surgeons throughout the country were known for their capabilities in special fields of plastic surgery. There were also those who were close to the border of being ethical, if not unethical, in their practice, and some were definitely below that level. Blair felt that those slightly below the ethical line could be raised if given proper recognition, and that those with special abilities should be recognized and their qualities brought to bear for the good of the specialty of plastic surgery. Accordingly Blair, on his own time and at his own expense, traveled about the country getting to know the various men in each locality and their accomplishments.

At the first annual meeting in Galveston, Feb. 2, 1938, a list was made of those who were to be included in the Founders' Group. Standards for training were set up which would eventually require all future diplomates of the Board to receive experience as interns for one year, assistant residents in general surgery, or the equivalent, for two years, and finally two years of training as residents in plastic surgery, or a longer time under a preceptor.

The Board as formed was recognized by the Advisory Board for Medical Specialists as an affiliate of the American Board of Surgery. But inasmuch as the problems of plastic surgeons differed from those of general surgeons, and the members of that Board could not be thoroughly familiar with such problems, the American Board of Plastic Surgery was given independent status in May of 1941. This was accomplished largely through Blair's efforts alone, and was done with the understanding that the requirements for certification by the Board of Plastic Surgery would never be lowered as regards the requisite two years of residency training in general surgery prior to training in plastic surgery, and that the

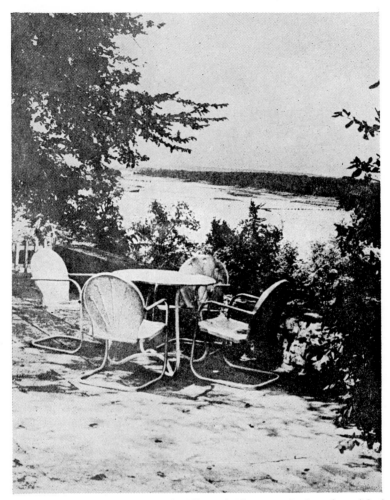

Fig. 8. View from the terrace across the Missouri River near its junction with the Mississippi.

candidates should be examined on plastic surgery for all parts of the body. Some of the younger men performing plastic surgery who could not be expected to fulfill all these requirements were admitted by examination as an interim group until such time as it was possible for the requirements to become known and complied with.

Many were the problems that arose during those early days of formation of the Board, and Dr. Blair worked assiduously and with a quiet firmness and tact that kept the organization on an even keel. The Executive Committee, consisting mainly of Blair and those members of the Board who lived on the Eastern seaboard, met several times a year to try to solve the many perplexing problems that arose. Whenever the meeting was held in St. Louis, this small group was stimulated by informative clinical sessions put on by Dr. Blair and his staff. Blair remained as Secretary of the Board until 1942, when he was succeeded by his associate, James Barrett Brown, and later by Byars, Cannon and McDowell, all trained under him. Mrs. Estelle Hillerich, a former secretary to Dr. Blair, has been Clerical Secretary of the Board from its inception to the present day. Dr. Blair remained as a member of the Board until 1946. As a result of Blair's successful efforts to organize the American Board of Plastic Surgery, great strides forward were made in the education and training of scores of plastic surgeons, and the standards of plastic surgery were raised in this country and abroad.

Blair established a summer home at Fish Creek, Wisconsin, where he exercised his ingenuity in construction and reconstruction to his heart's content in various buildings around the place. He also acquired River View Farm above the Missouri River, ten miles north of St. Louis near the Portage des Sioux, where Lewis and Clark passed on their way to the West. Of this place, which he made his home until a month before he died, he wrote (24):

The place we have on the Missouri River was first used to furnish wood to the steamboats going up the river. Most of the timber was cut and then they started raising wheat on it. The people we bought it from had built, first, a log cabin, then additions to it, starting now nearly a hundred years ago. We have fixed it up with air-conditioning, etc., and now we get quite a bit of our food from there. We have been living in an apartment in town in the winter for six years or more.

Dr. Blair had a very happy family life and was devoted to his beloved wife' Kathryn, and their five children. Two sons and two daughters survive him, a third daughter having died in 1931 at the age of 20. Dr. Blair was deeply stricken emotionally when Mrs. Blair suffered a stroke in 1942, but with characteristic vigor and imagination he attacked the problem of making life bearable for her. He wrote of her illness (25):

Kathryn never did forgive me for going into the army.... When her two boys were taken from her in World War II, one in Africa and the other in New Zealand, while sitting in a movie one evening she did not get up when I did to leave. I turned around and she had slumped down in her seat. With help she stood up and we walked out of the theater together, and the chauffeur who had been nurse to all our children and lady's maid to her, a tremendously stout nigger, carried her from the foyer to the car, and on the way home I made up my mind against taking her to a hospital which was a good "bet." That was five and a half years ago and she has been confined to bed and wheelchair since. You know she was crippled but had, when young, ridden horseback, bicycled, swam, and never let it interfere with anything, and her good side is the one affected. She had a "heck" of a time for four years, pain and everything but now is fairly comfortable. I have a thirty-foot bus rigged up as a hospital, with an elevator for taking her chair in and out (Fig. 9). It is equipped for cooking, sleeping, etc. In addition to Kathryn's compartment, there are sleeping accommodations for her two nurses, the chauffeur and myself. We have traveled around some in this bus; in Canada, Florida, New England States, and we wanted to go up to Banff last summer but it was too hot to go over the plains. But she gets out too little, so now I am getting her a small station wagon—a jeep—which has an elevator so the chair can be put into the car from the back. The elevator

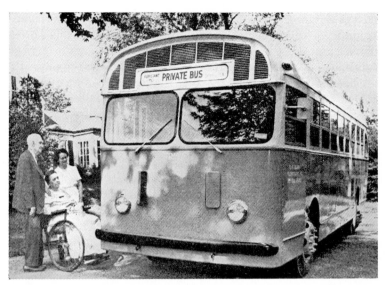

FIG. 9. Dr. and Mrs. Blair and her nurse and the bus "Kathryn" which he had constructed to provide a traveling home and hospital.

will get the power from the engine so it is a very simple affair, and the girls can
carry her around in town in this. . . .The bus is kept out at our country place
. . . . Under no circumstances has she ever complained except about my going
to the war.

Dr. Blair's devotion to his "Missus," as he called her, was exceptionally deep
and enduring. He tried to be with her as much as possible to give her every care
and attention and to permit her to extend her outlook from a bed or wheelchair.
When she finally died in 1950 he was so distraught by his loss that he never fully
recovered.

Dr. Blair's writings cover more than half a century, his first independent
article being published in 1898 and his last paper in 1950. In the early years he
wrote almost entirely on problems of the mouth and jaws, with surprising excur-
sions in several articles on the care of premature infants, including the construction of an incubator, and an apparatus for the application of hot, dry air to
various parts of the human body. Both of these articles (26) show his inventive
flair for construction. Others were on the operative treatment of the thyroid
and of tuberculosis.

He wrote three classic volumes in the field of plastic surgery, the first of which,
"Surgery and Diseases of the Mouth and Jaws," was published in three editions
from 1912 to 1917. The second, "Essentials of Oral Surgery" (1923), was written
with Dr. Robert H. Ivy and, for the second, third and fourth editions (1936,
1944, 1951) with James Barrett Brown as co-author. His third book, "Cancer of
the Face and Mouth," appeared in 1941, with Sherwood Moore and Louis T.
Byars as co-authors. He also provided chapters for various textbooks, such as
Evarts Graham's "Surgical Diagnosis;" Dean Lewis' "Practice of Surgery;"
Mock, Pemberton and Coulter's "Principles and Practice of Physical Therapy;"

Brenneman's "Practice of Pediatrics;" and Christopher's "Textbook of Surgery" (27).

Blair had five of his important papers bound together in what is now a collector's item entitled "Some Tool Subjects of Surface Repair (28)." The first of these, "The Influence of Mechanical Pressure on Wound Healing," is a model of conciseness and is filled with pithy statements of principles and technic. In "The Full Thickness Skin Graft," he stressed the importance of this comparatively little used tissue for small and large denuded areas, while in "The Surgical Restoration of the Lining of the Mouth" he utilized both pedicle flaps and free grafts with the so-called "outlay" of free grafts on Stent mold, for it was found that these grafts would take in the midst of secretions and bacteria. In "The Delayed Transfer of Long Pedicle Flaps in Plastic Surgery" he demonstrated the principle of increasing the blood supply of a flap which was to be raised by preliminary undermining and resuture in the original bed. This was of great value to fellow plastic surgeons and to patients in the prevention of catastrophic losses of raised pedicle flaps. Blair had a happy way of expressing himself and provided a refreshingly new viewpoint to what might be considered a worn subject. He started another admirable article of this group, the one on "The Deep Scar," by saying "A scar is the epitaph of lost tissue; the problem of its removal should be approached as one of restoration and not of simple excision." Indeed, throughout Blair's writings, one finds many statements that could be collected in a book of aphorisms.

Other important papers (29) of the approximately two hundred articles that he contributed to the improvement of surgical technic and an understanding of the anatomy and principles of various conditions encountered in plastic surgery are: "Operative Treatment of Ankylosis of the Mandible;" "Pyogenic Infections of the Parotid Ducts;" "The Correction of Ptosis and Epicanthus" (with James Barrett Brown and William G. Hamm); and "'Hits, Strikes and Outs' in the Use of Pedicle Flaps for Nasal Restoration or Correction" (with Louis T. Byars).

Blair did not hesitate to go into such detail of the various steps of his operations as to enable the reader to understand and later to carry out his procedures successfully.

While Halsted and his school, including John Staige Davis, who was the first man to limit his practice to plastic surgery, used split skin grafts extensively, these were placed only on clean wounds. All granulating wounds, invariably contaminated by bacteria, were grafted with small deep grafts which, although they gave an unsightly appearance to the grafted area and the donor site, did hasten healing. In "The Use and Uses of Large Split Skin Grafts of Intermediate Thickness (30)," Blair and his co-author, James Barrett Brown, brought to the profession the concept that large split skin grafts could also be used for the immediate covering of satisfactorily prepared granulating surfaces, no matter how large. Although the authors cannot be given the credit of being the first to use these grafts in this way, this paper did much to popularize the procedure and to bring about the speedy covering of large areas of granulating surfaces in distressing cases of burns. This method even today is not sufficiently known to the general surgeon who may be called upon to treat such cases, and we still see unhealed burns of over a year's duration. The first paragraph of this paper reads: "Early, quick, and permanent surfacing of burns and other cutaneous defects conserves health, comfort, function, time and money; while unnecessary waiting spells economic waste." Such an opening sentence in many of Blair's papers concisely summarized the whole raison d'être of the paper and expressed the accumulated wisdom of years of thought and experience.

The positions Dr. Blair held and the honors that were showered upon him were too many to be enumerated now, but are appended to this paper together with a bibliography of his writings. Suffice it to say here that he was an Honorary Member of the American Association of Plastic Surgeons, the American Society of Plastic and Reconstructive Surgery, and the British Association of Plastic Surgeons, the three great societies of this specialty in the English speaking world.

Blair's place is assured as having done more than anyone in this country to advance the art and practice of plastic surgery, to have it recognized as a distinct specialty, and to formulate means of educating on-coming generations of plastic surgeons in the principles and technic of reconstructive surgery that mean so much for the function, appearance and happiness of innumerable individuals. Those who have taken or will take the examinations of the Board may be thankful to Blair for his insistence that high standards be maintained in this specialty. You and I and those to come should be grateful for what Blair accomplished and for what he thought, taught and fought for during his lifetime.

> So when a great man dies,
> For years beyond our ken,
> The light he leaves behind him lies
> Upon the paths of men.
>
> (Longfellow, Charles Sumner, Stanza IX)

CURRICULUM VITAE

Born: June 15, 1871 in St. Louis, Missouri
   Father: Edmund Harrison Blair (Born March 13, 1840; died Feb. 8, 1906)
   Mother: Mary Clementine Papin (Born Oct. 15, 1850; died Feb. 12, 1934)

Education:

   Christian Brothers' College: A.B., 1890; A.M., 1894
   Medical Department of Washington University: M.D., 1893
Married: Kathryn Lyman Johnson of St. Louis, April 22, 1907
   Children: Kathryn Lyman (Mrs. George A. Lane); Nancy Lucas (Mrs. James L. O'Leary); Mary Papin (dec.); Vilray Papin, Jr.; John Bates Johnson

Religion: Catholic

Professional Record

   1893: Licensed to practice medicine in Missouri

Hospital Positions:

St. Louis Mullanphy Hospital
  Intern: 1893–1895
  Visiting Surgeon: 1922–1928
St. Louis City Hospital
  Visiting Staff: 1910–1922
St. Luke's Hospital
  Visiting Staff: 1905–1948
  Honorary Staff: 1948 to date of death
Barnes Hospital
St. Louis Children's Hospital } Associate Surgeon: 1915–1949
St. Louis Maternity Hospital   Asso. Surgeon Emeritus: 1949 to death
De Paul Hospital
  Courtesy Staff: 1930–1932
  Visiting Staff: 1932–1947
  Honorary Staff: 1947 to date of death

Academic Positions:

Washington University School of Medicine
  Instructor in Practical Anatomy
  Associate Professor of Anatomy } 1894–1912
  Clinical Professor of Surgery

  Associate in Surgery
  Associate in Clinical Surgery } 1912–1922

  Asst. Prof. of Clinical Surgery: 1922–1927
  Professor of Clinical Surgery: 1927–1941
  Professor Emeritus of Clinical Surgery: 1941 to date of death
Washington University School of Dentistry
  Professor of Oral Surgery: 1927–1941
  Prof. Emeritus of Oral Surgery: 1941 to date of death
Retired from active practice: June 30, 1947

Military Record

Ashanti War:

1900: Surgeon, British Mercantile Marine, and Acting Troop Surgeon

World Wars I and II:

In Service June 1917 to June 24, 1919.
Entered as Captain, discharged as Lt. Colonel
July 1917—March 1918 } Chief of Section, Oral and Plastic Surgery,
Jan. 1919—June 1919   U.S.A.

March 1918–Dec. 1918: Sr. Consultant in Maxillo-Facial Surgery, A.E.F.

Oct. 1, 1922–June 1946: Attending Specialist in Plastic Surgery, Veterans Hospital, Jefferson Barracks, Mo.

June 19, 1946–June 30, 1947: Consultant in Plastic Surgery, Jefferson Barracks, Mo.

Colonel, Medical Reserve Corps (Inactive); Honorable Discharge, April 1, 1953.

Died: Nov. 24, 1955

PROFESSIONAL AFFILIATIONS

Honorary Member or Fellow:

Amer. Assn. of Plastic Surgeons
Amer. College of Dentists
Amer. Society of Plastic & Reconstructive Surgery
British Assn. of Plastic Surgeons
Dental Forum of Milwaukee, Wisconsin
Los Angeles Surgical Society
Missouri State Medical Assn.
Mississippi Valley Medical Society
St. Louis Medical Society
Southeastern Surgical Congress
Southern Medical Assn.
Washington University Dental Alumni Assn.

Member or Fellow:

Amer. Assn. for the Advancement of Oral Diagnosis (1939–41)
Amer. Assn. for the Advancement of Science
Amer. Assn. for the Surgery of Trauma (Sr. Fellow)
Amer. Assn. of Anatomists
Amer. Coll. of Surgeons (Founder Fellow)
Amer. Laryngological Assn. (Corresponding Fellow)
Amer. Medical Assn.
Amer. Society for the Control of Cancer
Amer. Surgical Assn. (Sr. Fellow)
Archeological Institute of America (1924–27)
Assn. of Military Surgeons
Gulf Coast Clinical Society
Missouri Historical Society
National Institute of Social Science
St. Louis Academy of Science (Oct. 18, 1909 to resignation Feb. 3, 1955)
Société Internationale de Chirurgie
Southern Surgical Assn. (Sr. Fellow)
Western Surgical Assn. (Sr. Member)

FRATERNITIES

Alpha Omega Alpha (Honorary Medical Fraternity)
Pi Gamma Nu: National Social Science Honor Society
Theta Kappa Psi Medical Fraternity

SPECIALTY BOARDS

Amer. Board of Otolaryngology: 1928
Amer. Board of Plastic Surgery (Founders' Group): 1939

AWARDS

American Medical Association: Bronze medal for exhibit: 1927
Mississippi Valley Medical Society: Distinguished Service Award: 1938
American Dental Assn. and the Maryland State Dental Assn.: Certificate of
achievement for Centenary of Dentistry: March 18–20, 1940
St. Louis Medical Society: Gold medal and certificate of merit for scientific accomplishment: 1947
American Society of Plastic and Reconstructive Surgery: Certificate in recognition of his leadership in the organization and development of the specialty of
plastic surgery and his outstanding contributions to the advancement of its
practice: Nov. 19, 1948.

HONORARY DEGREE

Washington University: Sc.D.: 1949

BIBLIOGRAPHY OF DR. BLAIR'S WRITINGS*

BOOKS

1. Blair, Vilray P. A textbook for the modeling of the human bones in clay. St. Louis, Cooperative Association of the Medical Department of Washington University, 1906.
2. Blair, Vilray P. Surgery and diseases of the mouth and jaws; A practical treatise on the surgery and diseases of the mouth and allied subjects. St. Louis, Mosby, 1912 (1st ed.); 1914 (2nd ed.); 1917 (3rd ed.).
3. Blair, Vilray P. and Ivy, Robert H. (and with James Barrett Brown as co-author of the 2nd, 3rd and 4th editions). Essentials of oral surgery. St. Louis, Mosby, 1923 (1st ed.); 1936 (2nd ed.); 1944 (3rd ed.); 1951 (4th ed.)
4. Blair, Vilray P., Moore, Sherwood, and Byars, Louis T. Cancer of the face and mouth; diagnosis, treatment, surgical repair. St. Louis, Mosby, 1941.

CHAPTERS IN BOOKS

1. Blair, Vilray P. Plastic repair of wounds of the face and jaws. *In:* Oxford loose-leaf surgery, vol. 5: 615–662; New York, Oxford Univ. Press, 1921.
2. Blair, Vilray P., Padgett, Earl C., and Brown, James Barrett. Diseases of the face, mouth and jaws. *In:* Graham, Evarts A. (ed.): Surgical diagnosis by American authors, vol. 2: 209–414; Philadelphia, Saunders, 1930.
3. Blair, Vilray P. and Olch, Isaac Yale. The salivary glands. *In:* Lewis, Dean (ed.): Practice of surgery, vol. 4, chap. 5; Hagerstown, Md., W. F. Prior Co., [1930].
4. Blair, Vilray P. and Brown, James Barrett. Deformities of the nose; remodeling and repair. *In:* Sajous, Charles E. de M. and Sajous, Louis T. de M. (eds.): The cyclopedia of medicine, vol. 9: 920–936; Philadelphia, Davis, 1934.
5. Blair, Vilray P. and Brown, James Barrett. Physical therapy in plastic surgery. *In:* Mock, Harry E., Pemberton, Ralph, and Coulter, John (eds.): Principles and practice of physical therapy, vol. 2, chap. 12: 1–15; Hagerstown, Md., W. F. Prior Co., 1934.
6. Blair, Vilray P. and Brown, James Barrett (and with Louis T. Byars as co-author in the 4th and 5th editions). Repair of defects of the face, hands and feet. *In:* Christopher, Frederick (ed.): A textbook of surgery. Philadelphia, Saunders, 1936, (1st ed.: pp. 743–760); 1939 (2nd ed.: pp. 1534–1553); 1942 (3rd ed.: pp. 1598–1616); 1945 (4th ed.: pp. 1382–1399); 1949 (5th ed.: pp. 1422–1438).
7. Blair, Vilray P. and Brown, James Barrett. Diseases of the mouth and adnexa. Anomalies of development. *In:* Brenneman, Joseph (ed.): Practice of pediatrics by various authors, vol. 3, chap. 1; Hagerstown, Md., W. F. Prior Co., 1937.
8. Blair, Vilray P. and Byars, Louis T. Diseases of the salivary glands. *In:* Lewis, Dean (ed.): Practice of surgery, vol. 4, chap. 5; Hagerstown, Md., W. F. Prior Co., [1942–1951].

ARTICLES

1897

1. Tupper, Paul and Blair, Vilray P. Two practical wrinkles in through-and-through drainage. Med. Rec. 51: 418–419, March 20, 1897.

1898

2. Blair, Vilray P. An apparatus for the application of dry hot air to different portions of the human body. Med. Rev., St. Louis, 37: 422–424, June 4, 1898; [Discussion: 433–435].

1902

3. Blair, Vilray P. (Late Surgeon in African Royal Mail S. S. Co., of London, Eng.) Some personal observations of malarial and blackwater fever on the West Coast of Africa. Courier of Med., St. Louis, 26: 9–22, Jan. 1902.
4. Blair, Vilray P. Three anomalies of thoracic blood vessels. [Abstract] Amer. J. Anat. 1: 513, Sept. 15, 1902.

1903

5. Blair, Vilray P. An incubator for delicate or premature infants. Med. Fortnightly, St. Louis, 23: 464–471, June 25, 1903.

1904

6. Blair, Vilray P. Some notes on the care of premature infants. Med. Rev., St. Louis, 49: 321–326, May 21, 1904. Cf. No. 7.

---

* Arranged in chronological sequence.

7. Blair, Vilray P. Some notes on the care of premature infants. Am. J. Obst. 49: 771–780, June 1904. Cf. No. 6.
8. Blair, Vilray P. Fixation of the kidney with regard to its physiological excursion. Interstate Med. J. 11: 302–306, 1904.

1905

9. Blair, Vilray P. Conservation of the parietal motor nerves in abdominal section. Surg. Gyn. & Obst. 1: 152–157, Aug. 1905.
10. Blair, Vilray P. Premature infants. The necessity for and the difficulty of formulating a general plan for their care. Med. Courier, St. Louis, 33: 207–211, Oct. 1905; [Discussion: 240–249].
11. Blair, Vilray P. Osteology and the general practitioner. Interstate Med. J. 12: 536–540, 1905.

1906

12. Blair, Vilray P., Elisha H. Gregory, M.D., of St. Louis. (Obituary) Med. Rev., St. Louis, 53: 133–334, Feb. 17, 1906. Cf. No. 113.
13. Blair, Vilray P. Report of a case of double resection for the correction of protrusion of the mandible. Dental Cosmos 48: 817–820, Aug. 1906. Cf. No. 14.
14. Blair, Vilray P. A report of a case of double resection for the correction of protrusion of the lower jaw. Interstate Med. J. 13: 712–717, Sept. 1906. Cf. No. 13.

1907

15. Blair, Vilray P. Operations on the jaw-bone and face: A study of the etiology and pathological anatomy of developmental malrelations of the maxilla and mandible to each other and to the facial outline, and of their operative treatment when beyond the scope of the orthodontist. Surg. Gyn. & Obst. 4: 67–78, Jan. 1907. Cf. No. 16.
16. Blair, Vilray P. Operations on the jaw-bone and face: A study of the etiology and pathological anatomy of developmental malrelations of the maxilla and mandible to each other and to the facial outline, and of their operative treatment when beyond the scope of the orthodontist. The Dental Era 6: 169–192, 1907. Cf. No. 15.

1908

17. Blair, Vilray P. The angle splint (Fractures). Dental Items of Interest 30: 829–832, 1908.
18. Blair, Vilray P. Exophthalmic goiter plus other surgical lesions. Interstate Med. J. 15: 723–727, 1908.

1909

19. Blair, Vilray P. Underdeveloped lower jaw, with limited excursion. Report of two cases with operation. J.A.M.A. 53: 178–183, July 17, 1909.
20. Blair, Vilray P. Points in the anatomy and surgery of the hard palate of the infant. Interstate Med. J. 16, no. 3: 191–199, 1909.
21. Blair, Vilray P. and Senseney, E. T. a. Presentation of a patient five and one-half years after partial laryngectomy for recurrent carcinoma. b. Report of an unusual case for which an external unilateral pan-sinus operation was performed; presentation of patient. Weekly Bull., St. Louis Med. Soc., 3: 106–110, 1909.

1910*

22. Blair, Vilray P. Facial and palate clefts, their origin and supposed causes. Weekly Bull., St. Louis Med. Soc., 4: 53, 1910 [Read Jan. 8, 1910].
23. Blair, Vilray P. Ideal age for cleft palate operations. Interstate Med. J. 17, no. 2: 118–119, 1910.
24. Blair, Vilray P. Notes on trifacial neuralgia treated by deep injection. Weekly Bull., St. Louis Med. Soc., 4: 87–88, 1910 [Read Jan. 22, 1910]. Cf. Nos. 25 and 28.
25. Blair, Vilray P. Treatment of trifacial neuralgia by deep injection. Weekly Bull., St. Louis Med. Soc., 4: 199, 1910. Cf. Nos. 24 and 28.
26. Blair, Vilray P. and McGuigan, Hugh. A suggestion for the treatment of air embolism. Weekly Bull., St. Louis Med. Soc., 4: 267–269, 1910. Cf. No. 27.
27. Blair, Vilray P. and McGuigan, Hugh. A suggestion for the treatment of air embolism. Ann. Surg. 52: 471–486, Oct. 1910. Cf. No. 26.

1911

28. Blair, Vilray P. Notes on trifacial neuralgia treated by deep injections. J.A.M.A. 56: 335–339, Feb. 4, 1911. Cf. Nos. 24 and 25.

* An article, "The action of the psoas magnus muscle," is said by Miss Cooper and Dr. Robert J. Terry, formerly Professor of Anatomy at Washington University, to have been published by Dr. Blair around 1910 or 1911, but so far all efforts to trace the place of publication of such an article have been unavailing.

29. Blair, Vilray P. Operative treatment of difficult cases of palate defect after infancy. Surg. Gyn. & Obst. 12: 289–294, March 1911. Cf. No. 30.
30. Blair, Vilray P. Operative treatment of difficult cases of palate defect after infancy. Trans. South. Surg. & Gyn. Assn. 23: 479–483, 1911.* Cf. No. 29.
31. Blair, Vilray P. Vein to vein transfusions. Weekly Bull., St. Louis Med. Soc., 5: 201, 1911.

1913

32. Blair, Vilray P. A case of naso-pharyngeal polyp. Weekly Bull., St. Louis Med. Soc., 7: 270, 1913.

1914

33. Blair, Vilray P. Dental disorders and peridental infections: Their relation to neighboring organs. Surg. Gyn. & Obst. 18: 470–476, April 1914.
34. Blair, Vilray P. The diagnosis and treatment of tic douloureux. Lancet-Clinic, Cincinnati, 111: 443–445, April 11, 1914.
35. Blair, Vilray P. The treatment of a case of birth fracture of the shaft of the femur. Surg. Gyn. & Obst. 18: 640, May 1914.
36. Blair, Vilray P. Treatment of unlocalized intracranial injuries by drainage through a subtemporal approach. J.A.M.A. 63: 863–866, Sept. 5, 1914.
37. Blair, Vilray P. Operative treatment of ankylosis of the mandible, with a history of the operation and an analysis of two hundred and twelve cases. Surg. Gyn. & Obst. 19: 436–451, Oct. 1914. Cf. No. 38.
38. Blair, Vilray P. Operative treatment of ankylosis of the mandible, with a history of the operation and an analysis of two hundred and twelve cases. Trans. South. Surg. & Gyn. Assn. 26: 435–465, 1914. Cf. No. 37.
39. Blair, Vilray P. Surgical treatment of pulmonary tuberculosis. Interstate Med. J. 21: 902–906, 1914.

1915

40. Blair, Vilray P. Importance of early diagnosis of malignant tumors of the mouth. Dental Rev. 29: 545–556, June 1915.
41. Blair, Vilray P. Indications for operative interference in goiter. J.A.M.A. 64: 1896–1898, June 5, 1915.
42. Blair, Vilray P. Instances of operative correction of mal-relation of the jaws. Internat. J. Orthodontia 1: 395–421, Aug. 1915.
43. Blair, Vilray P. Factors of safety in goiter operations. J. Missouri State Med. Assn. 12: 446–449, Oct. 1915.
44. Blair, Vilray P. Personal observation of the Brophy plan of dealing with complete clefts of the lip and palate. Dental Cosmos 56: 1141–1142, Oct. 1915.
45. Blair, Vilray P. Operative indications for goiter. Weekly Bull., St. Louis Med. Soc., 9: 59–64, 1915.

1916

46. Blair, Vilray P. Tumors of the mouth. Internat. Abstract of Surg. 22: 117–142, Feb. 1916.
47. Blair, Vilray P. Implantation of the trigonum into the segregated lower end of the ileum. Surg. Gyn. & Obst. 22: 352–353, March 1916. Cf. No. 48.
48. Blair, Vilray P. Implantation of the trigonum into the segregated lower end of the ileum. Trans. South. Surg. & Gyn. Assn. 28: 90–92, 1916. Cf. No. 47.
49. Blair, Vilray P. The treatment of cleft palate and harelip in early infancy. Internat. Clinics 4 (ser. 26): 211–222, 1916, Cf. No. 50.
50. Blair, Vilray P. The treatment of cleft palate and harelip in early infancy. Trans. South. Surg. Assn. 29: 70–85, 1917. Cf. No. 49.

1917

51. Blair, Vilray P. The present status of the treatment of carcinoma of the mouth in this locality. J. Missouri State Med. Assn. 14: 101–105, March 1917.
52. Blair, Vilray P. Septic parotitis. Med. & Surg., St. Louis, 1: 34–37, March 1917.
53. Blair, Vilray P. The treatment of carcinoma of the mouth. Texas State Med. J. 13: 205–208, Oct. 1917.
54. Blair, Vilray P. The aims of the Sub-Section of plastic and oral surgery. Surg. Gyn. & Obst. 25: 730–731, Dec. 1917.

1919

55. Blair, Vilray P. The maxillofacial service of the American Army in the war. J.A.M.A. 73: 325–328, Aug. 2, 1919. Cf. No. 56.

* Dates on the various "Transactions" are dates of publication and not necessarily the dates of the meetings of the societies.

56. Blair, Vilray P. The maxillofacial service of the American Army in the war. Dental Reg., Cincinnati, 73: 352–360, 1919. Cf. No. 55.

1920

57. Blair, Vilray P. Cleft palate and harelip. Internat. J. Orthod. & Oral Surg. 6: 43–54, Jan. 1920.
58. Blair, Vilray P. Operation for advanced carcinoma of the tongue or floor of the mouth. Surg. Gyn. & Obst. 30: 149–153, Feb. 1920. Cf. Nos. 61 and 63.
59. Blair, Vilray P. Doctor Gilmer; The surgeon. Internat. J. Orthod. & Oral Surg. 6: 369–374, June 1920. Cf. No. 143.
60. Blair, Vilray P. Some observation [sic] on our war experiences with face and jaw injuries. Military Surgeon 47: 379–388, Oct. 1920.
61. Blair, Vilray P. Treatment of advanced carcinomata of the mouth. J. Missouri State Med. Assn. 17: 395–402, Oct. 1920. Cf. Nos. 58 and 63.
62. Blair, Vilray P. Report of two cases of Kroenlein operation. Am. J. Ophth. 3: 789–797, Nov. 1920.
63. Blair, Vilray P. Operation for advanced carcinoma of the tongue or floor of the mouth. Trans. West. Surg. Assn. 29: 405–413, 1920. Cf. Nos. 58 and 61.

1921

64. Blair, Vilray P. The anesthesia problem in goiter surgery from the surgeon's viewpoint. Am. J. Surg. 35: 5–6, Jan. 1921, Anesthesia supplement.
65. Blair, Vilray P. The delayed transfer of long pedicle flaps in plastic surgery. Surg. Gyn. & Obst. 33: 261–272, Sept. 1921. Cf. No. 69.
66. Blair, Vilray P. A note on the treatment of secondary hemorrhage from the branches of the common carotid artery. Ann. Surg. 74: 313–315, Sept. 1921. Cf. No. 70.
67. Blair, Vilray P. The repair of major defects of the face. Texas State Med. J. 17: 301–302, Oct. 1921.
68. Blair, Vilray P. Rhinoplasty, with special reference to saddle nose. J.A.M.A. 77: 1479–1482, Nov. 5, 1921.
69. Blair, Vilray P. The delayed transfer of long pedicle flaps in plastic surgery. Trans. South. Surg. Assn. 33: 202–210, 1921. Cf. No. 65.
70. Blair, Vilray P. A note on the treatment of secondary hemorrhage from the branches of the carotid arteries. Trans. Am. Surg. Assn. 39: 402–406, 1921. Cf. No. 66.

1922

71. Blair, Vilray P. Reconstruction surgery of the face. Surg. Gyn. & Obst. 34: 701–716, June 1922.
72. Blair, Vilray P. Saddle nose. Trans. South. Surg. Assn. 34: 524–527, 1922.

1923

73. Blair, Vilray P. and Moskowitz, Morris J. Cancer of the mouth and jaws. Internat. J. Orthod., Oral Surg. & Radiog. 9: 218–226, March 1923.
74. Blair, Vilray P. and Moskowitz, Morris J. Cancer of the tongue, lips and cheek. A résumé of recent literature. Internat. J. Orthod., Oral Surg. & Radiog. 9: 302–305, April 1923; 384–387, May 1923; 468–470, June 1923.
75. Blair, Vilray P. Intra-oral support of the ramus in fractures of the lower jaw. Dental Cosmos 65: 589–595, June 1923.
76. Blair, Vilray P. An opportunity. Washington Univ. Dental J. 2, no. 1: 3–4, June 1923.
77. Blair, Vilray P. Prevention of carcinoma of the mouth. J. Am. Dental Assn. 10: 463–470, June 1923.
78. Blair, Vilray P. Ranula. Ann. Surg. 77: 681–684, June 1923. Cf. No. 83.
79. Blair, Vilray P. and Padgett, Earl C. Pyogenic infection of the parotid glands and ducts. Arch. Surg. 7: 1–36, July 1923.
80. Blair, Vilray P. Restoration of the burnt child. South. Med. J. 16: 522–525, July 1923.
81. Blair, Vilray P. Congenital facial clefts. Surg. Gyn. & Obst. 37: 530–533, Oct. 1923.
82. Blair, Vilray P. The "ulcerated tooth." (Editorial) Surg. Gyn. & Obst. 37: 845–846, Dec. 1923.
83. Blair, Vilray P. Report of a case of ranula, with comments on the Thompson theory of origin. Trans. South. Surg. Assn. 35: 268–271, 1923. Cf. No. 78.
84. Blair, Vilray P. Rhinoplasty: A preliminary report. Trans. Am. Surg. Assn. 41: 200–206, 1923.
85. Blair, Vilray P. Radical operation for extrinsic carcinoma of the larynx. Trans. Am. Laryngol. Assn. 45: 228–251, 1923. Cf. No. 86.

1924

86. Blair, Vilray P. Radical operation for extrinsic carcinoma of the larynx. Ann. Otol. Rhin. & Laryng. 33: 373–387, June 1924. Cf. No. 85.

87. Blair, Vilray P. The full thickness skin graft. Ann. Surg. 80: 298–324, Sept. 1924. Cf. No. 90.
88. Blair, Vilray P. Restoration of the function of the mouth. Ann. Clin. Med. 3: 242–244, Sept. 1924.
89. Blair, Vilray P. The influence of mechanical pressure on wound healing. Illinois Med. J. 46: 249–252, Oct. 1924.
90. Blair, Vilray P. The full thickness skin graft. Trans. Am. Surg. Assn. 42: 335–368, 1924. Cf. No. 87.

1925

91. Blair, Vilray P. Nasal deformities associated with congenital cleft of the lip. J.A.M.A. 84: 185–187, Jan. 17, 1925.
92. Blair, Vilray P. The surgical restoration of the lining of the mouth. Surg. Gyn. & Obst. 40: 165–174, Feb. 1925.
93. Blair, Vilray P. The deep scar. (Editorial) Surg. Gyn. & Obst. 40: 436–438, March 1925.
94. Blair, Vilray P. Total and subtotal restoration of the nose. J.A.M.A. 85: 1931–1935, Dec. 19, 1925.
95. Blair, Vilray P. and Brown, James Barrett. Personal observations on the course and treatment of simple osteomyelitis of the jaws. Surg. Clin. No. Am. 5: 1413–1436, 1925. Cf. No. 96.

1926

96. Blair, Vilray P. and Brown, James Barrett. Personal observations on the course and treatment of simple osteomyelitis of the jaws. Internat. J. Orthod., Oral Surg. & Radiog. 12: 52–68, Jan. 1926. Cf. No. 95.
97. Blair, Vilray P. The problem of bringing forward the retracted upper lip and nose. Surg. Gyn. & Obst. 42: 128–132, Jan. 1926.
98. Blair, Vilray P. Notes on the operative correction of facial palsy. South. Med. J. 19: 116–120, Feb. 1926.
99. Blair, Vilray P. Surgical correction of various types of malrelation of the jaws. Internat. J. Orthod., Oral Surg. & Radiog. 12: 453–466, May 1926.
100. Blair, Vilray P. Operations for relief of harelip and cleft palate. Hygeia 4: 325–326, June 1926.
101. Blair, Vilray P. The restoration of function and appearance after certain injuries or in deformities of the jaw bones and mouth. J. Am. Dent. Assn. 13: 1511–1529, Nov. 1926.

1927

102. Blair, Vilray P. Repair of defects caused by surgery and radium in cancers of the hand, mouth and cheek. Am. J. Roent. & Rad. Ther. 17: 99–101, Jan. 1927. Cf. No. 119.
103. Blair, Vilray P. and Brown, James Barrett. Septic osteomyelitis of the bones of the skull and face. A plea for conservative treatment. Ann. Surg. 85: 1–26, Jan. 1927.
104. Blair, Vilray P. and Dameron, E. P. Coordination of dental and medical services in the treatment of battle casualties. J. Am. Dental Assn. 14: 573–581, April 1927.
105. Blair, Vilray P. Face, neck and chest skin losses. Trans. Am. Surg. Assn. 45: 190–198, 1927; [Discussion: 199].

1928

106. Blair, Vilray P. The consideration of contour as well as function in operations for organic ankylosis of the lower jaw. Surg. Gyn. & Obst. 46: 167–179, Feb. 1928. Cf. Nos. 109 and 117.
107. Blair, Vilray P. Paul Yoer Tupper—1858–1928. In Memoriam. St. Louis Med. Soc. Bull. 22, no. 25, March 1, 1928.
108. Blair, Vilray P. The why and how of harelip correction. Ann. Otol. Rhin. & Laryng. 37: 196–205, March 1928. Cf. No. 115.
109. Blair, Vilray P. The consideration of contour as well as function in operations for organic ankylosis of the lower jaw. Chicago Dental Soc. Bull. 8: 8–14, July 6; and 5–14, July 13, 1928. Cf. Nos. 106 and 117.
110. Blair, Vilray P., Brown, James Barrett and Womack, Nathan A. Cancer in and about the mouth. A study of two hundred and eleven cases. Ann. Surg. 88: 705–724, Oct. 1928. Cf. No. 118.
111. Blair, Vilray P. The not-pleasing nose. Trans. Am. Laryng. Assn. 50: 36–40, 1928.
112. Blair, Vilray P. Plastic surgery of the nose—The patient's viewpoint. Trans. Am. Acad. Ophth. & Otolaryng. 33: 436–444, 1928.

1929

113. Blair, Vilray P. Master surgeons of America. Elisha H. Gregory. Surg. Gyn. & Obst. 48: 714–716, May 1929. Cf. No. 12.

114. Blair, Vilray P. and Brown, James Barrett. The use and uses of large split-skin grafts of intermediate thickness. Surg. Gyn. & Obst. 49: 82–97, July 1929. Cf. No. 116.
115. Blair, Vilray P. The why and how of harelip correction. Internat. J. Orthod. 15: 1112–1119, Nov. 1929. Cf. No. 108.
116. Blair, Vilray P. and Brown, James Barrett. The use and uses of large split-skin grafts of intermediate thickness. Trans. South. Surg. Assn. 41: 409–424, 1929. Cf. No. 114.

1930

117. Blair, Vilray P. The consideration of contour as well as function in operations for organic ankylosis of the lower jaw. Internat. J. Orthod., Oral Surg. & Radiog. 16: 62–80, Jan. 1930. Cf. Nos. 106 and 109.
118. Blair, Vilray P., Brown, James Barrett and Womack, Nathan A. Cancer in and about the mouth. A study of two hundred and eleven cases. Internat. J. Orthod., Oral Surg. & Radiog. 16: 188–209, Feb. 1930. Cf. No. 110.
119. Blair, Vilray P. Repair of defects caused by surgery and radium in cancers of the hand, mouth and cheek. Internat. J. Orthod., Oral Surg. & Radiog. 16: 326–328, March 1930. Cf. No. 102.
120. Blair, Vilray P., Brown, James Barrett and Moore, Sherwood. Osteomyelitis of the jaws. J. Missouri State Med. Assn. 27: 173–176, April 1930. Cf. No. 126.
121. Blair, Vilray P. and Brown, James Barrett. Mirault operation for single harelip. Surg. Gyn. & Obst. 51: 81–98, July 1930. Cf. Nos. 128 and 135.
122. Blair, Vilray P. Further observation upon the compensatory use of live tendon strips for facial paralysis. Ann. Surg. 92: 694–703, Oct. 1930. Cf. No. 123.
123. Blair, Vilray P. Further observation upon the compensatory use of live tendon strips for facial paralysis. Trans. Am. Surg. Assn. 48: 369–378, 1930. Cf. No. 122.
124. Blair, Vilray P. Hypospadias and epispadias, indications for and technique of their operative correction. Trans. South. Surg. Assn. 42: 163–165, 1930.

1931

125. Blair Vilray P. and Brown, James Barrett. A plea for better average harelip repairs. Dallas Med. J. 17: 4–9, Jan. 1931. Cf. No. 130.
126. Blair, Vilray P., Brown, James Barrett and Moore, Sherwood. Osteomyelitis of the jaws. Internat. J. Orthod., Oral Surg. & Radiog. 17: 169–175, Feb. 1931. Cf. No. 120.
127. Blair, Vilray P. Facial abnormalities, fancied and real; the reaction of the patient; their attempted correction. [The Seventh Lewis Linn McArthur Lecture of the Billings Foundation delivered at the joint meeting of the Institute of Medicine and the Chicago Surgical Society, Feb. 27, 1931.] Proc. Inst. Med. Chicago 8: 217–223, April 15, 1931. Cf. Nos. 133 and 137.
128. Blair, Vilray P. and Brown, James Barrett. Mirault operation for single harelip. Internat. J. Orthod., Oral Surg. & Radiog. 17: 370–396, April 1931. Cf. Nos. 121 and 135.
129. Blair, Vilray P. and Brown, James Barrett. Early and late repair of extensive burns. Dallas Med. J. 17: 59–70, May 1931.
130. Blair, Vilray P. and Brown, James Barrett. A plea for better average harelip repairs Internat. J. Orthod., Oral Surg. & Radiog. 17: 472–483, May 1931. Cf. No. 125.
131. Blair, Vilray P. The treatment of burns. The promotion of early healing and correction and prevention of late complications. J. Oklahoma Med. Assn. 24: 271–272, Aug. 1931.
132. Blair, Vilray P. Congenital atresia or obstruction of the nasal air passages. Ann. Otol. Rhin. & Laryng. 40: 1021–1035, Dec. 1931. Cf. Nos. 134 and 138.
133. Blair, Vilray P. and Brown, James Barrett. Nasal abnormalities, fancied and real; the reaction of the patient: their attempted correction. Surg. Gyn. & Obst. 53: 797–819, Dec. 1931. Cf. Nos. 127 and 137.
134. Blair, Vilray P. Congenital atresia or obstruction of the nasal air passages. Trans. Am. Laryng. Assn. 53: 229–246, 1931. Cf. Nos. 132 and 138.
135. Blair, Vilray P. and Brown, James Barrett. Mirault operation for single harelip. Trans. Western Surg. Assn. 40: 299–347, 1931. Cf. Nos. 121 and 128.

1932

136. Blair, Vilray P., Brown, James Barrett and Hamm, William G. The early care of burns and the repair of their defects. J.A.M.A. 98: 1355–1359, April 16, 1932.
137. Blair, Vilray P. and Brown, James Barrett. Nasal abnormalities, fancied and real; the reaction of the patient: their attempted correction. Internat. J. Orthod., Oral Surg. & Radiog. 18: 363–401, April 1932. Cf. Nos. 127 and 133.
138. Blair, Vilray P. Congenital atresia or obstruction of the nasal air passages. Internat. J. Orthod., Oral Surg. & Radiog. 18: 516–526, May 1932. Cf. Nos. 132 and 134.
139. Blair, Vilray P. Correction of losses and deformities of the external nose, including those associated with harelip. Calif. and Western Med. 36: 308–313, May 1932.

140. Blair, Vilray P., Brown, James Barrett and Hamm, William G. Correction of ptosis
     and of epicanthus. Arch. Ophth. 7: 831–846, June 1932.
141. Blair, Vilray P., Brown, James Barrett and Hamm, William G. Surgery of the inner
     canthus and related structures. Am. J. Ophth. 15: 498–507, June 1932.
142. Blair, Vilray P. Types of contour repair. South. Surgeon 1: 162–166, July 1932.
143. Blair, Vilray P. Master surgeons of America. Thomas L. Gilmer. Surg. Gyn. & Obst.
     55: 670–672, Nov. 1932. Cf. No. 59.
144. Blair, Vilray P., Brown, James Barrett and Hamm, William G. The surgical treatment
     of post-radiation keratosis. Radiology 19: 337–344, Dec. 1932.
145. Blair, Vilray P. Repairs and adjustments of the eyelids. J.A.M.A. 99: 2171–2176.
     Dec. 24, 1932. Cf. No. 146.
146. Blair, Vilray P. Repairs and adjustments of the eyelids. Trans. Sect. Ophth., A.M.A.,
     pp. 328–341, 1932. Cf. No. 145.

                                        1933

147. Blair, Vilray P., Brown, James Barrett and Hamm, William G. Types of reconstruc-
     tive surgery of the orbital region. South. Surgeon 1: 293–300, Jan. 1933.
148. Blair, Vilray P., Brown, James Barrett and Hamm, William G. Radical treatment of
     carcinoma of the lip. Am. J. Roent. & Rad. Ther. 29: 229–233, Feb. 1933.
149. Blair, Vilray P. Summary of sixty-five "cures" of cancer about the mouth. Surg. Gyn.
     & Obst. 56: 469, Feb. 15, 1933.
150. Brown, James Barrett, Blair, Vilray P. and Hamm, William G. Release of axillary
     and brachial scar fixation. [Presented by Dr. Blair at the Southern Surgical Asso-
     ciation, Dec. 14, 1932.] Surg. Gyn. & Obst. 56: 790–798, April 1933. Cf. No. 153.
151. Blair, Vilray P. and Brown, James Barrett. The treatment of cancerous or potentially
     cancerous cervical lymph-nodes. Ann. Surg. 98: 650–661, Oct. 1933.
152. Blair, Vilray P., Brown, James Barrett and Hamm, William G. The correction of
     scrotal hypospadias and of epispadias. Surg. Gyn. & Obst. 57: 646–653, Nov. 1933.
153. Blair, Vilray P., Brown, James Barrett and Hamm, William G. Release of axillary and
     brachial scar fixation. Trans. South. Surg. Assn. 45: 258–274, 1933. Cf. No. 150.

                                        1934

154. Blair, Vilray P. and Brown, James Barrett. The Dieffenbach-Warren operation for
     closure of the congenitally cleft palate. Surg. Gyn. & Obst. 59: 309–320, Sept. 1934.
     Cf. No. 162.
155. Blair, Vilray P. Presidential address: Ruminations of a journeyman surgeon. Trans.
     South. Surg. Assn. 46: 1–11, 1934.

                                        1935

156. Brown, James Barrett and Blair, Vilray P. The repair of defects resulting from full
     thickness loss of skin from burns. Surg. Gyn. & Obst. 60: 379–389, Feb. 15, 1935.
157. Brown, James Barrett, Blair, Vilray P. and Byars, Louis T. The repair of surface
     defects, from burns and other causes, with thick split grafts. South. Med. J. 28:
     408–415, May 1935; 529–531, June 1935.
158. Blair, Vilray P., Brown, James Barrett and Byars, Louis T. Cancer of the cheek and
     neighboring bone. Am. J. Surg. 30: 250–253, Nov. 1935. Cf. No. 159.

                                        1936

159. Blair, Vilray P., Brown, James Barrett and Byars, Louis T. Cancer of the cheek and
     neighboring bone. Internat. J. Orthod., Oral Surg. & Radiog. 22: 183–189, Feb.
     1936. Cf. No. 158.
160. Blair, Vilray P. Plastic surgery of the face, head and neck; the psychic reactions. J.
     Am. Dental Assn. 23: 236–240, Feb. 1936.
161. Blair, Vilray P. Surgery, specialty surgery, and "plastic" surgery. (Editorial) Surg.
     Gyn. & Obst. 62: 895–898, May 1936.
162. Blair, Vilray P. and Brown, James Barrett. The Dieffenbach-Warren operation for
     closure of the congenitally cleft palate. Internat. J. Orthod., Oral Surg. & Radiog.
     22: 853–868, Aug. 1936. Cf. No. 154.
163. Brown, James Barrett, Byars, Louis T. and Blair, Vilray P. A study of ulcerations of
     the lower extremity and their repair with thick split skin grafts. Surg. Gyn. & Obst.
     63: 331–340, Sept. 1936.
164. Blair, Vilray P. A plastic surgery board. Is its formation now desirable and opportune?
     [1936 and 1937] (Published in: Ivy, Robert H.: Some circumstances leading to or-
     ganization of the American Board of Plastic Surgery.) Plas. & Recons. Surg. 16:
     77–82, Aug. 1955.

                                        1937

165. Blair, Vilray P. Address made before the American Board of Surgery. [1937] (Published

in: Ivy, Robert H.: Some circumstances leading to organization of the American Board of Plastic Surgery.) Plas. & Recons. Surg. 16: 82–84, Aug. 1955.

166. Blair, Vilray P., Brown, James Barrett and Byars, Louis T. Plantar warts, flaps and grafts. J.A.M.A. 108: 24–27, Jan. 2, 1937.

167. Blair, Vilray P., Brown, James Barrett and Byars, Louis T. Early local care of face injuries. Surg. Gyn. & Obst. 64: 358–371, Feb. 15, 1937. Cf. No. 168.

168. Blair, Vilray P., Brown, James Barrett and Byars, Louis T. Early local care of face injuries. Internat. J. Orthod. 23: 515–533, May 1937. Cf. No. 167.

169. Blair, Vilray P., Brown, James Barrett and Byars, Louis T. Treatment of fracture of the upper jaw. Surgery 1: 748–760, May 1937.

170. Blair, Vilray P., Brown, James Barrett and Byars, Louis T. Observations on sinus abnormalities in congenital total and hemi-absence of the nose. Ann. Otol. Rhin. & Laryng. 46: 592–599, Sept. 1937. Cf. No. 173.

171. Blair, Vilray P., Brown, James Barrett and Byars, Louis T. Our responsibility toward oral cancer. Ann. Surg. 106: 568–576, Oct. 1937.

172. Blair, Vilray P. Cleft palate—Its surgery. J. Speech Disorders 2: 195–198, Dec. 1937.

173. Blair, Vilray P., Brown, James Barrett and Byars, Louis T. Observations on sinus abnormalities in congenital total and hemi-absence of the nose. Trans. Am. Laryng. Assn. 59: 223–229, 1937. Cf. No. 170.

1938

174. Blair, Vilray P. and Byars, Louis T. Treatment of wounds resulting from deep burns. J.A.M.A. 110: 1802–1804, May 28, 1938.

175. Blair, Vilray P., Brown, James Barrett and Byars, Louis T. Treatment of cancer of the tongue. Surg. Clin. No. Am. 18, no. 5: 1255–1274, Oct. 1938.

176. Blair, Vilray P. and Byars, Louis T. Hypospadias and epispadias. J. Urol. 40: 814–825, Dec. 1938.

177. Blair, Vilray P., Brown, James Barrett and Byars, Louis T. The prevention and correction of facial disfigurement. Am. J. Surg. 42: 536–541, Dec. 1938.

1939

178. Blair, Vilray P. Distortions accompanying congenital single lip cleft. Nebraska Med. J. 24: 41–43, Feb. 1939.

179. Brown, James Barrett, Blair, Vilray P. and Byars, Louis T. Ulceration of lower extremities and skin grafts. Am. J. Surg. 43: 452–457, Feb. 1939.

180. Blair, Vilray P. John Roberts Caulk, 1881–1938. Ann. Surg. 110: 151–152, July 1939.

1940

181. Blair, Vilray P. and Byars, Louis T. Paralysis of the lower lid and scleral scars and grafts. Surg. Gyn. & Obst. 70: 426–437, Feb. 15, 1940.

182. Blair, Vilray P. and Byars, Louis T. Cancer of the face. Mississippi Valley Med. J. 62: 90–93, May 1940.

183. Blair, Vilray P. and Byars, Louis T. Current treatment of cancer of the lip. A clinical speculation. Surgery 8: 340–352, Aug. 1940.

184. Blair, Vilray P. and Byars, Louis T. Toe to finger transplant. Ann. Surg. 112: 287–290, Aug. 1940.

185. Blair, Vilray P. The gingival operculum and the erupting lower third molar. Arch. Clin. Oral Path. 4: 283–284, Sept.–Dec. 1940.

1941

186. Blair, Vilray P. The role of the plastic surgeon in the care of war injuries. Ann. Surg. 113: 697–704, May 1941.

1943

187. Blair, Vilray P. and Byars, Louis T. The desirability of early proper treatment of face injuries. Texas State J. Med. 38: 533–537, Jan. 1943.

188. Blair, Vilray P. Relation of the early care to the final outcome of major face wounds in war surgery. Military Surgeon 92: 12–17, Jan. 1943. Cf. No. 190.

189. Blair, Vilray P. and Byars, Louis T. Cancer of the face and mouth. Texas State J. Med. 38: 641–645, March 1943.

190. Blair, Vilray P. Relation of the early care to the final outcome of major face wounds in war surgery. Cincinnati J. Med. 24: 121–127, May 1943. Cf. No. 188.

191. Blair, Vilray P. Uses of transplanted pedicle flaps for nasal restoration or correction. Trans. Am. Soc. Plas. & Recons. Surg. 12: 23–24, 1943.

1944

192. Blair, Vilray P. Symposium on plastic surgery; treatment of battle casualties or industrial wounds of the face. Surgery 15: 16–21, Jan. 1944.

1946

193. Blair, Vilray P. and Byars, Louis T. "Hits, strikes and outs" in the use of pedicle flaps for nasal restoration or correction. Surg. Gyn. & Obst. 82: 367–385, April 1946.
194. Blair, Vilray P. Cancer of the mouth. [Radio address, July 23, 1946] *In:* The'Doctors Talk it Over, Lederle Laboratories, vol. 4, pp. 133–140, 1946.
195. Blair, Vilray P. Foreword. Plas. & Recons. Surg. 1: 1–2, July 1946.

1947

196. Blair, Vilray P. In Memoriam—John Staige Davis, 1872–1946. Surgery 22: 158–159, July 1947.

1948

197. Blair, Vilray P. and Robinson, Robert R. Primary closure of harelip. (Editorial) Surg. Gyn. & Obst. 86: 502–504, April 1948.

1950

198. Blair, Vilray P. and Letterman, Gordon S. The role of the switched lower lip flap in upper lip restorations. Plas. & Recons. Surg. 5: 1–25, Jan. 1950.

REFERENCES

1. See Bibliography, Articles, Nos. 12, 113.
2. Letter of Dr. Blair, June 23, 1944, to Mr. Max Safron.
3. Letter of Dr. Blair, March 21, 1940, to Brother J. Austin, Christian Brothers' College.
4. Letter of Dr. Blair, Jan. 27, 1948, to Dr. E. H. Gregory, Jr.
5. See Bibliography, Books, No. 1.
6. See Bibliography, Articles, No. 1.
7. See Bibliography, Articles, No. 107.
8. Letter of Dr. Blair to Dr. E. H. Gregory, Jr., Jan. 27, 1948.
9. BROOKS, BARNEY. The making of a surgeon yesterday and today. J. Missouri State Med. Assn. **44:** 578–584, Aug. 1947.
10. See Bibliography, Articles, No. 3.
11. Letter of Dr. Blair, Jan. 27, 1948, to Dr. E. H. Gregory, Jr.
12. See Bibliography, Books, No. 2.
13. Letter of Dr. Blair, Jan. 27, 1948, to Dr. E. H. Gregory, Jr.
14. GILLIES, H. D. Plastic surgery of the face, p. x. London, Frowde, 1920.
15. GILLIES. H. D. AND MILLARD. RALPH. The art and principles of plastic surgery, p. 30. Boston, Little, Brown & Co., 1957.
16. See Bibliography, Articles, No. 193.
17. LOGAN, WILLIAM H. G. (1) Surgical correction of complete congenital cleft of palate. Report presented at the VIIIth Dental International Congress, Paris, Aug. 2–8, 1931; (2) Development of the human jaws and surrounding structures from birth to the age of fifteen years. J. Am. Dental Assn. **20:** 379–427, March 1933.
18. See Bibliography, Articles, No. 121.
19. See Bibliography, Articles, Nos. 121, 125.
20. BROWN, JAMES BARRETT AND McDOWELL, FRANK. Simplified design for repair of single cleft lips. Surg. Gyn. & Obst. **80:** 12–26, Jan. 1945.
21. Letter of Dr. Blair, Feb. 24, 1937, to Dr. Jerome P. Webster.
22. Idem.
23. IVY, ROBERT H. Some circumstances leading to the organization of the American Board of Plastic Surgery, pp. 77–82; 82–84. Plas. & Recons. Surg. **16:** 77–85, Aug. 1955.
24. Letter of Dr. Blair, Jan. 27, 1948, to Dr. E. H. Gregory, Jr.
25. Idem.
26. See Bibliography, Articles, Nos. 5, 2.
27. See Bibliography under "Books" and "Chapters of Books."
28. No date or place of the binding of these reprints together is indicated in this volume. The items included are Nos. 65, 89, 87, 92 and 93 of the Bibliography of Blair's articles.
29. See Bibliography, Articles, Nos. 37, 140, 193.
30. See Bibliography, Articles, No. 114.

INDEX